AF720631

The Handbook of Ornamental Fish Health and Welfare

Dedicated to my family:
Judy, Victoria, Alexandra, and Rachel

Cover photographs by Nicholas Saint-Erne, DVM, CertAqV

The Handbook of Ornamental Fish Health and Welfare

Edited by

Nicholas Saint-Erne, DVM, CertAqV

Certified Aquatic Veterinarian
Distinguished Fellow of the World Aquatic Veterinary Medical Association
Phoenix, Arizona USA

CABI

CABI is a trading name of CAB International

CABI
Nosworthy Way
Wallingford
Oxfordshire OX10 8DE
UK

Tel: +44 (0)1491 832111
E-mail: info@cabi.org
Website: www.cabi.org

CABI
200 Portland Street
Boston
MA 02114
USA

Tel: +1 (617)682-9015
E-mail: cabi-nao@cabi.org

© CAB International 2025. All rights, including for text and data mining, AI training, and similar technologies, are reserved. No part of this publication may be reproduced in any form or by any means, electronically, mechanically, by photocopying, recording or otherwise, without the prior permission of the copyright owners.

The views expressed in this publication are those of the author(s) and do not necessarily represent those of, and should not be attributed to, CAB International (CABI). Any images, figures and tables not otherwise attributed are the author(s)' own. References to internet websites (URLs) were accurate at the time of writing.
CAB International and, where different, the copyright owner shall not be liable for technical or other errors or omissions contained herein. The information is supplied without obligation and on the understanding that any person who acts upon it, or otherwise changes their position in reliance thereon, does so entirely at their own risk. Information supplied is neither intended nor implied to be a substitute for professional advice. The reader/user accepts all risks and responsibility for losses, damages, costs and other consequences resulting directly or indirectly from using this information.

CABI's Terms and Conditions, including its full disclaimer, may be found at https://www.cabidigitallibrary.org/terms-and-conditions.

A catalogue record for this book is available from the British Library, London, UK.

Library of Congress Cataloging-in-Publication Data

Names: Saint-Erne, Nicholas, editor.
Title: The handbook of ornamental fish health and welfare / edited by Nicholas Saint-Erne.
Description: Boston, MA : CAB International, [2024] | Includes bibliographical references and index. | Summary: "This book forms a complete resource covering ornamental fish health and welfare. It covers all the key elements of care, including water quality testing and maintenance, filtration systems, nutrition, husbandry, handling and transportation, disease diagnosis, treatments and medications, and disease prevention"-- Provided by publisher.
Identifiers: LCCN 2024030889 (print) | LCCN 2024030890 (ebook) | ISBN 9781789246018 (hardback) | ISBN 9781789246025 (ebk) | ISBN 9781789246032 (epub)
Subjects: LCSH: Ornamental fishes--Handbooks, manuals, etc. | Marine aquarium fishes--Handbooks, manuals, etc. | Fish culture--Handbooks, manuals, etc. | Handbooks and manuals.
Classification: LCC SF457.1 .H36 2024 (print) | LCC SF457.1 (ebook) | DDC 639.34/2--dc23/eng/20240916
LC record available at https://lccn.loc.gov/2024030889
LC ebook record available at https://lccn.loc.gov/2024030890

ISBN-13: 9781789246018 (hardback)
9781789246025 (ePDF)
9781789246032 (ePub)

DOI: 10.1079/9781789246032.0000

Commissioning Editor: Alexandra Lainsbury
Editorial Assistant: Emma McCann
Production Editor: Rosie Hayden

Typeset by Straive, Pondicherry, India
Printed and bound in the UK by CPI Group (UK) Ltd, Croydon, CR0 4YY

Contents

Contributors

Azureen Erdman, DVM, CertAqV
New River, Arizona USA
az.erdman@gmail.com

Sharmie Johnson, DVM, CertAqV
Wildlife World Zoo & Aquarium
Veterinary Medical Department
16501 W. Northern Avenue
Litchfield Park, Arizona 85345, USA
vetdept@wildlifeworld.com

Robert Martinez, DVM, CertAqV
Aquatic Veterinary Consulting, PLLC.
Salt Lake City, Utah, USA
drrobmartinez@aquaticvetconsulting.com

Lily Parkinson, DVM, DACZM, DACVECC, CertAqV, CWR
Brookfield Zoo
3300 Golf Road
Brookfield, Illinois 60513, USA
lilyparkinson@gmail.com

Nicholas Saint-Erne, DVM, CertAqV
WAVMA Distinguished Fellow
Dr. Saint-Erne Consulting, PLLC.
Phoenix, Arizona
DrSaintErne@gmail.com

Chris Walster, BVMS, MVPH, CertAqV
WAVMA Distinguished Fellow
C&J Walster Ltd.
Stafford, Staffordshire, United Kingdom
chris.walster@btconnect.com

Foreword

When I graduated from veterinary school in 1988, there was not easy access to a single comprehensive text on ornamental fish medicine written by veterinarians. A lot has changed in the last 36 years, and there are now over three dozen fish medicine books written by veterinarians in circulation. While these books are all great resources, providing valuable information on fish medicine and health, most do not focus on ornamental fishes. Nicholas Saint-Erne, the editor and primary author, has over 40 years of experience as a fish veterinarian and is a WAVMA Distinguished Fellow. Dr. Saint-Erne and I have been friends and colleagues for almost three decades, and I can say without hesitation that he truly is a pioneer in the field of aquatic animal medicine with a wealth of experience in both corporate and private practice.

From anabantid to zebrafish, ammonia to zeolite, this marvel of a book is truly the A-Z of ornamental fish health and welfare. Written entirely by a carefully selected team of World Aquatic Veterinary Medical Association (WAVMA) certified aquatic veterinarians, the contents provide the reader with all the information needed to handle any ornamental fish health challenge competently and effectively. Best of all, this resource is in a handbook format, with pertinent and easy-to-find information at the reader's fingertips. The text is richly illustrated in color with figures that highlight key points and guide the reader in performing diagnostic and medical procedures accurately and safely. The handbook also contains numerous tables, including a comprehensive formulary, which provides valuable information quickly for the busy clinician with limited time. The book is very easy to navigate, with concise and accurate knowledge nuggets just a few page-turns away.

Readers will be happy to see that in addition to the essentials of husbandry, water quality, disease diagnostics, infectious diseases, environmental diseases, neoplasia, therapeutics, analgesia, anesthesia, and surgery, this book also addresses important topics like animal welfare, biosecurity, and zoonotic diseases.

Dr. Saint-Erne and his contributing authors have seamlessly meshed their many decades of personal experience with a rich survey of the fish health literature to provide a reference on ornamental aquarium fishes that all practitioners of aquatic animal medicine should have on their bookshelves.

Gregory A. Lewbart, MS, VMD, DACZM, DECZM (ZHM)
WAVMA Distinguished Fellow
Professor of Aquatic, Wildlife, and Zoological Medicine
North Carolina State University
College of Veterinary Medicine
Raleigh, North Carolina
Editor of the *Self-Assessment Color Review of Ornamental Fish* (1998), *Ornamental Fishes and Aquatic Invertebrates; A Self-Assessment Color Review* (2017), *Invertebrate Medicine* (2006, 2012, 2022), and co-author of *The Aquarium Fish Medicine Handbook* (2024).

Preface

It was a great honor to be asked by CABI to compile a book on Ornamental Fish Health and Welfare and to work with some very talented veterinarians who have contributed material for this book, as well as working with the staff at CABI publishers, who were patient during the prolonged process of bringing it together.

When I published the book *Advanced Koi Care* in 2002, it was the culmination of my aquatic veterinary work with those amazing fish: Nishikigoi—the Japanese colored carp. It took all the knowledge and reference material that I had acquired in my 20 years of veterinary practice working with koi and other fish species to make a practical guide for veterinarians who wanted to care for these beautiful fish. Now, after another 20 years of aquatic veterinary medicine, it is time to make a complete veterinary reference book for tropical aquarium fish!

In recent years, there has been a surge in interest among veterinarians in aquatic veterinary medicine, including food fish production, marine mammal care, aquatic animals in the care of public aquariums and zoos, and in the ornamental fish industry. The growing interest by veterinarians ultimately produced organizations to help spread knowledge among veterinarians working with fish and other aquatic animals, including the International Association of Aquatic Animal Medicine, Fish Veterinary Society in the United Kingdom, the American Association of Fish Veterinarians, and the World Aquatic Veterinary Medical Association (WAVMA.org).

WAVMA is an international organization of aquatic veterinarians and holds an annual meeting and conference that rotates in locations throughout the world. It publishes a quarterly journal, *The Aquatic Veterinarian*, which contains news, research articles, case reports, book reviews, meeting announcements, and other material of interest to its members. It has student chapters in many veterinary colleges around the world. Their website has links to educational videos on various fields of aquatic veterinary medicine, listings of upcoming veterinary meetings, and a search section where fish keepers can find a local veterinarian that treats fish or other aquatic animals. And, most importantly, WAVMA has a credentialing program that certifies veterinarians who have knowledge, skill, and experience working with aquatic animals. These veterinarians are given the honorific title Certified Aquatic Veterinarian (CertAqV) to list after their veterinary degree initials. This handbook has been edited and written exclusively by veterinarians who have been awarded this certification.

In this handbook, you will find information about the history of keeping fish in aquariums, the pet fish industry, how to maintain an aquarium and proper water quality, fish diseases and treatments, anesthesia, surgery, and a plethora of fish-keeping information. It is our hope that this will be a useful handbook for aquatic veterinarians and anyone wanting to learn more about keeping tropical aquarium fishes and maintaining their good health and welfare.

Nicholas Saint-Erne, DVM, CertAqV
WAVMA Distinguished Fellow
Certified Aquatic Veterinarian
Phoenix, Arizona USA

1 A Brief History of Keeping Fish in Aquariums

NICHOLAS SAINT-ERNE

Dr. Saint-Erne Consulting, PLLC, Phoenix, Arizona

Abstract

Keeping fish in artificial ponds for food dates back to antiquity. In the late Middle Ages through the Renaissance period, interest in keeping fish for ornamental purposes began to flourish as well, first in Asia, then in Europe. By the 19th century, keeping fish in glass aquariums was a popular pastime.

1.1 Early Aquarists

The ancient Egyptians kept fish in hollowed-out stone bowls; however, this was to keep the fish alive until they could be cooked and eaten. Other ancient and medieval cultures—such as the Romans, Chinese, and Hawaiians—kept fish in man-made ponds to harvest them as needed for food. Keeping fish for strictly ornamental reasons was most notably done in the Chinese culture as early as AD 1369, breeding goldfish that were kept in porcelain bowls (Fig. 1.1) and even in glass aquariums. Glass bowls began to be used in Europe in 1572, and in 1666, Leonhard Baldner, a Strasbourg fisherman and naturalist, produced a handwritten illustrated book on birds, fishes, and mammals titled *Vogel, Fisch und Thierbuch*, which discussed using glass bowls to study fish. The book *Der See im Glasse*, published in Germany in 1856, increased interest in keeping fish for scientific observation (Hoedeman, 1974).

On May 21, 1853, the first public aquarium was opened as part of the London Zoo. First called the "Fish House" in Regent's Park Zoological Gardens, it was made possible by English naturalist Philip Henry Gosse, who is credited with promoting the glass tank as a novel way of housing marine creatures and was also responsible for using the word "aquarium" for this glass vessel (Ganesh, 2023). Forty years later, it was written that "every European city and town of consequence has a public aquarium" (Samuel, 1894).

Nature in the home, including plants and birds, was very popular in Victorian England, and bringing fish indoors in glass bowls and aquariums became common. A book published in 1894, *The Amateur Aquarist* (Fig. 1.2), described the care of goldfish, paradise fish, and three-spined sticklebacks in glass aquariums without any filtration or aeration. However, it was noted that fishes all gasping with their noses partly out of the water was due to a lack of oxygen, with too many fish in the aquarium, and the cure was to dip water up and let it splash back many times and to reduce the number of fishes. A summary of the advice given in the book follows:

"The self-sustaining aquarium is arranged so that the water need be changed but once a year. Under favorable conditions even this time may be extended. The modern iron-framed aquarium (Figs 1.3 and 1.4) is made with the sides, ends, and bottom of glass so arranged that the plates just unite inside the frame, while the amount of cement necessary to insure its being watertight is placed between the metal and glass where the even pressure of water serves to make it more secure. A self-sustaining aquarium may be fitted for either marine or fresh water, but I shall in this preliminary work confine myself to the fresh water, it being a little easier to maintain and for that reason better to start with.

Corresponding author: DrSaintErne@gmail.com

© CAB International 2025. *The Handbook of Ornamental Fish Health and Welfare* (ed. N. Saint-Erne)

DOI: 10.1079/9781789246032.0001

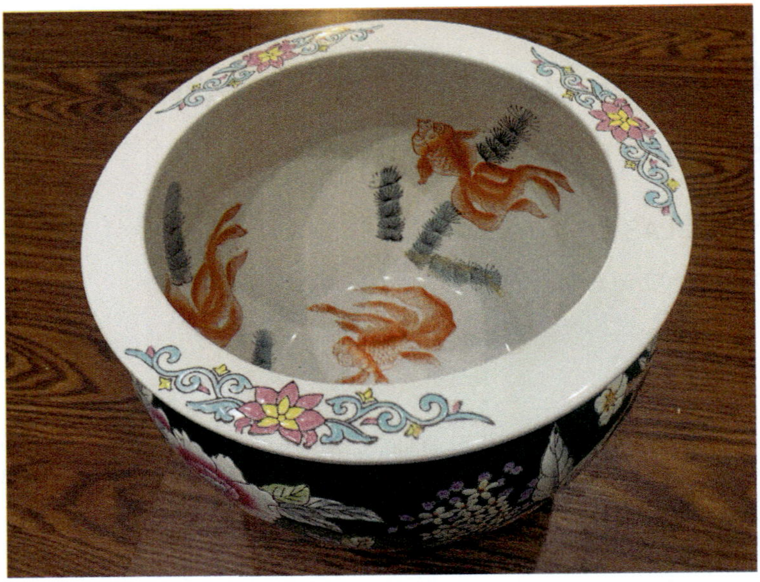

Fig. 1.1. Chinese porcelain bowl for maintaining goldfish. The inside painting depicts aquatic plants as well as a Chinese Fringetail Telescope Goldfish. (Photograph by N. Saint-Erne.)

"The thing to be done is to supply air to the water in the aquarium as rapidly as the fishes exhaust it. Water-plants under the action of daylight give off oxygen and absorb the carbonic-acid gas exhaled by the creatures in the pond. Place the aquarium on a steady table . . . opposite a northern exposure if possible, and if not, near the window having the least direct sunlight. The main point being to obtain sufficient light to stimulate the growth of aquatic plants without allowing the sun to shine directly on the water. In a few words then, a self-sustaining aquarium simply means "balancing," to use a technical term, the animals and vegetable life, with the addition of certain little water-creatures to act as scavengers" (Samuel, 1894).

1.2 Aquarium Societies

As a way of exchanging knowledge about fishkeeping, interested people gathered to discuss techniques, and this resulted in the formation of aquarium societies. The first aquarium society was called the *Gotha Aquarium*, founded in Germany in 1882 (Bleher, 2004, p. 13). The first aquarium society organized in America was established in New York City in 1892, which held its meetings at the American Museum of Natural History, located in Central Park (Ferdenzi, 2019). The oldest continuous aquarium club still in existence is the Boston Aquarium Society, founded in 1916 (Meserve and Meserve, 1973). The Brooklyn Aquarium Society in New York City was founded in 1911, but disbanded mid-century, and later reformed in the 1950s with the same name (Wikipedia.org, 2023). Aquarium societies hold monthly meetings and have lectures and newsletters with current information to educate members about fishkeeping. Some even have fish shows to exhibit fish and aquariums, where prizes are awarded. Today, there are aquarium societies in most major cities, along with koi pond societies and even aquatic plant societies. There are also several umbrella organizations for the organized hobby, including the International Federation of Online Clubs and Aquatic Societies (IFOCAS.net), the Federation of British Aquatic Societies, formed in 1932 (fbas.co.uk), the Northeast Council of Aquarium Societies, formed in 1956 (NorthEastCouncil.org), and the Federation of American Aquarium Societies (FAAS). Find these organizations' websites or Facebook pages to locate aquarium societies in local areas.

1.3 The 20th Century

In the early 20th century, home aquarium keeping continued its popularity, and techniques gradually became more advanced. However, mechanical aeration had not been introduced, and it was still essential

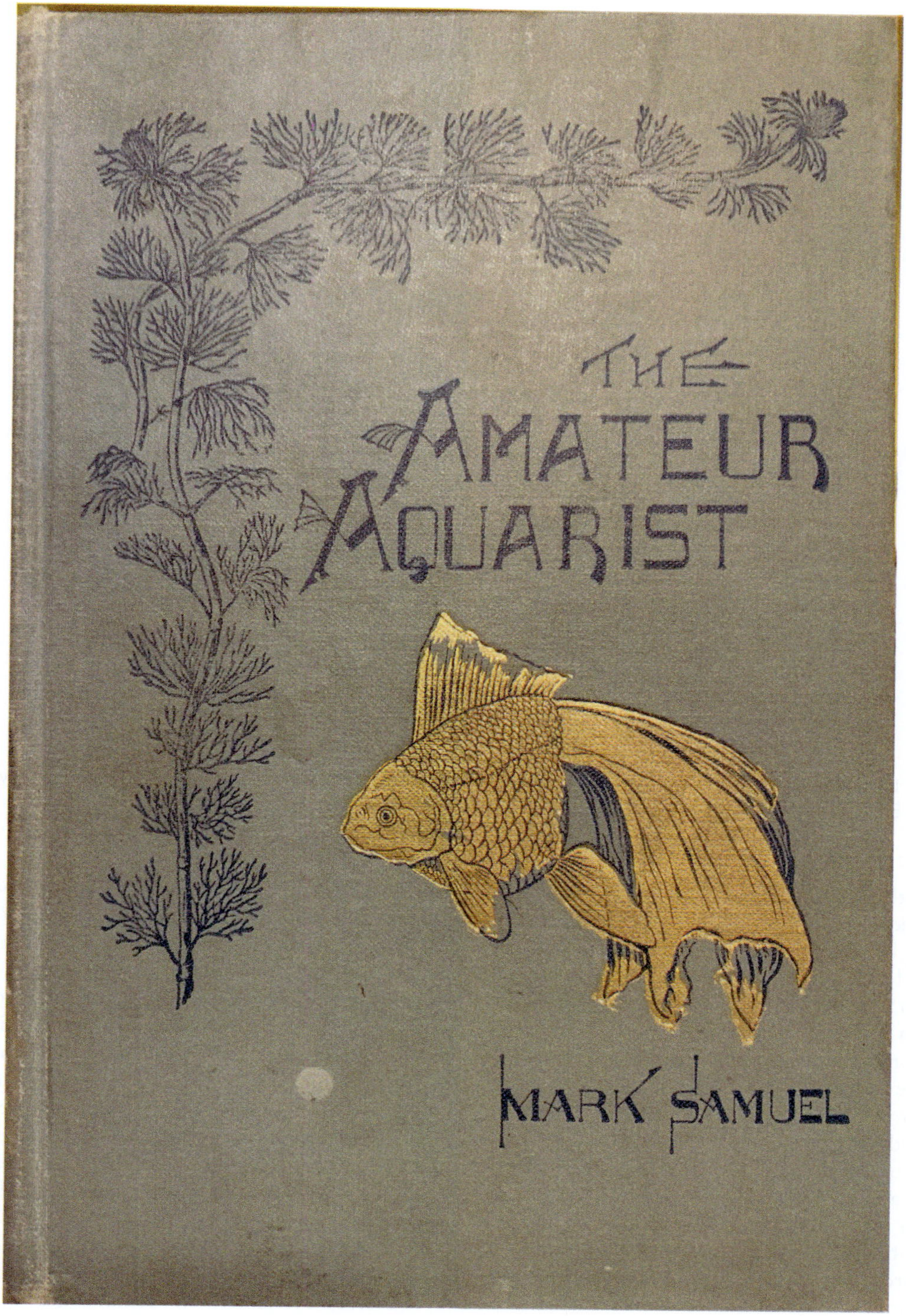

Fig. 1.2. Cover of the book *The Amateur Aquarist*, by Mark Samuel (1894). The illustration on the cover is a fringetail goldfish. (Photograph by N. Saint-Erne.)

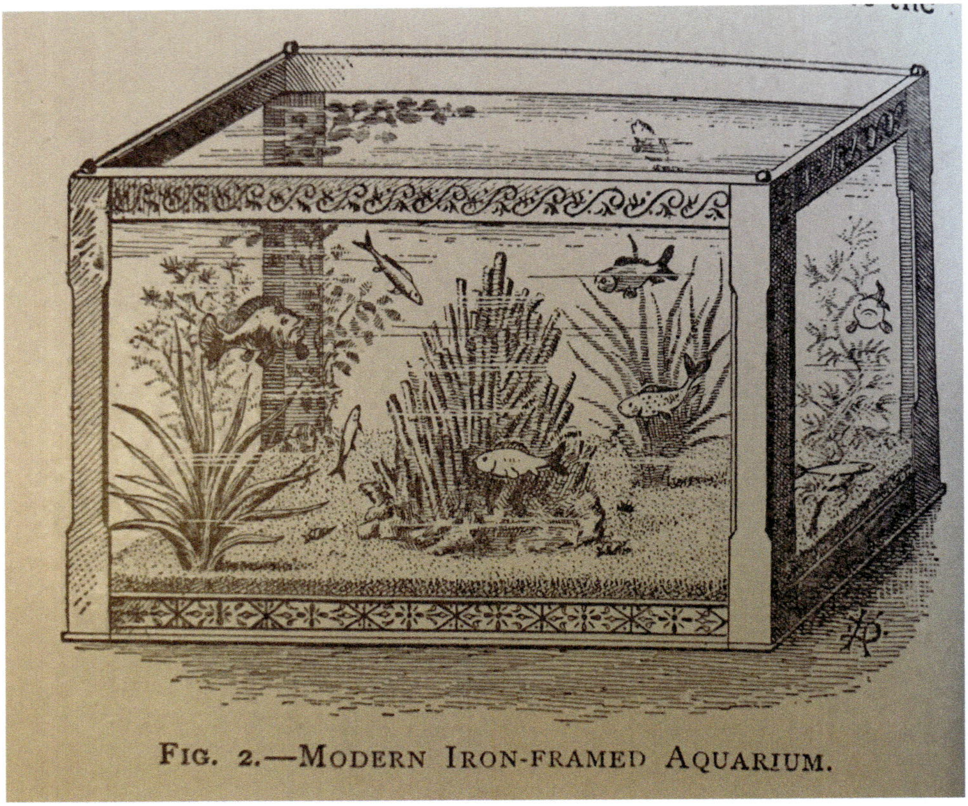

Fig. 1.3. Late 19th century metal-framed, glass aquarium illustration from *The Amateur Aquarist*. (Photograph by N. Saint-Erne.)

that if "the relations of plant to animal life correctly proportioned, the aquarium is virtually self-sustaining or balanced, and the water need only be changed at long intervals, often of a year or more" (Wolf, 1908). This same book also listed forms of aeration available at the time: a stream of water under pressure of a considerable elevation poured into the aquarium; use of a pressure tank filled with air by a bicycle pump and the compressed air admitted into the aquarium by a small tin pipe buried under the pebbles; by use of an elevated bucket and a rubber hose above the water line to create a fountain in the aquarium that would run for probably an hour. Despite the simplicity, a few hardy fish specimens could survive in these aquariums.

Today, one rarely sets up an aquarium for just one or two fish. In 1900, the fishkeeper had no choice. Today, we can keep many more fish in our tanks. The common rule of thumb for stocking aquariums is "one inch of fish to one gallon of water." This rule was already in print by 1921 (Innes, 1921, p. 7). Also, in the early part of the 20th century, one did not set up an aquarium without plants. Plants were required because they provided oxygen for the fish and removed carbon dioxide, which was the result of fish respiration (Hovanec, 2000). In his later book, *Exotic Aquarium Fishes*, Innes writes, "This is one of the modern developments in aquarium convenience. A small electric pump forces the air through a tube connected to a liberator at the bottom of the aquarium, sending up a spray of small bubbles" (Innes, 1935, p. 8).

As mechanical filters and air pumps were developed, the use of live plants in the aquarium decreased. However, one could argue that the increased use of filters and subsequent decline in the use of live plants resulted in the aquariums of the late 20th century having poorer water quality than the aquariums of the 1920s and 1930s,

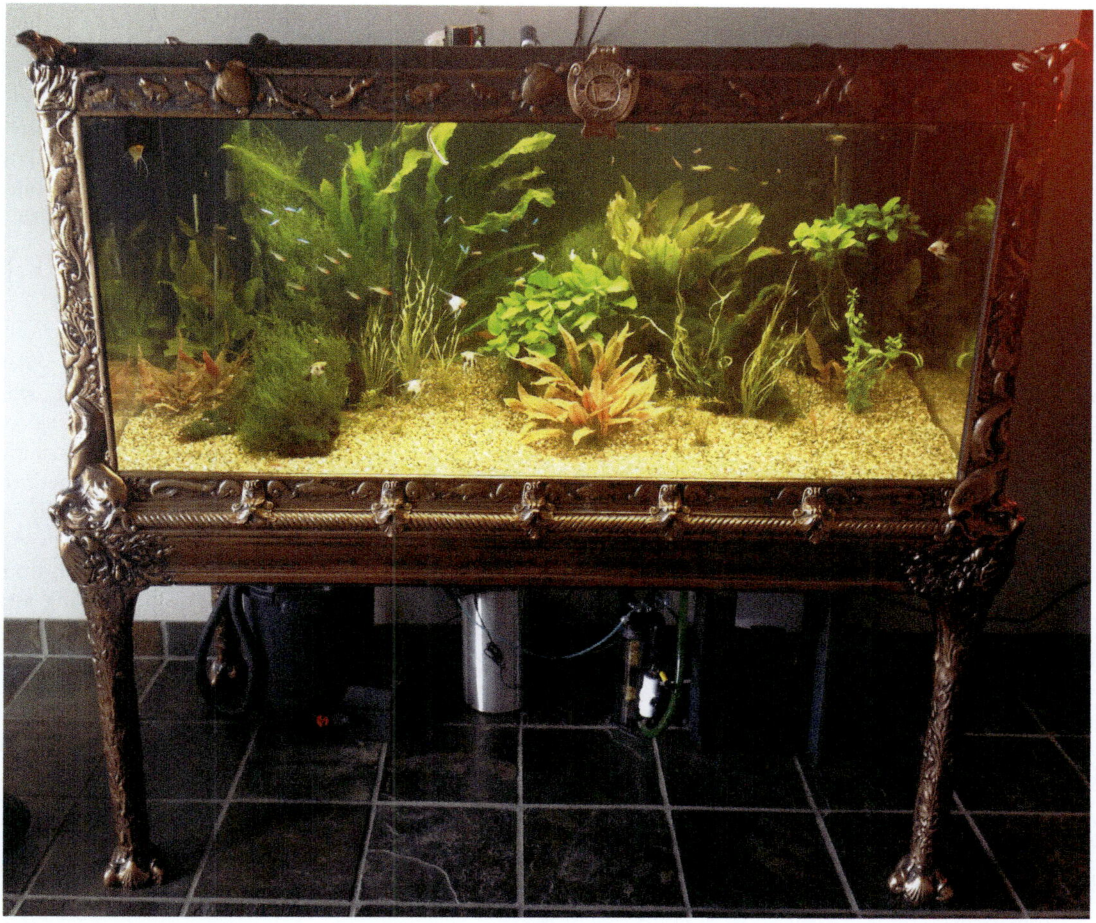

Fig. 1.4. Brass-framed antique aquarium in the collection of ZooMed/The Museum of Aquarium and Pet History in San Luis Obispo, California. (Photograph by N. Saint-Erne.)

because the plants remove many things that filters do not, including carbon dioxide and nitrate (Hovanec, 2000).

In the 1950s, the undergravel Miracle Filter was introduced and became the most common filter in an aquarium in the United States. The gravel at the bottom of the aquarium became the filter media for biofiltration, and water was drawn through the gravel by use of an air pump blowing air through uplift tubes in the corners of the undergravel plate. The undergravel filter became so popular that for years, just about every aquarium was set up with one (Hovanec, 2000). When the "power head"—an underwater motorized pump that drew water through the undergravel filter plate and up the airlift tube—was added, the undergravel filter became even more effective than when it was operated using air bubbles from an air pump outside of the aquarium.

By the 1960s and 1970s, the tropical fish hobby had grown rapidly. Thermostatically controlled aquarium heaters, plastic canister filters, and power filters (also called the "hang on the back" filter) were developed, as well as many books and magazines published to spread the latest information about fishkeeping. All glass and acrylic aquariums became affordable, replacing the leaky metal-framed aquariums. The New England Aquarium opened in Boston in 1969 and started a trend of large public aquariums, which is still going strong today (Hovanec, 2000). There are now even more public aquariums, at least one in every US state and major European city, just as described by Samuel in 1894. Aquarium keeping became not only a thing of beauty to have in a home but also became an active hobby. In the 1970s, it became the second-largest hobby, second to stamp collecting. It topped photography and coin collecting (Jailer, 1973, p. 112).

In the 1980s and 1990s, the cutting edge of the hobby became the marine reef tank (Hovanec, 2000). Keeping a variety of corals, anemones, and other marine invertebrates in a natural-looking aquarium became common. The "Nature Aquarium" became the craze in Asia and Europe with the publication of Takashi Amano's book in 1994. Reminiscent of the early aquariums from the 1800s, Nature Aquaria are full of plants, with only a few fish, usually a small school of one species (Fig. 1.5). These waterscapes attain one of the main goals of Zen Buddhist gardening: to create the impression of a great space in a small area (Amano, 1994, p. 17).

In the 1990s through 2010, koi ponds were a major growth area in fishkeeping. Koi and pond clubs were common in large cities, with monthly meetings and annual springtime pond tours of the members' ponds. The economic crisis and housing market collapse of 2010 brought an end to the rapid growth of pond keeping. The COVID-19 pandemic of 2020–2022 also affected pond keeping, with the largest US magazine for koi enthusiasts, *KOI USA*, ceasing publication one issue shy of 45 full years, the last and final issue was March/April 2020 (Chandler, 2020). To end on a positive note, during the COVID-19 pandemic, when many people were spending more time at home, keeping pets of all kinds became even more popular, with a resurgence of interest in fishkeeping.

1.4 Conclusion

Even as early as 1935, the theory that water changes are necessary more than once a year was documented. Innis wrote, "It is the experience of many leading aquarists that a systemic replenishing of water in small quantities is of marked benefit to most aquarium fishes—say 10 per cent weekly in winter and 25 per cent in summer" (Innes, 1935). Modern LED lighting, powerful canister filtration, water treatment chemicals, and water testing kits have made aquarium maintenance easier today than ever before. And once again, live plants are plentiful in aquariums, thanks to the Nature Aquarium concept. But one should still do partial water changes on the aquarium every month, not yearly!

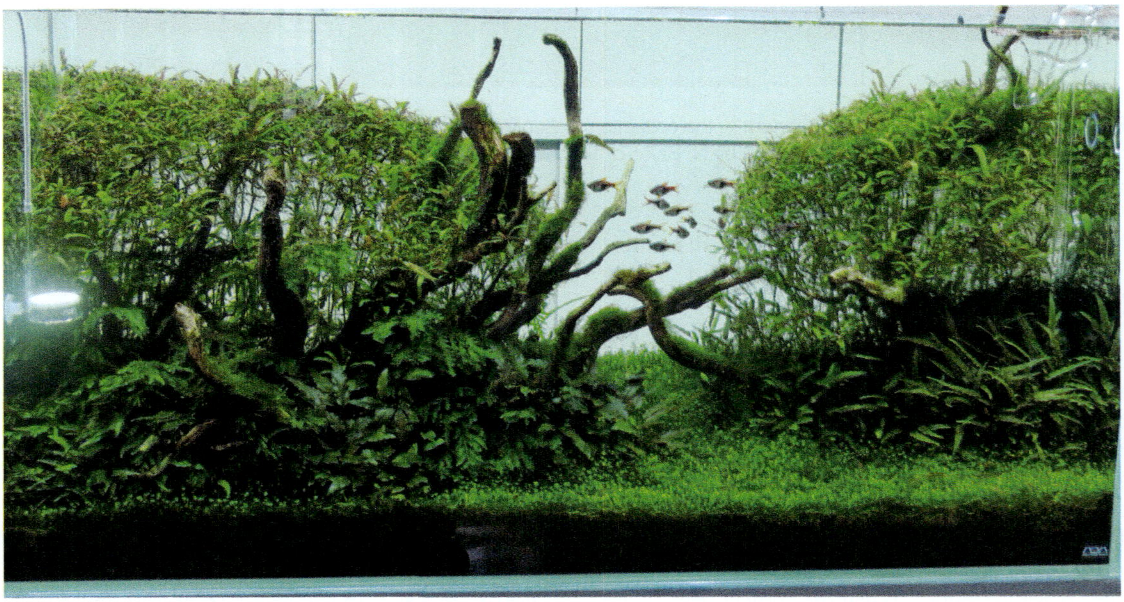

Fig. 1.5. Nature aquarium displayed in Takashi Amano's studio in Japan. (Photograph by N. Saint-Erne.)

References

Amano, T. (1994) *Nature Aquarium World*. T.F.H. Publications, Neptune City, New Jersey.

Bleher, H. (2004) Aquarium history. *Nutrafin Aquatic News*, Issue #4, p. 13. Available at: http://www.hagen.com/pdf/aquatic/Nutrafin_No4_English.pdf (accessed 20 June 2023).

Chandler, D. (2020) Letter to advertisers and consumers. KOIUSA. Available at: https://www.koi-bito.com/forum/forum/koi-hobbyists/main-forum/269129-koiusa-ceased-operations (accessed 1 August 2024).

Ferdenzi, J. (2019) Pioneering aquarist: the legacy of William Holbein. In: Redenbaugh, D. (ed.) *Modern Aquarium*. Vol. 26, No. 7. Greater City Aquarium Society, New York, New York, pp. 7–10.

Ganesh, A.S. (2023) Gosse gets the ocean home. *The Hindu*, 21 May 2023. Available at: https://www.thehindu.com/children/gosse-the-man-behind-the-worlds-first-public-aquarium/article66841544.ece (accessed 1 August 2024).

Hoedeman, J.J. (1974) *Naturalists' Guide to Fresh-Water Aquarium Fish*. Sterling Publishing, New York.

Hovanec, T.A. (2000) 100 years of fishkeeping: good advice never grows old. *Aquarium Fish Magazine*, January 2000. Available at: http://www.drtimsaquatics.com/resources/library-presentations/aquarium-hobby/history-fishkeeping (accessed 1 August 2024).

Innes, W.T. (1921) *Goldfish Varieties and Tropical Aquarium Fishes*. Innes & Sons, Philadelphia, Pennsylvania.

Innes, W.T. (1935) *Exotic Aquarium Fishes*. Innes & Sons, Philadelphia, Pennsylvania.

Jailer, M. (1973) A Snakeskin Guppy wins at fish show. *The New York Times*, 8 April 1973, p. 112.

Meserve, G. and Meserve, F. (1973) History of the Boston Aquarium Society, Inc. *Boston Aquarium News*. Vol. 25, No. 1. Available at: https://bostonaquariumsociety.org/about/ (accessed 1 August 2024).

Samuel, M. (1894) *The Amateur Aquarist*. The Baker & Taylor Co., New York.

Wikipedia.org. (2023) Aquarium fish clubs. Available at: https://en.wikipedia.org/wiki/Aquarium_fish_clubs (accessed 1 August 2024).

Wolf, H.T. (1908) *Goldfish Breeds and Other Aquarium Fishes*. Innes & Sons, Philadelphia, Pennsylvania.

2 Overview of the Ornamental Fish Industry

NICHOLAS SAINT-ERNE

Dr. Saint-Erne Consulting, PLLC, Phoenix, Arizona

Abstract

The largest number of animals kept in homes as pets are fish, followed by cats and then dogs. Fish were originally collected from the wild to be kept in ponds and aquariums, but now, the vast majority of aquarium fish are bred in commercial aquaculture facilities. From these farms, they are transported around the world to fish stores, where they can be sold to aquarium keepers.

2.1 Fish Keepers in the USA

According to the 2021–2022 American Pet Products Association National Pet Owners Survey (APPA, 2022), 70% of the U.S. households own some type of pet, up from 67% in the 2019–2020 survey. The Pet Ownership Statistics (Spots.com, 2023) indicated that in 2020, there were 139.3 million freshwater fish kept in homes in the United States, more than any other type of animal, and 18.8 million saltwater fish were also kept in home aquariums (Table 2.1).

2.2 Fish Production

The majority of freshwater tropical fish sold in the United States are produced on fish farms. About 40% of those are from the USA fish farms, primarily in Florida, and about 60% are imported, mostly from Asian countries such as China, Indonesia, Malaysia, Singapore, Sri Lanka, Taiwan, Thailand, or Vietnam. Nishikigoi (koi) are also bred in Japan, Israel, the United States, and South Africa as well. A very small percentage of freshwater fish are still collected from the wild in Africa, Asia, and South America. The South American fisheries in the Amazon Basin, supported by Project Piaba (Project Piaba, 2023), have been extensively studied and found to be very sustainable for the wild populations of fish. The tropical fish collectors in this area catch the fish by hand nets, and their fishing supports local communities in the rainforests, where other activities such as farming, cattle ranching, and logging would be destructive to the environment.

Marine fish are still mostly collected from coral reefs; however, over 400 species from 43 families of marine fish have been captive bred (Sweet and Pedersen, 2023). Many of these successful fish breedings have only been one time, experimental accomplishments, but several hundred species of marine fish are available for sale as captive-bred specimens in fish stores, and 106 species were available for online sale (LiveAquaria, 2023). The most abundant species were in the families: Angelfish, Blennies, Damselfish, Cardinal fish, Clown fish, Dottybacks, Gobies, and Seahorses. In order to sustain marine fishkeeping in aquariums, it is important that more species of fish and invertebrates are captive bred, as they are in the freshwater fish industry. More facilities dedicated to breeding ornamental marine fish are being built to provide an alternative to collecting fish from the ocean for the aquarium trade (Figs 2.1 and 2.2). The Rising Tide Conservation organization is dedicated to enhancing sustainability in the marine aquarium industry by funding and promoting marine ornamental fish aquaculture research (Rising Tides, 2023).

Corresponding author: DrSaintErne@gmail.com

 © CAB International 2025. *The Handbook of Ornamental Fish Health and Welfare* (ed. N. Saint-Erne)
DOI: 10.1079/9781789246032.0002

Table 2.1. Number of pets in U.S. households in 2022 (APPA, 2022; Spots.com, 2023).

393.3 million pets live in 84.9 million households in the United States.
139.3 million freshwater fish are kept as pets in 11.5 million households.
94.2 million cats live in 42.7 million households.
89.7 million dogs are kept as pets in 63.4 million households.
20.3 million pet birds live in 5.7 million households.
18.8 million saltwater fish are kept in 1.6 million households.
9.4 million reptiles are kept as pets in 4.5 million households.
7.6 million horses are kept in 1.6 million households.
14 million other types of small animals are kept as pets in 5.4 million households.

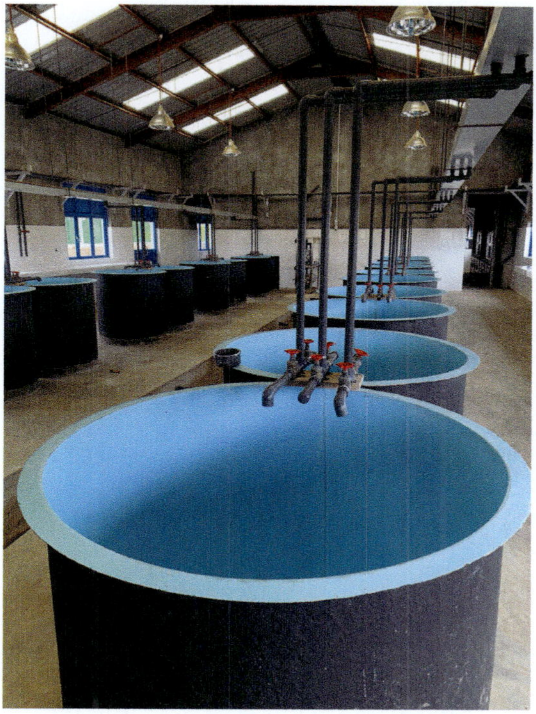

Fig. 2.1. Indoor holding tubs at marine ornamental fish breeding facility being built in Sri Lanka. (Photograph by N. Saint-Erne.)

Freshwater tropical fish traditionally have been bred in outdoor ponds (Figs. 2.3 and 2.4). This production method is cost-effective if done in areas with warm weather, inexpensive land, abundant water, and low-cost labor. Florida has been the primary site in the USA for aquarium fish aquaculture. Ponds dug in the sandy soil there naturally fill with water; however, the increased value of land and lowered underground water tables have caused some small ornamental fish farms to close and sell the land to developers due to the increased value of land versus the revenue from fish farming. The larger farms have more efficiently increased capacity to make up for the growing demand and decreasing domestic supply. Modern techniques, such as covered ponds (Figs. 2.5 and 2.6) and indoor intensive culturing (Figs. 2.7, 2.8, and 2.9), have increased the ability to produce more fish in less space and using less water. This efficiency comes with an increased cost of materials, though it is ultimately offset by greater production capacity. Large amounts of capital are needed for this endeavor, making it practical for only farms with high production (Saint-Erne, 2013).

The cost of covering a pond is initially expensive, but it protects the fish from predation by frogs, turtles, snakes, and especially birds, which can consume half to two-thirds of the fish stocked in the pond. Plus, access of water birds to the pond can lead to digenean trematodes infestation in the fish as the second intermediate host. In tropical climates, the shade cloth used to cover the pond can also reduce the water temperature and lower evaporation.

There is considerably more expense invested with lining a pond with Ethylene Propylene Diene Monomer (EPDM) rubber and covering it with shade cloth over steel frames, but it allows for better water control (no seepage into or out of the ground), and the lack of weeds at the pond edge eliminates hiding areas for predators. These ponds have no filtration but do have aerators at one end to keep the water oxygenated. Some fresh water is added each day and the excess water overflows into the standpipe. This method has allowed for greater production in a smaller overall space than the traditional open, dirt-bottom ponds.

The next level of production comes from indoor aquaculture. This involves considerable expense in building costs, vats or containers for fish production, and filtration systems for water quality control. Most of these use recirculating water rather than

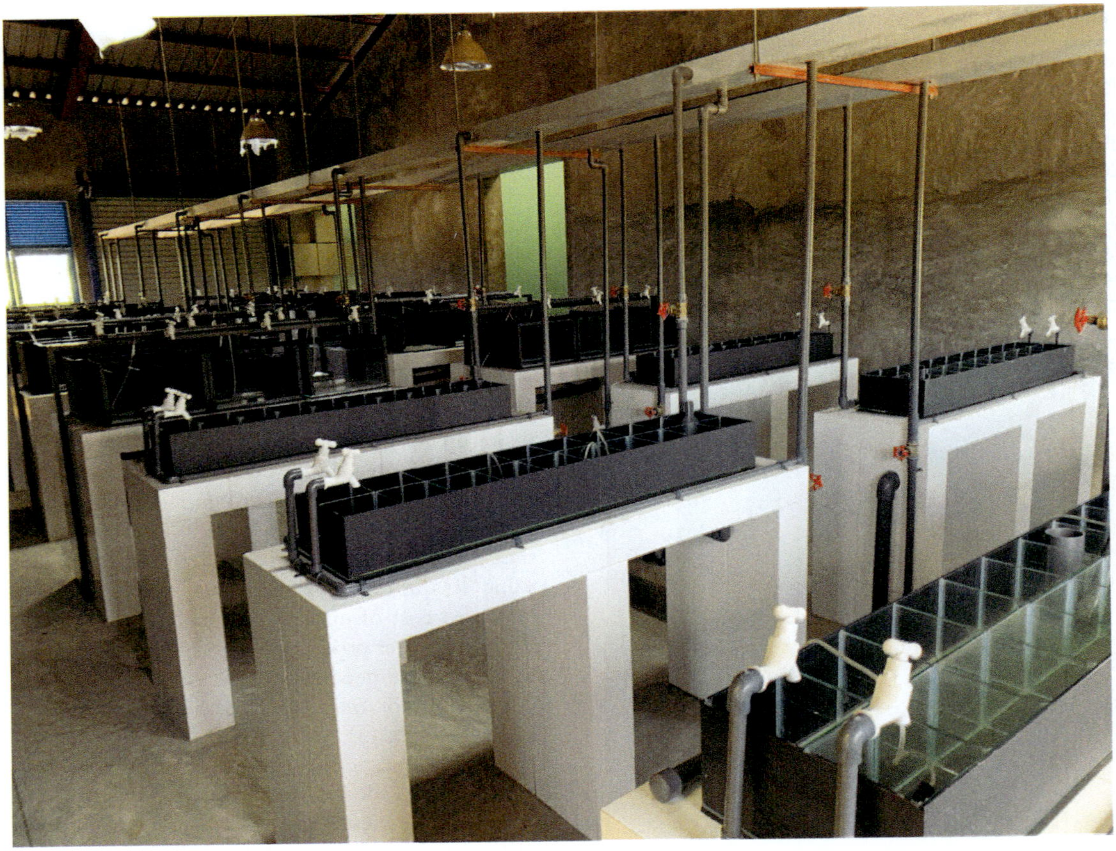

Fig. 2.2. Glass aquariums for growing ornamental marine fish and invertebrates. (Photograph by N. Saint-Erne.)

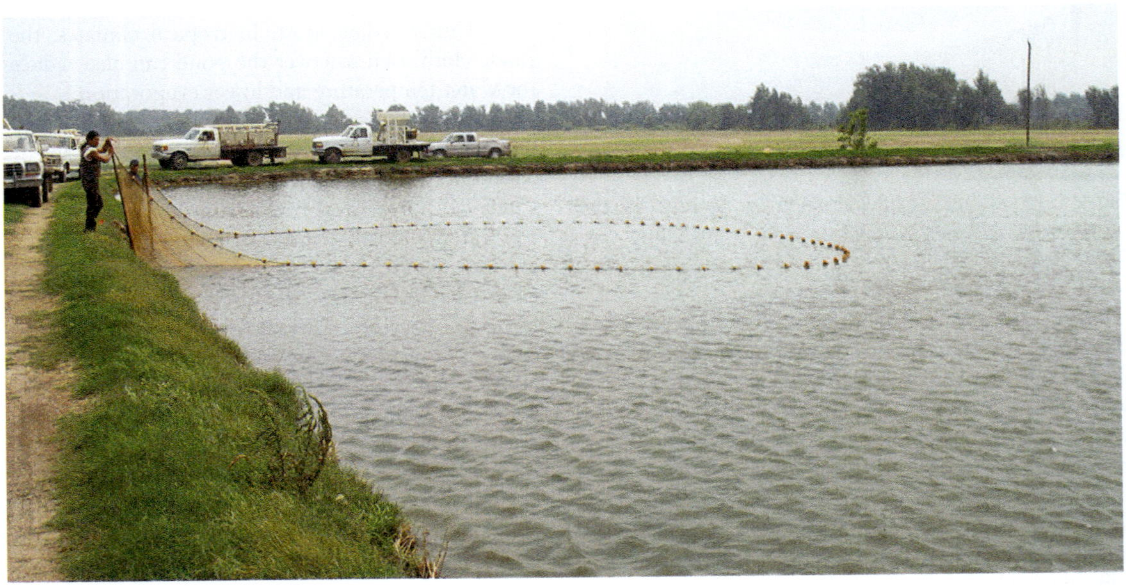

Fig. 2.3. Seining to catch goldfish in a dirt-bottomed fishpond. (Photograph by N. Saint-Erne.)

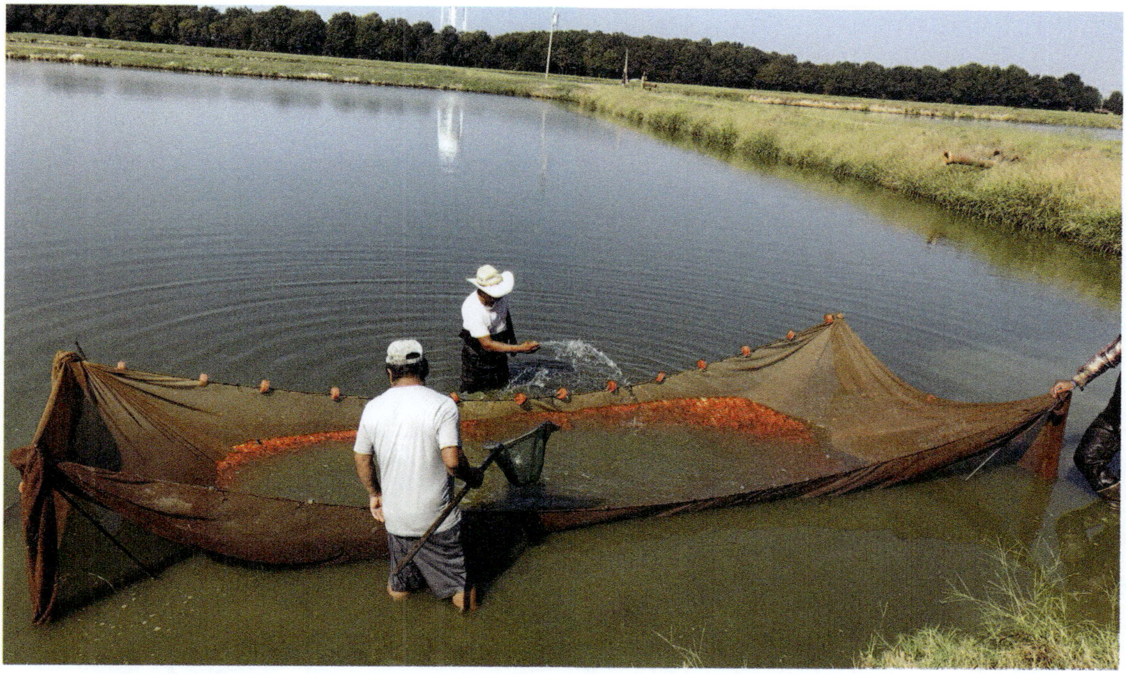

Fig. 2.4. Netting the goldfish out of the seine. (Photograph by N. Saint-Erne.)

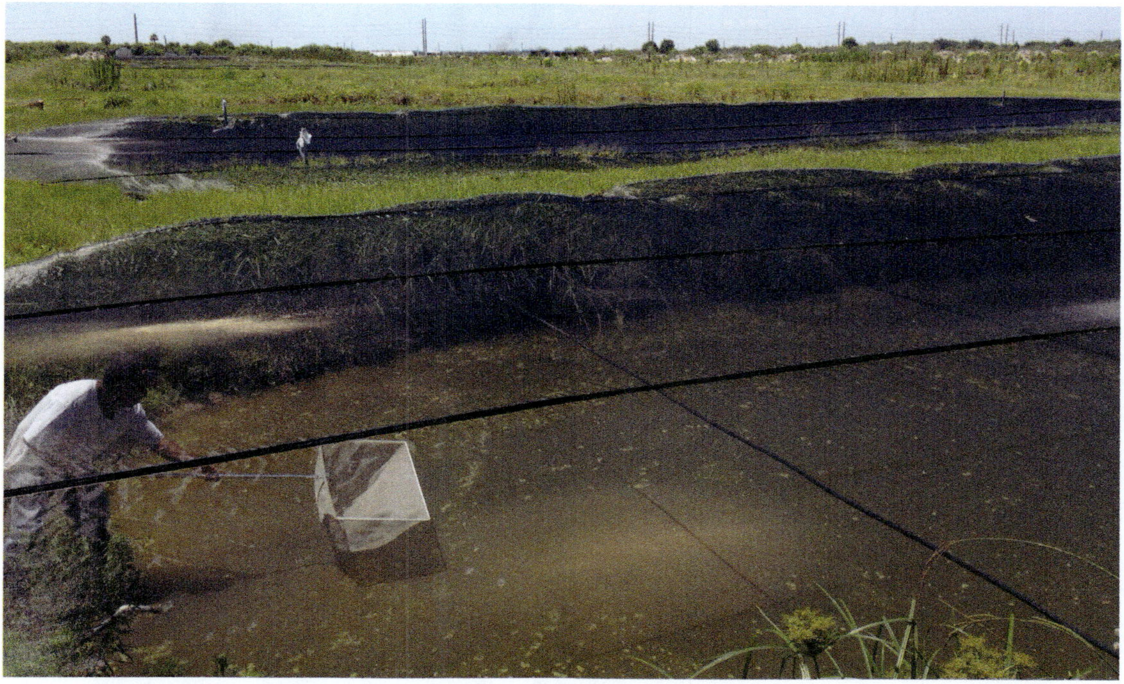

Fig. 2.5. A shade cloth covering a dirt-bottom pond. (Photograph by N. Saint-Erne.)

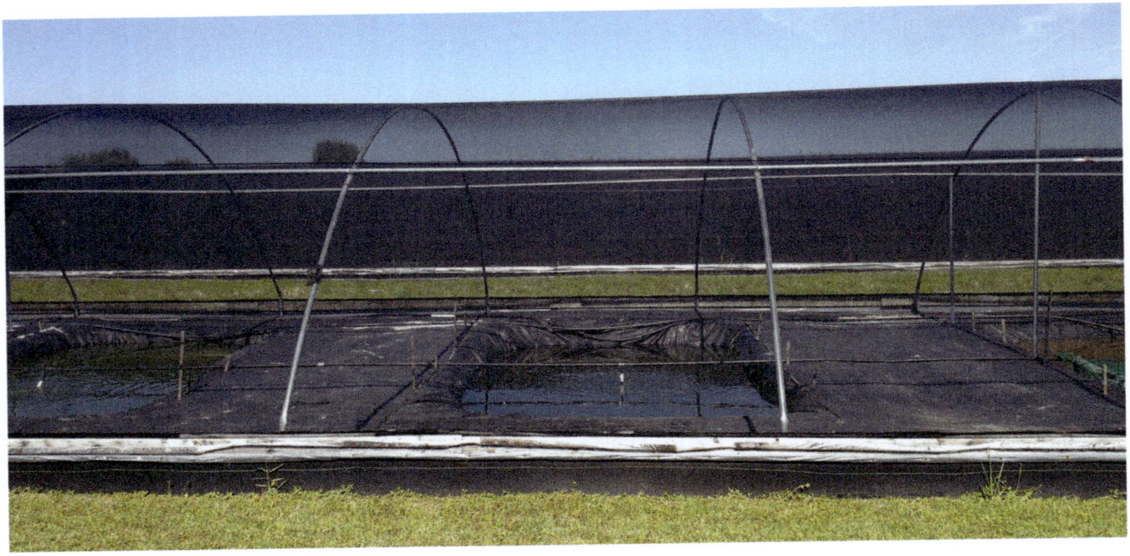

Fig. 2.6. A covered pond that is completely lined to eliminate predators, weeds, and water loss. (Photograph by N. Saint-Erne.)

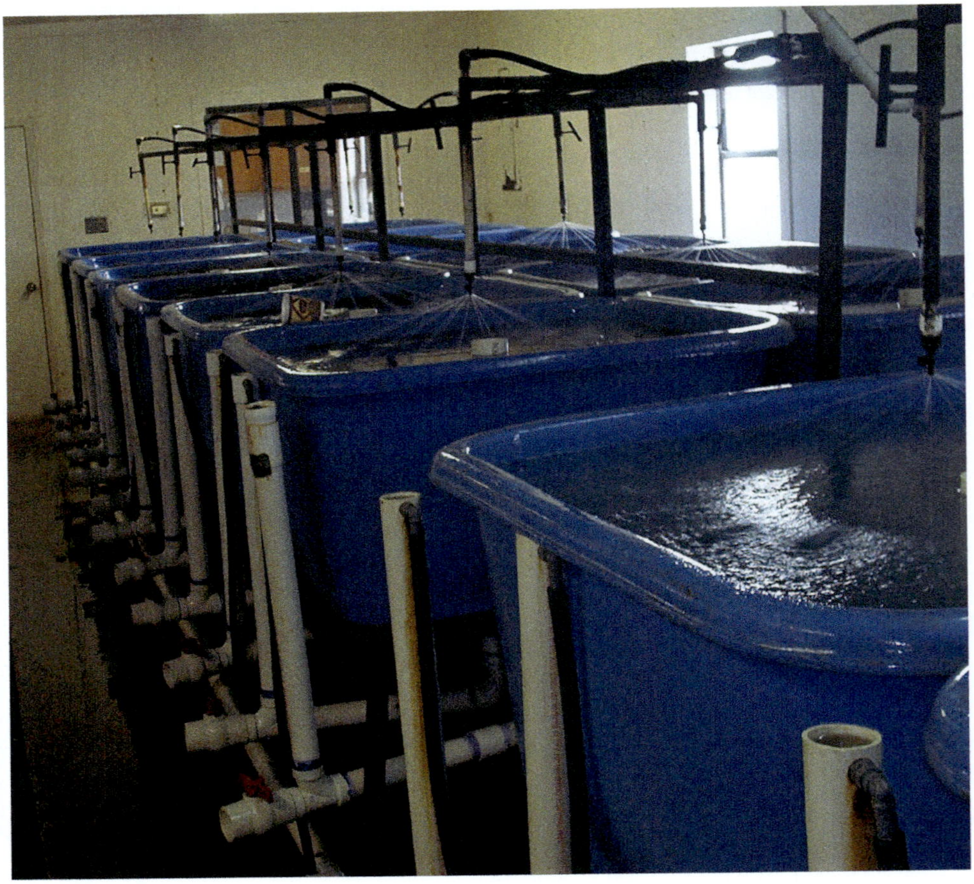

Fig. 2.7. Indoor breeding operations: Plastic vats for hatching eggs and raising fry. (Photograph by N. Saint-Erne.)

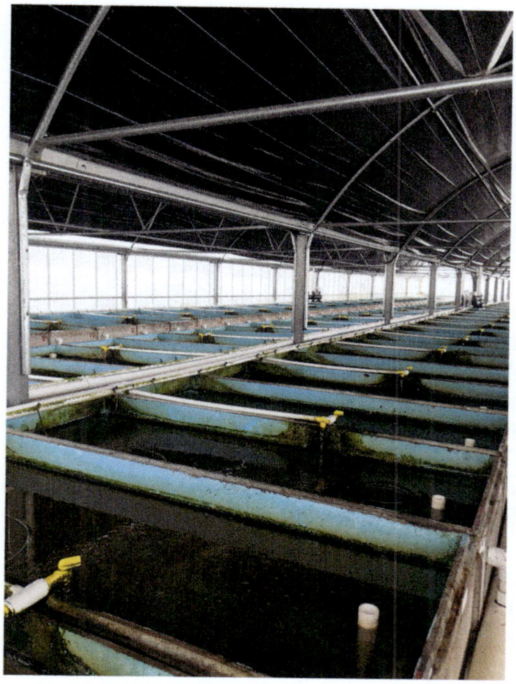

Fig. 2.8. Freshwater fish raised indoors in cement vats. (Photograph by N. Saint-Erne.)

the flow-through water that outdoor ponds use. This allows for proper water quality by mechanical and biological filtration without using as much water. Smaller indoor tanks with proper filtration can produce or hold more fish per water unit compared with outdoor ponds with no filtration, helping to reduce the overall cost of operation by comparison to traditional pond methods.

2.3 Transportation

From the fish farms, the fish are transported by truck to an exporter location, if farmed overseas, or to a domestic wholesale facility. The fish may be held in aquariums at that facility for a period of time or may be immediately repacked with fresh water in plastic bags and shipped in insulated cardboard boxes (Figs. 2.10 and 2.11) to the next destination. When a retail pet store or fish store places an order for the fish from a wholesaler or distributor, they are packed and shipped again. It may be as few as three or as many as seven stops for the fish to go from the farm to the home aquarium. In each step, the fish are netted, counted, packed in plastic bags, shipped, and then put in aquariums again, until they finally are home.

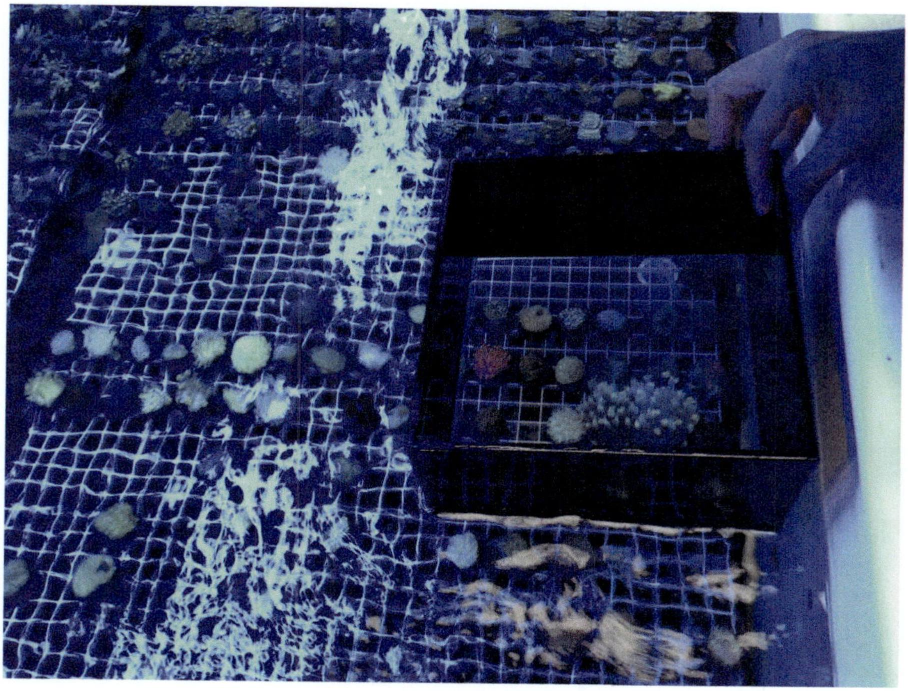

Fig. 2.9. Tank for culturing marine invertebrates. (Photograph by N. Saint-Erne.)

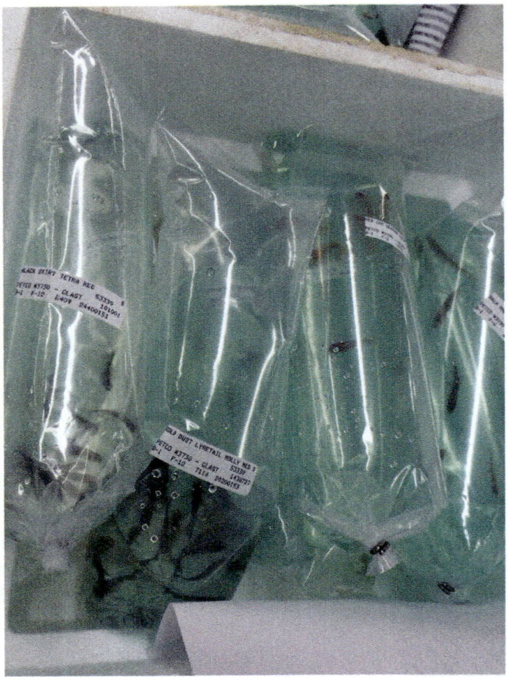

Fig. 2.10. Fish in shipping bags in styrene cartons. (Photograph by N. Saint-Erne.)

The stress of this process can cause adverse effects on the fish's immune system, as well as physical damage to its skin and fins. It is important for the health and welfare of the fish that the handlers are as gentle as possible when netting and moving fish, that the transportation methods are rapid in climate-controlled vehicles, and that the water quality in each facility is tested and maintained at the appropriate parameters for the fish species. Better breeding and wholesale facilities will perform physical examinations and diagnostic tests for fish diseases and provide appropriate treatments for any ailments discerned, but in many cases, only minimal testing and random preventative treatments are given.

Prior to each shipment of fish, the water quality and temperature should be monitored, and the fish checked for signs of disease (Fig. 2.12). The appropriate treatments should be administered, and the fish fed during the quarantine period. Food is withheld for 24 h before packing the fish for shipping to prevent waste accumulation in the shipping water. The shipping water is often medicated to reduce diseases associated with stress from handling. The water for freshwater fish may be treated

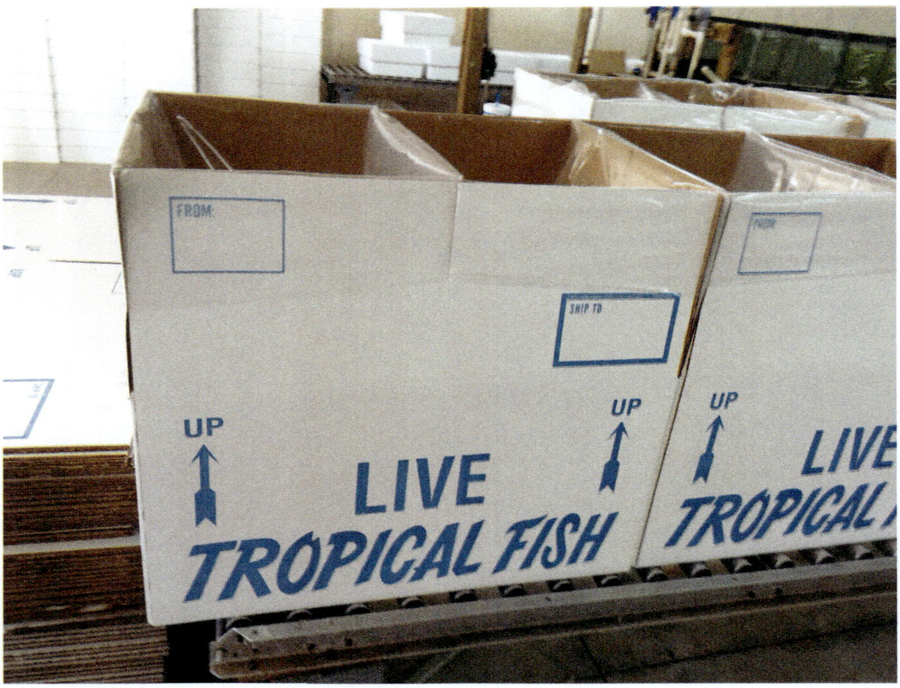

Fig. 2.11. Plastic-lined shipping boxes. (Photograph by N. Saint-Erne.)

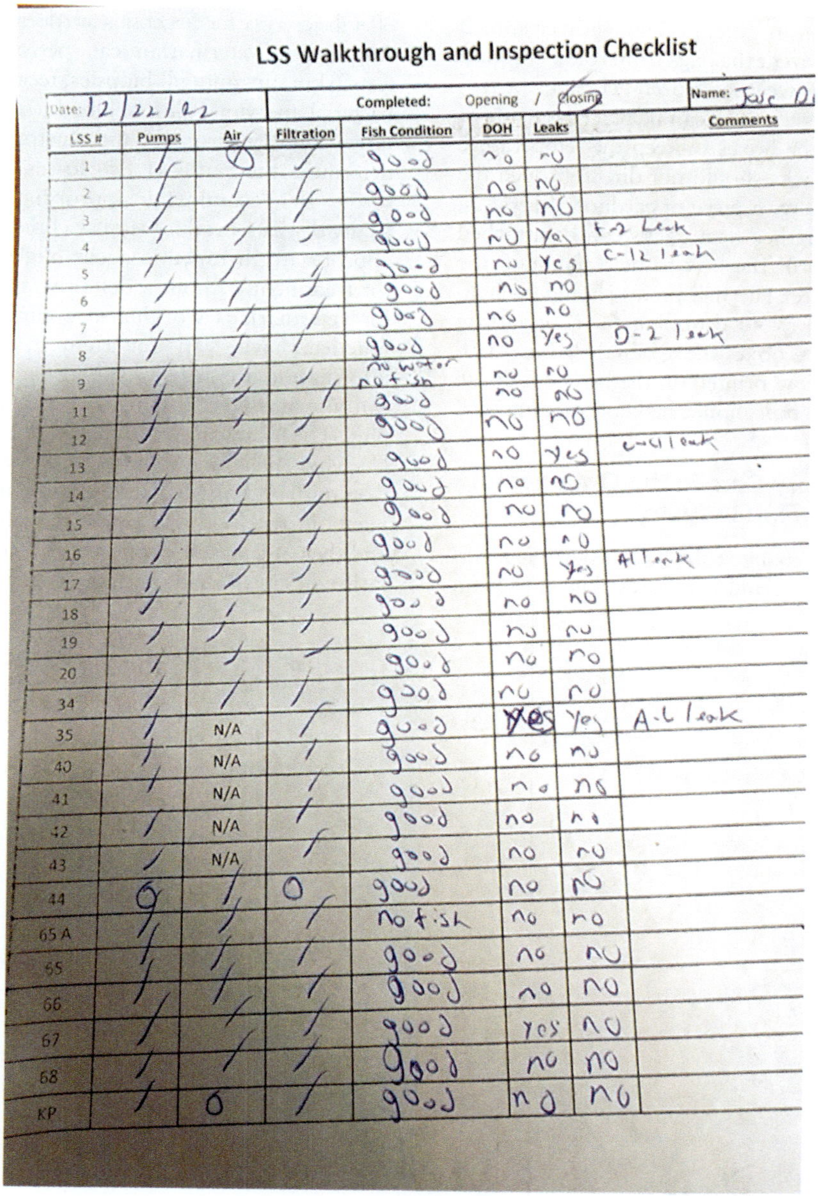

LSS Walkthrough and Inspection Checklist

Date: 12/22/22 | Completed: Opening / Closing | Name: Jose D

LSS #	Pumps	Air	Filtration	Fish Condition	DOH	Leaks	Comments
1	/	O	/	good	no	no	
2	/	/	/	good	no	no	
3	/	/	/	good	no	no	
4	/	/	/	good	no	Yes	t-2 Leak
5	/	/	/	good	no	Yes	C-12 leak
6	/	/	/	good	no	no	
7	/	/	/	good	no	no	
8	/	/	/	good	no	Yes	D-2 leak
9	/	/	/	no water no fish	no	no	
11	/	/	/	good	no	no	
12	/	/	/	good	no	no	
13	/	/	/	good	no	yes	C-11 leak
14	/	/	/	good	no	no	
15	/	/	/	good	no	no	
16	/	/	/	good	no	no	
17	/	/	/	good	no	Yes	Al leak
18	/	/	/	good	no	no	
19	/	/	/	good	no	no	
20	/	/	/	good	no	no	
34	/	/	/	good	no	no	
35	/	N/A	/	good	Yes	Yes	A-L leak
40	/	N/A	/	good	no	no	
41	/	N/A	/	good	no	no	
42	/	N/A	/	good	no	no	
43	/	N/A	/	good	no	no	
44	O	/	O	good	no	no	
65 A	/	/	/	no fish	no	no	
65	/	/	/	good	no	no	
66	/	/	/	good	no	no	
67	/	/	/	good	Yes	no	
68	/	/	/	good	no	no	
KP	/	O	/	good	no	no	

Fig. 2.12. Checklist used when examining the fish and the life-support systems (filtration) in a fish wholesale facility. (Photograph by N. Saint-Erne.)

with non-iodized salt at 1–3 g/l (0.12–0.36%), methylene blue (2 mg/l), ammonia binder to neutralize excreted ammonia during shipping or even some form of tranquilizer (MS-222, eugenol, or quinaldine).

The fish should be placed into plastic bags with enough water to comfortably accommodate all the fish, so they are not injuring each other from crowding. The remainder of the bag is filled with air for trips of short duration (a few hours maximum) or pure oxygen for longer time in transport (Saint-Erne, 2015). The amount of oxygen should be 50–66% of the volume of the bag. The plastic bags of fish are placed into a cardboard box and insulated with styrene sheeting to help maintain a constant temperature and packed with crumpled newspapers to prevent the bags from rolling around in the box. In hot weather, frozen gel packs or frozen plastic bottles of water can be placed outside of the fish bags in the boxes to keep the temperature cool. The cold packs should not directly touch the bags of fish but have a piece of cardboard between them. In cold weather, heat packs can be attached inside at the top of the box to help maintain the water temperature. The fish boxes should be handled carefully to avoid dropping them or jarring unnecessarily. The boxes must be labeled as LIVE FISH, and an arrow printed on the box to indicate which end of the box should be kept uppermost.

2.4 Veterinary Care in the Ornamental Fish Industry

Veterinarians can contact fish farms, wholesale facilities (Fig. 2.13), or retail pet stores (Fig. 2.14) and offer their service for diagnosing fish diseases (Table 2.2). An aquatic veterinarian can perform diagnostic tests (skin, fin, and gill biopsies, fecal examination, bacterial and viral cultures, blood tests, radiographs, ultrasound, necropsy, and histopathology) to determine the cause of fish losses and then prescribe or recommend appropriate treatments. Many diseases produce similar clinical signs, so the appropriate therapeutic agent might not be used for treatment without a definitive diagnosis. Also, for veterinarians working in a clinical veterinary practice, having an aquarium in the lobby, or information about fish hanging on the clinic wall can inform clients that fish are treated at the hospital. The American Veterinary Medical Association (AVMA) has an Aquatic Veterinary Medicine Committee (AqVMC) that advises it on developments in the food and ornamental fish industries, and they also review proposed governmental regulations. The World Aquatic Veterinary Medical

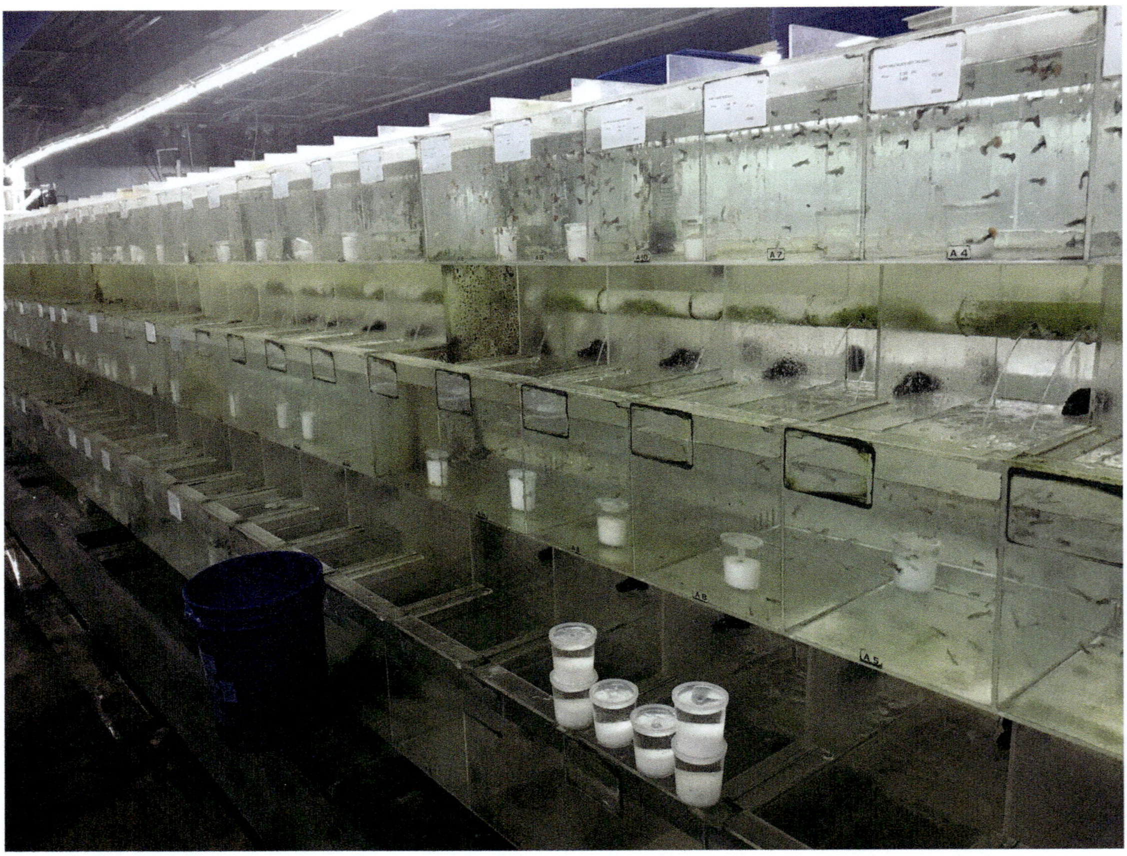

Fig. 2.13. Holding tanks at a fish wholesaler. (Photograph by N. Saint-Erne.)

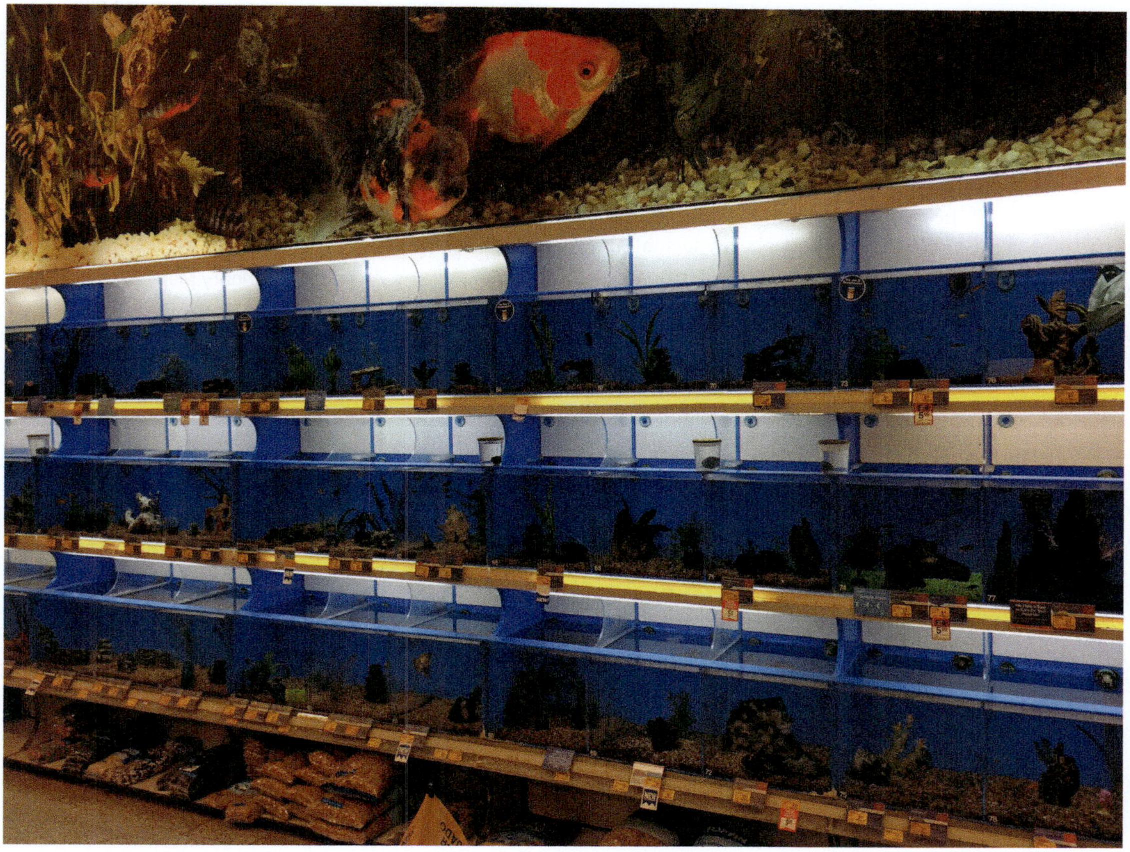

Fig. 2.14. Freshwater fish display in an aquarium store. (Photograph by N. Saint-Erne.)

Table 2.2. Veterinarian's role in ornamental aquaculture (Saint-Erne, 2013).

Fish Farms, Distributors, Retailers

- Visit facilities to examine fish and perform biopsy or other diagnostic tests
- Administer vaccinations and medications
- Water analysis/lab tests
- Biosecurity and disease prevention training
- Health certificates for shipping fish

Private Practice Clinic/House Calls

- Health check-ups/house call services
- Examine fish and perform diagnostic tests
- Water quality analysis
- Quarantine facilities for sick fish or new purchases
- Aquarium maintenance services referrals

Fish and Koi Clubs

- Lectures/Seminars to educate hobbyists
- Health checks at Koi and Fish shows or auctions

Association (WAVMA.org) has on their website a search engine to locate aquatic veterinarians: https://www.wavma.org/find-a-fish-vet.

2.5 Conclusion

The number of people keeping aquariums in the USA is the third-highest number of pet owners, after dogs and cats. There are more pet fish in more households than rodents, birds, and reptiles combined. Fishkeeping has been a way to bring nature into the home for more than a century. The fish go through many stages from farm to home aquarium, and veterinarians are important contributors to the health and welfare of fish in the aquarium industry. The lack of fish clients is not necessarily due to a lack of demand for veterinary care but an inability of pet owners to find a veterinarian who cares for fish.

References

APPA (American Pet Products Association) (2022) National pet owners survey. Available at: https://americanpetproducts.org/Uploads/NPOS/21-22_BusinessandFinance.pdf (accessed 8 May 2023).

LiveAquaria (2023) Captive bred marine fish. Available at: https://www.liveaquaria.com/category/15/marine-fish (accessed 8 May 2023).

Project Piaba (2023) Available at: https://projectpiaba.org/ (accessed 8 May 2023).

Rising Tides (2023) Available at: https://www.risingtideconservation.org/ (accessed 8 May 2023).

Saint-Erne, N. (2013) *Freshwater and Marine Ornamental Fish Industry*. American Veterinary Medical Association Convention, Lecture Event #14338, Chicago, Illinois.

Saint-Erne, N. (2015) *Culture Shock—Understanding and Managing Stress among Globetrotting Ornamental Fish*. World Small Animal Veterinary Association Congress, Bangkok, Thailand.

Spots.com (2023) Pet ownership statistics. Available at: https://spots.com/pet-ownership-statistics/#:~:text=Pet%20Ownership%20Statistics%201%2084.9%20million%20or%2067%25,9.6%25%20of%20households%20own%20freshwater%20fish.%20More%20items (accessed 8 May 2023).

Sweet, T. and Pedersen, M. (2023) *CORAL* Magazine Special Report: The State of the Marine Breeder's Art, 2023. *CORAL Magazine*. Available at: https://www.coralmagazine.com/?s=the+state+of+marine+breeders/ (accessed 1 August 2024).

3 Fish Taxonomy, Anatomy, and Physiology

Nicholas Saint-Erne

Dr. Saint-Erne Consulting, PLLC, Phoenix, Arizona

Abstract

Most ornamental fish kept in home aquariums are teleost fish, but in public aquariums, Elasmobranchs are also maintained. All fish are adapted to living in an aquatic environment, with gills and fins, rather than lungs and legs that terrestrial vertebrates have. Reviewing the anatomy of fish helps understand the differences and similarities between them and other vertebrates.

3.1 Fish Taxonomy

A fish is an aquatic, gill-bearing, vertebrate animal (Table 3.1). Bony fishes and cartilaginous fishes (the plural of "fish" when referring to more than one species) are typically divided into three groups: Superclass Agnatha (jawless fishes), Class Chondrichthyes (cartilaginous fishes), and Grade Osteichthyes (bony fishes). The latter two groups are included within the Superclass Gnathostomata, a category containing all jawed vertebrates (Britannica, 2023). Approximately 95% of living fish species are ray-finned fish, belonging to the class Actinopterygii, with around 99% of those being teleosts (bony fishes). Tetrapod vertebrates (amphibians, reptiles, dinosaurs, birds, and mammals) emerged from lobe-finned fishes (Nelson, 2016). There are over 32,000 documented species of bony fish and over 1100 species of cartilaginous fish (sharks, rays, and chimeras), and about 108 species of hagfish and lampreys (Nelson, 2016; Betancur *et al.*, 2017).

3.2 External Anatomy

Body shape: The shapes of bony fish include fusiform, laterally flattened, ventrally flattened, eel or ribbon-like, and spheroid (Mylniczenko, 2021).

Mouth: The upper jaw consists of the premaxilla and maxilla bones, and the lower jawbone is the mandible. The angle of the mouth can indicate the feeding habits of the fish: superior mouth types eat food from the surface, terminal mouths eat from directly ahead, inferior position mouths (Fig. 3.1) feed on the bottom, and protrusible jaws are used to suck in food, often by predators to gulp prey.

Tongue: Fish tongues have limited mobility and are used to move food into the esophagus.

Nostrils: Some fish have one pair of nostrils (nares), some two pairs, and cyprinids have one pair of nostrils with each nostril divided by a septum into an anterior inlet and posterior outlet. Water enters an olfactory sac filled with scent-detector cells within the nostril.

Barbels: Some fish have barbels attached to their lips or around the mouth. The barbels, lips, and oral mucosa have taste buds on their surfaces.

Eye: The sclera, the outer fibrous coat, connects to three pairs of muscles innervated by the third cranial nerve (oculomotor nerve), allowing it to move within the orbital bone. The cornea has a similar refractive index to water. The lens of the eye is spherical (Fig. 3.2)—giving fish a wide angle of vision—and protrudes slightly through the iris into the anterior chamber. The iris is round with a fixed pupil in most fish species. The iris contains striated muscles under voluntary control in fish that can change the shape of their iris. Fish have both rod

Corresponding author: DrSaintErne@gmail.com

© CAB International 2025. *The Handbook of Ornamental Fish Health and Welfare* (ed. N. Saint-Erne)
DOI: 10.1079/9781789246032.0003

Table 3.1. Taxonomy of fishes (Nelson, 2016; Britannica, 2023).

- Kingdom: Animalia
- Phylum: Chordata
- Clade: Olfactores
- Subphylum: Vertebrata (Craniata)
- Superclass Agnatha (jawless fish): having a suctorial or filter-feeding mouth; no true jaws
  - Class Cyclostomata (hagfish and lampreys)
    - Subclass Myxini (hagfish)
    - Subclass Petromyzontidae (lampreys)
    - Subclass Ostracodermi (extinct armored jawless fish)
- Superclass Gnathostomata (jawed vertebrates)
  - Class Chondrichthyes (cartilaginous fish)
    - Subclass Elasmobranchii (sharks, skates, rays)
      - Order Selachii (sharks)
      - Order Batoidei (rays, sawfishes, guitarfishes, skates, stingrays)
    - Subclass Holocephali (chimeras and extinct relatives)
      - Order Chimaeriformes (chimeras)
  - Class Placodermi (extinct armored fish)
  - Class Acanthodii (spiny sharks, sometimes classified under Actinopterygii)
- Grade Osteichthyes (bony fish)
  - Class Actinopterygii (ray-finned): Fins supported by bony spines or cartilage rays
    - Subclass Chondrostei
      - Order Acipenseriformes (sturgeons and paddlefishes)
      - Order Polypteriformes (reedfish and bichirs)
    - Subclass Neopterygii (new finned fishes)
      - Infraclass Holostei (gars and bowfins)
        - Order Lepisosteiformes (gars)
        - Order Amiiformes (bowfins)
      - Infraclass Teleostei (advanced bony fishes)
        - Superorder Osteoglossomorpha (bonytongues)
          - Order Osteoglossiformes (freshwater butterfly fish, mooneyes, knife fish, mormyrids)
        - Superorder Elopomorpha (eels, tarpons, bonefish)
          - Order Elopiformes (tarpons, ten-pounders)
          - Order Albuliformes (bonefishes, halosaurs, deep-sea eels)
          - Order Anguilliformes (eels)
          - Order Saccopharyngiformes (gulper eels)
        - Superorder Clupeomorpha (herrings, anchovies)
          - Order Clupeiformes (herrings, anchovies)
        - Superorder Ostariophysi
          - Order Gonorynchiformes (milkfish, sandfishes, mudheads)
          - Order Characiformes (hatchetfish, pencil fish, piranha, tetras)
          - Order Cypriniformes (carps and minnows)
          - Order Siluriformes (catfishes)
          - Order Gymnotiformes (knifefishes, gymnotid, and electric eels)
        - Superorder Protacanthopterygii
          - Order Esociformes (pikes and pickerels)
          - Order Osmeriformes (argentines and smelts)
          - Order Salmoniformes (salmons, trouts)
        - Superorder Stenopterygii
          - Order Stomiiformes (barbeled dragonfishes, bristlemouths)
          - Order Ateleopodiformes (highfin tadpole fish)
        - Superorder Cyclosquamata
          - Order Aulopiformes (barracudinas, lizard fishes, greeneyes)
        - Superorder Scopelomorpha
          - Order Myctophiformes (lantern fishes)

Continued

Table 3.1. Continued.

Superorder Lampridiomorpha
- Order Lampriformes (opahs, oarfish)

Superorder Polymixiomorpha
- Order Polymixiiformes (barbudos, beardfish)

Superorder Paracanthopterygii
- Order Percopsiformes (trout-perches, pirate perches, cave fish)
- Order Gadiformes (cods, hakes, grenadiers, rattails)
- Order Batrachoidiformes (toadfishes)
- Order Lophiiformes (goosefish, anglerfish, frogfish, batfish)
- Order Ophidiiformes (cusk eels, brotulas, pearlfish)

Superorder Acanthopterygii (spiny-rayed fishes)
- Order Atheriniformes (silversides)
- Order Cyprinodontiformes (killifish and live-bearers)
- Order Beloniformes (medakas, needlefish, halfbeaks)
- Order Mugiliformes (mullets)
- Order Stephanoberyciformes (whalefish, bigscale fish)
- Order Beryciformes (squirrelfish)
- Order Zeiformes (dories, boarfish)
- Order Gasterosteiformes (sticklebacks, tube snout fish, seahorses)
- Order Synbranchiformes (swamp eels, spiny eels)
- Order Scorpaeniformes (scorpion fishes, sculpins, flying gurnards)
- Order Perciformes (perch-like fishes): the largest group of fishes, represented by more than 6000 species placed in about 160 families, including tunas, mackerels, bonitos, skipjacks (family Scombridae), sea basses (Serranidae), sunfishes (Centrarchidae), cichlids (Cichlidae), perches, and walleyes (Percidae).
- Order Istiophoriformes (billfishes, marlins, swordfish)
- Order Carangiformes (pompanos, jacks, cavallas, scads, remoras)
- Order Pleuronectiformes (flounders, soles, halibuts)
- Order Syngnathiformes (trumpet fish, pipefish, seahorses)
- Order Tetraodontiformes (puffer fish, boxfish, filefish, triggerfish)
- Order Anabantiformes (snakeheads, fighting fish, gouramis)

Class Sarcopterygii (lobe-finned fish and tetrapods)
- Subclass Actinistia (Crossopterygii)
  - Order Coelacanthiformes (coelacanths)
- Subclass Dipnoi (lungfish)
  - Order Ceratodontiformes (Australian lungfishes)
  - Order Lepidosireniformes (South American and African lungfishes)
- Subclass Tetrapodomorpha (four-limbed vertebrates)

and cone cells in the retina, allowing them to see colors. However, cones and color vision are absent in fish living at depths where limited light produces only monochrome illumination (Roberts and Ellis, 2012). Fish have no eyelids.

Operculum: This is a hinged bony plate covered with epithelium that opens and closes to pull water from the mouth and across the gills, and out the gill slit. It consists of the preopercle, interopercle, opercle, and subopercle bones and the branchiostegal membrane.

Lateral line: This is a groove on each side of the fish, lined with neuromast receptors that can detect low-frequency vibrations in water, caused by sound or motion. This vibration detection allows the fish to be aware of objects near it in the water, even if it is too dark or muddy to see. Scales directly over the lateral line may contain perforations through them to allow vibrations to pass through.

Scales: Calcified flexible plates, consisting of collagen fibers, albuminoid materials, and hydroxyapatite crystals. Growth rings are added continuously as the fish grows, and not annually. The scales come from the dermis layer of the skin, and the exposed distal third is covered with a thin layer of epidermis (Fig. 3.3). Most fish do not have scales on the head. The scales over the lateral line have holes in them to allow vibrations to pass through. Scale shapes vary by fish taxonomy and include placoid, cosmoid,

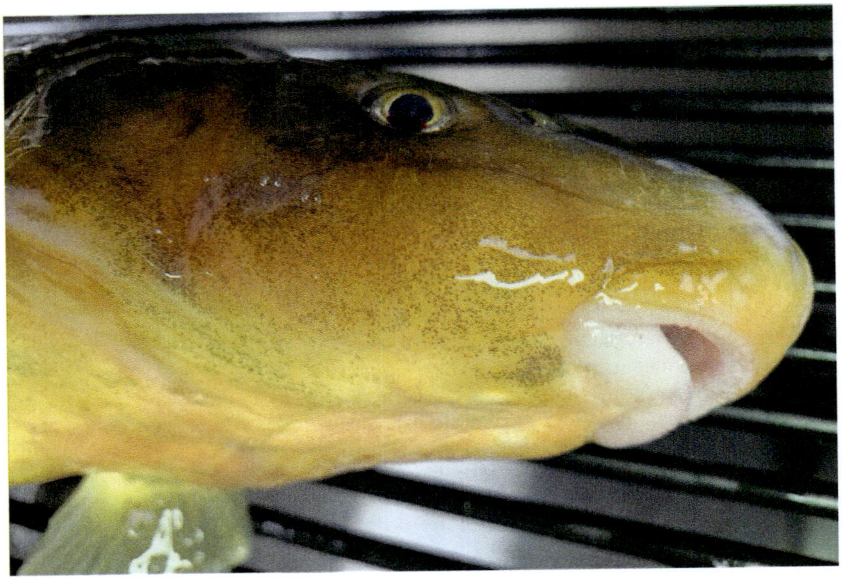

Fig. 3.1. Inferior mouth position of a razorback sucker (*Xyrauchen texanus*), a bottom-feeding fish. (Photograph by N. Saint-Erne.)

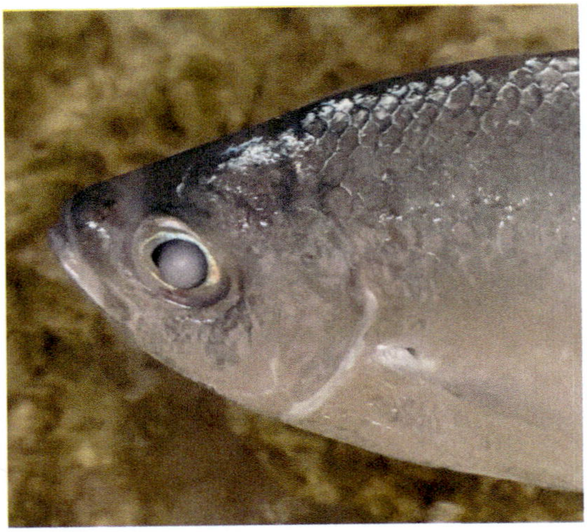

Fig. 3.2. Fivebar flagtail fish (*Kuhlia mugil*) with a cataract, showing the round shape of fish lenses. (Photograph by N. Saint-Erne.)

ganoid, cycloid, and ctenoid. Not all species of fish have scales, and scaleless fish may be more sensitive to toxins and medications in the water, as well as to trauma (Stoskopf, 1993).

Skin: The skin is made of three layers: hypodermis, dermis, and epidermis. The hypodermis, or subcutaneous tissue, is a vascularized fatty layer covering the muscles. The dermis consists of mast cells, fibrous connective tissue, blood vessels, nerves, osteogenic cells for scale production, scales, and chromatophores (pigment cells). The thin epidermis consists of a basal cell layer, fibrous epithelial cells, mucus-secreting goblet cells, leukocytes in the intracellular spaces, and some pigment cells. Fish skin is inelastic.

Mucus: The skin is coated with a cuticle, or glycocalyx, which is a slimy layer of mucus made from mucopolysaccharides, immunoglobulins, lysozymes, fatty acids, and sloughed epidermal cells. It protects the skin from pathogens, aids osmoregulation by reducing the permeability of the skin, and helps the fish glide through the water by reducing friction.

Chromatophores: These are pigmented cells that produce the fish's coloration. There are several types of pigment cells: melanophores, erythrophores, xanthophores, and iridophores (Saint-Erne, 2010). Melanophores contain black melanin granules and can expand or contract under neurological control to darken or lighten the skin color. Erythrophores contain red and orange carotenoid and pteridine pigments that are obtained from the diet (Fig. 3.4). Xanthophores contain yellow carotenoid pigments. The iridophores (also called iridocytes, or guanophores) contain crystalline deposits of guanine that produce the silvery glitter by reflecting light.

Wen: Certain varieties of goldfish, especially the Oranda, have been genetically selected to have a thickened skin on the head, called a *wen*. It consists of

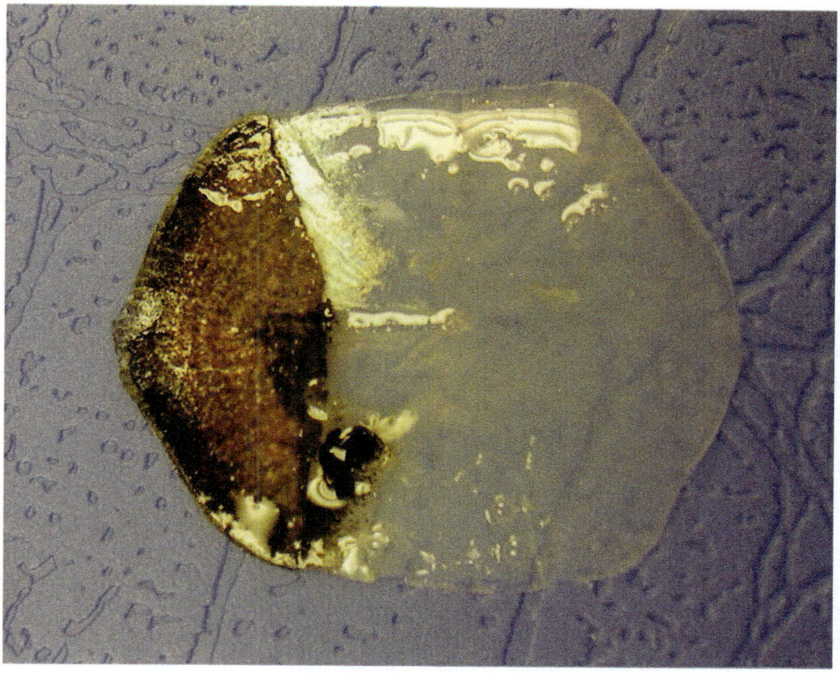

Fig. 3.3. Cycloid scale from a koi fish (*Cyprinus rubrofuscus*) showing the exposed portion covered with epidermis; the clear portion is buried in the dermis and covered by other scales. (Photograph by N. Saint-Erne.)

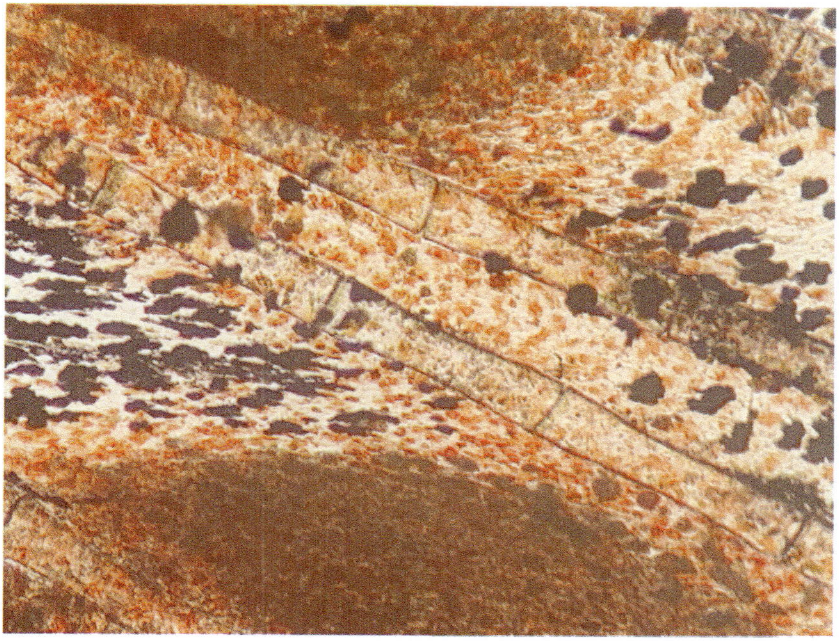

Fig. 3.4. Melanophore and erythrophore pigment cells in fish epithelium from a caudal fin biopsy. (Microphotograph by N. Saint-Erne.)

a non-ciliated epithelium with goblet cells covering a mucinous stroma (Mylniczenko, 2021). This growth can become enlarged to obscure the eyes or mouth and may require surgical trimming under anesthesia.

Caudal peduncle: the portion of the tail before the caudal fin, which contains the spine and the dorsal epidural and ventral hypural bones, which are flat articulated plates that support the caudal fin.

Fins: The limbs of fish are fins (Fig. 3.5) and vary in shape and location by species and function. The pectoral fins and pelvic fins are paired, analogous to front and rear legs of tetrapod vertebrates. The median dorsal and ventral fins are articulated to the pterygiophoral muscles along the vertebral neural and hemal spines. The caudal fin is articulated on a series of flat plates from the distal spine, the dorsal epural, and ventral hypural bones. Fins may have bony spines at the anterior portion followed by cartilaginous rays, or just cartilage for support. Some fish have fins modified into suckers for climbing, or leglike fins that allow them to walk on the substrate. Lobe-finned fish, lungfish, and coelacanths have muscular pectoral fins with articulating bones.

Caudal fin: Tail fin consisting of cartilaginous fin rays. Depending on the species, the caudal fin may be rounded, squared (truncated), emarginated, lunate, forked, or elongated. Sharks have a heterocercal tail. The caudal fin functions in rapid forward propulsion of the fish by strong side-to-side motions.

Dorsal fin: A median fin on the top of the fish that stabilizes the fish during forward motion. There may be one or more sections to the dorsal fin, and it can have stiff bony spines and softer cartilaginous branched fin rays, or just cartilaginous rays for support.

Pectoral fins: Paired fins behind the gill plates that may have bony spines and soft rays. The multifunctional pectoral fins stabilize and steer the body when swimming forward, moving it up and down. They are also used for braking and swimming backward and can propel the fish forward slowly when searching for food.

Pelvic (ventral) fins: Paired fins that may have bony spines and soft rays or just cartilaginous rays. They stabilize the body against pitch and are used to counterbalance lift.

Anal fin: Single median fin behind the vent, which may have bony spines and soft rays. It serves as a stabilizer during forward motion. Some species, such as male live-bearing fish, have modified anal fins (gonopodium) that act to pass sperm into the female's vent (Fig. 3.6).

Adipose fin: The single adipose fin is found on the dorsal caudal peduncle in approximately 6000

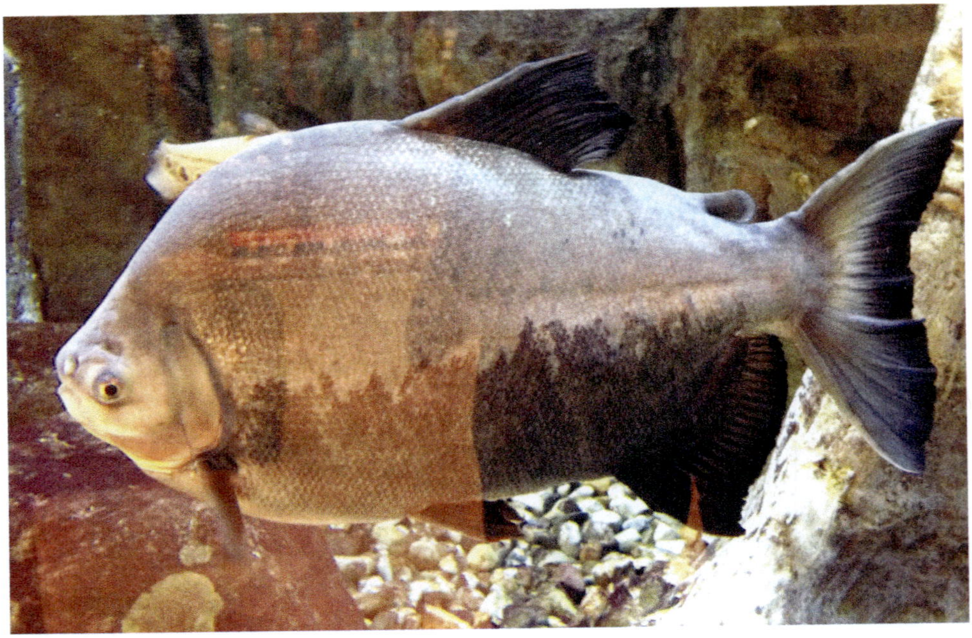

Fig. 3.5. Fins visible on this a black pacu fish (*Colossoma macropomum*), named in clockwise fashion starting at the top, include the dorsal fin, adipose fin, caudal fin, anal fin, pelvic fins (paired), and pectoral fins (paired). Also visible is the nasal septum anterior to the eye and above the mouth. (Photograph by N. Saint-Erne.)

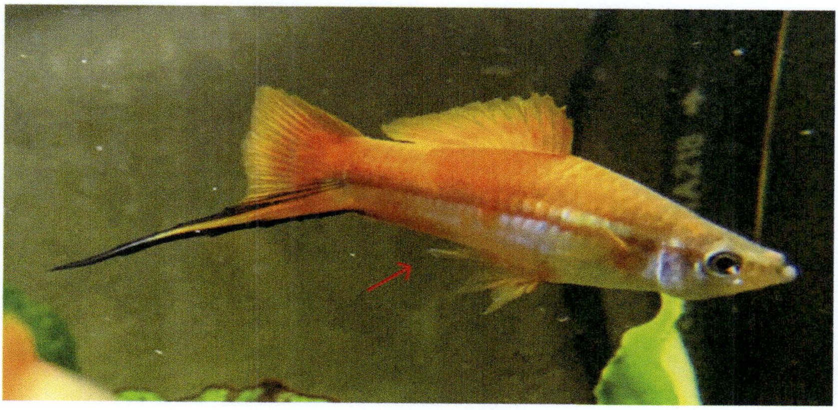

Fig. 3.6. Red swordtail (*Xiphophorus helleri*) and platinum sailfin molly (*Poecilia latipinna*) males showing the anal fin modified to a gonopodium. (Photograph by N. Saint-Erne.)

species of teleost fishes. The adipose fin is smaller than other fins and lacks musculature and cartilaginous rays but has sensory innervation. The adipose fin functions as a "precaudal flow sensor," detecting fluid flow anterior to the caudal fin (Aiello *et al.*, 2016). Adipose fins are found more commonly on fish species that live in high-flow habitats (streams and rivers) than those species occupying no-flow habitats (lakes and ponds).

Vent: External opening for the anus to excrete digestive waste and for the urogenital papilla.

Urogenital papilla: This is a small, fleshy tube behind the anus present in some fishes, from which the sperm or eggs are released (Fig. 3.7). In some species, such as cichlids, the gender of a fish can be determined by the shape of its papilla; with a male having a pointed tip and a female a rounded tip to the papilla. The papilla usually extends from the vent only during breeding.

Nuptial tubercles: During the reproductive season, males of some fish, such as cyprinids, present dermal structures on their head and pectoral fin spines called nuptial (or breeding) tubercles (Fig. 3.7). Nuptial tubercles are tiny keratinized epidermal structures that grow on the body parts of males that contact the females during courtship and spawning (Gallego and Sousa-Santos, 2022) and are used to stimulate egg laying in the female in species whose courtship involves chasing and pressing the head against the urogenital area of the female by the males. Their development is stimulated by hormones secreted by the pituitary and intrarenal glands, being induced shortly before the reproductive period.

3.3 Internal Anatomy

Teeth: Dentition varies by feeding method. Not all species of fish have teeth. Some fish have many teeth that are attached to the jaw by fibrous tissue, some teeth can bend inward by elastic ligaments to hold prey. Parrotfish and pufferfish have fused teeth that form a beak that grows continuously and needs to be worn down by chewing hard substances. Cyprinids have ventral pharyngeal teeth in the back of the mouth (Fig. 3.8) that masticate food against a fibrous pad situated on the roof of the pharynx before swallowing. In many fish species, teeth can be shed and replaced when lost.

Pharynx: The pharynx is the throat that opens into the esophagus. In koi and other carp, there are three rows of pharyngeal teeth in each of the lower pharyngeal ceratobranchial bones (modified fifth gill arches). These teeth grind against a thick masticating plate on the roof of the pharynx, attached to the basioccipital bone.

Gills: Most bony fish have four gill arches on each side of the pharynx. Gill filaments project in pairs from the gill arches. Each filament contains two rows of semicircular lamellae through which blood flows in short lamellar arteries (Fig. 3.9). These small "leaves" have a very high surface area across which the water passes in a countercurrent direction to the blood flow. Oxygen diffuses from the water into the blood as the water passes over the gill lamellae. The red blood cells in the blood are very efficient oxygen transporters and 1 ml of blood will be able to carry the amount of oxygen

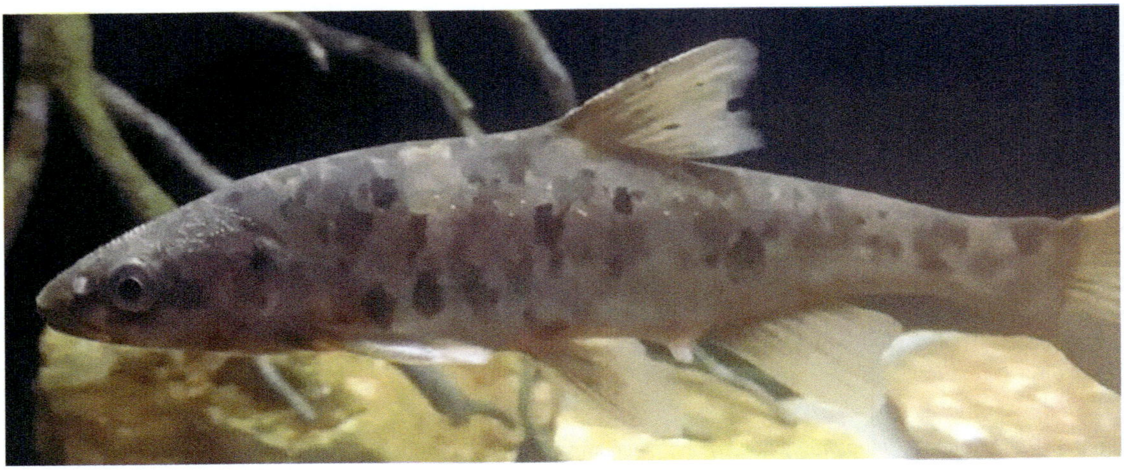

Fig. 3.7. Nuptial tubercles (raised white spots) on the head of a male roundtail chub (*Gila robusta*) that also has an extended genital papilla. These can be confused with white spots on the skin from *Ichthyophthirius* protozoa infestation. (Photograph by N. Saint-Erne.)

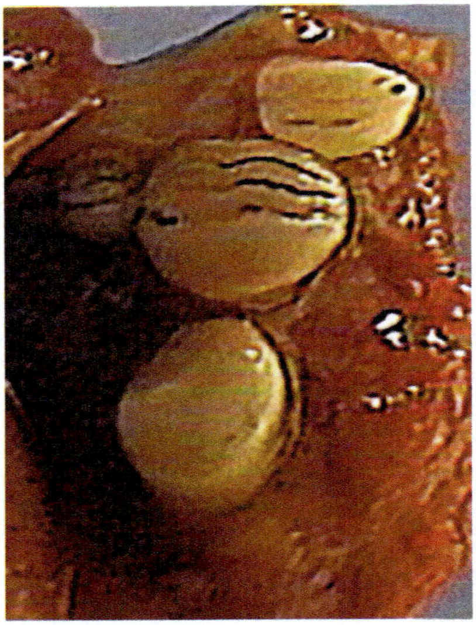

Fig. 3.8. Pharyngeal teeth of a koi (*Cyprinus rubrofuscus*) in three rows. The teeth fall out as they wear down and are replaced by new teeth. (Photograph by N. Saint-Erne.)

contained in 15–25 ml of water. The gills also release carbon dioxide and ammonia from the blood into the water. The gills are the main sites of ammonia and urea excretion in fish, rather than the kidneys. Gill rakers protrude from each of the gill arches into the pharynx, and their shape is specialized for the mode of feeding in each fish species (Hoole *et al.*, 2001).

Thymus: Paired glands located in the branchial cavity below the gills in fish other than Agnatha.

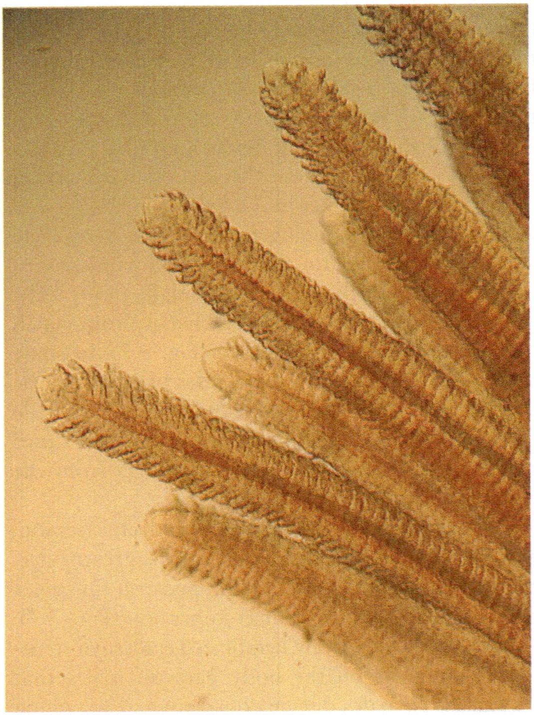

Fig. 3.9. Angelfish (*Pterophyllum scalare*) gill filaments with normal lamellae observed on a microscopic examination of a gill biopsy. (Microphotograph by N. Saint-Erne.)

This gland originates from the pharyngeal pouches and ontogenically is the first lymphoid organ to be infiltrated with lymphoid cells. Each gland is surrounded by an epithelial capsule. Within the gland, a framework of reticuloepithelial cells supports the lymphocytes (Chilmonczyk, 1992).

Esophagus: Food passes down the muscular esophagus into the stomach, or in some fish species directly into the intestines. Fish with no glandular stomach do not secrete digestive acids. In physostomous fish, the pneumatic duct arises from the dorsal surface of the anterior esophagus and connects to the gas bladder.

Stomach: Fish may have no glandular stomach or a stomach that varies in size based on its feeding habits. The cardia of the stomach consists of striated muscles, and the pylorus has smooth muscles. Pyloric caeca are diverticula of the stomach in salmonids and many other teleost fishes that increase absorptive surface area in the stomach.

Intestine: The intestinal length varies by species and the type of diet a fish consumes. Carnivorous fish have shorter intestines, and herbivorous fish have longer intestines that coil within the coelom. A long recurving intestine allows better digestion of fibrous food in herbivores. The intestines empty through the anus in the vent, anterior to the urogenital opening.

Adipose tissue: Fats and lipids occur in bony fish around the organs in the coelom, within the muscles, and in the liver. Visceral adipose tissue is the main lipid storage site in vertebrates (Fig. 3.10). The primary function of adipose tissue is to control energy balance by storing triacylglycerol in periods of energy excess and mobilizing it during energy deprivation (Ali *et al.* 2013). Besides the classical function of storing fat, adipocytes secrete numerous lipid and protein factors. Collectively they are considered to constitute a major endocrine organ, which has a profound impact on the metabolism of other tissues, the regulation of appetite, insulin sensitivity, immunological responses, and vascular disease. In aquaculture, the excessive fat deposition experienced in some fish species may compromise both their welfare and longevity, due to obesity and hepatic lipidosis (Salmerón, 2018).

Heart: The heart is below and just caudal to the gills in the pericardial cavity. It consists of two chambers, with four distinct regions: the sinus venosus, atrium, ventricle, and bulbus arteriosus (Fig. 3.11). The ventricle is triangular, muscular, and red colored; the atrium is softer and darker red colored. Blood flows through two sinoatrial valves

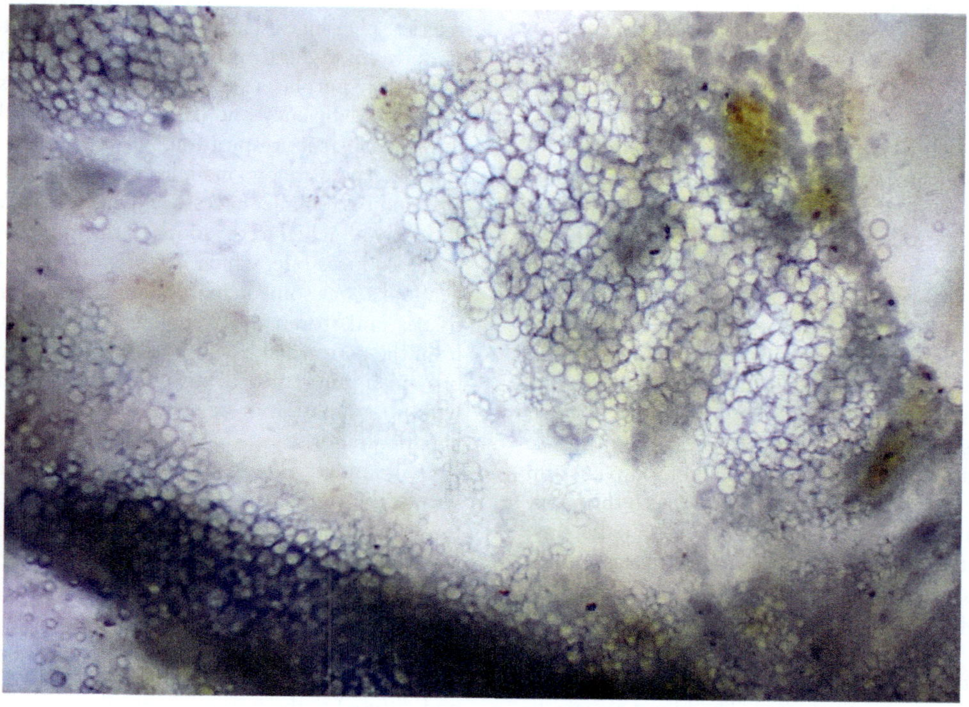

Fig. 3.10. Microscopic photograph of Sonora chub (*Gila ditaenia*) adipocytes, each containing a lipid droplet. (Microphotograph by N. Saint-Erne.)

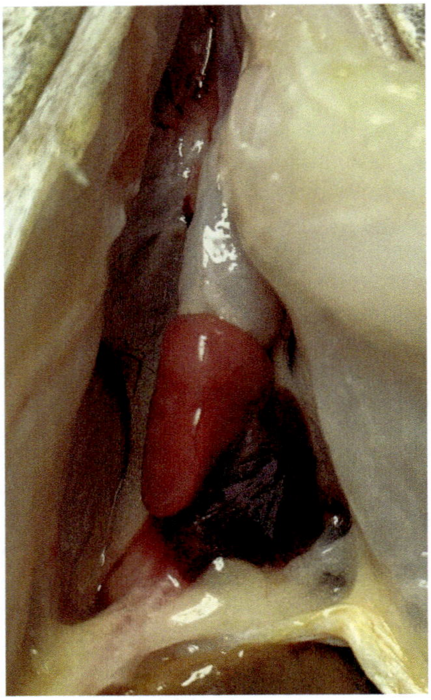

Fig. 3.11. Heart of a Colorado pike minnow (*Ptychocheilus lucius*) showing the bulbus arteriosus (white tube above ventricle) attached to the triangular ventricle, with the dark red, flaccid atrium to the right of the ventricle. (Photograph by N. Saint-Erne.)

from the sinus venosus into the atrium. Diastolic contraction of the thin-walled atrium forces blood through atrioventricular valves into the muscular ventricle. Systolic contraction of the ventricle pushes blood through a pair of semilunar ventriculobulbar valves into the bulbus arteriosus. The bulbus arteriosus stretches as blood enters, then slowly contracts to allow a continuous flow of blood through the arteries between heartbeats. Blood leaves the elastic bulbus arteriosus through the ventral aorta and goes to the gills to absorb oxygen and release carbon dioxide and ammonia. The blood passes up through the afferent branchial arteries to the capillaries in the gill lamellae (Fig. 3.12) to become oxygenated. The efferent branchial arteries join to form the dorsal aorta, which then circulates the oxygenated blood through the body via lateral arteries: the mesenteric arteries go to the coelomic organs, the carotid artery goes to the head, and the caudal artery goes to the tail. The blood returns to the heart through the hepatic portal system and cardinal veins and enters the sinus venosus.

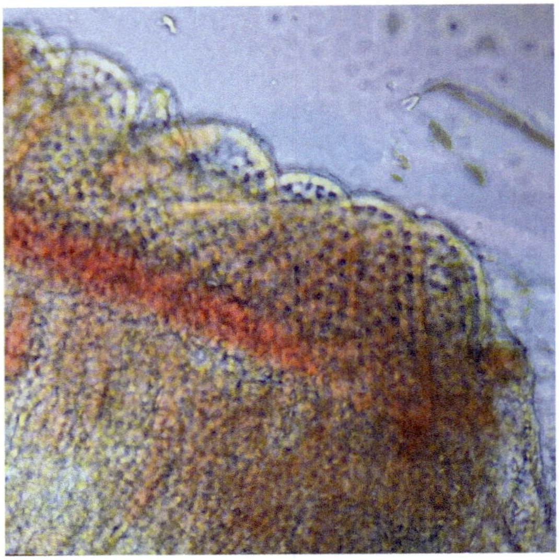

Fig. 3.12. Capillaries visible in lamellae of the gill filaments. Each capillary is just larger than the diameter of a red blood cell. (Microphotograph by N. Saint-Erne.)

Thyroid gland: This endocrine gland is usually diffuse in the area between the pharynx and the heart, with follicles along the ventral aorta, branchial arteries, pharyngeal cavity, and retro-orbital tissues. The thyroid gland produces growth hormones. Thyroid hyperplasia (goiter) can occur in fish due to iodine deficiency and causes a pharyngeal mass that can obstruct respiration.

Liver: There are two main liver lobes, united cranially, and two smaller accessory liver lobes. The liver is closely attached to the loops of the intestines. The liver produces bile, which is stored in the gallbladder. It also has some hematopoietic (blood forming) tissues and stores glycogen. The liver is separated from the pericardial cavity by a septum. It is usually brownish-pink colored but may become reddened with inflammation or be yellow-tan colored due to hepatic lipidosis.

Gallbladder: The greenish-colored gallbladder is within the right liver lobe. It stores bile produced by the liver and empties it into the intestines through the common bile duct.

Spleen: The spleen is covered by the left liver lobe. It is usually dark red in color. It contains phagocytic and hematopoietic tissues.

Pancreas: The pancreatic tissue is cream colored and diffused in the mesenteric membranes surrounding the intestines, or it may be incorporated within the liver tissue (hepatopancreas). It produces exocrine digestive enzymes (trypsin) and endocrine hormones (insulin).

Swim (gas) bladder: Not all fish have swim bladders, and those that do may have one, two, or three chambers to the swim bladder. The bladder may be physoclistous or physostomous (attached to the esophagus by the pneumatic duct). If there are two gas chambers, air can pass from the caudal chamber into the cranial chamber through the isthmus (Fig. 3.13). Guanine crystals impart a silvery appearance to the swim bladder. The volume of the swim bladder compared with body weight is under 5% in marine fish and under 7% in freshwater fish species. Cartilaginous fish and some bottom-dwelling fish species lack any gas bladder. Some fish species have modified gas bladders that can be used like a lung.

Pneumatic duct: In fish with a physostomous gas bladder, there is an air tube connecting the lower front end of the caudal swim bladder to the esophagus (Fig. 3.13). Swallowed air is forced into the gas bladder, or air can be released from the bladder through this tube.

Rete mirabile: Fish with physoclistous swim bladders exchange gas through the network of blood vessels on the cranial and ventral surface of the bladder, called the rete mirabile.

Kidney: The kidneys are dark red colored and attached ventral to the backbone. There is a right and a left kidney, each divided into an anterior (pronephros) section that is hematopoietic (blood forming), and a posterior (mesonephros) portion that is excretory (urine-producing). The anterior kidney also contains lymphoid tissue and chromaffin tissue, which produces corticosteroids. The kidneys filter blood through glomeruli, which are a series of capillaries in the excretory tubules (Bowman's capsule). The nephron empties into the ureter. The ureter ducts carry the urine from the kidneys to the urinary papilla that is in the vent caudal to the anus. Creatine is the main nitrogenous waste excreted through the posterior kidneys of fish and in lesser amounts ammonia, uric acid, and creatinine. Urine production in freshwater fish is primarily for osmoregulation, as it removes excess water from the body as dilute urine. The glomeruli of freshwater fish kidneys retain salts to maintain the body's osmotic pressure. Freshwater fish are hyperosmotic (greater salt concentration) compared with the surrounding water, so constantly need to conserve salt and eliminate water. Marine fish swallow water to keep the body from becoming dehydrated, since they are hypo-osmotic to their environment. They excrete excess salt from the blood through glands in their gills.

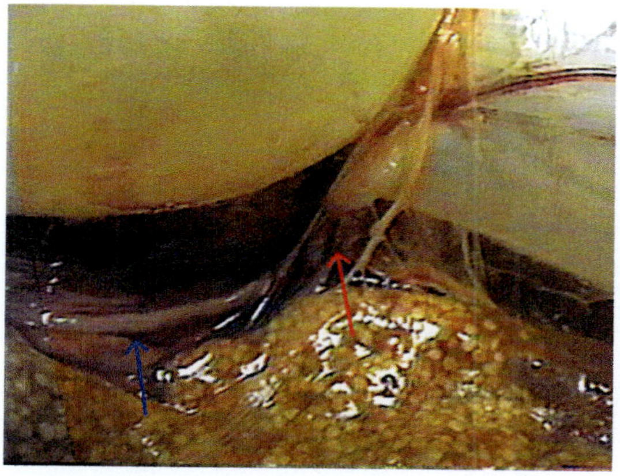

Fig. 3.13. Pneumatic duct (indicated by small blue arrow) in a female koi (*Cyprinus rubrofuscus*), extending from the pharynx to the anterior portion of the caudal chamber of the gas bladder (red arrow), where the caudal chamber connects to the anterior chamber by the isthmus. The ovary full of roe has been reflected ventrally to expose the pneumatic duct. (Photograph by N. Saint-Erne)

Interrenal glands: these glands are in the anterior portion of the kidneys (pronephros) and function similar to adrenal glands, producing adrenaline and norepinephrine.

Gonads: The male's cream-colored testes are paired and attached to the mesentery below and caudal to the kidneys. Each vas deferens carries spermatozoa from the testis to an excretory meatus at the urogenital papilla in the vent. The female's paired ovaries are suspended in mesentery lateral to the viscera, contain ova, and are usually tan to orange colored with a granular appearance (Fig. 3.13). The eggs pass through the oviduct and out the genital opening in the vent. In addition to gametogenesis, the gonads produce androgen and estrogen hormones. Fish species vary in reproductive methods. Some species are sexually dimorphic. Hermaphroditism and parthenogenesis also occur among fish species. Some fish are egg layers (oviparous), and some have internal fertilization of the eggs and hold the eggs until they hatch (ovoviviparous), giving birth to live young. In most ovoviviparous species the female holds the eggs, but in seahorses, the male holds them in a pouch. Some species hold the eggs in their mouth until the eggs hatch. Some fish species, notably anemonefish (Genus *Amphiprion*), have both male and female gonads and can change genders, depending on the availability of an appropriate mate. All anemonefish are protandrous sequential hermaphrodites, meaning they develop into males first, and when they mature, one from the shoal will become a female if there is not another dominant female present.

Muscles: The muscle myomeres are separated into right and left sides by the median septum and into upper (epaxial) and lower (hypaxial) muscle by the transverse horizontal septum. There are two types of muscle fibers: most muscles have white fibers, with a thin strip of red muscle fibers that runs horizontally along the side of the white muscle mass. The white muscle fibers are anaerobic, fast-contracting fibers for short-term, and rapid swimming. The red fibers are aerobic, slow-contracting fibers capable of slow, sustained activity. The red muscles have greater vascularization and a higher lipid content than do the white muscles.

Skeleton: Teleost fish have skeletons (Fig. 3.14) made of true bone (osteocytes). Fish bones may be cellular, as in most bony fish, or acellular in perch, bass, and sunfish. Elasmobranchs have cartilaginous skeletons. There is no hematopoietic tissue (marrow) in the bones of fish.

Spine: The cylindrical vertebral bodies, or centra, are connected to each other by longitudinal elastic ligaments and have a cushioning intervertebral pad between them. Each centrum has a neural arch and neural spine dorsally. The spinal cord runs through the neural arch. The anterior (coelomic) vertebrae have ventral pleural ribs, and the posterior (caudal) vertebrae have ventral hemal arches and spines. The caudal artery, which is the continuation of the dorsal aorta, along with the caudal vein, runs through the hemal arches. In many fish species, intermuscular bones radiate from the vertebrae in the septa between the muscle myotomes (Roberts and Ellis, 2012).

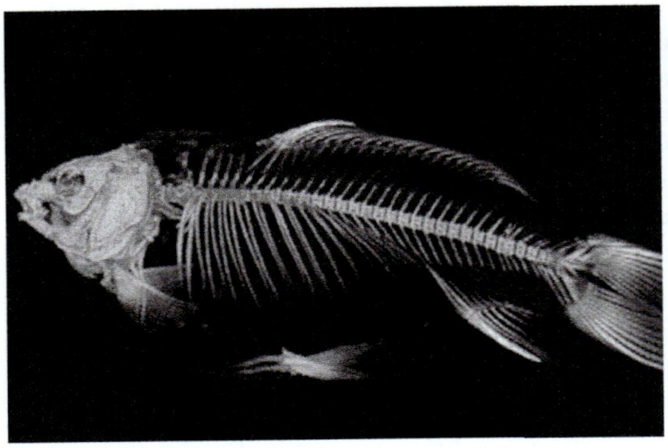

Fig. 3.14. Computed tomography (CT) image of a skeleton of a koi (*C. rubrofuscus*). (Photograph by Gregory Lewbart.)

Weberian Apparatus: In some fish species, there is a series of four bones under the first three vertebrae that connect the inner ear to the swim bladder to aid in sound perception (Fig. 3.15). The first vertebra produces the claustrum and scaphium, the second the intercalarium, and the third the tripus. These bones are interconnected by ligaments, and together are called the Weberian apparatus, or Weber's ossicles.

Skull: The skull of teleost fish has 185 bones, more than in any other vertebrate. The skull consists of a rigid cranium, attached to which are the bones of the jaws, and the branchial and operculum bones.

Nervous System: The nervous system in fishes consists of the brain, spinal cord, and peripheral nerves.

Brain: The brain is divided into the telencephalon (rhinencephalon, amygdala, hippocampus), the diencephalon (epithalamus containing the pineal body, thalamus, hypothalamus, pituitary), the mesencephalon (containing the two optic lobes), the metencephalon (cerebellum), and myelencephalon (medulla oblongata). Olfactory bulbs in the nares are connected to the telencephalon (forebrain) by the olfactory tract axons. The optic lobes connect to the optic nerve from each eye. The cerebellum is behind the optic lobes, and generally is associated with reception and coordination of proprioceptive and balance stimuli (Roberts and Ellis, 2012). The medulla oblongata attaches to the spinal cord. Fish have ten pairs of cranial nerves: the olfactory, optic,

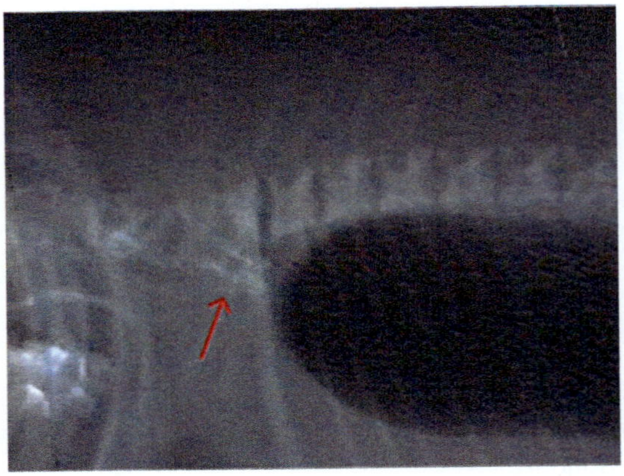

Fig. 3.15. Radiograph of a koi (*C. rubrofuscus*) showing the Weber's ossicles (red arrow) below the vertebrae at the anterior end of the cranial chamber of the gas bladder. (Photograph by N. Saint-Erne.)

oculomotor, trochlear, trigeminal, abducens, facial, acoustic, glossopharyngeal, and vagus nerves.

Pineal body: Part of the epithalamus, this is a light receptor with endocrine functions that control the pigmentation in some fish species.

Pituitary Gland: Located beneath the hypothalamus, it is divided into the anterior part (adenohypophysis) and posterior part (neurohypophysis). The former comprises several endocrine cell types that produce and release peptide hormones to regulate the endocrine system, controlling the fish's reproduction, growth, homeostasis, metabolism, stress responses, and coloration (Royan *et al.*, 2021).

Spinal Cord: the spinal cord runs from the medulla oblongata through the vertebrae the length of the body and terminates, in sharks and teleosts, in an endocrine structure, the urophysis. The urophysis hormones are peptides that are principally concerned with osmoregulation, and the smooth muscles of the reproductive tract (Roberts and Ellis, 2012).

Internal Ear: Fish have no external ears but have an inner ear on each side of the skull consisting of three semicircular canals, plus the utriculus (pars superior), and a sacculus and lagena (pars inferior). There is a calcareous otolith in each of the utriculus, sacculus, and lagena chambers. The pars superior functions in maintaining equilibrium, while the pars inferior functions in sound detection. In some fish species, this inner ear is connected to the air bladder by a series of bones called Weber's ossicles that increase their ability to hear.

3.4 Blood Cells

Red blood cells (Erythrocytes): An ellipsoid cell with an oval to round central nucleus. These are the most abundant cells in the blood. These cells transport oxygen and carbon dioxide through the bloodstream. They also transport ammonia to the gills for excretion. Erythropoiesis (red blood cell production) occurs in fish in the anterior kidneys and the spleen. Hemophagocytosis, the removal of worn-out red blood cells, also occurs in the anterior kidneys and the spleen.

White blood cells (Leukocytes): There are several types of these, each with its own structure and function. The granulocytes include neutrophils, eosinophils, and basophils, and are named by the color they take on when stained with dyes prior to microscopic examination.

Neutrophils (Heterophils): An oval to round cell with an eccentric lobed nucleus and containing small granules in its cytoplasm (Fig. 3.16). Their function is the phagocytosis of foreign material at sites of inflammation. The number of neutrophils increases in disease conditions. Band neutrophils are immature cells that have a band-shaped nucleus, rather than lobed. An increase in band neutrophils indicates new cell formation in response to an ongoing infection or inflammation.

Eosinophils: These round cells are not always present in peripheral blood samples. They appear similar to neutrophils, with a small, eccentric, condensed nucleus. The cytoplasm contains large refractile granules that stain red with eosin stains.

Basophils: These cells have round eccentric nuclei with large refractile granules in their cytoplasm that stain blue. Their function is similar to neutrophils.

Lymphocytes: These are small white blood cells (4.5–12 μm) with an irregular-shaped cytoplasmic membrane. The nucleus fills most of the cell and is round to oval shaped. The nucleus stains dark purple and the scant cytoplasm stains blue with blood stains (Fig. 3.17). Lymphocytes are the most abundant white blood cells in the peripheral blood of fish. The larger lymphocytes are immature cells and are released

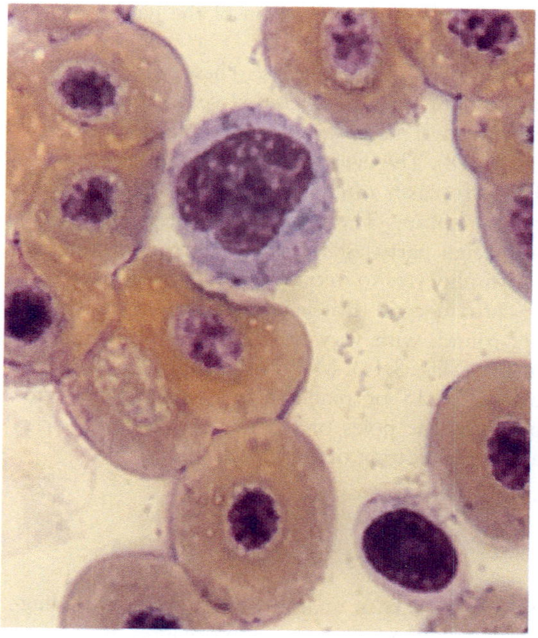

Fig. 3.16. Cownose ray (*Rhinoptera bonasus*) blood treated with Romanowsky stain showing nucleated red blood cells around a neutrophil (top center blood cell), and a smaller, immature thrombocyte near the bottom right of the microphotograph. (Microphotograph by N. Saint-Erne.)

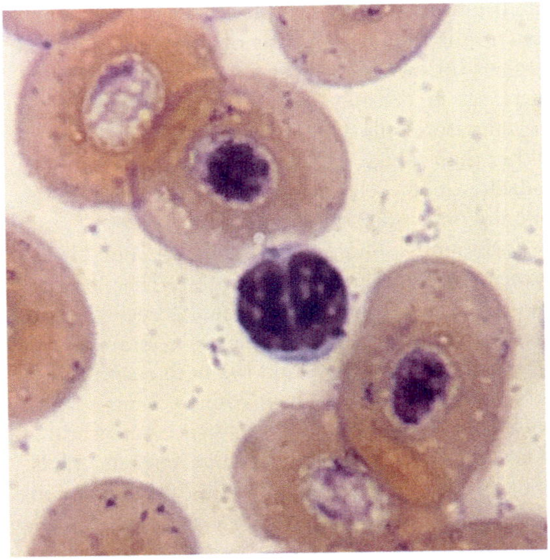

Fig. 3.17. Round lymphocyte surrounded by red blood cells in Cownose Ray (*R. bonasus*) blood treated with Romanowsky stain. (Microphotograph by N. Saint-Erne.)

in response to inflammation. Lymphocyte counts decrease in conditions of chronic stress or inflammation. One important function of the lymphocyte is antibody production.

Monocytes (Macrophages): These cells are slightly larger than other white blood cells. They have an eccentric oval nucleus with coarse, granular chromatin (Fig. 3.18). The cytoplasm has abundant vacuoles. The cytoplasm often has pseudopodia along the cell membrane. Their function is the phagocytosis of foreign particles. These cells introduce antigens to lymphocytes to initiate antibody responses.

Thrombocytes (Platelets): Immature thrombocytes are round, with very little cytoplasm around the nucleus (Fig. 3.16). Mature thrombocytes are more oval (Fig. 3.18) or spindle shaped, with minimal cytoplasm at the poles of the nucleus. Thrombocytes aid in the clotting of the blood.

3.5 Conclusion

Knowing the basic anatomy of fish helps with diagnostic techniques and surgical procedures. With more species of fishes than all the other vertebrates combined, there are many differences among fish species. However, the basic organs and their functions are similar among fish species, not too different from the organs of other vertebrate species.

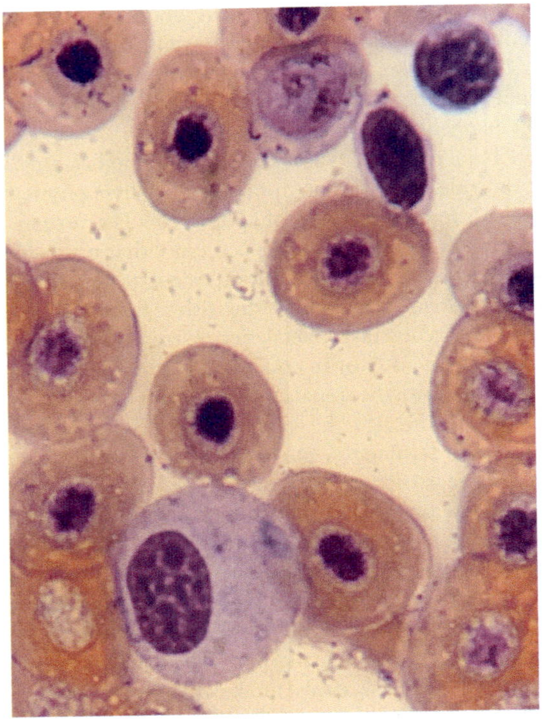

Fig. 3.18. Cownose ray (*R. bonasus*) blood treated with Romanowsky stain showing nucleated red blood cells, a neutrophil (top center blood cell), a thrombocyte next to it, and a lymphocyte to the far right, and near the bottom is a monocyte. (Microphotograph by N. Saint-Erne.)

References

Aiello, B.R., Stewart, T.A. and Hale, M.E. (2016) Mechanosensation in an adipose fin. *Proceedings of the Royal Society B: Biological Sciences* 283, 20152794. doi:10.1098/rspb.2015.2794.

Ali, A., Hochfeld, W., Myburgh, R. and Pepper, M. (2013) Adipocyte and adipogenesis. *European Journal of Cell Biology* 92(6–7), 229–236. doi:10.1016/j.ejcb.2013.06.001.

Betancur, R., Wiley, E.O., Arratia, G., Acero, A., Bailly, N. *et al.* (2017) Phylogenetic classification of bony fishes. *BMC Evolutionary Biology* 17:162. doi:10.1186/s12862-017-0958-3.

Britannica (2023) Annotated classification. Available at: https://www.britannica.com/animal/fish/Annotated-classification (accessed 1 August 2024).

Chilmonczyk, S. (1992) The thymus in fish: development and possible function in the immune response. *Annual Review of Fish Diseases* 2, 181–200.

Gallego, V. and Sousa-Santos, C. (2022) Nuptial tubercles in fish: what are they for? *FiSHMED*. Available at: https://fishmedjournal.sibic.org/10.29094/FiSHMED.2022.002.pdf (accessed 1 August 2024).

Hoole, D., Bucke, D., Burgess, P. and Wellby, I. (2001) Cyprinid biology. In: Hoole, D., Bucke, D., Burgess, P. and Wellby, I. (eds) *Diseases of Carp and Other Cyprinid Fishes*. Blackwell Science, Oxford, pp. 8–20.

Mylniczenko, N. (2021) Anatomy and taxonomy. In: Hadfield, C. and Clayton, L. (eds) *Clinical Guide to Fish Medicine*. Wiley, Hoboken, New Jersey, pp. 3–34.

Nelson, J.S. (2016) *Fishes of the World*. Wiley. Hoboken, New Jersey.

Roberts, R.J. and Ellis, A.E. (2012) The anatomy and physiology of teleosts. In: Roberts, R.J. (ed) *Fish Pathology*. 4th edn. Wiley, West Sussex, UK. pp. 17–61.

Royan, M.R., Siddique, K., Csucs, G., Puchades, M.A., Nourizadeh-Lillabadi, R. *et al.* (2021) 3D Atlas of the pituitary gland of the model fish Medaka (*Oryzias latipes*). *Frontiers in Endocrinology* 12, 719843. doi:10.3389/fendo.2021.719843.

Saint-Erne, N. (2010) Anatomy of Koi. In: Saint-Erne, N. (ed.) *Advanced Koi Care*. 2nd edn. Erne Enterprises, Glendale, Arizona, pp. 27–34.

Salmerón, C. (2018) Adipogenesis in fish. *Journal of Experimental Biology* 221(Pt. Suppl. 1): jeb161588. doi:10.1242/jeb.161588.

Stoskopf, M. (1993) *Fish Medicine*. Saunders, Philadelphia, Pennsylvania.

4 Aquarium Care

NICHOLAS SAINT-ERNE

Dr. Saint-Erne Consulting, PLLC, Phoenix, Arizona

Abstract

Setting up and maintaining an aquarium requires more knowledge than typically required for the care of other pets. Following the appropriate steps when starting an aquarium will lead to better health of the fish and more success with the aquarium.

4.1 Choosing an Aquarium and Equipment

4.1.1 The aquarium and stand

When selecting an aquarium, one needs to determine if a freshwater or saltwater aquarium is preferred. Saltwater aquariums require slightly more equipment than freshwater aquariums, require more maintenance, and marine fish generally cost more than freshwater fish. The size of the aquarium should be based on the location where it will be set up and the type and quantity of fish that are desired. Larger aquariums are actually easier to maintain than small ones; for the beginning aquarist, a minimum size of 10 gallons (38 l) is recommended, and 30 gallons (114 l) is preferable (Gratzek, 1992a).

The next necessary item that is often neglected is an aquarium stand (see Table 4.1 for equipment list). Water weighs 8.34 pounds (3.785 kg) per gallon, or 1 kg per liter. A proper aquarium stand needs to be used to support the weight of an aquarium filled with water. Typical household furniture and cabinets are not strong enough to use as a stand for a large aquarium. Aquarium stands are designed to support the weight of the aquarium, and usually provide housing for the filtration system and other equipment inside a cabinet in the stand (Fig. 4.1). Place the aquarium on the stand on level flooring, and not in direct sunlight or drafts. Be sure it is located near a power source.

4.1.2 Filtration and heating

The filter system depends on the size of the aquarium and the budget of the aquarist. "The bigger the better" is the general rule for aquarium filtration. Filters should be able to move the water volume in the aquarium through the filter media 3–5 times per hour; so, a 40-gallon (150 l) aquarium should have a water pump that moves 120–200 gallons (450–750 l) per hour. Filters can include undergravel filters, hang-on-the-back power filters, or canister filters (See Chapter 6 Filtration Systems of this volume for more information on filtration). The filtration system traps particulate waste from the water and provides biological filtration that turns the toxic ammonia that the fish produce into nitrite and then nitrate.

Aquarium heaters are specifically designed to maintain a constant temperature in an aquarium. Do not use any other heater around water; only use submersible aquarium heaters. The heater size is based on 5 watts per gallon (3.785 l) of water in the aquarium; so, a 40-gallon (150 l) aquarium would need a 200-watt heater. For large aquariums, it is better to use two heaters, one at each end of the tank, rather than using a single large heater. The aquarium heater should be placed close to the water outflow from the filter so that the heated water is dispersed around the aquarium by the filter outflow. Most tropical aquariums are maintained at 72–78°F/22–26°C. Use an aquarium thermometer to monitor the water temperature.

Corresponding author: DrSaintErne@gmail.com

© CAB International 2025. *The Handbook of Ornamental Fish Health and Welfare* (ed. N. Saint-Erne)
DOI: 10.1079/9781789246032.0004

Table 4.1. Aquarium equipment list

- Aquarium (glass or acrylic)
- Aquarium stand
- Filter system
- Aquarium hood with lighting
- Aquarium heater and thermometer
- Gravel (2″–3″/5–8 cm layer, or about 1.5 pounds per gallon/179 g per l)
- Decorative rocks (be sure they are chemically inert and safe for use in aquariums)
- Décor (driftwood/ornaments/plastic plants/background)
- Live aquarium plants
- Water conditioner/dechlorinator
- Biological filter starter
- Water test kit/strips
- Fish food (flakes/pellets)
- Fish treats (frozen/freeze-dried)
- Gravel vacuum with tubing (Fig. 4.4)
- Bucket for use with water changes
- Fish net
- Algae scrubbing pads
- Fish reference book

Once the heater is set at a specific temperature, it thermostatically maintains that set temperature within 1–2 degrees.

4.1.3 Aquarium cover and lighting

Most aquariums should have a tight-fitting cover (hood) over them to keep the fish from jumping out, prevent splashing, and reduce water loss through evaporation. The hood typically contains lighting. Older aquariums used incandescent and fluorescent lighting, but newer ones use light-emitting diode (LED) lighting. The LED lights are brighter than other lights, do not produce as much heat, use less energy, and can be controlled to change colors. They often can be set to turn on and off at specific times and can be controlled remotely. Lights should be on for 8–12 h a day.

4.1.4 Substrate and décor

For freshwater fish, quartz or silica gravel is commonly used as an aquarium substrate. Many of the commercial aquarium gravels are covered with epoxy to color them. These can be used in aquariums, but over time the colored epoxy coating may flake off the gravel. Do not use limestone or calcium carbonate gravels in freshwater aquariums, unless for species of fish that require high water hardness and alkalinity such as African cichlids, as these minerals will dissolve in low pH water and increase the hardness and alkalinity. Marine aquariums often have sand or crushed coral as a substrate. Rinse the substrate in a clean container before adding it to the aquarium. Use 1.5 pounds (680 g) of gravel for every gallon (4 l) of tank capacity to make a 2–3″ (5–8 cm) layer on the bottom. If using an undergravel filter, place the filter plate on the bottom of the tank first and cover it with the gravel.

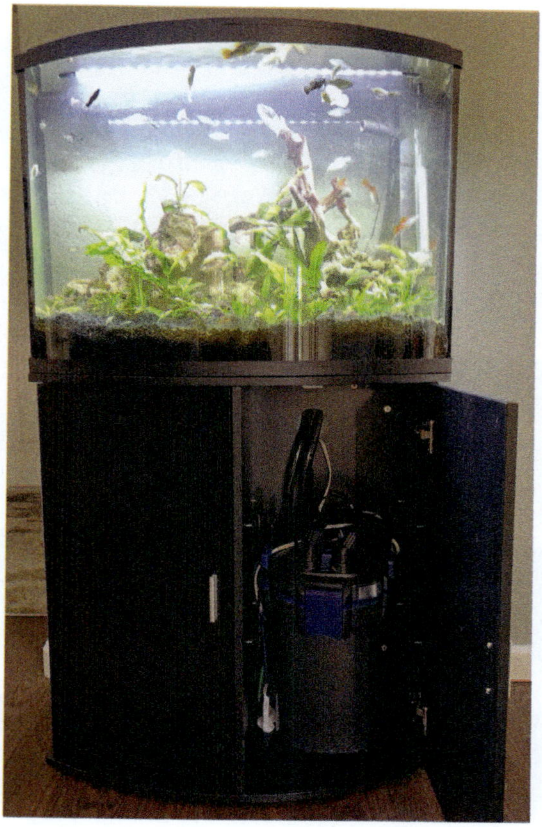

Fig. 4.1. A bowfront glass aquarium on a commercial aquarium stand, with cabinet door open to show the canister filter. (Photograph by N. Saint-Erne.)

Décor is useful to create hiding places for the fish. All decorations should be rinsed before adding them to the aquarium. There are aquarium décor items available at pet stores that look like logs or rocks, plastic plants, and ornaments such as sunken ships or scuba divers (Fig. 4.2). Only use products specifically made for use in an aquarium to prevent adding décor items that contain lead, zinc, copper, or other minerals that could affect the water quality.

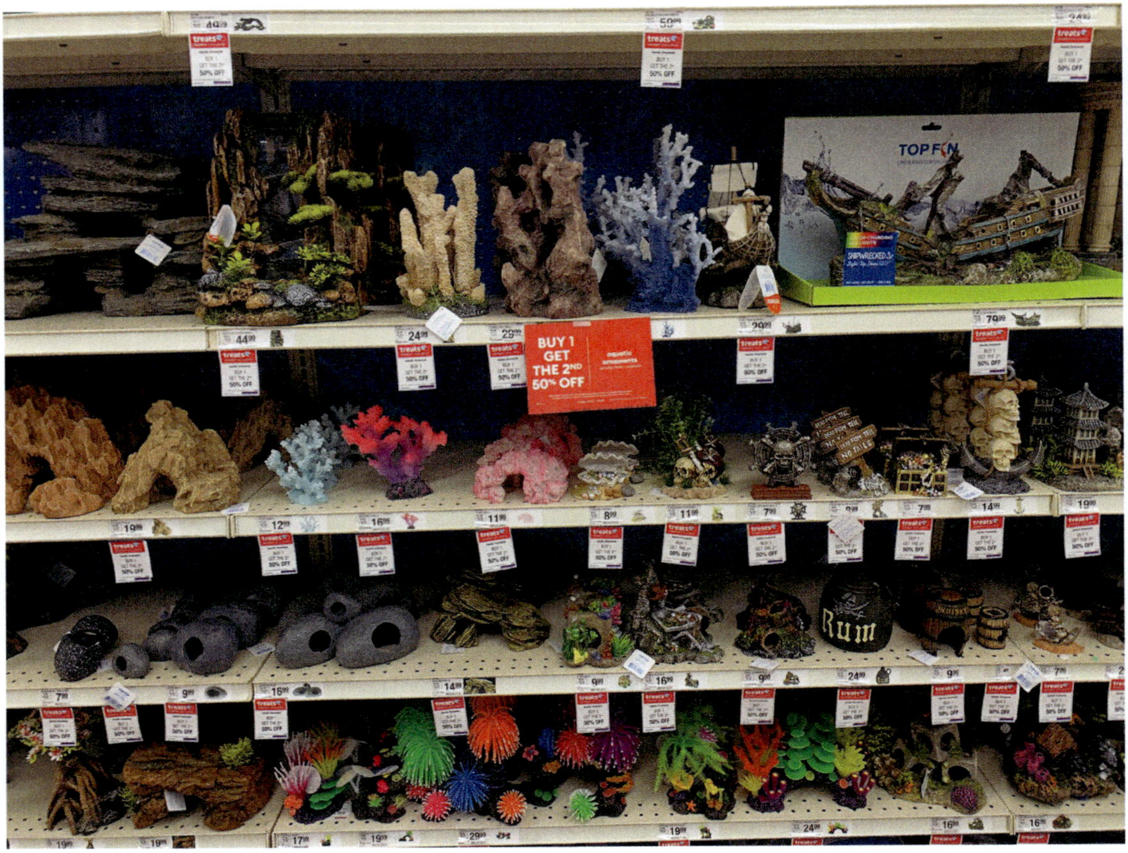

Fig. 4.2. Variety of aquarium décor available in aquarium stores. (Photograph by N. Saint-Erne.)

The décor items should give the fish places to hide but leave enough space in the middle of the aquarium for them to have a swimming area.

4.1.5 Fish food

Choose a flake or pelleted food of the appropriate size for your fish as its staple diet (Fig. 4.3). Feed your fish as much food as they will consume in 3 minutes, twice daily. Young, growing fish may need to be fed three to four times daily until mature. Be sure all the fish are eating, and not being chased away from the food by more aggressive fish. Bottom-feeding fish may need to be fed sinking pellets, rather than flakes or floating pellets. Fish that prefer to feed at night should be fed right before turning the lights out. Vary the fish's diet by giving them frozen or freeze-dried brine shrimp, bloodworms, tubifex worms, or algae sheets or wafers, every few days.

4.2 Setting up the Aquarium

Once all the necessary aquarium equipment and supplies are available, they should be rinsed with clean water and set up BEFORE obtaining any fish. Do not buy fish at the same time as buying an aquarium. The aquarium should be set up and filled with water for at least a day before adding any fish (Saint-Erne, 2008). It is preferable to set up the aquarium and filtration and "seed" the aquarium to get the beneficial bacteria in the biofilter growing before adding the fish. This process can take days to weeks! Adding bacteria supplements available at pet stores will reduce the time necessary to get the bacteria colony in the biofilter established. Here are steps to follow when setting up the aquarium:

1. Determine the size and location of your aquarium.
2. Place the rinsed-out tank on an aquarium stand designed to support the weight of a filled aquarium.

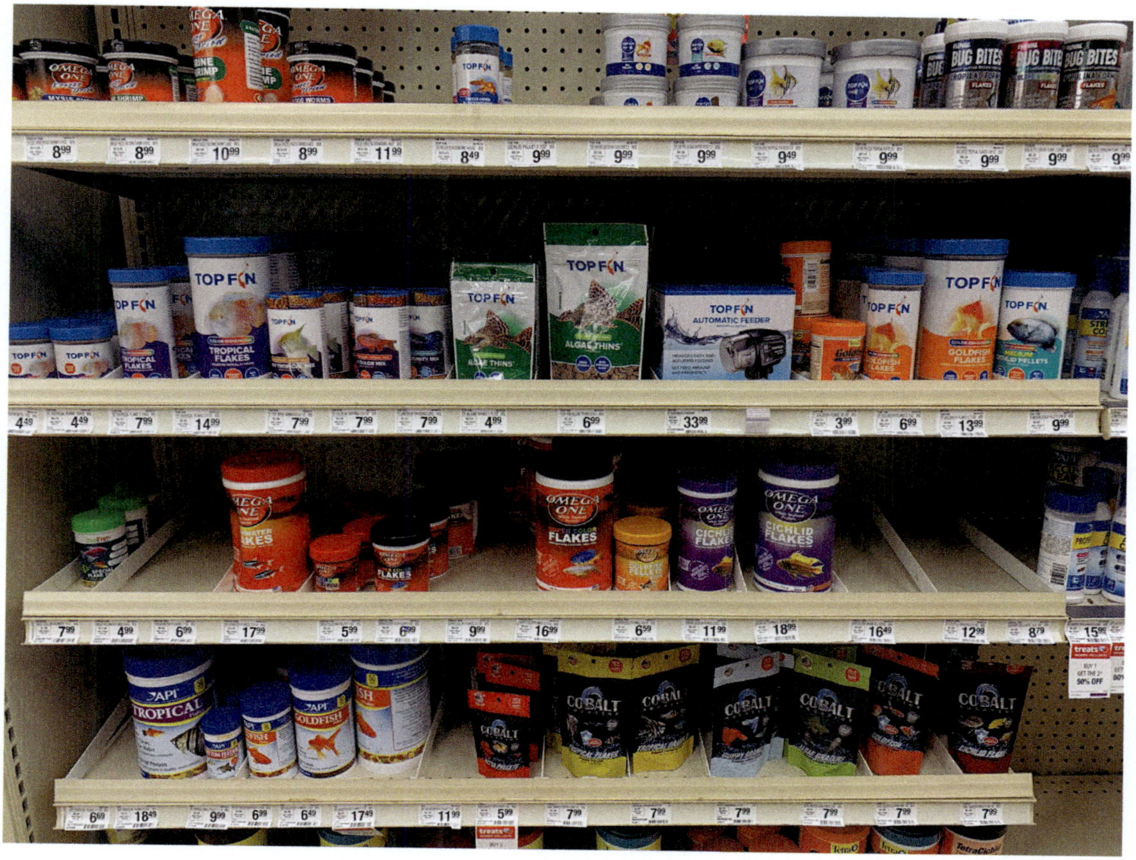

Fig. 4.3. A variety of fish food brands are available at an aquarium store. (Photograph by N. Saint-Erne.)

If using an undergravel filter, place it in the bottom of the tank now.

3. Pour rinsed gravel or marine sand into the tank.

4. Fill one-third of the tank with water that has been treated with dechlorinator to remove the harmful chlorine or chloramine from the tap water. Use your hand or place a small bowl on the substrate to prevent it from being disturbed when the water is poured in (Fig. 4.5). For marine aquariums, mix the sea salt in a bucket of water to the correct salinity before adding the water into the aquarium. Use a hydrometer or refractometer to measure the specific gravity of the salt water.

5. Place decorations, plants, aquarium heater, thermometer, and filter tubes in the desired locations. If necessary, connect the air pump and airline tubing to the appropriate attachments. Place the aquarium water heater where water flows from the filter, this will mix the heated water throughout the aquarium.

6. Follow the manufacturer's instructions to set up the filtration system. The water intake should be close to the substrate and the water return should be at the surface of the water.

7. Fill the remaining two-thirds of the tank with dechlorinated fresh water, or mixed salt water for marine aquariums.

8. Let the heater stand in the water for at least 15 min after filling the tank before plugging it in and turning it on to equilibrate its internal temperature to the water temperature.

9. Add a biological supplement to help the beneficial bacteria start growing. The beneficial bacteria need to have time to grow in the new aquarium and can make the water initially become cloudy. The beneficial bacteria will slowly be filtered out of the water and colonize the media in the biofilter.

10. Place the hood/light on the tank and plug it in. The lighting can be connected to a timer to automatically turn it on in the morning after dawn and turn it off at night.

11. Run the filter for 24–48 h and adjust the heater to the appropriate temperature for the species of

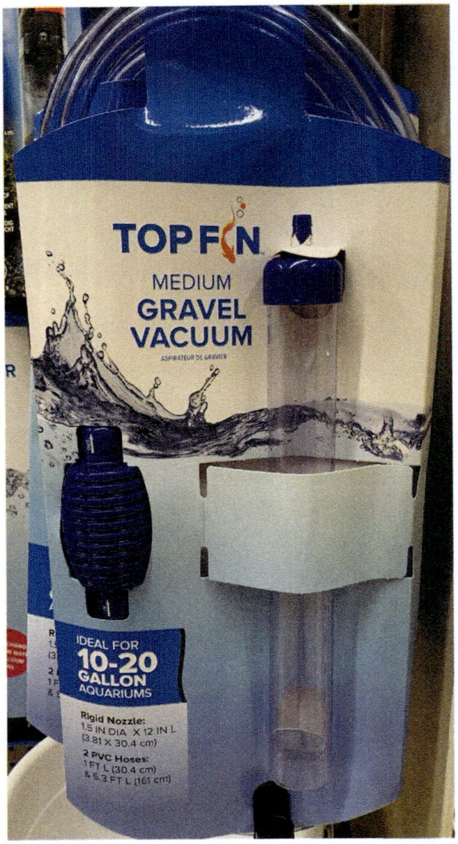

Fig. 4.4. Gravel vacuums for cleaning aquarium substrate come in various tube sizes and hose lengths. (Photo by N. Saint-Erne.)

fish you will be adding. This is to ensure that all the equipment is working properly before adding any fish and that there are no leaks in the tank.

12. Test the water quality daily for the first few weeks. Perform a partial water change if the ammonia or nitrite levels are elevated. Use ammonia-binding water conditioners if any ammonia or nitrite is detected still after the water change. Monitor and adjust the salinity as needed for marine aquariums. Add more sea salt mix to the water being replaced to keep it at the correct salinity level.

4.3 The Aquarium Nitrogen Cycle

4.3.1 Heterotrophic bacteria and fungi

In soils as well as in the substrates of aquatic environments, there are microorganisms, including bacteria, fungi, protozoa, and larger organisms such as nematodes, which break down organic matter, or detritus. This process is what causes decomposition, and releases chemicals into the environment. In aquatic environments, the main waste by-products include ammonia and phosphate. The heterotrophic bacteria in aquariums grow more rapidly than the nitrifying bacteria and are also more stable. Many of the bacterial supplements that are available for purchase at aquarium stores contain heterotrophic bacteria, rather than nitrifying bacteria. Still, they can help a new aquarium establish a beneficial bacterial colony to break down fish waste, uneaten food, or other debris.

4.3.2 Nitrifying bacteria

It was originally assumed that *Nitrosomonas* were the bacteria responsible for breaking down ammonia in aquatic systems, and *Nitrobacter* was responsible for oxidizing nitrite. That's because when aquarium bacteria were cultured in the laboratory, those two species tended to predominate. Other species of bacteria, most notably *Nitrospira*, may actually be handling much of the nitrification in fish tanks (Muha, 2007). But in new tanks, there won't be enough of the nitrifying bacteria to process the waste produced by a full load of fish; that is why fish need to be added gradually over a period of several weeks into newly established aquariums. This allows time for the beneficial bacteria in the biofilter to multiply, and as they break down the toxic fish waste (ammonia), they produce nitrite, which provides an energy source for the second group of bacteria, the nitrite oxidizers, which also multiply. Those bacteria convert toxic nitrite into nitrate, which is much less toxic. When both colonies are large enough to handle all the waste produced in the tank, it is considered "cycled," meaning the biofilter has been established. This is the aquarium nitrogen cycle (Fig. 4.6), and it is an important part of maintaining healthy fish in a closed aquatic environment, like an aquarium or fish pond.

How long it takes to cycle an aquarium varies considerably, from as little as 21 days to as long as 6 weeks, but under any circumstances, nitrifiers are slow growers compared to many other bacteria species. For instance, *E. coli* bacteria double in number every 20 min, but the fastest-growing nitrifiers take 8 h to do the same (Muha, 2007). Each species also has a temperature range for optimum growth. If the temperature is outside that range, bacterial growth slows down. Fish ponds in colder

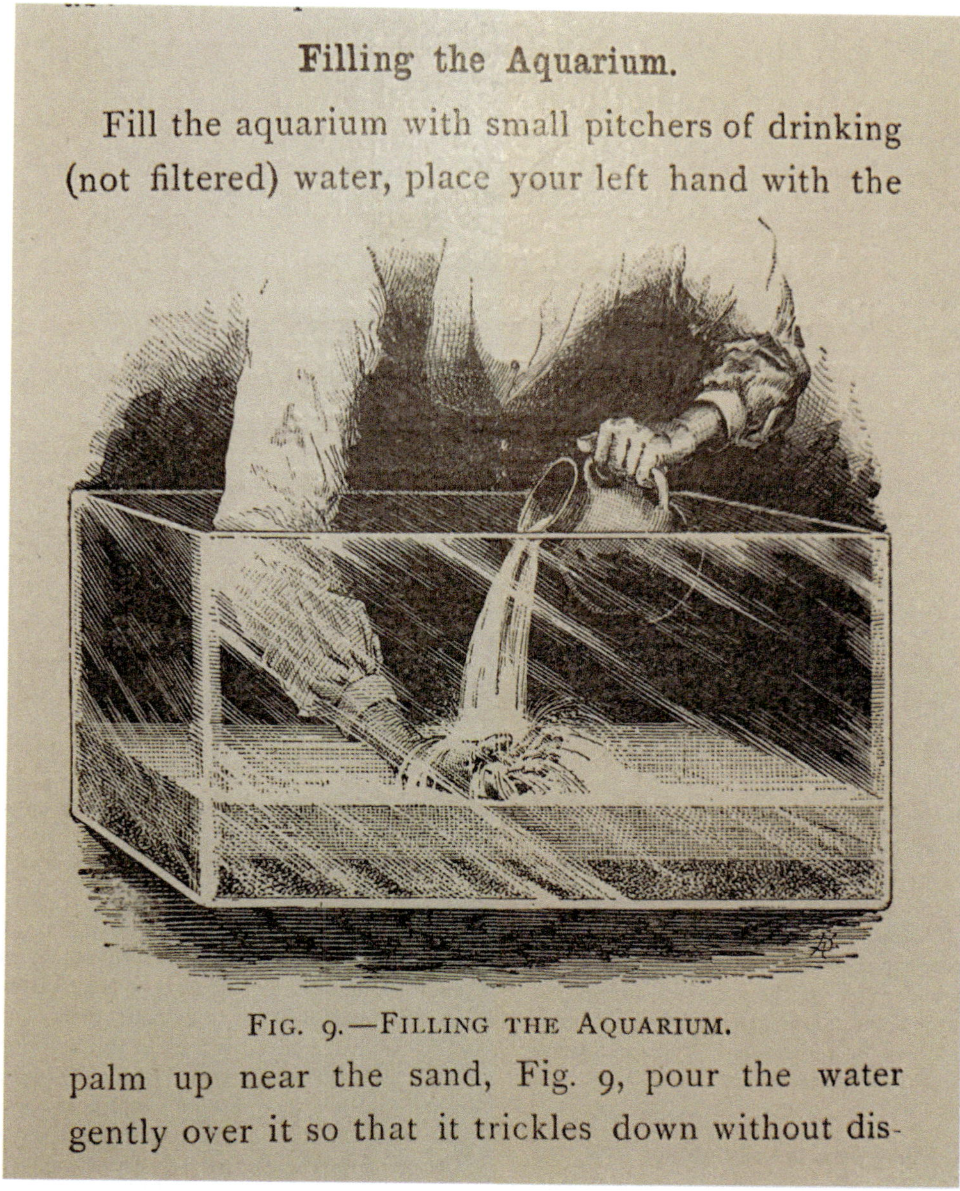

Filling the Aquarium.

Fill the aquarium with small pitchers of drinking (not filtered) water, place your left hand with the

FIG. 9.—FILLING THE AQUARIUM.

palm up near the sand, Fig. 9, pour the water gently over it so that it trickles down without dis-

Fig. 4.5. An illustration from the 1894 book, *The Amateur Aquarist*, showing how to add water into an aquarium. (Photograph of the book page by N. Saint-Erne.)

climates may lose most of the nitrifying bacteria over the winter, so the biofilter must be re-established each spring. Likewise, a drop in oxygen—which can occur if the water becomes too warm or a power outage disrupts water circulation—can destroy some of the nitrifying bacteria. Debris in the filter can cause slow water flow through it, decreasing oxygen and ammonia (food for the bacteria), resulting in a decrease in the biofilter bacterial population (Muha, 2007). Poor tank maintenance can affect bacteria in another way. Over time, the bacteria utilize the carbonate in the water, lowering the alkalinity and allowing the water pH to decrease, as the acids that are a

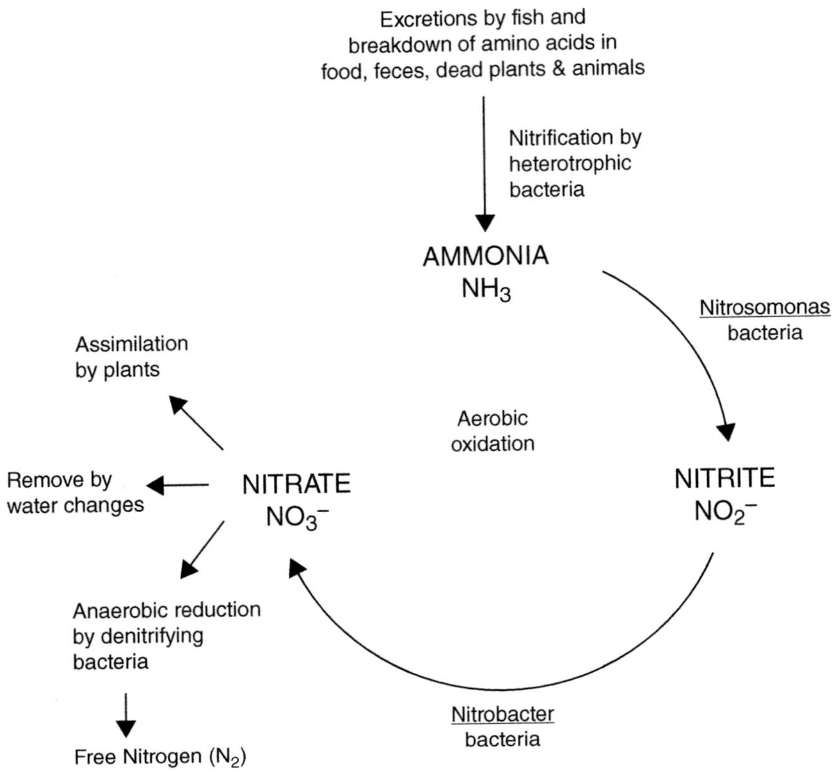

Fig. 4.6. The aquarium nitrogen cycle, where beneficial bacteria convert fish wastes and ammonia into nitrite and then nitrate. (Saint-Erne, 2010, p.97.)

by-product of nitrification build up in the water. If the buffering capacity (alkalinity) is not replenished through a water change, the decreased pH stresses not only the fish but also the bacteria. A pH below 6.5 slows down bacterial nitrification and below 5.5 inhibits nitrifying bacteria.

4.3.3 New tank syndrome

Beneficial bacteria require many weeks to establish in a new aquarium. "New Tank Syndrome" occurs when too many fish are added to the aquarium when first set up because a person is reluctant to wait to add all the fish or is unaware of the nitrogen cycle. This leads to disaster as ammonia is produced faster than it is broken down, killing the fish, and the new aquarium owner might give up keeping fish without ever knowing why they were unsuccessful.

To help prevent "New Tank Syndrome," add fish to the aquarium gradually. Don't rush and purchase all the fish for the new aquarium at once. Let the tank run for at least a day before adding any fish. Establishing an adequate level of beneficial bacteria in the biological filter usually takes about 3–6 weeks. Add fish a few at a time, preferably no more than three fish per week, while frequently testing the water quality. Make partial water changes to keep the ammonia, nitrite, and nitrate levels down. Add bacteria supplements to the water to provide beneficial bacteria for the biological filter, helping the system cycle faster. After the initial cycling period, water tests and water changes may only be necessary every few weeks. Each week, add a few more fish until you reach the appropriate number of fish for the aquarium size.

4.3.4 Starting the nitrogen cycle

Starting the nitrogen cycle involves introducing nitrifying bacteria into the biofilter media. Nitrifying bacteria can be introduced with water or biofilter media from an already operating filtration system, or by adding commercial nitrifying bacterial supplements. A more desirable method is to develop the nitrifying bacteria within the biofilter before stocking the aquarium with fish species to be cultured (Banrie, 2013). This is sometimes called "Fishless Cycling." The advantages of cultivating nitrifying bacteria before adding fish are:

1. Reducing stress on the newly introduced fish when added to the aquarium.
2. Shortening the growing cycle with higher feed rates from the first day of stocking.
3. Creating better water quality, which improves health, growth rates, and survival.

Prepare the water chemistry of the aquarium before introducing either nitrifying bacteria or fish. The aquarium water should be at the temperature, pH, salinity, alkalinity, and hardness appropriate for the fish species to be kept. Nitrifying bacteria require carbonates to convert ammonia to nitrite and nitrate. If the alkalinity is too low, add a carbon source to increase the alkalinity. Add sodium bicarbonate ($NaHCO_3$), or common baking soda, to increase the alkalinity to 150–250 mg/l to start the biofilter. As a rule, to raise the alkalinity by 10 mg/l, add 5 g (one teaspoon) of sodium bicarbonate for every 378.5 l (100 gallons) of water. With the alkalinity at 150–250 mg/l, the pH is usually within the range of 6.8–7.8, which is appropriate for freshwater nitrifying bacteria.

To provide the initial ammonia to start the bacteria growing, add ammonium chloride (NH_4Cl) at 12 mg/l to raise the total ammonia level to 3–4 mg/l. An alternative to using powdered ammonium chloride is using clear, unscented household ammonia (10% ammonia). Using 12 ml of liquid ammonia will raise the ammonia concentration of 378.5 l (100 gallons) of water to about 3.2 mg/l. Adjustments will be necessary if using a different concentration of liquid ammonia solution. After adding the ammonium chloride or ammonia to the water, allow enough time for thorough mixing through the aquarium or pond, and then test the ammonia level. Add more incrementally if needed to increase the concentration of ammonia in the water to 3–4 mg/l. Do not exceed 4 mg/l or the nitrifying bacteria growth will be inhibited.

Once the ammonia is at the appropriate concentration, introduce the nitrifying bacteria. If using commercial preparations of bacteria, follow the manufacturer's recommendations. An alternative way to introduce bacteria is to move media from a cycled aquarium's biofilter. Monitor the water quality parameters of ammonia, nitrite, nitrate, pH, temperature, and alkalinity. Initially, ammonia concentration increases to a high point and then declines as the nitrifying bacteria convert it to nitrite. After a lag period, the nitrite concentration begins to increase and then declines, as the nitrate increases. Use water changes as needed to lower the nitrate level. Once the nitrite and ammonia levels are reduced, fish can be added to the aquarium.

4.4 Adding Fish to the Aquarium

Stock the aquarium with fish slowly; never add more than three fish to your aquarium per week. For freshwater aquariums, a good starting point is to add a few hardy fish such as danios, gouramis, or live-bearers that can cope with the presence of low levels of ammonia and nitrite. For marine aquariums, add a few hardy fish such as damsels or clown fish as your first aquarium inhabitants. After adding the fish, test the water's pH, ammonia, nitrite, and nitrate levels daily. If levels are elevated, perform a partial water change. For marine aquariums, add more sea salt mix to the water being replaced to keep it at the correct salinity level. Once the ammonia and nitrite levels are decreased, a few more fish can be added (Saint-Erne, 2008).

The size of the aquarium and the species of fish wanted to be kept will help determine how many fish the tank can hold safely. A traditional guide is 1 gallon (3.8 l) of water for every 1″ (2.5 cm) of full-grown tropical fish; 2 gallons (7.5 l) of water for every 1″ (2.5 cm) of full-grown goldfish, cichlids, other large-bodied fish, and marine fish species. Fish that may grow up to a meter in length, such as arowanas and koi, may need 5 gallons (19 l) of water per inch of body length. Be sure when purchasing fish from an aquarium store that the adult size of the fish is taken into consideration, not the current size it is at the store. Do not overcrowd the tank, as this may lead to toxic ammonia levels.

After purchasing new fish, take the bags of fish home immediately. Do not expose the bag to hot or cold temperatures. If the weather is very hot or cold, the fish bags can be transported in a Styrofoam box or ice chest to help maintain the proper water temperature. At home, remove the aquarium hood and float the bag of fish in the tank for 15 min to allow water temperatures to equalize. Remove the bag and use a net to take the fish out of the bag, or slowly pour the fish into a net over a bucket (this is to prevent adding the water in the bag to the aquarium). Carefully add the fish from the net to their new home. Feeding the fish when you add new ones can distract them from the new fish, allowing the new ones to become acclimated to the aquarium. Do not overfeed the fish. That can cause an increase in ammonia and is a common cause of fish loss. Feed twice daily and only as much food as can be consumed within 3 minutes. Retest the pH, ammonia, nitrite, and nitrate levels 24–48 h after adding new fish. More often if any abnormal water conditions are detected. Test for each of these at least every other day for the first 4 weeks after setting up your aquarium.

4.5 Water Quality Testing

It is important to have consistent water quality at the optimum parameters. Since water changes are the main method of improving water conditions in the aquarium, it is important to test the local tap water to ensure it is safe for use with fish. Tap water that contains high levels of ammonia, nitrite, nitrate, phosphate, copper, zinc, or lead may not be suitable for use with fish. Additives are available to remove chlorine, chloramine, ammonia, and copper from the tap water. Bottled water may be an option instead of local tap or well water if that water is not safe for the fish. Use a good water quality test kit or test strips (Fig. 4.7) to monitor water quality, and water conditioners to adjust the aquarium water to the desired parameters. Here are the water quality parameters that should be tested and their normal ranges for aquarium fish:

pH (acid/base balance)—normal range: freshwater 6.5–8.2; marine 8.0–8.4

This is the measure of the activity (power) of the hydrogen ions in the water. Water that has a pH of 7.0 is considered neutral, and pH less than 7.0 is acidic, and more than 7.0 is basic. The stability of

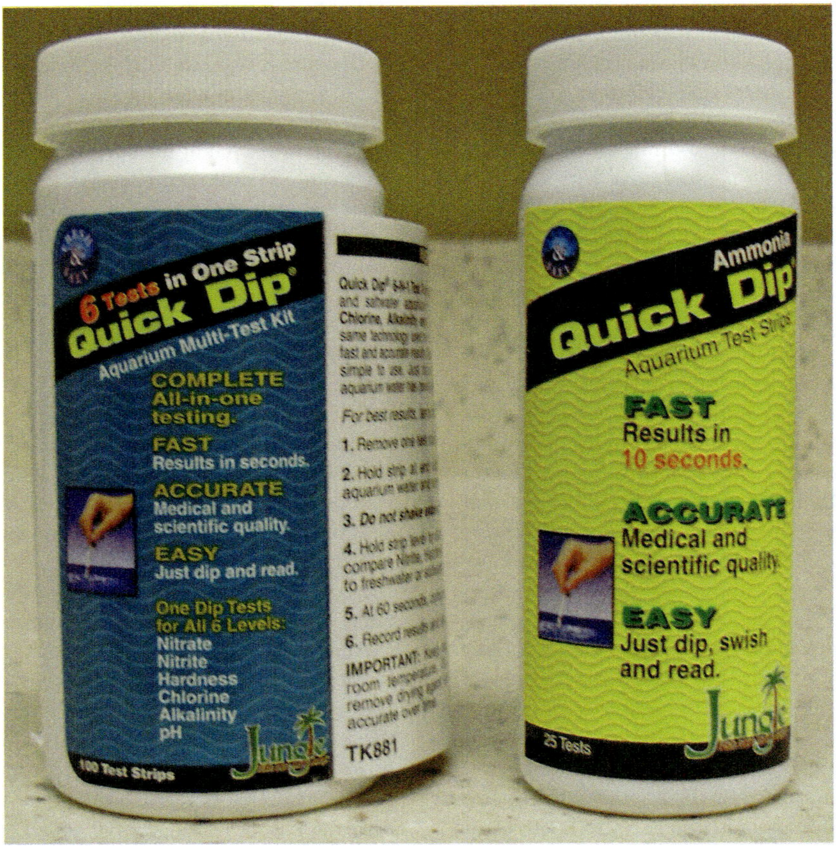

Fig. 4.7. Aquarium water quality testing strips are easy to use and provide rapid results. (Photograph by N. Saint-Erne.)

the pH is related to water alkalinity and hardness. Rapid changes in pH are detrimental to fish.

Chlorine and Chloramine—normal range: 0.0 mg/l

These are added to city water supplies to make the water supply safe for human use. Be certain to always use a dechlorinator when adding tap water to an aquarium as any amount of chlorine is toxic to fish.

Ammonia—normal range: 0.0–0.25 mg/l

Aquariums with properly operating filtration systems should have no ammonia present (after they have been cycled). In new aquariums, ammonia-binding chemicals can be used to decrease ammonia toxicity, along with performing partial water changes.

Nitrite—normal range: 0.0–0.5 mg/l

Nitrite reduces the ability of the fish's blood to carry oxygen. Lower the nitrite level by performing a partial water change. For a freshwater aquarium, adding salt to the water at 0.1–0.3% (1–3 teaspoons of aquarium salt per gallon of water) also reduces nitrite toxicity.

Nitrate—normal range: 0–40 mg/l

If nitrate levels exceed 40 mg/l, water changes can be used to lower the concentration. High levels of nitrate are harmful to marine invertebrates and can also cause increased algae growth.

General Hardness—normal range: 100–250 mg/l

Water with high hardness usually has a high pH. Softening the water through a home water softener will lower the hardness. Most fish will adapt to moderate hardness levels.

Carbonate Hardness (Alkalinity)—normal range: 100–300 mg/l

With low alkalinity water, your aquarium may experience sudden and deadly pH shifts. Increase the alkalinity of the water, if necessary, to stabilize the pH.

Salinity—normal range: freshwater 0–0.3%, marine 3.0–3.5%

Salinity in marine aquariums is most easily measured using a hydrometer or refractometer, which measures the specific gravity of the water. Saltwater at 3.0–3.5% will have a specific gravity of about 1.020–1.026.

Temperature—normal range: 72–78°F/22–26°C

Use an aquarium heater to maintain stable water temperatures. Rapid temperature changes are harmful to tropical fish. Most tropical fish are comfortable in this temperature range. Cool water fish such as goldfish may prefer temperatures of 66–73°F/19–23°C, while some tropical fish like discus, angelfish, and bettas, prefer warmer water temperatures of 78–84°F/26–29°C.

4.6 Aquarium Maintenance

Avoiding problems is preferable to correcting them, and preventive measures will increase the success of maintaining a trouble-free aquarium (Gratzek, 1992b). A new aquarium requires more frequent monitoring, with daily water quality testing, and water changes if indicated by the test results. After the aquarium has been established for a month or two, the maintenance decreases, with most tasks being performed monthly (see Table 4.2 for a standard aquarium maintenance schedule).

Table 4.2. Aquarium maintenance schedule. Author's own table.

Daily	• Feed fish twice daily • Check the water temperature and general health of fish • Test water quality in new aquariums
Weekly	• Test water quality in recently established aquariums • Remove 10% of the water and replace it with dechlorinated water if any abnormal water conditions are found • Scrub glass to remove algae, if necessary
Monthly	• Test water quality in established aquariums • Scrub glass to remove algae, if necessary • Prune live plants, if necessary • Vacuum the gravel and replace 25% of the water with dechlorinated water • Perform filter maintenance (e.g. replace filter cartridge, replace carbon, rinse prefilter) • Replace the air stone if the volume of air output is decreasing (allows for more aeration and makes the air pump last longer) • Remove artificial plants/decorations and clean, if necessary • Wipe the exterior and hood of aquarium with a damp cloth

Add an aquarium dechlorinator or water conditioner to the tap water before adding it to the aquarium. Do not use any soaps or detergents to clean the aquarium or décor, as they are toxic to fish. Always wash your hands before and after handling fish or cleaning the aquarium.

Do not clean aquariums or equipment in the kitchen sink or near food preparation areas.

4.7 Conclusion

Having the right equipment makes aquarium keeping easier and more enjoyable. Selecting the aquarium size that is appropriate for the species and quantity of fish planned to be kept is important for the fish's health and welfare. Proper filtration of the appropriate size for the aquarium and the number of fish will reduce water quality concerns. An efficient biological filtration system and regular water changes, with simultaneous cleaning of the gravel using a gravel vacuum, should keep the water conditions optimal (Gratzek, 1992b).

References

Banrie (2013) Using ammonium chloride to start a biofilter. Southern Regional Aquaculture Center (SRAC). Available at: https://thefishsite.com/articles/how-to-start-a-biofilter (accessed 1 August 2024).

Gratzek, J.B. (1992a) Getting started with aquaria. In: Gratzek, J.B. and Matthews, J.R. (eds) *Aquariology: The Science of Fish Health Management*. Tetra Press, Morris Plains, New Jersey, pp. 3–19.

Gratzek, J.B. (1992b) Maintaining aquaria. In: Gratzek, J.B. and Matthews, J.R. (eds) *Aquariology: The Science of Fish Health Management*. Tetra Press, Morris Plains, New Jersey, pp. 21–33.

Muha, L. (2007) The skeptical fishkeeper: nitrifying bacteria. *Tropical Fish Hobbyist*, January 2007. Available at: http://www.tfhmagazine.com/aquarium-basics/columns/nitrifying-bacteria.htm (accessed 1 August 2024).

Saint-Erne, N. (2008) *Saltwater Care Manual*. PetSmart Store Support Group, Phoenix, Arizona.

Saint-Erne, N. (2010) *Advanced Koi Care*. Erne Enterprises, Glendale, Arizona.

5 Water Quality

AZUREEN ERDMAN

New River, Arizona

Abstract

Maintaining proper water quality is the most important part of the health and well-being of aquarium fish. The water parameters should be tested regularly, daily in newly set up aquariums, and then weekly or every few weeks in established aquariums. At a minimum, the water should be tested for ammonia, nitrite, nitrate, acid-base balance, general hardness, alkalinity, and temperature. Water tests for other compounds can be conducted as needed.

5.1 Water Quality Testing

When working with aquatic species, the most important aspect of management is monitoring and testing the environment in which these individuals reside. This is performed through water quality testing. In private veterinary practice, many medical problems present in fish patients stem from improper water quality. Water quality testing should be performed with every aquatic animal exam. Owners and aquarists should be testing water quality at home weekly, or at least monthly in an established aquarium. Water temperature should be monitored daily. The hospital water testing kit should include the following parameters: temperature, ammonia, nitrite, nitrate, pH, hardness, alkalinity, salinity or specific gravity, iron, copper, phosphate, and dissolved oxygen. Water test strips (Fig. 5.1) are rapid and easy to use, but the results are not as accurate as when using a water test kit (Fig. 5.2) with liquid reagents. Electronic meters (Fig. 5.3) are best for measuring temperature, pH, salinity, and dissolved oxygen but need to be calibrated for accuracy.

For the most accurate reading, testing should be performed tank side. If an owner is transporting a fish to the clinic, request a separate container of water be brought along for testing. A fish in a small transport container will continue to respire and perform normal physiologic functions, decreasing the pH and oxygen, and increasing the ammonia and CO_2, affecting the water test results in the transport water. This provides an inaccurate representation of the water quality within the aquarium at home.

5.2 Filtration

To maintain optimum water quality, a healthy aquatic environment requires both mechanical and biological filtration. Mechanical filtration removes solids from the water and provides further surface area for colonization of the bacteria that form the biofilter. In addition, mechanical filters often agitate the water to increase aeration and gas exchange. Biofiltration involves nitrogenous waste product removal by the bacteria that colonize the surface of the filter media. Ammonia within an aquarium is created during fish metabolism and by decomposition of organic material, such as dead plants, fecal material, and excess fish food (Boyd, 2020). During the nitrification process, *Nitrosomonas* bacteria convert ammonia to nitrite. Then the *Nitrobacter* and *Nitrospira* bacteria convert nitrite to nitrate. Nitrate leaves the water through absorption by plants, water changes, or denitrification. Denitrification is the anaerobic microbial process of reducing nitrate to gaseous forms of nitrogen, principally nitrous oxide and nitrogen (Andrews *et al.*, 2011).

Corresponding author: az.erdman@gmail.com

© CAB International 2025. *The Handbook of Ornamental Fish Health and Welfare* (ed. N. Saint-Erne)
DOI: 10.1079/9781789246032.0005

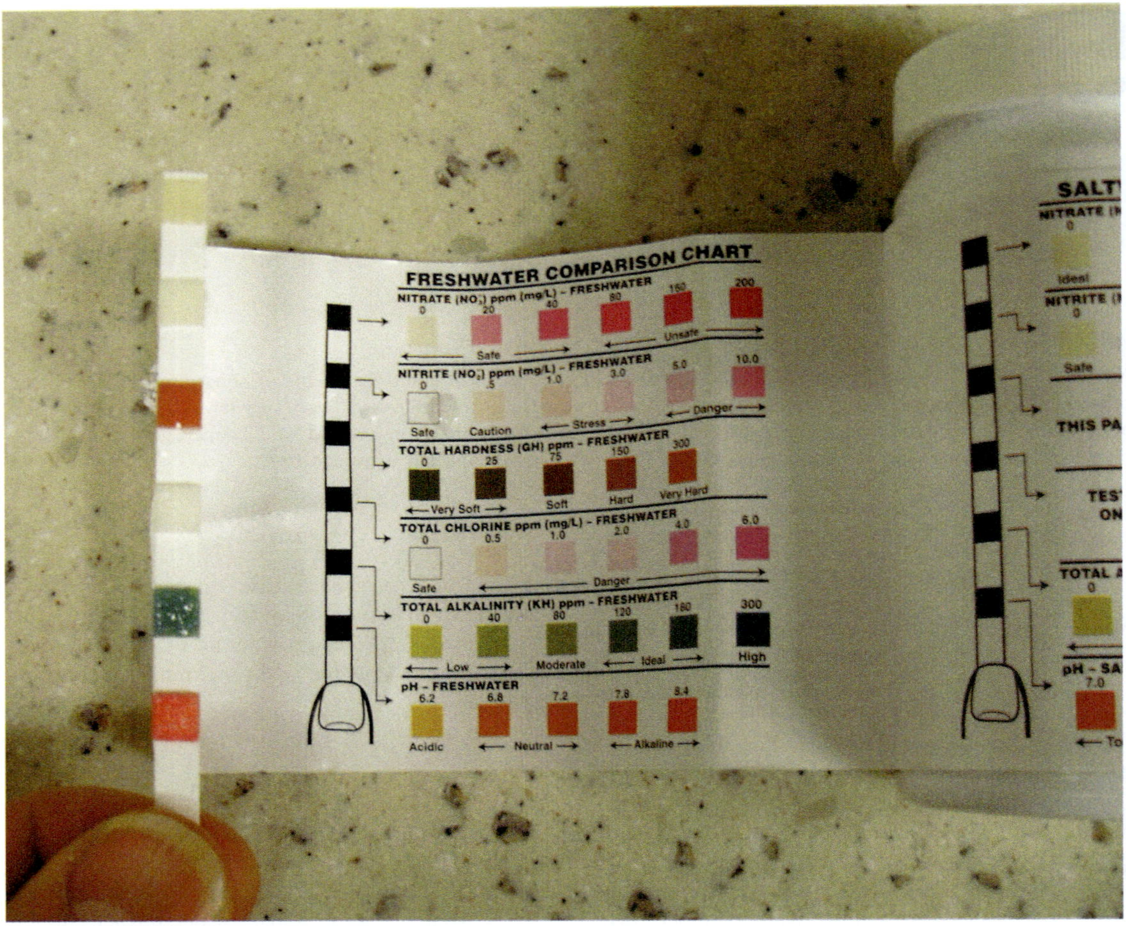

Fig. 5.1. Water test strips are easy to use and provide rapid results. (Photo by N. Saint-Erne.)

5.3 Ammonia/Ammonium

Ammonia is excreted by fish across the gills and in the feces and urine (Wildgoose, 2001). It is also a product of the breakdown of organic material like uneaten food, feces, and dead plant matter within the aquarium (Durborow *et al.*, 1997a). Ammonia can be present in the water in two forms: ionized ammonium (NH_4^+) and unionized ammonia (NH_3). Unionized ammonia is more toxic than ionized ammonium because it reduces the passive transfer of ammonia from the gills into the water as it accumulates. The conversion of toxic ammonia to ammonium is dependent on water pH, salinity, and temperature. Ammonium decreases and ammonia levels increase with more basic pH, higher temperatures, and lower salinity. At a neutral pH and ambient temperature, almost all free ammonia exists as NH_4^+. As the pH and temperature increase, the amount of NH_3 increases and the amount of NH_4^+ decreases. In general, a water test kit will give a total ammonia level that will include the sum of the concentration of ammonia and ammonium. An ammonia level above 0.05 mg/l is considered toxic (Noga, 2010). Ammonia levels should be measured daily in new aquariums and every 2–3 days for up to 2 weeks after the addition of new fish. Once an aquarium is set up and the biofilter nitrifying bacteria are established, ammonia levels should be tested once weekly (Calado *et al.*, 2017).

Ammonia levels are dependent on a functional and established biofilter within an aquarium. Ammonia levels will spike in situations where a biofilter has not had time for the beneficial bacteria to become established, the biofilter is inadequate for the bioload, or

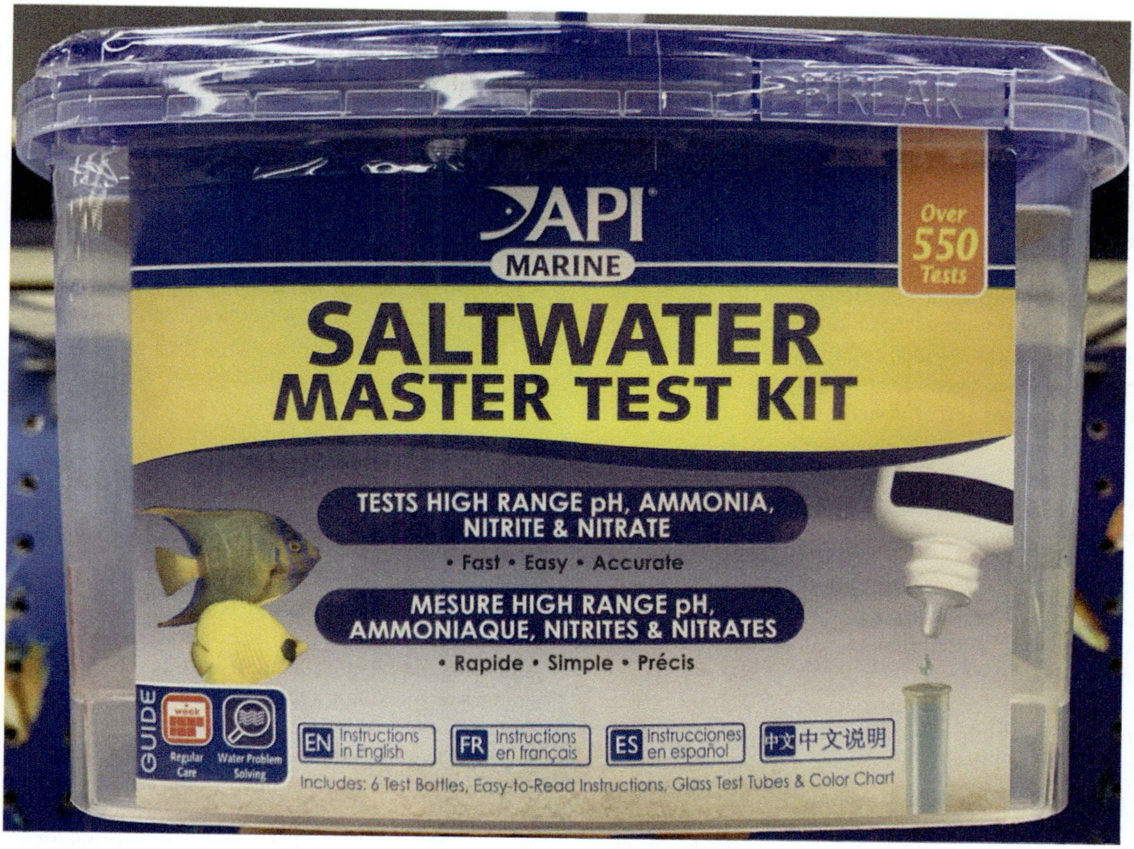

Fig. 5.2. Water test kits with powdered and liquid reagents provide reliable results. (Photo by N. Saint-Erne.)

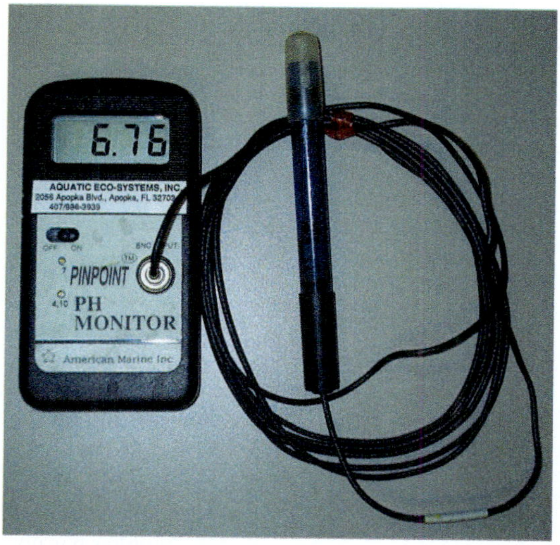

Fig. 5.3. Electronic pH meter results are accurate once the unit is calibrated. (Photo by N. Saint-Erne.)

if the biofilter stops functioning. Biofiltration is due to the beneficial nitrifying bacteria that colonize the surface areas around the tank, filter, and the décor within. Those bacteria require a few weeks to fully colonize a biofilter and increase in numbers high enough to process ammonia within the aquarium. New tanks without sufficient time for the bacteria to establish will have a spike in ammonia levels once fish and plants are added to the aquarium. Those initial fish may die due to ammonia accumulation in the water. Other situations can involve tanks with overfed fish, with too high of stocking density, and with large algae or plant die-offs. Often, a patient will get ammonia toxicity when the owner has over-cleaned the tank and filter, removing large amounts of the beneficial bacteria. Another situation that causes an increase in ammonia involves the decreased function or the death of the biofilter bacteria. This can occur when the aquarium is placed through a hypoxic situation, the pH drops below 6.0, the alkalinity drops too low, or the tank is treated with certain chemicals or medications.

High ammonia levels can be physically irritating to the gills and skin, causing hyperplasia and hypertrophy of the gill filaments as well as excessive production of the protective mucous layer. Ammonia can destroy the mucous barrier causing an increase in permeability and changes to the fish's ability to osmoregulate, creating electrolyte imbalances in the bloodstream (Noga, 2010). Increases in ammonia within the bloodstream also cause alkalosis of the blood, resulting in a decrease in hemoglobin-oxygen-carrying capacity. Ammonia will then cross into the nervous system and cause signs associated with neurotoxicity. Clinically, a patient suffering from elevated levels of ammonia will present with hyperexcitability, congregating near aeration, gasping at the surface, anorexia, and immunosuppression with secondary infections. At lethal levels, the patient will present with neurologic signs due to effects on the central nervous system (unable to swim or uncoordinated swimming) or acute death (Durborow *et al.*, 1997a).

Treatment for elevated levels of ammonia can involve multiple steps. First, it is important to check the pH level of the water and remember that higher pH will cause higher toxicity of ammonia. The lower the pH, the higher the concentration of ionized ammonium (NH_4^+), which is the less toxic form of ammonia (Table 5.1). To determine the concentration of toxic ammonia, multiply the test result value of total ammonia nitrogen (TAN) by the number in Table 5.1 at the intersection between the pH value and the water temperature. This will give the percentage of toxic ammonia (NH_3) present out of the total ammonia test result. For example, if the water pH is 7.8 and the water temperature is 75°F/24°C, the chart indicates that the percentage of the total ammonia that is toxic NH_3 is 0.0322 (3.22%). If the water test found a level of 3.0 mg/l total ammonia present, then multiply the total ammonia by this number from the chart: 3.0 mg/l × 0.0322 = 0.0966 mg NH_3/l. This is higher than the toxic level of 0.05 mg/l, so the fish would be subject to ammonia toxicity and water changes should be performed, or ammonia-binding treatments containing sodium hydroxymethanesulfonate should be added to the aquarium.

Elevated ammonia and pH must be addressed together carefully; if the pH is raised by adding a buffer, the ammonia will become more toxic. Ammonia can be reduced using 25–30% water changes or by adding zeolite to the filtration system. Zeolite is a clay that binds ammonia and removes it from the water. Zeolite can be added to a filtration system, or it can be suspended in the water column in a net bag where water will flow through it. Once the absorptive ability of the zeolite is at capacity, it

Table 5.1. Percentage of total ammonia that is toxic unionized ammonia (NH_3) (Saint-Erne, 2010).

	Temperature													
	42.0 (°F)	46.4	50.0	53.6	57.2	60.8	64.4	68.0	71.6	75.2	78.8	82.4	86.0	89.6
pH	6 (°C)	8	10	12	14	16	18	20	22	24	26	28	30	32
7.0	.0013	.0016	.0018	.0022	.0025	.0029	.0034	.0039	.0046	.0052	.0060	.0069	.0080	.0093
7.2	.0021	.0025	.0029	.0034	.0040	.0046	.0054	.0062	.0072	.0083	.0096	.0110	.0126	.0150
7.4	.0034	.0040	.0046	.0054	.0063	.0073	.0085	.0098	.0114	.0131	.0150	.0173	.0198	.0236
7.6	.0053	.0063	.0073	.0086	.0100	.0116	.0134	.0155	.0179	.0206	.0236	.0271	.0310	.0369
7.8	.0084	.0099	.0116	.0135	.0157	.0182	.0211	.0244	.0281	.0322	.0370	.0423	.0482	.0572
8.0	.0133	.0156	.0182	.0212	.0247	.0286	.0330	.0381	.0438	.0502	.0574	.0654	.0743	.0877
8.2	.0210	.0245	.0286	.0332	.0385	.0445	.0514	.0590	.0676	.0772	.0880	.0998	.1129	.1322
8.4	.0328	.0383	.0445	.0517	.0597	.0688	.0790	.0904	.1031	.1171	.1326	.1495	.1678	.1948
8.6	.0510	.0593	.0688	.0795	.0914	.1048	.1197	.1361	.1541	.1737	.1950	.2178	.2422	.2768
8.8	.0785	.0909	.1048	.1204	.1376	.1566	.1773	.1998	.2241	.2500	.2774	.3062	.3362	.3776
9.0	.1190	.1368	.1565	.1782	.2018	.2273	.2546	.2836	.3140	.3456	.3783	.4116	.4453	.4902
9.2	.1763	.2008	.2273	.2558	.2861	.3180	.3512	.3855	.4204	.4557	.4909	.5258	.5599	.6038
9.4	.2533	.2847	.3180	.3526	.3884	.4249	.4618	.4985	.5348	.5702	.6045	.6373	.6665	.7072
9.6	.3496	.3868	.4249	.4633	.5016	.5394	.5762	.6117	.6456	.6777	.7078	.7358	.7617	.7929
9.8	.4600	.5000	.5384	.5778	.6147	.6499	.6831	.7140	.7428	.7692	.7933	.8153	.8351	.8585
10.0	.5745	.6131	.6498	.6844	.7166	.7463	.7735	.7983	.8207	.8408	.8588	.8749	.8892	.9058
10.2	.6815	.7152	.7463	.7746	.8003	.8234	.8441	.8625	.8788	.8933	.9060	.9173	.9271	.9389

will start leaching ammonia back into the system. In order to remove the ammonia from the clay and replenish its absorptive capacity, the clay can be soaked in a 3% saltwater solution overnight. Once the ammonia levels are addressed, correct the pH and the inciting cause of the high ammonia. This could involve reseeding the biofilter, decreasing the stocking density, decreasing the plant matter, reducing overfeeding, or educating the client on proper tank cleaning and water-changing protocols.

5.4 Nitrite

Nitrite is produced through the oxidation of ammonia by *Nitrosomonas* bacteria within the biofiltration system. Nitrite is toxic in a freshwater aquarium because nitrite enters the blood through the gills. In the presence of chloride ions, less nitrite is absorbed into the gills. Therefore, in a saltwater aquarium where chloride ions are higher in concentration, nitrite is less of a concern (Shinn *et al.*, 2013). In levels as low as 0.5 mg/l, nitrite can cause immunosuppression and stress in a patient (Stamper and Semmen, 2012). At higher levels, varying by the species, it is considered toxic.

Nitrite is absorbed through the gills and binds to the hemoglobin within the erythrocytes. This causes oxidation of the hemoglobin, converting it to methemoglobin, which disrupts the erythrocytes' ability to carry oxygen. Oxidation of the hemoglobin will turn the blood cells brown, causing nitrite toxicosis to also be known as "brown blood disease" (Durborow *et al.*, 1997b). Clinically, a fish patient will present as listless, anorexic, dyspneic, and gasping at the water surface. On examination, the patient will appear to have brown discolored gills. Blood tests will show brown blood with anemia secondary to hemolysis.

Treatment for high nitrite level involves a 25–30% water change and addressing the underlying cause of the nitrite elevation. Since both nitrite and chloride compete to travel across the gills, sodium chloride can be added to freshwater aquariums to minimize further absorption of nitrite (Shinn *et al.*, 2013). In a freshwater aquarium, 6 mg/l of chloride ion (Cl-) is needed to prevent nitrite toxicity for every 1 mg/l of nitrite present. Sodium chloride is 60% chloride, so 6 mg of chloride ion is contained in 10 mg of sodium chloride. It is safe to add one teaspoon (5 g) of salt per gallon (3.8 l) of water to increase the chloride ion by 3000 mg/l. This will bring the salinity to 0.12%, and the chloride ion level is enough to treat 500 mg/l of nitrite (Saint-Erne, 2010). Sodium chloride (NaCl) concentration should not exceed 5 mg/l (0.5% salinity) in freshwater aquariums.

Nitrite levels will spike with insufficient biofiltration. The same causes for high ammonia, as mentioned above, will affect the nitrite concentrations as well. Biofiltration that hasn't had time to grow adequate bacterial colonies, isn't functioning properly, or is inadequate for the aquarium size or bioload should all be differentials when determining the cause of high nitrite levels within an aquarium.

5.5 Nitrate

Nitrate is produced by the oxidation of nitrite by *Nitrobacter* and *Nitrospira* bacteria. Generally, nitrate is considered non-toxic unless in very high concentrations. Nitrate is absorbed across the gills and, like nitrite, binds with hemoglobin causing methemoglobin formation. However, for nitrate, this occurs at much higher concentrations. Less than 50 mg/l is considered an ideal level (Stamper and Semmen, 2012). Levels higher than that can cause stunted growth, immunosuppression, and delayed wound healing. At levels 200 mg/l or greater lethal toxicities have occurred. It is important to note that nitrate can compete with and decrease the uptake of iodine. In certain saltwater species, like elasmobranchs, this can cause goiter despite proper iodine supplementation.

Nitrate levels will increase gradually in an aquarium. Rapid increases can occur with an inadequately sized biofilter, high stocking densities, or from lack of water exchange. Nitrate is the final product of the nitrification process and leaves the system in three ways: (i) it is absorbed by aquatic plants as a nutrient source, (ii) through denitrification where nitrate is converted to nitrogen gas that then escapes the water through gas exchange on the surface, and (iii) through routine water changes. Aquariums that have high stocking densities will have nitrate increase faster as the nitrogenous waste is processed by the biofilter. In an enclosed system that does not have continuous water inflow and outflow, the environment is dependent on the aquarist performing water changes to decrease the nitrate level. It is recommended to test the nitrate level once a week. Though not always practical in a pond setting, an indoor aquarium should undergo a 10–20% water change once a week, or at least 25% water change every 3–4 weeks, to keep the nitrate low.

5.6 Hydrogen Concentration (pH)

The hydrogen ion concentration in an aquatic system plays a large role in many reactions. The hydrogen ion concentration is measured in a logarithmic equation (pH = $-\log_{10} [H^+]$) giving a "power of hydrogen" (pH) value. The pH value can range from 1.0 to 14.0, with 7.0 being neutral. Below 7.0 the water is acidic, and above 7.0 the water is basic. Because the units are logarithmic, a change of 0.1 unit in the pH value is a tenfold change in the actual concentration of the hydrogen ions in the water. Most freshwater fish species prefer to live in a pH of 6.5–8.5, with marine species preferring a more basic pH of 8.0–8.5. Acidophiles are species preferring a more acidic water, such as the Amazon River species; and alkaliphiles are species preferring a more basic pH, such as some African cichlids. However, most species will be raised and kept within the pH range of 7.0–8.5.

There are constant processes creating a more acidic or basic environment within an aquatic setting. The alkalinity or buffering capacity helps maintain a stable pH. This will be discussed in the carbonate hardness section. Carbon dioxide within the water will decrease the pH and make a more acidic environment (Wurts and Durborow, 1992). Carbon dioxide is often found in high concentrations in rainwater and is also released by organisms during respiration within the water. Nitrification by the biological filter will also produce a more acidic environment as the process utilizes carbonates. The carbonate concentration, or alkalinity, helps maintain the pH during these processes.

The pH plays a large role in the metabolism of living organisms within an aquarium. Too low or too high pH levels can be lethal or cause slow growth, immunosuppression, or stress. The bacteria within the biofilter operate within a specific pH range and a pH lower than 6 or higher than 9 causes the bacteria to stop functioning, which can cause a rise in the ammonia levels, creating a toxic situation.

Fluctuations in the pH are considered stressful. A change of 0.3 pH units or less within 24 h is considered safe for most fish species. Acidosis within a species is usually seen when the pH of the environment drops below 5.5 pH units. Alkalosis of a fish patient may occur at a pH above 8.0 in freshwater species and 9.0 in marine species. The clinical signs of either acidosis or alkalosis are similar. The patient can be highly excitable, jumping, and gasping at the surface due to reduced oxygen-carrying capacity of hemoglobin and may have excess mucous production over the gills and skin. Treatment for a drop in pH involves adding a buffer to counteract the acidity. Adding one teaspoon (5 g) of baking soda (sodium bicarbonate) per 10 gallons (38 l) of water, or in a pond using 1 lb (454 g) of baking soda per 1000 gallons (3800 l) of water, can be used to buffer the pH and raise the alkalinity. To help prevent further drops in pH, this same ratio of baking soda can be added with each water change, or crushed limestone can be added to the filter system, as it will slowly dissolve and release calcium and carbonate. Remember to monitor the ammonia level closely and do not change the pH by more than 0.3 units in a 24-h period.

Fluctuations of pH will occur due to high stocking densities, dysfunction of the biofilter, heavy plant loads, low buffering capacity, or low carbonate hardness within an aquarium. In general, biological processes within a tank shift the pH to a more acidic environment. High stocking densities with heavy organic loads and large numbers of respiring fish can quickly create an acidic environment. During daylight, aquatic plants will absorb carbon dioxide from the water, creating a more alkaline environment; however, once the carbon dioxide levels are depleted, as can occur in heavily planted aquatic environments, the plants will switch to absorbing bicarbonate from the water, depleting the buffering capacity. Measurements of pH should be taken weekly in most aquariums, but daily in new tanks or when adding new fish.

5.7 Oxygen

Every aquarium containing fish has oxygen requirements. The more living organisms within a system, the higher the oxygen demand. Oxygenation of the water is measured by quantifying the amount of dissolved oxygen using a cathode probe meter. Levels will vary depending on the temperature, salinity, elevation, surface area of the water, and water movement or turbulence. Temperature and salinity are inversely related to the solubility of oxygen (Table 5.2). This means that the solubility of oxygen decreases with warmer temperatures or higher salinity levels. Dissolved oxygen levels of less than 5 mg/l are considered very stressful. Lethal levels of hypoxia occur when oxygen falls below 1 mg/l. Levels should be measured tank or pond side for the most accurate reading (Fig. 5.4).

Table 5.2. Dissolved oxygen saturation chart (Saint-Erne, 2010).

Temperature		DO Saturation
(°F)	(°C)	(mg/l)
64.4	18	9.45
66.2	19	9.26
68.0	20	9.07
69.8	21	8.90
71.6	22	8.72
73.4	23	8.56
75.2	24	8.40
77.0	25	8.24
78.8	26	8.09
80.6	27	7.95
82.4	28	7.81
84.2	29	7.67
86.0	30	7.54

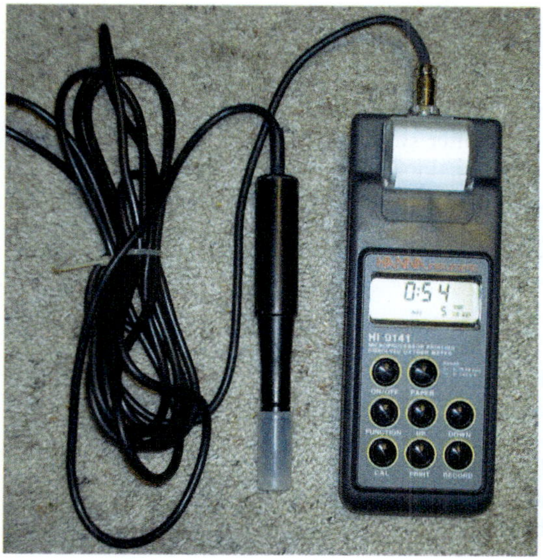

Fig. 5.4. An oxygen meter with print-out capability. (Photograph by N. Saint-Erne.)

Clinical signs of low oxygen include the fish open-mouth breathing and flaring its operculum, congregating at the surface (piping) or around aeration sources, anorexia, lethargy, and mortalities in severe hypoxic cases (Esmail *et al.*, 2015).

Hypoxic events often occur in heavily stocked ponds, heavily planted ponds, and during warm weather months. Warm weather increases the risk of hypoxic events as oxygen gas solubility decreases at higher temperatures. A heavily planted or stocked pond will have an increase in oxygen demand leading to depletion of the dissolved oxygen levels. Hypoxic events in heavily planted ponds or those with algae blooms are usually associated with mortalities overnight or in the morning. Throughout the day, the plants are photosynthesizing and releasing oxygen into the water. Once the sun goes down the plants switch to respiration and absorb oxygen and release carbon dioxide overnight (Pedersen *et al.*, 2006). This means that overnight and into the early morning prior to sunrise the oxygen levels will be at the lowest. It is important in these cases to measure the oxygen levels in the early morning rather than in the afternoon, as the plants will then have restored the oxygen in the water and the reading may not show hypoxia. In areas where the weather allows for a body of water to freeze, the oxygen that is present once the surface is fully frozen is all that is available until it thaws. If the winter months are longer or colder than usual, hypoxic events can be seen in the later winter or early spring.

Treatment and prevention for low oxygen levels usually focus on increasing agitation of the water and decreasing oxygen demand. Agitation and aeration can increase dissolved oxygen levels in the water by increasing the water surface contact with air. Decreasing the oxygen demand often means addressing the stocking density or plant and algae population. Removing plants and using a UV filter to kill algae can help. Algicide chemicals can be used in the case of large algae populations. However, remove or clean out as much debris as possible and monitor the ammonia levels closely for 1–2 weeks after treatment. Dead algae can increase ammonia and its decay can also reduce oxygen, causing fish mortality. For those living where a pond will freeze over entirely, a pond surface heater can be used to allow for one area of the pond to stay unfrozen and provide surface gas exchange through the winter. It is important to remember that the biofiltering bacteria require oxygen to function. If a hypoxic event were to occur, monitor ammonia and nitrite levels carefully afterward for 1–2 weeks until the biofilter returns to normal function.

5.8 General Hardness

General hardness (GH) is a measure of all divalent cations (ions having two positive charges) in the water. The majority of divalent minerals in water consist of calcium and magnesium (Swistock, 2015), but will include low levels of strontium, ferrous iron, and manganese. The calcium level is related to the carbonate level, which affects the measurement of alkalinity (Brightwell, 2007). In most freshwater, the calcium (Ca^{++}) from calcium carbonate ($CaCO_3$) is the largest component of hardness and is used to measure the hardness of the water. Hardness can be expressed in milligrams per liter (mg/l) of calcium carbonate, in grains of calcium carbonate per gallon of water, or in degrees of German hardness (°dH), which is the millimoles of calcium carbonate contained in each liter of water. The hardness of water is classified as soft, moderate, hard, to very hard (Table 5.3), depending on the amount of mineral cations present in the water.

Mineral cations are used for scale and skeletal growth and play an important role in photosynthesis for plants. In aquatic environments with hard water, the high calcium cations can cause nephrocalcinosis and other dystrophic mineralization. In addition, high levels of calcium can out-compete zinc ion absorption and cause zinc-deficiency-induced cataracts (Ketola, 1979). In low hardness, soft water situations, fish may show stunted growth or spinal curvature. GH is linked to carbonate hardness, so soft water has a decreased buffering capacity. To remove cations from hard water, it can be processed through a water softener, reverse osmosis filtration, or filtered through peat moss. To make soft water harder, crushed oyster shells or limestone can be added to the filtration system.

5.9 Carbonate Hardness

Carbonate hardness (KH) is also known as alkalinity or buffering capacity. Carbonate hardness is most commonly due to dissolved limestone or other environmental minerals that leach into the water. The measurement of carbonate hardness is the sum of the bicarbonate and carbonate ions in the water. These compounds provide both buffering capacity for the water as well as a carbon energy source for the biofilter bacteria, and plants when the carbon dioxide levels are low (Wurts and Duborow, 1992). The carbonate hardness is important for skeletal growth in fish and shell production in corals and invertebrates (Leewis and Janse, 2008).

Carbonate hardness is measured in "degree of carbonate hardness," and the measurement should remain greater than 4.5 dKH (1 dKH = 17.9 mg/l $CaCO_3$). In coral or invertebrate tanks, the hardness should be 7.0–9.8 dKH. The higher the carbonate hardness, the greater the buffering capacity of the water, and the greater the ability to bind H^+ ions to prevent pH fluctuations. If the buffering capacity is reduced and the carbonate hardness drops below 4.5 dKH, there will be a drop in the pH. This reduces the biofilter activity and causes the fish to become stressed and undergo changes due to acidic irritation. Adding crushed limestone to the filter system, or a measure of one teaspoon (5 g) of baking soda per 10 gallons (38 l) of water or 1 lb (454 g) of baking soda per 1000 gallons (3800 l) of pond water with each water change can help maintain the alkalinity level.

5.10 Phosphorus

Phosphorus is an important nutrient for plant growth and maintenance of life within an aquarium. It is found in the genetic material DNA and RNA. It is used for energy in the form of ATP, and it plays a key role in the formation of cell membrane phospholipids. It is vital for bone and shell

Table 5.3. Water hardness levels (Saint-Erne, 2010).

Classification	$CaCO_3$ mg/l (PPM)	Grains per Gallon	Degrees Hardness (°dH)
Very soft	0–17.0	<1	0–0.9
Soft/slightly hard	17.1–60	1–3.5	1–3.4
Moderately hard	61–120	3.6–7.0	3.5–6.7
Hard	121–180	7.1–10.5	6.8–10
Very hard	181–239	10.6–14	10.1–13.4
Extremely hard	>240	>14	>13.5

One part per million (PPM) is equal to 1 mg/l.
One grain per gallon = 17.1 mg $CaCO_3$/l.
One degree of German hardness (°dH) = 17.9 mg $CaCO_3$/l of water.

formation. Phosphorous can enter a pond through runoff of fertilizers and other chemicals, dissolution of minerals within the ground or sediment, or through production by microorganisms in the decay of organic material. In aquariums, it primarily comes from the food. Though important for the maintenance of life, high levels of phosphorus can lead to overgrowth of plants, algae, and cyanobacteria. Phosphorus levels should be maintained at less than 0.1 mg/l in the aquarium water.

Treatment to remove the phosphorus from the aquarium water should be aimed at addressing the source. Avoid overfeeding, and feed diets that contain no more than 1.0–1.4% phosphorus content. Clean the tank or pond of extra plants, algae, and debris. Water changes can be performed to lower phosphorus; however, the source water needs to be tested as some cities' tap water contains high levels of phosphorus. In that case, or in a large aquarium or pond, phosphate-binding filters or phosphate-binding chemicals can be used to lower the phosphorus.

5.11 Copper

Copper is important for many biological processes in animals including RNA and DNA synthesis, electron-transferring reactions, and photosynthesis (Ebrahimpour *et al.*, 2010). Low levels of copper can be tolerated by some fish species; however, high copper can be toxic, and the goal is to have a level of zero mg/l within aquarium water (Cardeilhac, 1979). Toxic levels of copper are considered over 2.0 mg/l but can be toxic even at lower levels depending on water hardness and alkalinity. Generally high levels will come directly from the water source, by treatment with a copper medication, or with some algicide treatments. The softer the water hardness, the more toxic the copper ions become. Calcium ions will compete with copper for receptors in the gills. A higher calcium level equates to harder water and therefore less ability for copper toxicity in the fish (Playle *et al.*, 1992; Meyer *et al.*, 1999). Copper causes dysfunction of the osmoregulatory system and acute kidney failure, immunosuppression, damage to lateral line organ, and generalized cell damage (Cardeilhac, 1979). High copper levels are physically irritating, causing hyperplasia of the gills and increased mucus, decreasing respiratory exchange, and causing hypoxia.

Copper toxicity can occur as an acute process or chronic process. Chronically, signs involve stunted growth, anorexia, immunosuppression with secondary infections, and incoordination or abnormal swimming patterns due to effects on the lateral line organ. Acute toxicity cases will exhibit gasping at the water surface, congregating around water inlets or aerators, lethargy, anorexia, and death from cardiac arrest due to high potassium (K^+) associated with acute renal failure and cell damage. Treatment for high copper levels involves using EDTA in the water or activated carbon in the filter to bind and remove it from the water. When using medications containing copper, the copper level in the water should be tested daily and the copper level maintained at no more than 0.2 mg/l.

5.12 Iron

Iron is a heavy metal used in many biological enzymes, anaerobic respiration, and photosynthesis. High levels of iron can become toxic. Ideally, the iron level in the water should be 0.1–0.3 mg/l. High levels of iron cause anemia, oxidative damage to gill tissue, and physical gill irritation from precipitation of iron complexes on the gills occurring when water has increased aeration. Iron in the aquarium generally doesn't reach high levels because constant aeration within the water helps expose iron ions to oxygen, creating ferric oxide (rust) that can be filtered out as a solid. Some well water is high in iron, and the water should be aerated in a storage tank to precipitate the iron before using this water in aquariums or ponds.

5.13 Temperature

Fish are poikilothermic animals, which means their body temperature will fluctuate with the environmental temperatures. A change of 4°F/2°C in temperature within 24 h, even if within a preferred temperature range for a species, is considered stressful (Esmail *et al.*, 2015). Fish in natural habitats can regulate their body temperature by moving to different areas within their environment that have differing water temperatures, such as sunny vs shaded areas or perhaps with cooler or warmer currents present. Metabolism rate, immune system, and other physiological processes of a species are affected by the temperature of the environment. Warm water fish tend to become more active in warmer weather and slower when it is cooler; however, cool water species will often slow and become stressed in warmer temperatures. Certain pathogens thrive in different temperature ranges, leading to outbreaks as the water temperature changes.

Temperature can also affect other water quality parameters, like the level of dissolved oxygen and toxicity of ammonia, making it an important parameter to monitor carefully. The temperature in an aquarium should be checked daily. Maintain the aquarium water temperature within the appropriate range for the fish species using a thermostatically controlled submersible aquarium water heater. For some marine species, a chiller may be required to keep the water cooler than room temperature.

5.14 Salinity

Salinity is a measure of the dissolved salts within water. Though sodium chloride is the main salt in seawater, there are 78 total inorganic elements in seawater (Table 5.4). Seawater has a salinity of 3.4–3.6% (34–36 g/l, or PPT), and a specific gravity (SG) of 1.025. The salinity of water can be measured with a hydrometer, refractometer, or conductivity meter. Salt mixtures can be purchased as premixed formulas and added to deionized water to mimic natural salt water. The ideal salinity for saltwater species is a SG of 1.021–1.026, though some species are kept at a lower SG. Brackish water ranges from 1.005 to 1.020 SG. Freshwater has a SG near 1.000 and typically contains less than 0.1% salt. To convert a specific gravity reading to salinity in parts per thousand (PPT), record the temperature of the water and then use Table 5.5 to find the SG on the left column, and the temperature across the top. The intersecting number is the salinity in g/l or PPT.

5.15 Conclusions

The aquarium or pond water should be tested on a regular basis to ensure the water quality is appropriate for the fish species present. Whenever fish are showing signs of stress or illness, always check the water quality. Take corrective action to return the water parameters to the proper ranges (Table 5.6) by performing water changes, correcting filtration, or adding chemical treatments (Fig. 5.5) to the pond or aquarium. The best health and welfare of the fish occurs when the water quality is maintained at ideal parameters.

Table 5.4. Constituents of sea water at 3.5% salinity (values vary in different ocean areas). Author's own table.

Element	Molecular weight	mg/l (PPM) in Seawater
Oxygen	16	85,840,000
Hydrogen	1	10,820,000
Chloride	35.4	18,980–19,980
Sodium	23	10,556–10,752
Magnesium	24.3	1272
Sulfur (as sulfate)	32	884–2701
Calcium	40	400–410
Potassium	39.1	380–402
Bicarbonate	12	145
Bromine/bromide	79.9	65
Carbon (inorganic)	12	28
Strontium	87.6	7.9–13
Boron	10.8	4.6
Silicon	28.1	4
Carbon (organic)	12	3
Aluminum	27	1.9
Fluorine/fluoride	19	1.4
Nitrogen (as nitrate)	14	0.7
Nitrogen (organic)	14	0.2
Rubidium	85	0.2
Lithium	6.9	0.1
Phosphorus (as phosphate)	31	0.1
Copper	63.5	0.09
Barium	137	0.05
Iodine	126.9	0.05
Nitrogen (as nitrite)	14	0.05
Nitrogen (as ammonia)	14	0.05
Arsenic	74.9	0.024
Iron	55.8	0.020
Phosphorus (as organic)	31	0.016
Zinc	65.4	0.014
Manganese	54.9	0.010
Lead	207.2	0.005
Selenium	79	0.004
Tin	118.7	0.003
Cesium	132.9	0.002
Molybdenum	95.9	0.002
Uranium	238	0.0016
Gallium	69.7	0.0005
Nickel	58.7	0.0005
Thorium	232	0.0005
Cerium	140	0.0004
Vanadium	50.9	0.0003
Lanthanum	139.9	0.0003
Yttrium	88.9	0.0003
Mercury	200.6	0.0003
Silver	107.9	0.0003
Bismuth	209	0.0002
Cobalt	58.9	0.0001
Gold	197	0.000008

Table 5.5. Conversion of specific gravity to salinity in parts per thousand (PPT). Author's own table.

	Temperature °F/°C									
SG	74/23.5	75.2/24	76/24.5	77/25	78/25.5	78.8/26	79/26.5	80/27	81/27.5	82/28
1.000	1.8	1.9	2.0	2.1	2.4	2.5	2.7	2.9	3.1	3.2
1.001	2.9	3.1	3.2	3.4	3.6	3.8	4.0	4.2	4.4	4.5
1.002	4.4	4.6	4.8	4.9	5.0	5.1	5.4	5.5	5.7	5.9
1.003	5.8	5.9	6.1	6.2	6.3	6.6	6.7	6.8	7.1	7.2
1.004	7.1	7.2	7.4	7.5	7.7	7.9	8.0	8.3	8.4	8.5
1.005	8.4	8.5	8.7	8.9	9.1	9.2	9.3	9.6	9.7	10
1.006	9.7	9.8	10.1	10.2	10.4	10.5	10.7	10.9	11.0	11.3
1.007	11.0	11.3	11.4	11.5	11.7	11.9	12.0	12.2	12.4	12.6
1.008	12.4	12.6	12.7	12.8	13.0	13.2	13.4	13.6	13.7	13.9
1.009	13.7	13.9	14.0	14.1	14.4	14.5	14.7	14.9	15.0	15.3
1.010	15.0	15.2	15.3	15.6	15.7	15.8	16.1	16.2	16.5	16.6
1.011	16.3	16.5	16.7	16.9	17.0	17.3	17.4	17.5	17.8	17.9
1.012	17.7	17.9	18.0	18.2	18.3	18.6	18.7	19.0	19.1	19.3
1.013	19.1	19.2	19.3	19.5	19.7	19.9	20.0	20.3	20.4	20.6
1.014	20.4	20.5	20.6	20.9	21.0	21.2	21.4	21.6	21.8	22.0
1.015	21.7	21.8	22.0	22.2	22.3	22.5	22.7	22.9	23.1	23.3
1.016	23.0	23.3	23.4	23.5	23.6	23.9	24.0	24.3	24.4	24.7
1.017	24.3	24.6	24.7	24.8	25.1	25.2	25.3	25.6	25.7	26.0
1.018	25.6	25.9	26.0	26.1	26.4	26.5	26.8	26.9	27.2	27.3
1.019	27.0	27.2	27.3	27.6	27.7	27.8	28.1	28.2	28.5	28.6
1.020	28.3	28.5	28.6	28.9	29.0	29.2	29.4	29.6	29.8	30.0
1.021	29.6	29.8	30.0	30.2	30.3	30.6	30.7	30.9	31.1	31.3
1.022	30.9	31.2	31.3	31.5	31.7	31.9	32.0	32.2	32.5	32.6
1.023	32.2	32.5	32.6	32.8	33.0	33.2	33.4	33.5	33.8	33.9
1.024	33.7	33.8	33.9	34.2	34.3	34.5	34.7	35.0	35.1	35.4
1.025	35.0	35.1	35.2	35.5	35.6	35.9	36.0	36.3	36.4	36.7
1.026	36.3	36.4	36.7	36.8	36.9	37.2	37.3	37.6	37.7	38.0
1.027	37.6	37.8	38.0	38.1	38.4	38.5	38.8	38.9	39.1	39.3
1.028	38.9	39.1	39.3	39.4	39.7	39.8	40.1	40.2	40.5	40.7
1.029	40.2	40.5	40.6	40.8	41.0	41.2	41.4	41.6	41.8	42.0

Table 5.6. Normal water parameters (optimum ranges) (Saint-Erne, 2010).

- Ammonia (0 mg/l)
  - highly toxic, aim for zero
- Nitrite (0 mg/l)
  - highly toxic, aim for zero
- Nitrate (0–20 mg/l)
  - <30 mg/l in fresh water, <10 mg/l in marine aquariums
  - <0.25 mg/l in marine tanks with coral or other invertebrates
- pH (6.0–8.5)
  - most fresh water 6–8 pH, marine 8–8.4, brackish 7.2–8.5
- Oxygen (6–9 mg/l)
  - >5 mg/l; compare level to saturation at the water temperature
  - measure pond water early in the morning when the reading will be lowest
- Temperature (73–80°F/23–27°C)
  - generally, tropical fish do best at 75–78°F/24–25°C, with other ranges that are species specific
- General hardness (magnesium and calcium salts in the water)
  - Measured in degrees of German hardness (°dH)
  - 4–12°dH in freshwater aquariums but can vary for different species
  - 1°dH = 17.9 mg/l $CaCO_3$

Continued

Table 5.6. Continued.

- Carbonate hardness/alkalinity (measures carbonates and bicarbonates)
  - Measured in degree of carbonate hardness (dKH)
  - 1 dKH = 17.9 mg/l $CaCO_3$
  - 7–10 dKH in marine aquariums
  - 4–8 dKH in freshwater aquariums
- Specific gravity (marine and brackish)
  - Marine: 1.021–1.026
  - Brackish: 1.005–1.020
- Iron (marine)
  - 0.1–0.3 mg/l
- Copper (<0.2 mg/l)
  - Monitor copper levels when using it as a parasite treatment
- Phosphorus (0–0.1 mg/l)
  - Less than 0.1 mg/l; causes algae growth at high levels

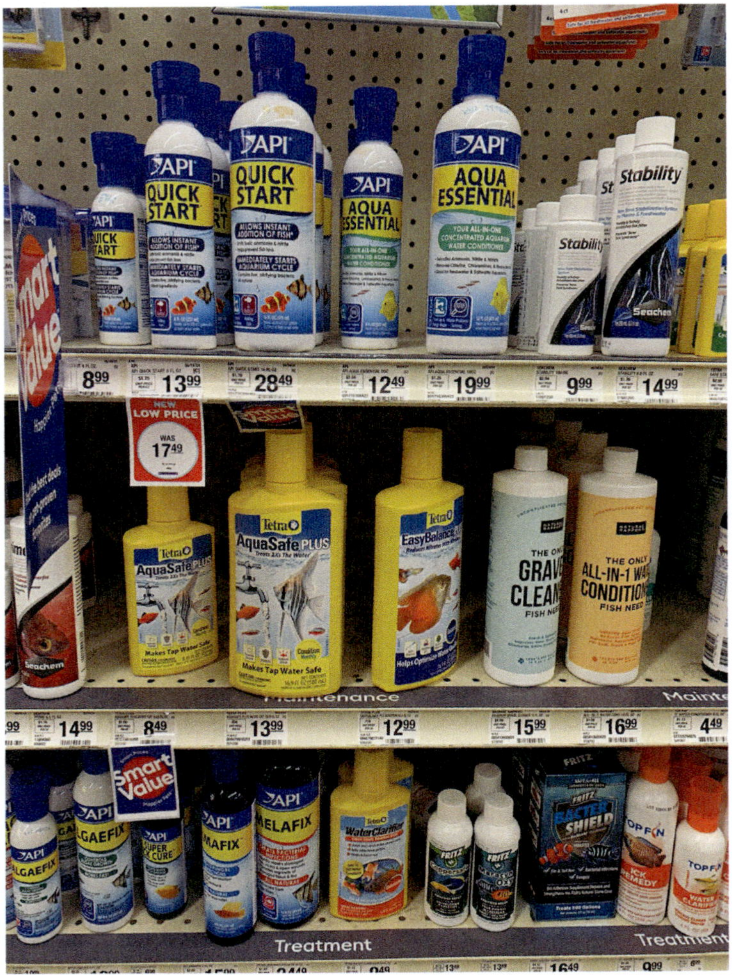

Fig. 5.5. There are many commercial water conditioners available to correct water quality problems. (Photograph by N. Saint-Erne.)

References

Andrews, C., Exell, A. and Carrington, N. (2011) *The Manual of Fish Health*. Interpret, Surrey, UK.

Boyd, C.E. (2020) *Water Quality: An Introduction*. Springer Nature, Cham, Switzerland.

Brightwell, C. (2007). *Marine Chemistry*. T.F.H. Publications, Neptune City, New Jersey.

Calado, R., Olivotto, I., Oliver, M.P. and Holt, J. (2017) *Marine Ornamental Species Aquaculture*. Wiley, Chichester, UK.

Cardeilhac, P. (1979) *Mechanisms of Copper Toxicity in Marine Fish*. International Association for Aquatic Animal Medicine conference, St. Augustine, Florida.

Durborow, R., Crosby, D. and Brunson, M. (1997a) *Ammonia in Fish Ponds*. Southern Regional Aquaculture Center. Available at: https://aquaculture.ca.uky.edu/sites/aquaculture.ca.uky.edu/files/srac_463_ammonia_in_fish_ponds.pdf (accessed 1 August 2024).

Durborow, R., Crosby, D. and Brunson, M. (1997b) *Nitrite in Fish Ponds*. Southern Regional Aquaculture Center. Available at: https://aquaculture.ca.uky.edu/sites/aquaculture.ca.uky.edu/files/srac_462_nitrite_in_fish_ponds.pdf (accessed 1 August 2024).

Ebrahimpour, M., Alipour, H. and Rakhshah, S. (2010) Influence of water hardness on acute toxicity of copper and zinc on fish. *Toxicology and Industrial Health* 26(6), 361–365.

Esmail, M.Y., Astrofsky, K.M., Lawrence, C. and Serluca, F.C. (2015) The biology and management of the zebrafish. *Laboratory Animal Medicine* 3, 1015–1062.

Ketola, H.G. (1979) Influence of dietary zinc on cataracts in rainbow trout (*Salmo gairdneri*). *The Journal of Nutrition* 109(6), 965–969.

Leewis, R.J. and Janse, M. (2008). *Advances in Coral Husbandry in Public Aquariums*. Burgers' Zoo, Arnhem, Netherlands.

Meyer, J.S., Santore, R.C., Bobbitt, J.P., DeBrey, L.D., Boese, C.J. *et al.* (1999) Binding of nickel and copper to fish gills predicts toxicity when water hardness varies, but free-ion activity does not. *Environmental Science and Technology* 33(6), 913–916.

Noga, E.J. (2010) *Fish Disease: Diagnosis and Treatment*. Wiley, Ames, Iowa.

Pedersen, O., Andersen, T. and Christensen, C. (2006) CO_2 in planted aquaria. *The Aquatic Gardener* 20(3), 24–33.

Playle, R.C., Gensemer, R.W. and Dixon, D.G. (1992) Copper accumulation on gills of fathead minnows: influence of water hardness, complexation and pH of the gill micro-environment. *Environmental Toxicology and Chemistry* 11(3), 381–391.

Saint-Erne, N. (2010) Water quality. In: Saint-Erne, N. *Advanced Koi Care*. Erne Enterprises, Glendale, Arizona, pp. 94–109.

Shinn, C., Marco, A. and Serrano, L. (2013). Influence of low levels of water salinity on toxicity of nitrite to anuran larvae. *Chemosphere* 92(9), 1154–1160.

Stamper, M. and Semmen, K. (2012) Basic water quality evaluation for zoo veterinarians. In: Fowler, M. and Miller, R.E. (eds) *Zoo and Wild Animal Medicine: Current Therapy*. Elsevier/Saunders, St. Louis, Missouri, pp. 177–186.

Swistock, B. (2015) Interpreting water tests for ponds and lakes. Penn State Extension. Available at: http://extension.psu.edu/interpreting-water-tests-for-ponds-and-lakes (accessed 26 October 2020).

Wildgoose, W.H. (2001) *BSAVA Manual of Ornamental Fish*. British Small Animal Veterinary Association, Gloucester, UK.

Wurts, W. and Durborow, R. (1992) *Interactions of pH, Carbon Dioxide, Alkalinity and Hardness in Fish Ponds*. Southern Regional Aquaculture Center. Available at: https://freshwater-aquaculture.extension.org/wp-content/uploads/2019/08/Interactions_of_pH_Carbon_Dioxide_Alkalinity_and_Hardness.pdf (accessed 26 October 2020).

6 Filtration Systems

Nicholas Saint-Erne

Dr. Saint-Erne Consulting, PLLC, Phoenix, Arizona

Abstract

Water filtration is the most important part of maintaining the health and welfare of fish in an aquarium. There are many types of filters that can be used in aquariums. Each has advantages and disadvantages. Factors including the size, cost, ease of maintenance, availability of media, and appropriateness for the size of the tank must be considered when selecting a filter for the aquarium.

6.1 Filtration Types

Filtration of the water in an aquarium is what allows it to support aquatic life, and the filtration system can recirculate the water, so a continuous flow of incoming water (as used in certain aquaculture facilities) is not required to maintain good water quality. With filtration, the aquarium will be cleaner, the water clearer, and it will support a greater density of fish. Without filtration, an aquarium may run out of oxygen, ammonia will accumulate, and the water may stagnate and become toxic to fish (Saint-Erne, 2010).

The size of the filter unit should be as large as is practical. Most filters are small plastic containers that are connected to the aquarium by pipes, and water is circulated through them by water pumps. The water passes through various filter media such as foam, gravel, lava rock, plastic beads, ceramic rings, and filter brushes. The flow rate of water through the filter should be three to five times the aquarium volume water every hour (Spotte, 1970). Therefore, a 20-gallon aquarium would need a water pump for the filter that pumps 60–100 gallons per hour. The water intake for the filters should be near the bottom of the aquarium to remove debris that settles on the substrate.

There are three main types of filtration that are used in recirculating systems. Biological filtration is the most important in making the water safe for fish, but mechanical filtration is necessary to keep the water clear and free of particulate matter, and chemical filtration is useful in removing contaminants such as ammonia, chlorine, copper, or other chemical compounds.

6.2 Mechanical Filtration

This is the process of removing suspended solids, detritus, and debris (total particulate matter) from the water. The water is pumped from the pond or aquarium into filter chambers, where it moves through the filter media and drains back into the pond or aquarium. The filter media is usually sand, ceramic or plastic beads, nylon brushes, foam, or fiber matting. The solid debris is trapped in the filter media, which needs to be cleaned frequently to prevent obstruction of the water flow. Mechanical filtration clears or "polishes" the water but does not remove dissolved wastes or toxic chemicals. Water should pass through the mechanical filter before the other filter stages to reduce sediment buildup in those filter chambers. Mechanical filters that are separate from the biological filtration units are often called "prefilters."

6.3 Chemical Filtration

This filtration uses chemical reactions to remove dissolved substances such as ammonia, chlorine, soluble heavy metals, dissolved organic carbon compounds,

Corresponding author: DrSaintErne@gmail.com

© CAB International 2025. *The Handbook of Ornamental Fish Health and Welfare* (ed. N. Saint-Erne)

DOI: 10.1079/9781789246032.0006

and other chemicals. The filter medium is placed into a separate chamber of the filter or placed into a removable mesh bag within the filter. Periodically, the media must be replaced. One commonly used filter medium is granular activated carbon, which contains a porous internal structure. This allows it to adsorb chemicals such as chlorine, copper, and other heavy metals into microscopic pores on its surface. Eventually, all the pores will be filled, and the activated carbon will need to be replaced. Activated carbon will also remove most medications from the water when the aquarium is treated, so it must be removed from the filter before treating diseases. It can be added to the filter system to remove excess medication when the aquarium is accidentally overdosed. Activated carbon does not remove ammonia, nitrite, or nitrate from the water.

Zeolite (clinoptilolite, an aluminosilicate clay) can be used to remove ammonia from the water by ion exchange. This occurs when the zeolite releases sodium chloride (NaCl) into the water and absorbs ammonia. This is only effective for freshwater aquariums, not marine. Periodically, the zeolite must be "recharged" by removing it from the filter and placing it in a plastic container of 3.5% salt water (3 lb salt per 10 gallons of water). After 24 h, rinse the zeolite in fresh water and return it to the filter. There it will gradually release the sodium chloride again in exchange for any ammonia. One precaution—if using salt to treat freshwater fish disease, remove the zeolite from the filter first. Otherwise, as the salt concentration in the water increases, the zeolite will recharge itself, releasing ammonia back into the water in exchange for the added sodium chloride.

In locales that have very soft, acidic water, using calcium carbonate (crushed oyster shells or limestone), or dolomite [calcium magnesium carbonate, $CaMg(CO_3)_2$] in the filter will increase the hardness and buffering capacity of the water. In locales with very hard water, the use of ion exchange resins may be necessary to lower the hardness of the water before adding it into the aquarium or pond. These units exchange the sodium cation from salt (NaCl) added to the unit for the calcium and magnesium cations in the hard water, producing softer water, since sodium does not contribute to water hardness. Potassium chloride (KCl) should never be used as the salt in water softeners used to soften the water for an aquarium or pond. This could cause an excessively high level of potassium ions in the water.

To decrease the pH of aquarium water or create a "blackwater" environment common in South American rivers such as the Rio Negro for discus, angelfish, and tetras, catappa leaves can be added to the aquarium. Catappa leaves (*Terminalia catappa*) contain tannins and humic acid (Mohale *et al.*, 2009). Punicalagin is the main tannin, and its extracts are helpful in decreasing heavy metal toxicity as well as decreasing the water pH (Khan *et al.*, 2023). The presence of the catappa leaf litter allows zooplankton to colonize the leaf surfaces. These organisms become food for the fish. One study observed that the catappa leaves that were simply laid on the bottom and allowed to decompose in the culture tanks resulted in a 48% survival of larval fish. Meanwhile, those tanks without the leaf substrate only achieved 27% larval survival rate (Aya *et al.*, 2019). The dried catappa leaves are added to the aquarium water or can be placed within a chamber in the filter. The catappa leaf usually floats for the first few days, so if placed into the aquarium it can be weighed down with a rock or decoration to stop it from floating. Use one large leaf for every 10–20 gallons of water in the aquarium. Most leaves last about 1–2 months in the aquarium until they break down. Once the leaf is mostly decayed, it can be removed from the aquarium and another leaf added. Monitor the pH of the water to ensure it is appropriate for the fish species being maintained in the aquarium. Water changes can be used to reduce the tannins and brown-colored water, as needed.

6.4 Biological Filtration

This is the most important filtration process for living organisms in an aquarium. There should be a mechanical filter prior to the biological filter (biofilter) to remove debris that may otherwise clog or impede the water flow through the biofilter. The biofilter requires living aerobic chemolithoautotrophic bacteria to function, so if the water flow is greatly diminished or stopped, even for a few hours, the oxygen levels to the bacteria will be reduced, and they will die. This will prevent the nitrification of the toxic ammonia waste in the water. It may take days or weeks to replace the live nitrifying bacteria and return the biofilter to normal function.

When setting up a new biofilter, it is relatively sterile, without any nitrifying bacteria (*Nitrosomonas*, *Nitrobacter*, *Nitrospira*, and other species). With water circulating through the filter, gradually the nitrifying bacteria will grow on the filter media, producing biological filtration. This process can take several weeks to develop at an adequate level to convert all the toxic ammonia and nitrite into nitrate. In the meantime, toxic conditions can occur in the aquarium or pond affecting the fish. This is called the "new tank syndrome" in aquariums or "new pond syndrome" in koi ponds. Adding nitrifying bacteria to the biofilter can reduce the time of inadequate biological filtration.

One way of doing this is to add some filter media (gravel, plastic beads, filter foam) from an established running biofilter. This provides large quantities of live nitrifying bacteria immediately. They will continue to grow and rapidly colonize the new filter media. There is a slight risk in doing this of spreading disease organisms from the old filter into the new filter, however. When changing biofilter media during routine cleaning, do not remove all the old material at the same time, but leave some to help seed the new material.

Another way of seeding the new biofilter is to add a commercially prepared bacterial supplement. These have bacterial spores or live bacteria in a suspension that become active when added to water in the filter. Some of these products work better than others, and all have a limited shelf life before they lose their efficacy. Be sure to buy fresh products that have been stored properly for the best results.

Ammonium chloride (NH_4Cl) can be added to a fishless aquarium to provide the initial ammonia source to get the nitrogen cycle started. Do not use this with any animals in the aquarium—only to get the biofilter bacteria growing before adding fish! Add 4.5 g (approximately one level teaspoonful) per 380 l (100 US gallons) of water (DeLong and Losordo, 2012). This dose (12 mg/l) will create an ammonia concentration of approximately 3–4 mg/l. Be careful not to use too much ammonium chloride. Raising ammonia levels above 5 mg/l may increase the cycle time due to bacterial inhibition. Unscented household ammonia used for cleaning, which is an aqueous solution of ammonia, can also be used. Add sufficient ammonia to raise the total ammonia level to 3–4 mg/l. This should allow for good detection by most testing methods. Generally, 60 ml (¼ cup) of clear household ammonia (10% aqueous ammonia) will raise the ammonia concentration of 3785 l (1000 gallons) of water by about 1.6 mg/l. Adjustments will be necessary if you are using a different concentration of aqueous ammonia. Start with a minimum amount, allow enough time for thorough mixing through the system, and then test for the ammonia concentration. If more is needed to increase the concentration in the system to 3–4 mg/l, add more incrementally (DeLong and Losordo, 2012). Once the ammonia is converted to nitrite and then nitrate, it will be safe to start adding a few fish to the aquarium. New fish should be added gradually, still. Do not add more than two or three new fish into an aquarium each week, as the bacteria need time to grow as the fish waste increases.

The optimum water temperature for biological filtration is 75–95°F/24–35°C. The rate of nitrification by bacteria decreases as the water temperature drops and is minimal below 50°F/10°C. Nitrification occurs most rapidly at pH levels of 7.1–7.8 and ceases at pH below 5.0 or above 9.0. Maximum saturation levels of dissolved oxygen are required for the most efficient nitrification by aerobic bacteria. Placing air stones connected to aquarium air pumps into the biofilter will ensure adequate oxygen levels.

An ideal biofilter setup would have shut-off valves on the pipes to the biofilter with a separate air or water pump in the biofilter. This way the biofilter could be bypassed when medicating the aquarium or koi pond, but it would still be oxygenated to keep the bacteria alive. The main pump would continue moving water through the mechanical filter (bypass the chemical filter as well when medicating) and back to the aquarium or pond through a spray bar, waterfall, or fountain to aerate the water.

When cleaning filter components, it is important to not harm the beneficial bacteria in the biofilter. Filter media housing the biofilter should be gently rinsed with aquarium water when performing a partial water change, rather than using tap water. That way, the bacteria will not be exposed to chlorinated water or high-pressure streams. Do not let the biofilter media dry out; keep it in clean, dechlorinated water while cleaning other parts of the filter. Keep it at the same temperature as the aquarium water. When replacing used filter media with new components, do not change all the biofilter media at once, or there will be too little bacteria in the filter when it is restarted. Only change part of the biofilter media at a time and leave some of the established media in the filter to restart the beneficial bacterial colony.

6.5 Aeration

Aeration is the movement of oxygen from air to water (Boyd and Tucker, 2014). Aeration allows oxygen absorption and waste gas release through turbulence at the air-water interface. Water that does not flow or move has a reduced capacity for exchanging gases and will often become stagnant and oxygen depleted. Aerobic bacteria in the biofilter can significantly reduce oxygen levels in the water passing through the filter, so aeration of the water returning to the aquarium or pond is essential. Water returning to an aquarium from the filter should gently break the surface of the water to mix with oxygen and circulate the oxygenated water throughout the aquarium. The additions of fountains, waterfalls, streams, and venturi jets increase oxygen in the water, as it returns from the filter. Aquarium air stones, attached to air pumps or compressors, can be placed in the aquarium or within filter chambers to increase aeration (Fig. 6.1). Adding air stones or water fountains strategically placed in large ponds may be necessary to prevent areas of stagnant water.

6.6 Channeling

Channeling occurs when the water follows a single path of least resistance around the filter media or through a small number of channels in media such as pea gravel. This significantly reduces the effectiveness of the filters. In filter media where channeling has occurred, the material that is bypassed may become anaerobic from lack of oxygenated water flow. Hydrogen sulfide production can occur in these areas. Regular backflushing, cleaning detritus from the filter media, and stirring the sand or gravel to reduce channeling are recommended for filters with media that can become filled with trapped debris. Some koi pond filters, including sand and bead filters, may have an air blower that stirs the media during a backflow to clean it and prevent packed media that would result in water channeling.

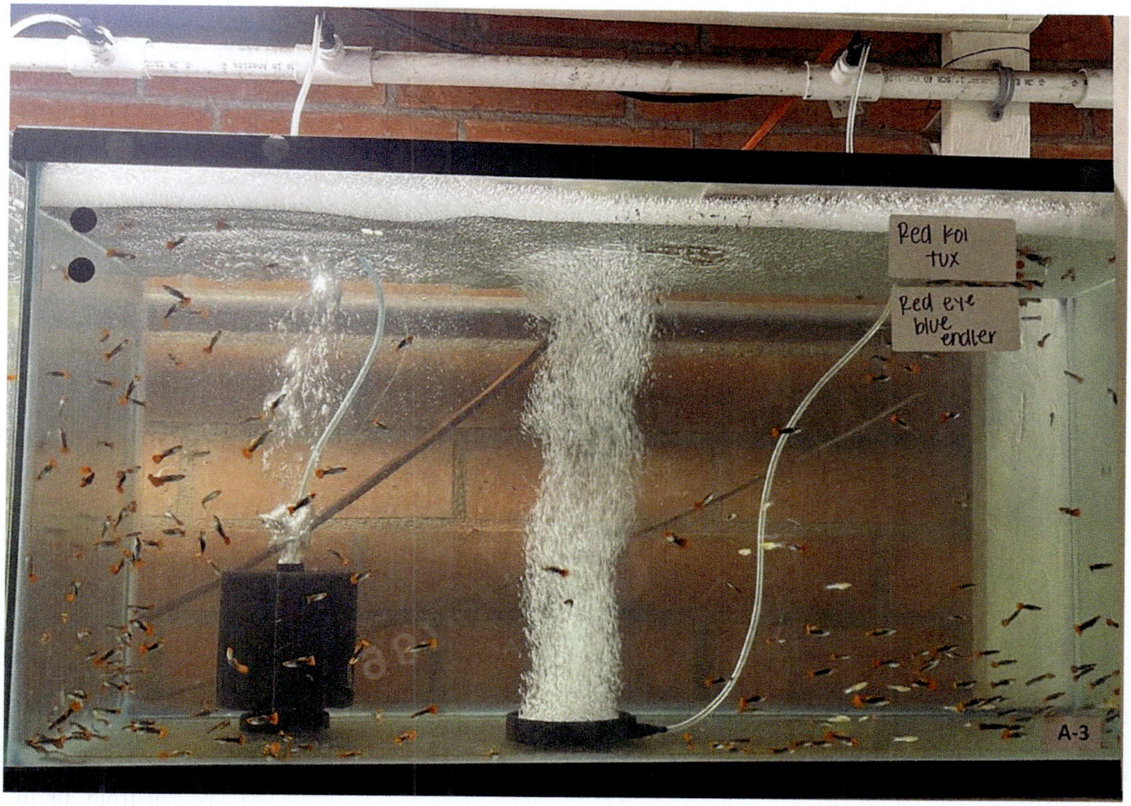

Fig. 6.1. Piping from an air pump brings air to a sponge filter and an air stone in an aquarium of guppies (*Poecilia reticulata*). (Photograph by N. Saint-Erne.)

6.7 Types of Filters

6.7.1 Internal aquarium filters

The most common early aquarium filters were box filters that were placed inside the aquarium and powered by an air pump. Air flowed through the tubing into the box, where it bubbled out the tube through the top of the filter. The bubbles created a vacuum inside of the box that drew water through the filter media as the bubbles pushed the water back out the top of the box. The bubbles rising through the water also circulated the water in the aquarium and caused surface agitation when they burst at the surface, resulting in water aeration. That is a very complex function for such a small filter. The concept was great, but the box filters were undersized for the work that needed to be done in an aquarium. The filter media consisted of fiberglass filter floss, along with activated carbon. The box filter needed to be removed from the aquarium to be cleaned or to change the media. Replacing the filter floss or carbon removed the beneficial bacteria that were growing on it, so the process was not efficient.

There are in-pond filters that are similar in design to the aquarium box filter but are not suitable for use in anything other than a water garden or small pond.

More recent internal aquarium filters move water by use of an electrical pump that is inside the filter box. These filters hang inside the aquarium on the back wall of the tank, and water is drawn in through the bottom slits, passes through filter media, including bioballs and foam pads, and then flows out across the surface of the water, providing aeration (Fig. 6.2). These are suitable for small aquariums and could be used in quarantine tanks, or in treatment tanks if they do not have carbon in the filter media.

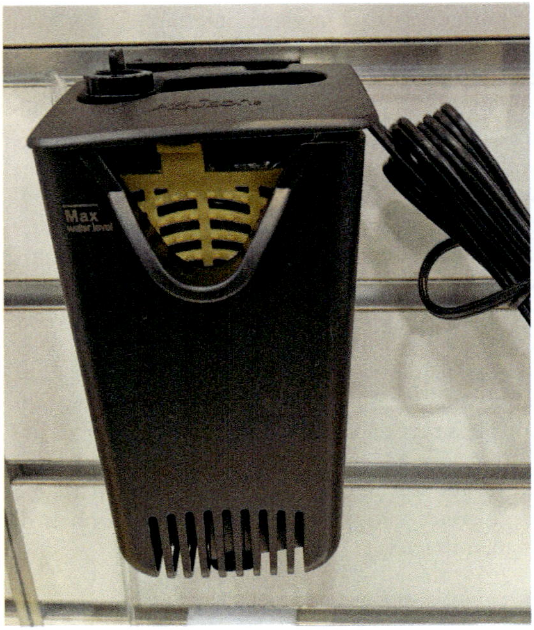

Fig. 6.2. Internal filter that uses an electrical water pump, rather than air, to move the water through the filter media. (Photograph by N. Saint-Erne.)

6.7.2 Undergravel filters

A huge improvement occurred in aquarium filtration with the introduction of the undergravel filter in the 1970s. In this filter, a perforated plastic plate covers the bottom of the aquarium, with airlift tubes in the back corners. The plate is covered with 1–3 inches (2.5–7.5 cm) of coarse substrate (aquarium gravel, not sand), which becomes the surface for the bacteria to colonize for the biofilter. An air pump pushes air through tubing into the uplift tubes, and bubbles coming from the tube draw water down through the gravel, underneath the filter plate, and up with the bubbles through the tubes. Water flowing through the gravel allows aerobic bacteria to perform nitrification. The water flow also draws solid debris through the gravel where it accumulates under the filter plate.

The undergravel filter works great initially. Then debris accumulates in the gravel and under the plate, which eventually impedes the flow of water. If the substrate is regularly cleaned with a gravel vacuum to remove trapped particles, an undergravel filter can work continuously. One way of cleaning the undergravel filter plate is to attach the inflow tube of a canister filter to the uplift tube. Place the outflow tube into a bucket and turn on the canister filter. This will suck all the accumulated debris out from under the filter plate and into the waste bucket, which effectively cleans the filter and does a water change at the same time (Sanders, 2022).

Replacing the air pump with a "power head," a small water pump that sits atop the uplift tube inside of the aquarium, greatly increases the flow of water and, therefore, the effectiveness of the undergravel filter. While undergravel filters have gone out of style in modern aquariums, they are still practical and inexpensive filters when cleaned regularly.

6.7.3 Hang-on-back filter

These are also called "power filters," since they run by a water pump rather than by air. They usually hang on the back of the aquarium, outside the tank, and so are called "Hang on Back" (HOB) filters (Fig. 6.3). They are the most common type of filter for smaller aquariums, largely because they offer excellent mechanical, chemical, and biological filtration simultaneously (Sharpe, 2022). Mechanical filtration is achieved by water flowing through a sponge pad or floss media. Chemical filtration is provided by the water flowing through an activated carbon insert, and biological filtration is produced by beneficial bacteria that grow on the media inside the filter cartridge. The filter inserts need to be periodically rinsed off or replaced. Be careful to not replace all the media at the same time or the biofilter bacterial population can be significantly reduced.

6.7.4 Canister filters

This filter consists of a plastic housing (the canister) fitted inside with trays that contain various filter components, such as foam pads, bioballs, ceramic beads, activated carbon, or other chemical media (Figs 6.4a and b). The removable top contains a water pump and two hoses. They are usually placed in the cabinet under the aquarium, with the tubing going into the aquarium for water intake and outflow. The intake tube should be near the substrate at the bottom of the aquarium, and the outflow at the top of the aquarium where the outflow will agitate the water surface. These large units provide very good mechanical, chemical, and biological filtration (Sharpe, 2022). On a periodic basis, the canister filter must be removed to open it and clean each of the trays of filter media, replacing any chemical media used. This chore is slightly more difficult than cleaning other filters, but the efficiency of the canister filter makes it the best filtration for home aquariums.

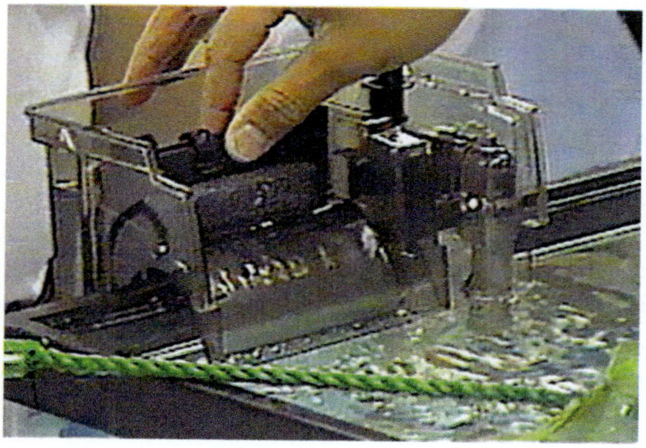

Fig. 6.3. External HOB power filter has media cartridge that can be removed to clean or change while the filter is still working. (Photograph by N. Saint-Erne.)

6.7.5 Sponge filters

This is the simplest and lowest-cost filter type. A large synthetic sponge is fitted over an uplift tube that receives air from an air pump or water from a power head (Fig. 6.5). The air or water forced through the tube in the sponge creates a suction that pulls water and debris into the sponge material providing mechanical filtration, and bacteria will grow on the sponge to establish biological filtration (Sharpe, 2022). Sponge filters clog quickly if there is excess debris, so they should be removed from the tank and rinsed with aquarium water when performing water changes. They are excellent for use in tanks with fry, as the sponge prevents young fry from being sucked into the filter. Sponge filters are good for a hospital isolation tank, as a sponge from an established aquarium quickly provides the tank with nitrifying bacteria.

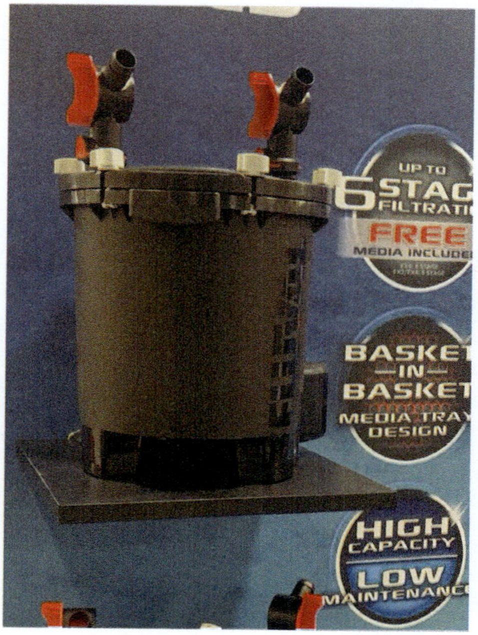

Fig. 6.4a. Canister filter. (Photograph by N. Saint-Erne.)

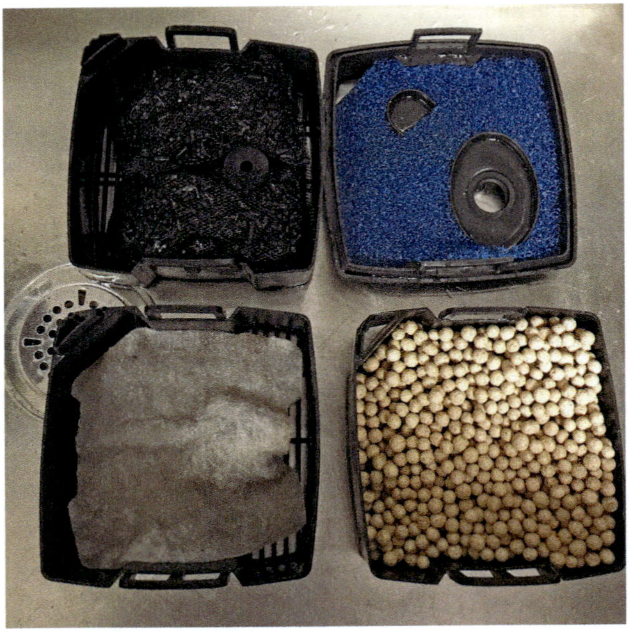

Fig. 6.4b. A canister filter opened to show the media trays containing bags of activated carbon, foam prefilter, fiber floss pad, and ceramic balls that act as a substrate for nitrifying bacteria. (Photograph by N. Saint-Erne.)

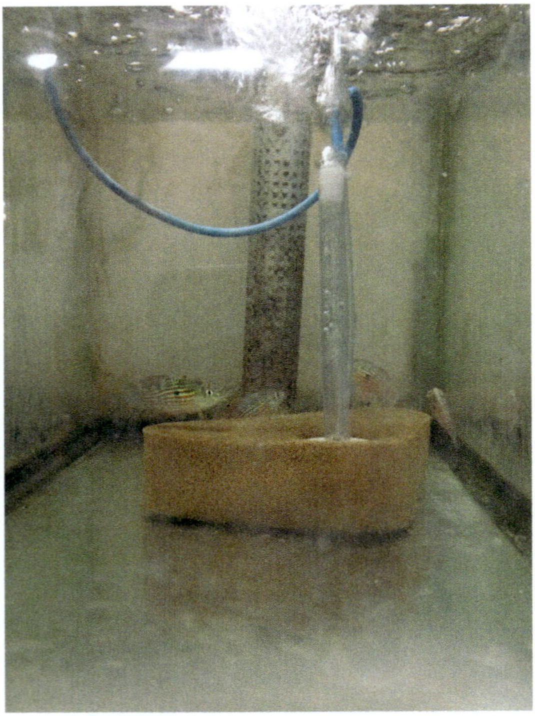

Fig. 6.5. Sponge filter in a quarantine tank with American Flag Fish (*Jordanella floridae*). (Photograph by N. Saint-Erne.)

6.7.6 In-pond filters

These are the least efficient of the filters, but in small ponds with only a few goldfish, they may be adequate. Basically, they consist of a submersible pump that draws water through filter media and pumps it out to a fountainhead or to a waterfall. This adds oxygen to the pond by circulating the water. The filter media may be as simple as an attached foam rubber pad, which serves as both a mechanical and biological filter, or it may be contained in a plastic box filled with lava rock, plastic balls, or fiber pads. These units must be frequently lifted out of the pond and be rinsed off or otherwise cleaned to keep them working properly. They do work well for hospital tanks or small goldfish ponds, and for breeding/fry-raising ponds, when only a small amount of fish waste is expected. Frequent partial water changes and cleaning debris from the pond bottom also help in maintaining ponds using these types of filters.

6.7.7 Pressurized sand filters

These are the swimming pool filters that are often used in koi ponds and public aquariums. They are large, oval fiberglass containers filled with sand (Fig. 6.6). Water is pumped through them under pressure and is filtered mechanically as the debris gets stuck in the sand. If the pressure gauge reading increases, then it is time to backflush the unit to remove accumulated waste trapped in the sand. The disadvantage of this system is that it clogs rapidly, so it requires frequent checks on the pressure gauge and backflushing. If they are not cleaned, the sand will compact with debris, and a channel will form allowing the water to bypass the sand.

6.7.8 Fluidized bed filters

These are both biological and mechanical filters in a single unit. Fluidized bed filters look similar to sand filters (Fig. 6.7), but they use fine silica sand or polyethylene beads that are "fluidized" in the filter by the flow of water and air bubbles, suspending them within the filter chamber. The small particles have a very large surface area. The sand or beads trap debris acting as a mechanical filter, and nitrifying bacteria colonize the bead surfaces providing biological filtration.

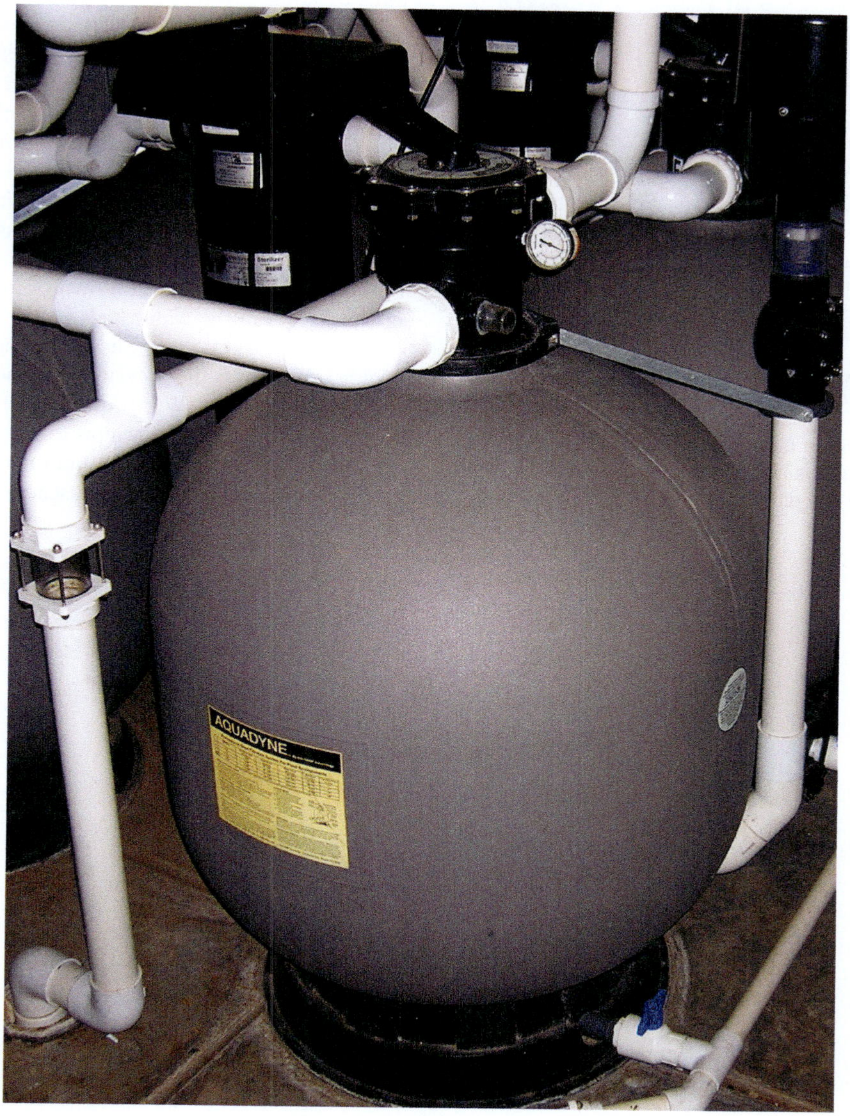

Fig. 6.6. Sand filters are being used in a public aquarium. (Photograph by N. Saint-Erne.)

Because of the constant motion of the fluidized media, no channeling or dead spaces occur, and biological filtration is increased. This results in highly efficient filtration. Periodic backflushing (temporary reversal of the flow of water through the filter to flush out waste) of the filter keeps the detritus from accumulating in the media. Since the sand or plastic beads are not tightly packed in a fluidized bed, as is the sand in standard sand filters, these filters are easier to clean when backflushing and use less water in the process.

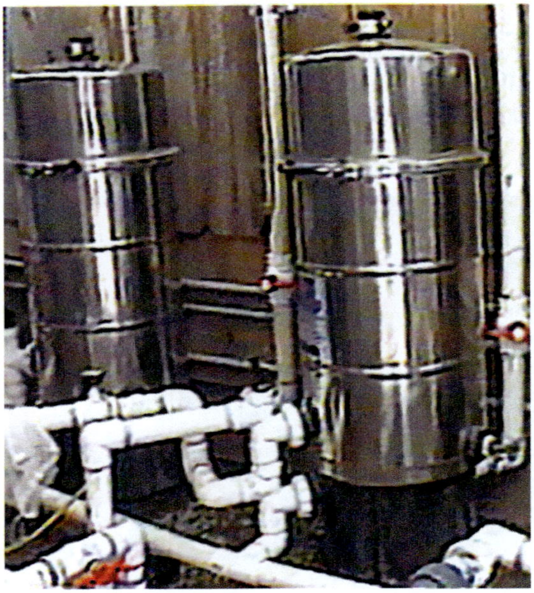

Fig. 6.7. Bead filters (fluidized filters containing plastic beads) are being used for filtering a koi pond. (Photograph by N. Saint-Erne.)

6.7.9 Wet/dry filtration (trickle filters)

This filtration system increases the air-water interface for improving biological filtration. Air contains 21% oxygen (210,000 mg/l), while aquarium water usually has 0.0006–0.0012% oxygen (6–12 mg/l, depending on temperature), therefore air contains 17,500–35,000 times more oxygen than does the water in a typical aquarium or pond. By trickling or spraying water onto a biofilter media that is not under the water but exposed to the high oxygen levels in the air, yet keeping the nitrifying bacteria wet, the bacteria have more accessible oxygen than if they were submerged in the water. This optimizes the aerobic breakdown of ammonia and nitrite wastes in the water.

The bakki shower is an inexpensive form of trickle filter. It was first developed at the Momotaro koi farm in Japan (Wikipedia, 2023). The bakki shower (Figs 6.8a and b) attempts to simulate nature's way of filtering water in a mountain stream where water becomes aerated as it cascades over rocks.

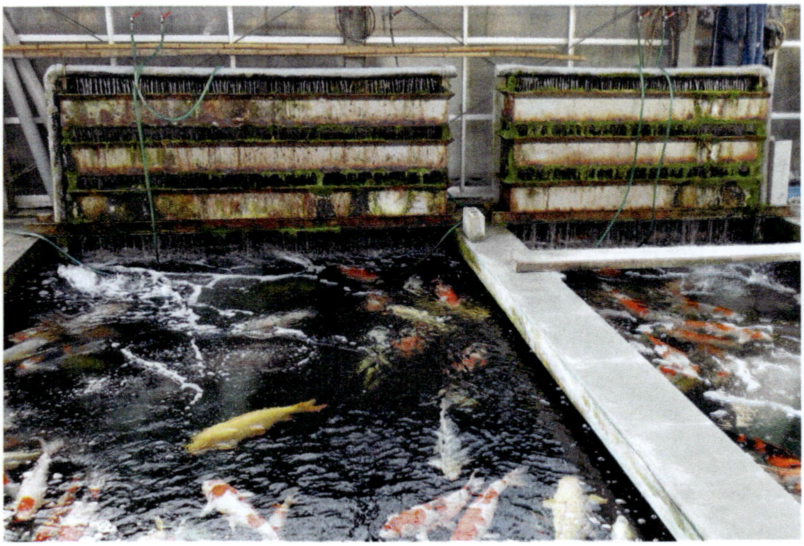

Fig. 6.8a. Bakki shower at koi farm in Japan. (Photograph by N. Saint-Erne.)

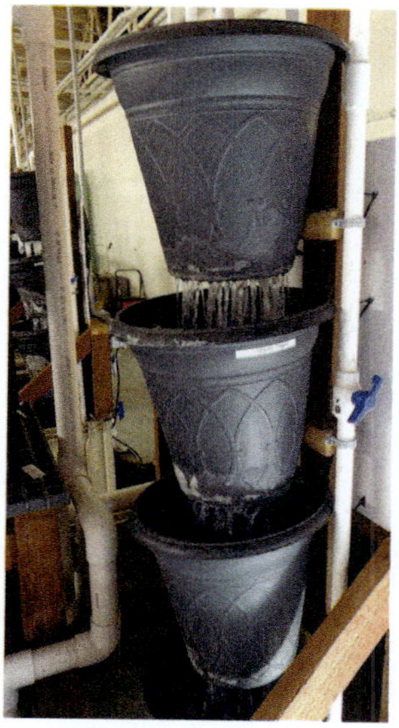

Fig. 6.8b. Bakki shower made from plastic flowerpots filled with bioballs at a tropical fish wholesale facility in California. (Photograph by N. Saint-Erne.)

The filter consists of three to four stainless steel or plastic containers with small holes throughout the bottoms. The containers are filled with lava rock, ceramic rings, plastic bioballs, or other porous material that will allow a high surface area for the biofilter bacteria. The containers are stacked vertically with a gap between each one. Aquarium or pond water is pumped into the top one, where it flows through the media and out the bottom without retaining any water inside of the container. The water is showered onto the surface of the next container, where it also flows through. The water flows through each container until leaving the bottom of the last one, when it flows into a filter sump or into the pond. Biofilms and algae grow on the media and utilize the nutrients, filtering the water. The bakki shower does not take up much space, is easy and inexpensive to construct, and requires very little maintenance. It only needs a water pump to bring the water to the top chamber, where the water flows back down by gravity. The free-falling water between the chambers oxygenates the water and off-gases carbon dioxide (CO_2). The oxygenated water flowing down the wet media inside of the chambers allows for the greatest level of nitrification by the biofilter bacteria. Algae, mosses, and other plants growing on the media also help remove nitrate and phosphate from the water.

6.7.10 Ultraviolet sterilizers

An ultraviolet (UV) sterilizer uses a fluorescent low-pressure mercury vapor bulb that produces electromagnetic radiation in the far UV wavelengths of 185–300 nm, most often 253.7 nm (Siegel, 1974). This is shorter than visible light wavelengths, which range from violet at 400 nm to red at 700 nm, and infrared light at 800 nm. This bulb is placed into a quartz sleeve that is inserted into the water pipes of the filtration system (Fig. 6.9). Water flows outside the sleeve past the UV bulb and any algae, fungi, viruses, bacteria, or protozoa exposed to the UV rays will be killed by irradiation of the microorganism's DNA or RNA. This is helpful in controlling algal blooms and in treating the free-swimming stages of parasites like *Ichthyophthirius*. The quartz sleeve must be kept clean of debris and the bulb needs to be replaced after 12–14 months of continuous operation. After this period, the amount of UV light produced will be ineffective, even though the lamp still produces visible light.

The UV dosage is measured in microwatt seconds per square centimeter of surface area ($\mu Ws/cm^2$). The effective dose of UV light varies depending on the organisms. The actual dosage level produced by the UV sterilizer is dependent on the power of the UV bulb and the water flow rate. If the water flow rate past the UV bulb is too rapid, the UV sterilizer will be less effective. It is better to use a UV sterilizer rated for more water volume than in the system for which it is being used, rather than one for a smaller-sized pond or aquarium.

The optimum operating temperature for the UV lamp is 104°F/40°C. Direct contact with cooler water will lower the lamp's efficiency. The quartz sleeve insulates the lamp from the water to allow it to operate at a higher temperature but still allows the UV rays to penetrate through the sleeve into the water (Fruland, 1977).

The UV sterilizer should be placed at the end of the filtration circuit so the water passing through it is relatively free of suspended particles that would block the UV rays. The UV sterilizer should be temporarily turned off when adding medications to the water to avoid loss of the medication's efficacy. It may not be necessary to run the UV sterilizer continuously but only when disease conditions or algal blooms occur. However, frequent on-off cycles of the UV lamp will shorten its useful life in comparison to continuous operation.

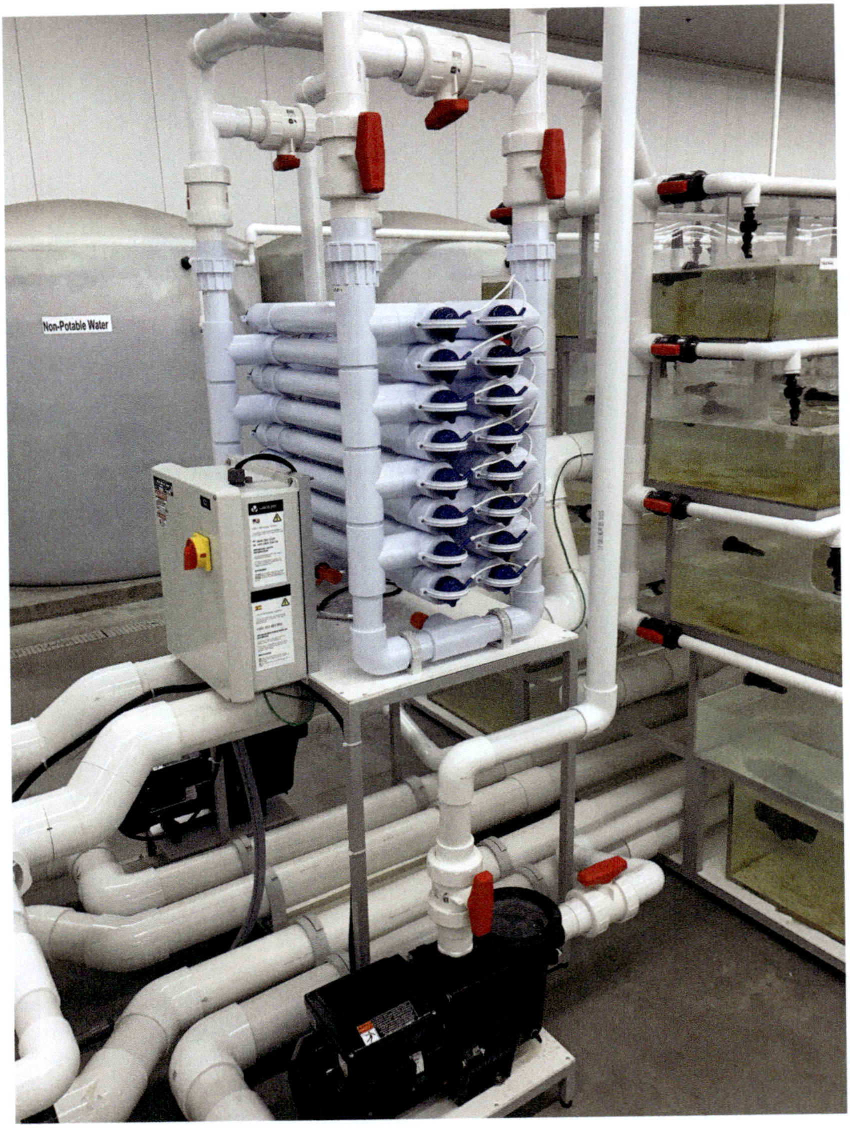

Fig. 6.9. Water returning from the filter to the fish tanks passes through UV light tubing. There are bypass valves so that the water can be shunted around the UV lights when medicating the system, or when changing the UV bulbs. (Photograph by N. Saint-Erne.)

6.7.11 Ozone

The unstable triatomic oxygen molecule ozone (O_3) is a potent oxidizing agent. It is used to prevent diseases by destroying viruses, bacteria, and protozoa and to improve water quality by oxidizing many organic compounds. An electric ozonator is necessary to produce ozone from air or oxygen (Summerfelt and Hochheimer, 1997). The ozone is added to the water after it has passed through the biological and other filters. It is important that all the ozone dissipates from the filtered water before it returns to the aquarium or pond to prevent oxidation burns on the gills and skin of the fish. Activated carbon can be used to remove residual ozone from the water. Passing the water through an ultraviolet filter will also break down the ozone. In pure water at 68°F/20°C, the half-life of ozone is 165 min. Ozone is dissociated (broken down) faster in hard water or basic pH water than in soft or acidic water. It also dissociates faster at higher temperatures and in water with high organic loads or inorganic ions.

Ozone is typically used in water at a concentration of 0.01–0.3 mg/l for a short period of up to 2 min. It has a distinct odor that can be smelled at concentrations above 0.02 mg/l. At high doses, it can be toxic if inhaled, with coughing the first sign to appear. When using an ozone generator, make sure it is in a well-ventilated area, or outside. A considerable amount of heat is also produced by the ozonator. Ozone can be used effectively in protein skimmer units, in place of air or oxygen.

6.7.12 Protein skimmers

Protein foam fractionation (protein skimming) is a process where air, pure oxygen (O_2), or ozone (O_3) is injected into a vertical column of water, producing foam made of proteinaceous compounds dissolved in the water that adsorb onto tiny bubbles. The foam rises into a narrow vertical tube and is collected in a chamber above the water line, which is periodically emptied and cleaned (Fig. 6.10). The treated water is returned from a spout below the top of the vertical tube to the filter. A strong flow of extremely fine bubbles is necessary to efficiently extract dissolved proteins from the water.

Dissolved proteins form bubbles more readily in saltwater than freshwater, so protein skimmers are less commonly used in freshwater filter systems, except when there may be a high density of fish, such as in public aquariums, fish farms, or wholesale facilities. The use of foam fractionation removes the dissolved organic carbons (DOC) from the water, which reduces toxic compounds, detritus, and yellow discoloration of the water. It can also remove medications, so the protein skimmer should be bypassed, or the airflow turned off when medicating the aquarium.

6.7.13 Refugium/bog filter/plant filter

This is a separate container that the filtered water flows through before returning to the aquarium or pond. It is filled with aquatic plants like anacharis, water hyacinth, water lettuce, or emerging plants like water irises, cattails, and rushes (Fig. 6.11). In saltwater aquariums, it is called a refugium and can contain macroalgae and live rock. The bog or refugium plants and algae will remove nitrates, the end result of bacterial biological filtration, as well as phosphate from the water. Settling of suspended particles into the soil of the bog filter will also help remove particulate debris from the water.

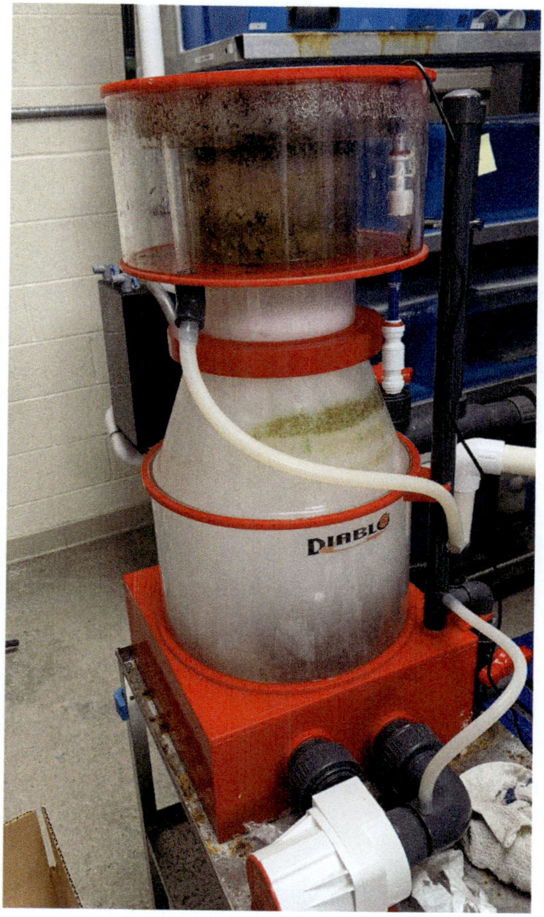

Fig. 6.10. Protein skimmer in use at a wholesale fish facility. (Photograph by N. Saint-Erne.)

6.7.14 Cartridge filters

Cartridge filters are commonly used to remove particulate matter from incoming tap water (Fig. 6.12). Cartridge filters utilize mechanical filtration in the form of a pleated membrane that the water passes

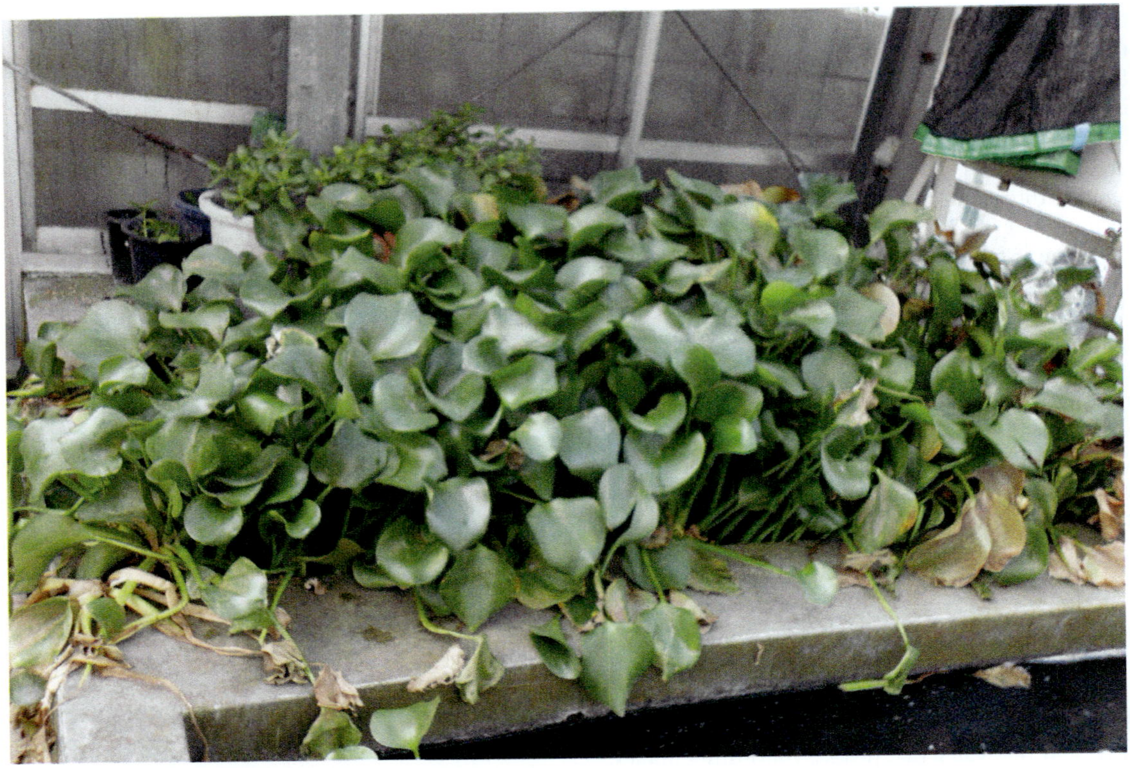

Fig. 6.11. Bog filter containing water hyacinths (*Eichhornia crassipes*) in a Japanese koi dealer's pond. (Photograph by N. Saint-Erne.)

through to trap suspended solids from the water supply. The pleated filter can be removed to be cleaned but periodically needs to be replaced. They are used in swimming pools and spas to filter and "polish" the water, removing suspended particles. Reverse osmosis filters, carbon filters, and UV sterilizers require clean water to operate efficiently. For this reason, cartridge filters are added inline prior to the water entering those units to ensure clean water enters the filtration system. Different membranes are available to use in the housing of the cartridge filter, including water filter cartridges that remove particle sizes ranging from 100 μm down to 0.2 μm.

6.7.15 Venturi device

If water flowing through a pipe is passed through a restricted tapered section and then the pipe is expanded again, a vacuum will form immediately beyond the restricted section. An air inlet pipe attached just beyond the restriction will suck in air and mix it with the flowing water, thus increasing the dissolved oxygen content. The amount of air entering the venturi can be adjusted by a valve on the air inlet pipe. This is commonly used to increase the oxygen in water returning to the pond from the filter system. In warm water conditions, it is possible to supersaturate the water with air using a venturi device, so the water must be observed for tiny bubbles that can be a sign of supersaturation.

6.7.16 Surface skimmer

A skimmer is a prefiltration device where water is taken from the aquarium or pond surface through the skimmer inlet and passes through a strainer before being pumped into the main filter. This

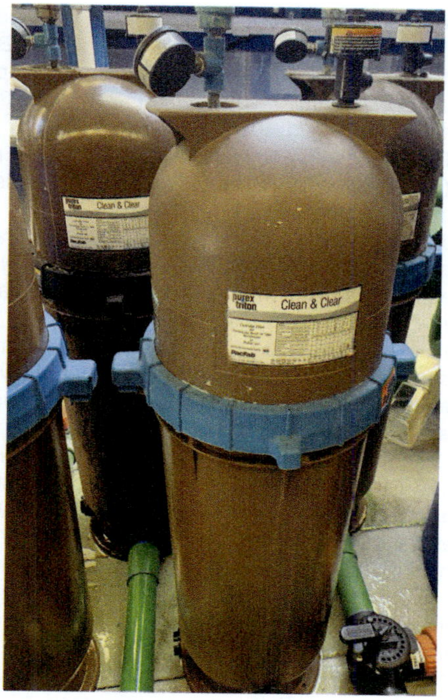

Fig. 6.12. Canisters that hold pleated membrane cartridges for removing particulate matter from the water. (Photograph by N. Saint-Erne.)

allows floating debris such as leaves to be trapped in a strainer basket or net and to be removed from the prefilter without having the large debris pass into the main filter. The strainer needs to be checked frequently and manually cleaned out.

6.8 Conclusion

Aquarium filtration can consist of a simple box filter to units that include a prefilter; a mechanical filter to remove particulate matter; a biofilter for nitrification of wastes; an ultraviolet sterilizer to kill algae, bacteria, and protozoa; and a protein skimmer, especially for a saltwater aquarium (Kasper *et al.*, 2022). Gas exchange occurs as the water is returned from the filter, or additional aeration such as air stones or venturi devices can be used. Fish wholesale facilities, public aquariums, and fish ponds use similar concepts for filtration, in just larger devices (Fig. 6.13). An appropriately sized filter system with adequate water flow is imperative for good water quality. And, as explained in other chapters, proper water quality is important for maintaining the health and welfare of fish and other aquatic animals.

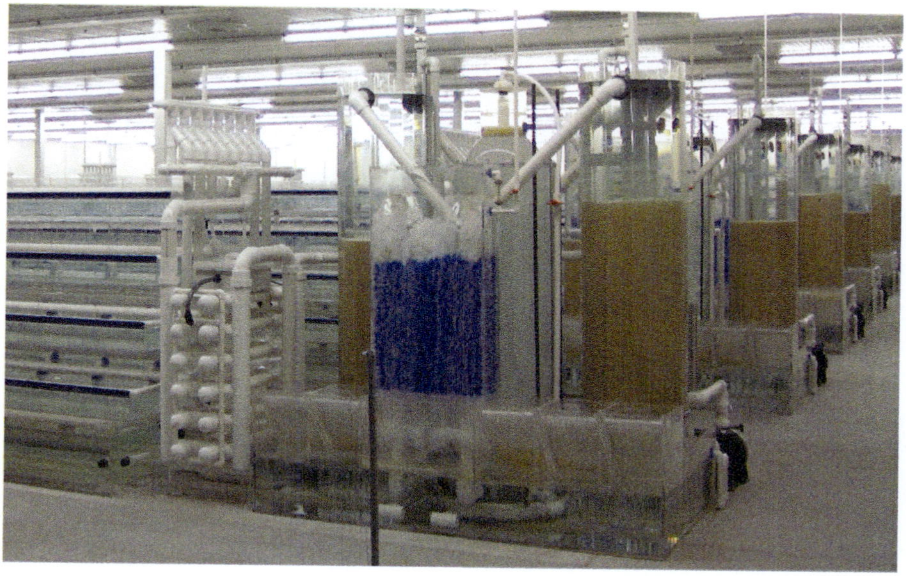

Fig. 6.13. Filtration system used in wholesale fish distribution facility includes fiber mats to trap particulate matter along the front lower level, a bioball tower to oxygenate the water and provide biological filtration, two fluidized bed towers containing suspended silica sand, a protein skimmer tower between them, and UV lights along the left side of the filter to treat the water going back into the fish tanks. (Photograph by N. Saint-Erne.)

References

Aya, F.A., Nillasca, V.S.N., Sayco, M.J.P. and Garcia, L.M.B. (2019) Improved survival, prey selectivity and diel feeding cycle of silver therapon *Leiopotherapon plumbeus* (Perciformes: Terapontidae) larvae reared in tanks with substrate. *Ichthyological Research* 66, 239–248.

Boyd, C.E. and Tucker, C.S. (2014) *Handbook for Aquaculture Water Quality*. Craftmaster Printers, Auburn, Alabama.

DeLong, D.P. and Losordo, T.M. (2012) How to start a biofilter. Southern Regional Aquaculture Center (SRAC) Publication No. 4502. Available at: https://srac.tamu.edu/fact-sheets (accessed 1 August 2024).

Fruland, R.M. (1977) *Ultraviolet Sterilization and the Serious Aquarist*. Hawaiian Marine Imports, Houston, Texas.

Kasper, S., Adeyemo, O., Becker, T., Scarfe, D. and Tepper, J. (2022) Aquatic environment and life support systems. In: Urdes, L., Walster, C. and Tepper, J. (eds) *Fundamentals of Aquatic Veterinary Medicine*. Wiley, Hoboken, New Jersey, pp. 1–27.

Khan, N.G., Panezai, M.A., Kakar, M.A., Achakzai, J.K., Kakar, A.M. *et al.* (2023) Biological activities and phytochemistry of tropical almond tree leaves extract from Gwadar, Balochistan (a review). *European Academic Research* XI(1), 122–134.

Mohale, D.S., Dewani, A.P., Chandewar, A.V., Khadse, C.D., Tripathi, A.S. and Agrawal, S.S. (2009) Brief review on medicinal potential of Terminalia catappa. *Journal of Herbal Medicine and Toxicology* 3(1), 7–11.

Saint-Erne, N. (2010) Filtration systems. In: Saint-Erne, N. (ed.) *Advanced Koi Care*. 2nd edn. Erne Enterprises, Glendale, Arizona, pp. 110–117.

Sanders, J. (2022) What to know about undergravel filters. The Spruce Pets. Available at: https://www.thesprucepets.com/what-to-know-about-undergravel-filters-5248625 (accessed 12 May 2023).

Sharpe, S. (2022) Basic types of aquarium filtration systems. The Spruce Pets. Available at: https://www.thesprucepets.com/before-you-buy-an-aquarium-filter-1378506 (accessed 13 May 2023).

Siegel, A.D. (1974) *Ultraviolet Purification of Aquarium Water*. Gull Manufacturing, Cheshire, Connecticut.

Spotte, S. (1970) *Fish and Invertebrate Culture*. Wiley, New York.

Summerfelt, S.T. and Hochheimer, J.N. (1997) Review of ozone processes and applications as an oxidizing agent in aquaculture. *The Progressive Fish-Culturist* 59, 94–105.

Wikipedia (2023) Bakki shower. Available at: https://en.wikipedia.org/wiki/Bakki_shower (accessed 12 May 2023).

7 Fish Pond Care

NICHOLAS SAINT-ERNE

Dr. Saint-Erne Consulting, PLLC, Phoenix, Arizona

Abstract

Filtration systems in a pond are similar to the methods used in aquariums but larger. However, being outdoors provides elements that do not occur in an aquarium, such as changes in the weather. Care of the pond may differ throughout the seasons. Being outside also exposes the pond to predators and other wildlife not seen in an indoor aquarium.

7.1 Water Filtration in a Pond

Filtration is what separates an artificial containment of water from a natural environment. With filtration, the pond will be cleaner, the water clearer, and will support a greater density of fish. Without filtration, a pond that does not have the natural inflow and outflow of a freshwater source—along with the associated plants, microflora and fauna, and aquatic animals—may stagnate and become a cesspool (Saint-Erne, 2010). Pond filtration uses similar techniques to aquariums but on a much larger scale (Fig. 7.1). The filter must be adequate for the number and size of the fish in the pond and allow for the effects of sunlight, which increases algae growth and exposure to the elements of wind, rain, and temperature changes. Variations in temperature throughout the year will alter a fish's activities and metabolic rate. The immune system becomes less effective at lower water temperatures, and stressful conditions can lead to an increase in diseases. Prevention of stress by proper pond care during each season will help reduce the incidence of disease.

It is advisable that the water pump moves the total volume of pond water through the filter system every hour. Therefore, a 1000-gallon pond would need a water pump for the filter that pumps 1000 gallons per hour. In larger ponds that are not highly stocked, a lower flow rate may suffice. The pipes used in the filter system should be the same diameter as the pump outflow port or only slightly bigger. Larger diameter pipes will cause low water pressure in the pipes, resulting in the settlement of debris within the pipes. Smaller pipes will cause increased pressure, possibly damaging the pump, or causing gas supersaturation, leading to "gas bubble" disease in the fish. Keep bends in the pipes and total pipe length to a minimum to reduce resistance. The water intake for the filters should be near the bottom of the pond to remove debris when the water is warm. In cold weather, the water should be removed near the surface to prevent stirring the denser warm water that settles to the bottom of the pond, which keeps the water from freezing.

7.2 Seasonal Variations

Variations in temperature throughout the year will alter a fish's metabolic rate, which affects activities such as feeding, growth, and reproduction. The immune system becomes less effective at lower water temperatures, and stressful conditions can lead to an increase in diseases (McDowall, 1989). Prevention of stress by proper pond care during each season will help reduce the incidence of disease in the fish.

7.2.1 Spring

In springtime, water temperatures will begin to rise but will fluctuate between colder and warmer days, sometimes with wide extremes between daytime and nighttime temperatures. Water quality can change

Corresponding author: DrSaintErne@gmail.com

© CAB International 2025. *The Handbook of Ornamental Fish Health and Welfare* (ed. N. Saint-Erne)
DOI: 10.1079/9781789246032.0007

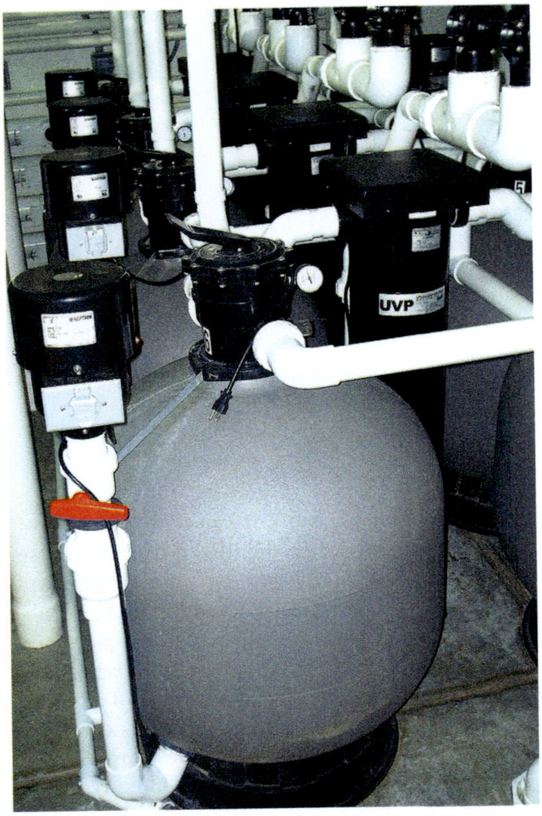

Fig. 7.1. This filtration system used for a koi pond includes a pressurized sand canister filter with an air blower for stirring the sand during the back wash to clean the sand. (Photograph by N. Saint-Erne.)

rapidly during this time, as bacterial and algal activity increases. This is the time to clean and backflush the pond filter to make sure it is functioning optimally. Make sure the water is being adequately aerated, as the fish and nitrifying bacteria will utilize more oxygen as the water warms, and warm water holds less dissolved oxygen.

Bacterial decomposition of organic debris (fallen leaves, dead algae, uneaten food) will reduce oxygen and increase ammonia concentrations in the water. Test the water frequently and change 20% of the water if ammonia or nitrite levels are elevated. Remove the debris from the pond as soon as possible (after the ice melts if the pond freezes over). Check aquatic plants, and prune, thin, or repot them as needed.

Gradually, the fish will come out of their winter dormant state and become active when the water temperature reaches about 40–45°F/4.4–7.2°C. They will start feeding at about 45–50°F/7.2–10°C. Do not overfeed at this point! Uneaten food will increase the ammonia levels in the water, as will the increase in fish waste (urine, feces). Feed the koi in the mornings when the water temperature is warm during the day, so the food will be properly digested. Do not feed them in the late afternoon or night yet if the water gets colder at night. Fish eating in cold water may be unable to completely digest the food due to decreased digestive enzyme activity at a low temperature. Bacterial decay of the ingested food can occur within the digestive tract causing gas formation and bloating.

Pathogenic bacteria also become more active as water warms, and since many fish are weakened during the winter, many cases of bacterial diseases occur in springtime, when fish are weak from winter dormancy and the water temperature is at the optimal level for the bacteria.

7.2.2 Summer

When the pond water is warmer, the fish will be active and grow. Feeding at this time requires food with more protein than would be used during the spring and fall. Feed as much food as the fish will eat in 5 min, twice daily for adults and 3–4 times daily for young, growing fish. Floating food is best to be used, so the fish can be observed while eating to ensure all the food has been consumed. Overfeeding will pollute the water by increasing ammonia and reducing oxygen. This is even more serious in warmer water, so test the water quality frequently.

As water evaporates from the pond in the summer, the dissolved minerals (calcium and magnesium carbonate) will remain behind, increasing the water hardness. Consequently, it is important to not just replace water, as it evaporates from the pond, but to drain out some of the high-mineral water and replace it with fresh water. When fresh water is being added manually, it is important to not let a hose run into the pond continuously, as that may cause the pond to overflow. It is helpful to use a device on the end of the hose that will automatically shut off the water after a certain volume has been delivered (Fig. 7.2). Always use a water dechlorinator when adding city water to the pond. Chlorine in the water will irritate the fish's gills and can lead to respiratory distress, secondary gill infections, or even death.

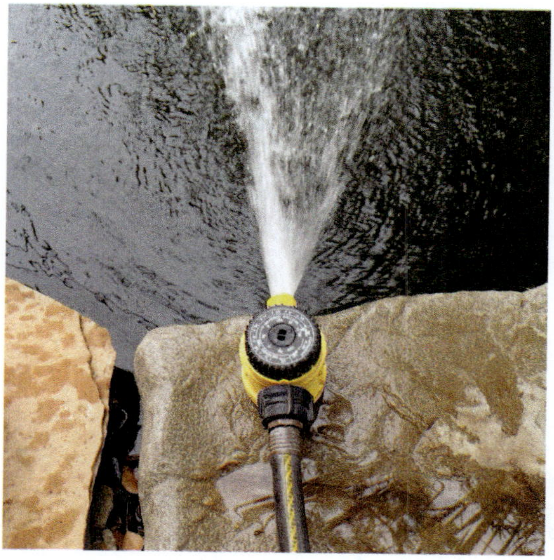

Fig. 7.2. Hose attachment that measures the volume of water added and shuts off automatically. (Photograph by N. Saint-Erne.)

If summertime temperatures are extreme (water temperature above 86°F/30°C), the pond may need to be partially shaded. Warmer water not only holds less oxygen but also increases parasite reproduction, which adds to the fish's stress. Treat with appropriate medications if the fish are seen scraping their sides on rocks (flashing), have increased mucus on their skin, or are breathing rapidly at the water surface (due to low dissolved oxygen and gill irritation from parasites). Be aware that many medications may also lower the oxygen level in the water. Bright sunlight in the summer in a shallow pond with clear water can even cause sunburn on the backs of white koi. Be sure adequate shade is provided over the pond or there is shade from floating plants or underwater hideouts.

Oxygen levels are lowest in the morning, as aquatic plants will use oxygen for respiration in the dark at night. During the day, they use carbon dioxide (CO_2) for photosynthesis and give off oxygen (O_2), but this process is reversed in the absence of sunlight. High levels of CO_2 in the water from plant respiration may lower the pH of the water. Adequate water agitation will cause the dissolved CO_2 to dissipate. Ensure that filters, waterfalls, and fountains remain on at night to oxygenate the water (Robinson, 2000).

7.2.3 Autumn

In the fall, prune dead aquatic vegetation, remove fallen tree leaves, and clean out organic debris from the pond and filters. Check the fish to ensure all are well fed and healthy in preparation for winter dormancy. Any thin, injured, or sick fish should be isolated and treated before winter. When the water temperature drops to 59°F/15°C decrease the quantity of food, as the fish will become less active. Perform water tests regularly along with partial water changes to maintain the correct water quality. Ensure that falling leaves do not impede water flow through the surface skimmers or filter (Fig. 7.3).

7.2.4 Winter

Pond fish should not be fed when the water temperature remains below 45°F/7.2°C. Once the temperature is below 40–45°F/4.4–7.2°C, the fish will become dormant. The pond water depth should be at least 3 ft (1 m) and, in cold climates, preferably 6 or more feet (2 m or more) deep. At this depth, the water will remain 39°F/4°C even if frozen solid at the surface.

Mild surface water agitation will keep the pond from freezing over completely. Solid ice covering the pond can cause damage to the sides of the pond and will trap toxic gasses underneath it. Holes can be drilled in the ice or melted through it, but the ice should never be smashed, as this will disturb the fish's dormancy, increasing the metabolic demands. Stock tank heaters, floating pond deicers, or similar safe water heaters can be used in locales with extreme winters to keep an area of the pond surface from completely freezing over (Fig. 7.4).

The filtration system should be adjusted so that it does not disturb the water at the bottom of the pond, only the surface water. If the denser water (39°F/4°C) that settles on the bottom is mixed with the colder water at the surface (32°F/0°C), it will chill all the water and can cause the fish to freeze. Cold water holds more oxygen than warm water, so waterfalls and fountains are not necessary for oxygenation during the winter months if the fish are not overcrowded. In ponds heavily planted with submerged aquatic plants, these plants will consume oxygen by respiration if thick ice or snow-covered ice prevents photosynthesis. The resulting low oxygen can cause fish deaths known as "winterkill" to fish farmers (Boyd and Tucker, 2014). In these cases, oxygenation is necessary to avoid hypoxia.

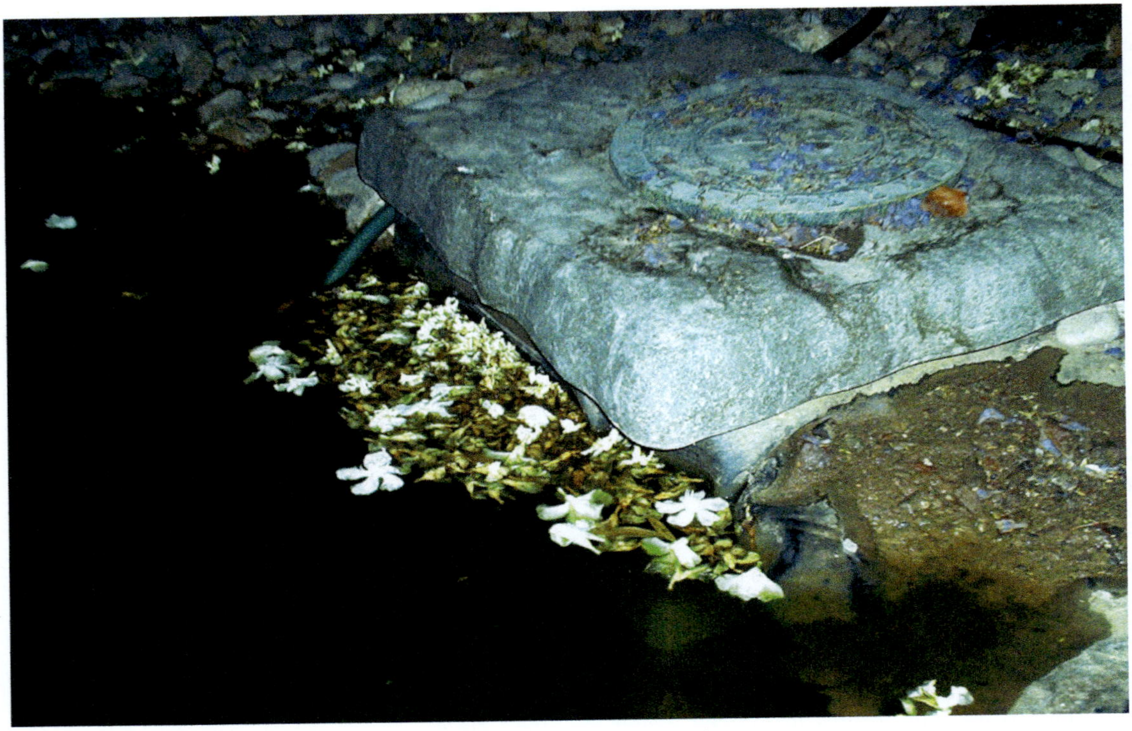

Fig. 7.3. Fallen leaves and flowers collecting at the surface skimmer entrance in a koi pond filter. (Photograph by N. Saint-Erne.)

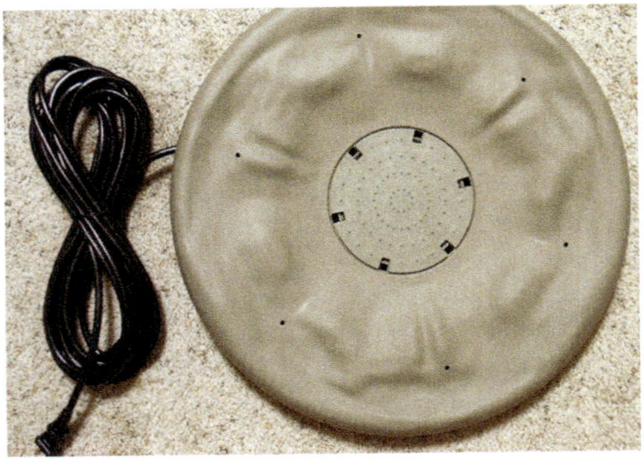

Fig. 7.4. A floating pond de-icer will keep an area of the pond's surface from freezing over in the winter, but does not heat the pond water. (Photograph by N. Saint-Erne.)

7.3 Pond Predation

Dogs, cats, raccoons, and herons can all prey on the pond population. Fencing around the pond may be necessary to keep out dogs and make it safe for children, and netting over the pond is required to deter raccoons, cats, and herons. Deep ponds with straight sides make it harder for predators to reach the fish than it is with shallow ponds that have sloping sides. Various bird-scaring devices are available, such as air cannons, metallic ribbons, noisemakers, fake owls, and big predator-eye balls. Another useful device is a motion-activated water sprayer that attaches to the garden hose (Fig. 7.5). When a predator gets near the pond in the motion-detection zone, the sprayer is activated and sprays a fan of water to scare off the predator.

Baby fish can be preyed upon by larger fish, frogs, water turtles, aquatic snakes, birds, and aquatic insects. Keep smaller fish in netted fry-rearing ponds for protection until they are large enough to safely go out in the main pond with the bigger fish.

7.4 Sunburn

Fish in shallow water less than 2 ft/26 cm deep that are in direct sunlight for extended periods of time each day (no shade) may suffer from sunburn (Fig. 7.6). The lesions appear as hyperemia (redness) of the skin, usually the white parts, and blistering along the margins of the scales on the dorsum. Severe cases may result in ulceration of the skin.

Treatment is to increase the depth of the water if possible and to provide shade over the pond. Temporarily using large pieces of Styrofoam or other floating objects in the pond will provide immediate sources of shade. Floating plants such as water hyacinth will also provide some shade for the fish. Antibiotic or antifungal treatments may be needed if a secondary infection of the skin occurs.

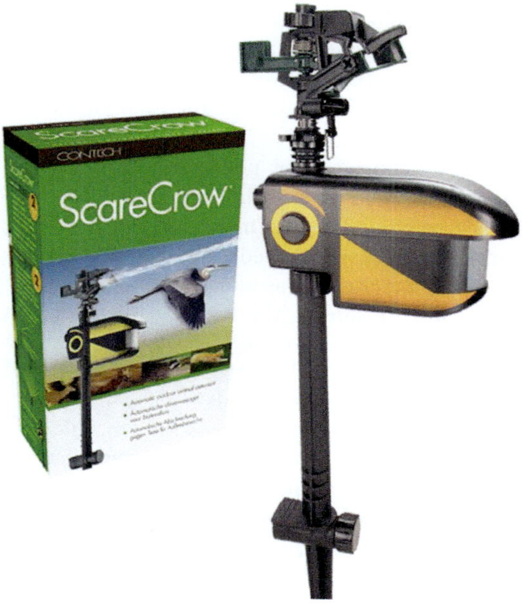

Fig. 7.5. Motion detector spray device used to deter predators from the pond. (Photograph from manufacturer.)

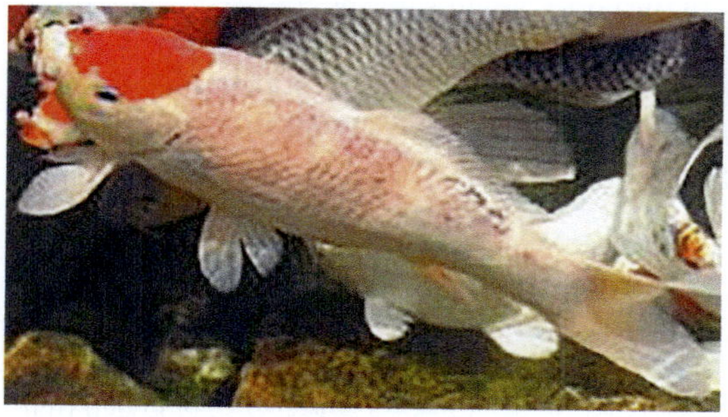

Fig. 7.6. Erythema on Tancho Kohaku Koi (*C. rubrofuscus*) from excessive UV exposure (sunburn). (Photograph by John Fornaro, courtesy of Hanover Koi Farm.)

7.5 Ova Retention in Female Koi

Koi have been selectively bred in Japan for centuries and are now one of the most popular species of ornamental fish. In natural pond situations, koi become torpid during the cold winter months and then, after the water warms above 63°F/17°C in the springtime, they breed and the female releases up to 100,000 eggs per pound of body weight, and large female koi can weigh 30 pounds. However, because koi are sometimes kept in heated ponds during the winter or kept in southern regions where the water never gets very cold, or even kept in an indoor pond or large aquarium, the female koi may not have a stimulus to spawn and release its large volume of eggs. This can lead to retention of the ova, or egg binding, which can cause pathological changes in the abdominal organs (Saint-Erne, 2012).

Over time, unspawned eggs are normally reabsorbed in a female koi, as egg production is at the expense of stored visceral fat. During the winter torpor, when the water temperature is below 45–50°F/7–10°C, the koi stop feeding and become dormant. At this time the female koi will utilize stored fat and the ovarian mass is reduced. But in an overfed female koi or one that is fed throughout the winter due to warmer water temperature, this reabsorption of the eggs may not occur. This can lead to many mature eggs in the ovary that are unable to be released. Eventually, the distended ovaries can become necrotic or impede normal hepatic or intestinal functions by causing physical compression (Fig. 7.7).

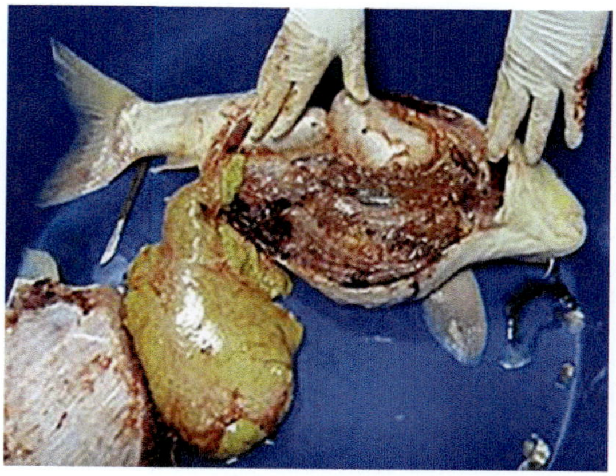

Fig. 7.7. Necropsy of a female koi showing the enlarged right ovary (removed from coelom) and congestion in the coelomic organs due to compression between the two ovaries. (Photograph by N. Saint-Erne.)

Ova retention is suspected when there is abdominal distention in a female koi after the typical springtime spawning season is over. Diagnosis can be confirmed with imaging techniques such as radiography, ultrasonography, or computed tomography (CT) imaging. The risk of ova retention may increase in overweight koi. Obesity is not uncommon in well-cared-for koi. The pond owners may tend to overfeed the fish to get them to come up to the surface for viewing or for rapid growth. Normal feed quantities should be 1–3% of the body weight daily, and a good rule of thumb is to feed only what the fish will consume in 3–5 min, once or twice daily. Reducing the feeding quantity after the normal spawning season so that female koi will reabsorb any remaining eggs may prevent egg binding.

Providing a cool-water period before spring can help produce a normal spawning cycle in fish that are otherwise kept in a warm pond in the winter. If cooling then increasing the water temperature does not stimulate spawning to relieve the egg binding, ovulation can also be induced by injections of carp pituitary extract (2–5 mg/kg intramuscularly, repeat in 9–12 h), human chorionic gonadotropin (20–30 IU/kg intramuscularly, given twice, 6 h apart), or Ovaprim® (Syndel; salmon gonadotropin-releasing hormone analog 20 µg/ml + domperidone 10 mg/ml). Ovaprim is dosed at 0.1–0.5 ml/kg of body weight, given intramuscularly or intracoelomically. Ovaprim is effective in fish that are within or near their natural spawning season. Ovulation may occur in as little as 4 h post-treatment, so fish should be monitored accordingly.

7.6 Medicating Fish Ponds

Before applying any chemicals or medications to the pond, be sure an accurate measurement of the water volume has been made. Underdosage of medications will reduce the effectiveness of the treatment and overdosage can cause additional stress to the fish, or even death. Pond volume can be calculated in a rectangular pond by multiplying the length times the width of the pond and then multiplying by the average water depth. Circular pond volumes are calculated by the pond's surface area (πr^2) times the average depth. That is the radius squared (r^2 = radius × radius) times 3.14 (π, or pi) times the pond's average depth. The average depth can be calculated by measuring the depth of the water in the pond at regular intervals throughout the pond's surface area, adding the depth measurements together, and then dividing the sum by the total number of depth readings taken. Irregularly shaped ponds can be measured in small sections at a time, and these calculations are added together for the total pond volume.

The final result will give you the total volume of water in the pond in cubic feet (if measured in feet) or cubic meters (if measured in meters). After measuring the pond, multiply the volume of water measured in cubic feet by 7.48 to get the total gallons of water in the pond. Multiply the measured pond volume in cubic meters by 1000 to get total volume in liters. Be sure to add to the volume of pond water the amount of water that is in the filtration system and pipes for the total volume of water.

It is recommended for pond owners to use the meter on the water main when filling a pond to get the beginning and ending meter reading. Then the numbers can be subtracted to find out the total volume of water that was added to the pond when it was filled, including the water in the filtration system. This number should be recorded for future reference when needed for treating the pond with medications or other chemicals.

Once the total pond volume is known, calculate the appropriate dosage of medications to apply to the pond. It is helpful to mix the measured medication quantity in a container of pond water to dilute it, then distribute the medication over the surface of the pond so it spreads through the pond, or pour it where the waterfall or filtration outflow will distribute it quickly throughout the pond. Be sure adequate aeration is present when medicating the pond, as many chemicals will lower the dissolved oxygen content. Remove carbon filtration media and turn off UV lights during the treatment period, as they will inactivate the medications. Use personal protective equipment, such as gloves and splash goggles, when handling chemicals that are being added to the pond.

7.7 Conclusion

Experience in keeping an aquarium is helpful for pond owners, as the water quality is just as important in a pond as it is in aquariums. The water quality should be tested on a regular basis, and water changes made when needed. Filtration systems for ponds must include both mechanical filtration to remove sediment and particulate matter and biological filtration to convert ammonia to nitrite and then nitrate. Many ponds also use ultraviolet light filters to reduce algae suspended in the water that would otherwise create green-colored water. Weather affects outdoor ponds in different ways throughout the year and varying steps need to be taken to keep the pond clean and the fish healthy all year around. Feeding schedules may change as the water temperature cools in the winter, and pond maintenance needs to be performed as appropriate for each season.

References

Boyd, C.E. and Tucker, C.S. (2014) *Handbook for Aquaculture Water Quality*. Craftmaster Printers, Auburn, Alabama.

McDowall, A. (1989) *The Tetra Encyclopedia of Koi*. Tetra Press, Morris Plains, New Jersey.

Robinson, P. (2000) *Pond Basics*. Sterling Publishing, New York.

Saint-Erne, N. (2010) *Advanced Koi Care*. Erne Enterprises, Glendale, Arizona.

Saint-Erne, N. (2012) *Diagnosis and Treatment of Ova Retention and other Reproductive Disorders in Koi*. American Veterinary Medical Association Convention Program, San Diego, California.

8 Fish Nutrition

Nicholas Saint-Erne

Dr. Saint-Erne Consulting, PLLC, Phoenix, Arizona

Abstract

Like the higher vertebrates, fish require proteins, fats, carbohydrates, vitamins, minerals, and water from their diet. The last of these is readily acquired by fish from their aquatic environment. Feeding fish sufficient quantities of the appropriate diet is paramount for their health and welfare. Food formulas may differ for carnivorous, omnivorous, or herbivorous fish species; however, commercial food preparations available are usually satisfactory for feeding aquarium fish.

8.1 Feeding Ornamental Fish

Fish are poikilothermic (cold-blooded); therefore, their rate of metabolism depends on the temperature of the surrounding water. Food consumption and nutritional requirements vary with their metabolic rates. The warmer the water temperature, the greater will be their nutritional requirements. In aquariums, the water should maintain a constant temperature throughout the year by use of a submersible electric aquarium water heater. Feeding should be once or twice daily, and more frequently for fry or juvenile fish. For outdoor ponds, feed fish more frequently during warm weather, and decrease feeding when the water temperature cools. For outdoor koi and goldfish ponds in cold climates, reduce the quantity and frequency of feeding when the temperature drops below 50°F/10°C and discontinue feeding when the water temperature remains below 45°F/7.2°C (Saint-Erne, 2010). Adding food when the fish are not eating will result in poor water quality.

Fish in the wild will eat plankton, insects, worms, crustacea, mollusks, other fish, fish eggs, algae, aquatic plants, and decaying organic matter. Fish diets vary by trophic category; some are carnivores, eating only other animals (piscivores if they only eat other fish), omnivores that will eat almost anything, or herbivores eating primarily plant matter. Even fish such as algae eaters are actually getting a wide variety of foods in their diet as the algae may contain many insects or other small invertebrates and zooplankton. The diets of fish in the wild have enough variety to meet their nutritional needs. In an aquarium, the wild diet of the fish must be considered to ensure adequate nutrition is provided (Fig. 8.1). Diets for carnivores and omnivores can be based on the known diet in the wild (Hoopes and Koutsos, 2021). For herbivores and detritivores (scavengers), the actual wild diet might not be known, but most fish will adapt to eating prepared diets (Fig. 8.2), including flakes and pellets, frozen and freeze-dried foods, dried algae wafers and sheets, and live food such as brine shrimp, copepods, and worms.

Feeding fish pelleted food or a floating flake (Fig. 8.3) makes it easier to see if the fish are eating and to tell how much to feed them. Some fish eat food off the substrate at the bottom of the aquarium, such as Corydoras catfish. It is important to be sure food is reaching the bottom for those fish. An adequate amount of food at each feeding is the quantity they will consume in about 3–5 min. If all the food is gone in less time, the fish should be given more. If there is food remaining after 5 min, they have been given too much. Cyprinids, such as minnows, goldfish, and koi, are grazers, and as they have no stomach to store large meals, they should eat small amounts frequently. Also, nocturnal fish may not eat during the day but hunt for their food at night, so feeding them and then turning out the

Corresponding author: DrSaintErne@gmail.com

© CAB International 2025. *The Handbook of Ornamental Fish Health and Welfare* (ed. N. Saint-Erne)
DOI: 10.1079/9781789246032.0008

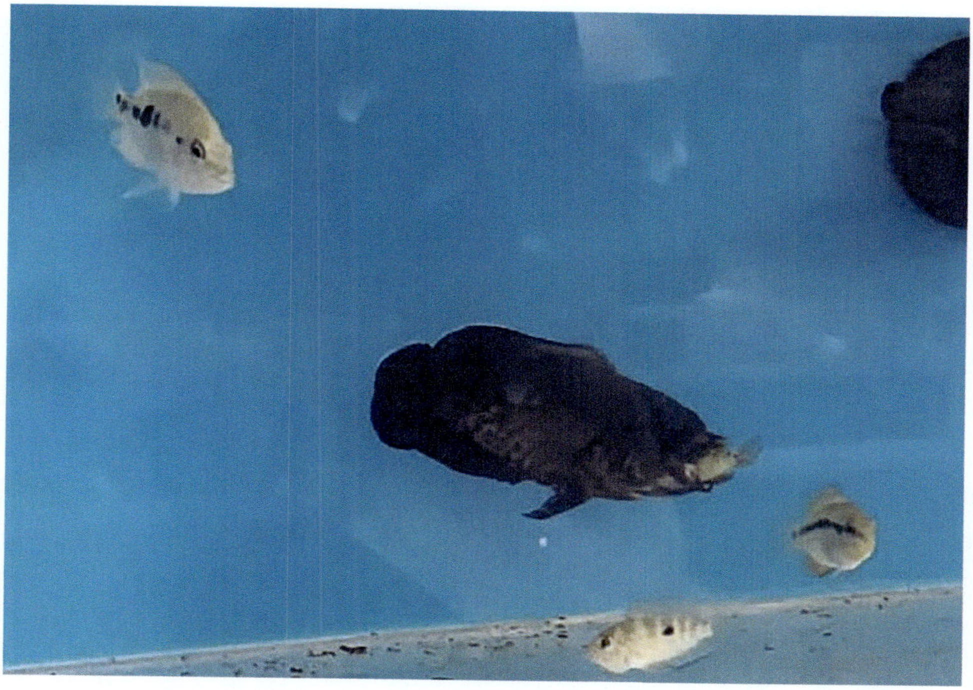

Fig. 8.1. Oscar (*Astronotus ocellatus*) eating a smaller cichlid in an aquarium. It is important to know the feeding habits of each fish species and to not mix incompatible fish. Hungry fish may attempt to eat things that they would not otherwise eat. (Photograph by N. Saint-Erne.)

light may be necessary. Young fish (fry) should be fed 3–6 times daily. Older fish can be fed once or twice daily. Overfeeding is as much a health risk as starvation. Older healthy fish can go for days or even weeks without being fed. However, overfeeding will cause obesity, fatty liver syndrome (Figs. 8.4 and 8.5) and can foul the water, producing toxic ammonia.

Overfeeding is especially a risk when neighbors take care of the fish while the owner is on vacation! In this situation, place the proper amount of food for each feeding in individual plastic ziplock bags and label the bags with the time and date they are to be used for feeding the fish. Secure all remaining food, so it is unavailable for the temporary caregivers to prevent additional feedings. Leave an emergency telephone number where the owner or the veterinarian can be reached, in case of fish health or water quality problems. An alternative for feeding fish while on vacation is to use an automatic fish feeder. Many types are commercially available (Fig. 8.6). The feeder should be set up and tested for several days prior to needing it during a vacation so that the correct amount of food to be dispensed can be calibrated, and then checked and adjusted after multiple feedings.

Besides commercially prepared diets, fresh foods should be fed to fish as well. Cooked or chopped raw vegetables, such as peas, kale, and zucchini, are relished by omnivores and herbivores such as algae eaters and plecostomus, as are leafy vegetables. Many fish species, such as koi, goldfish, Oscars, and other large cichlids can be trained to come to a certain spot when being fed and will even eat out of one's hand. In general, feed adult fish 1–3% of their body weight (BW) per day, growing fish 3–5% BW/day, and young fish (fry) 5–8% of their body weight per day. Young fish should be fed multiple small feedings throughout the day.

8.2 Protein

Protein makes up the major portion of a fish's diet on a dry matter basis. Young growing fish require up to 44–55% protein in their diet, while mature fish only need 28–38% protein in their diet (NRC, 2011). Many foods for adult fish have too much protein and can lead to overweight fish, fatty liver

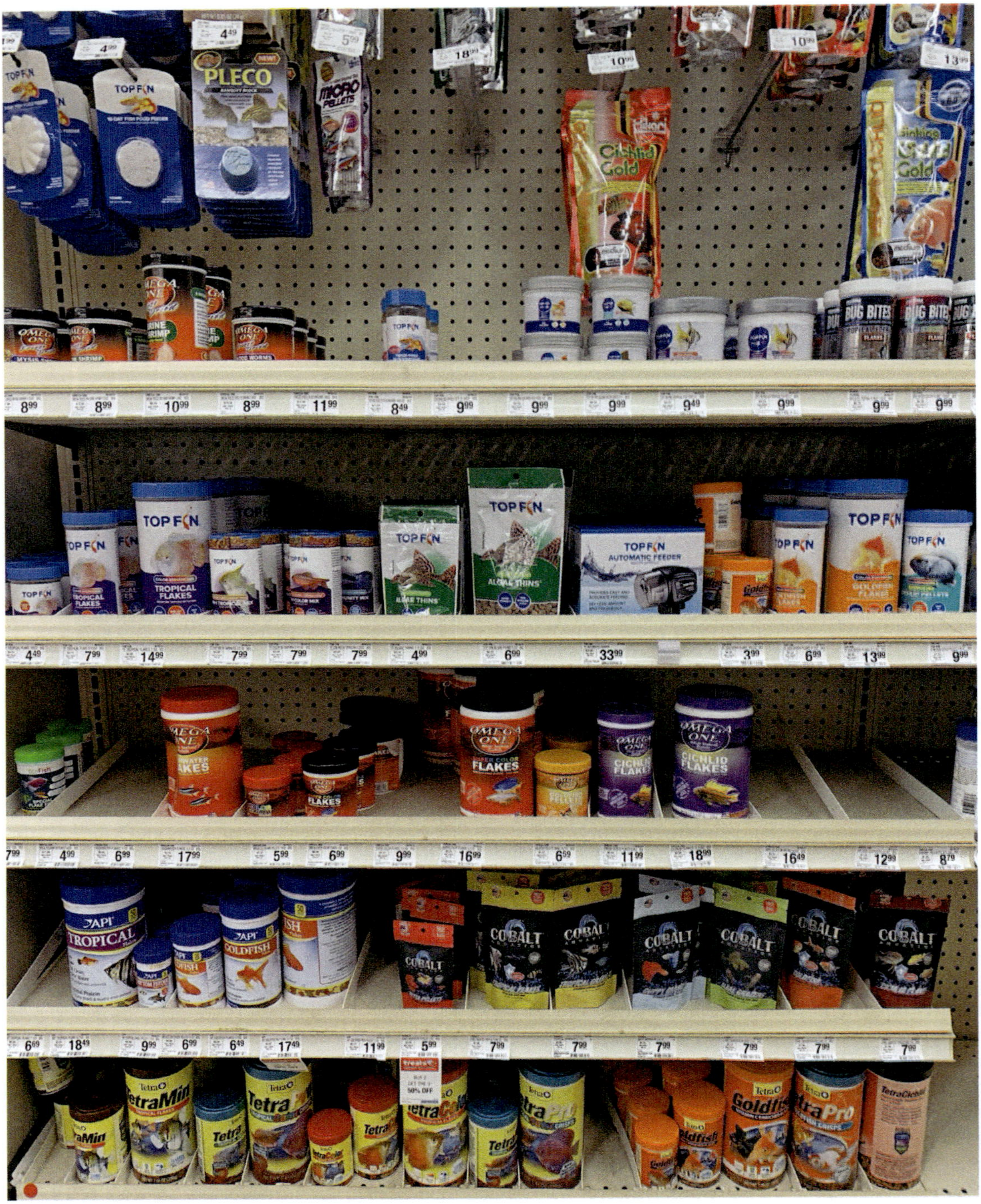

Fig. 8.2. There is a large variety of commercial fish foods available at pet stores. (Photograph by N. Saint-Erne.)

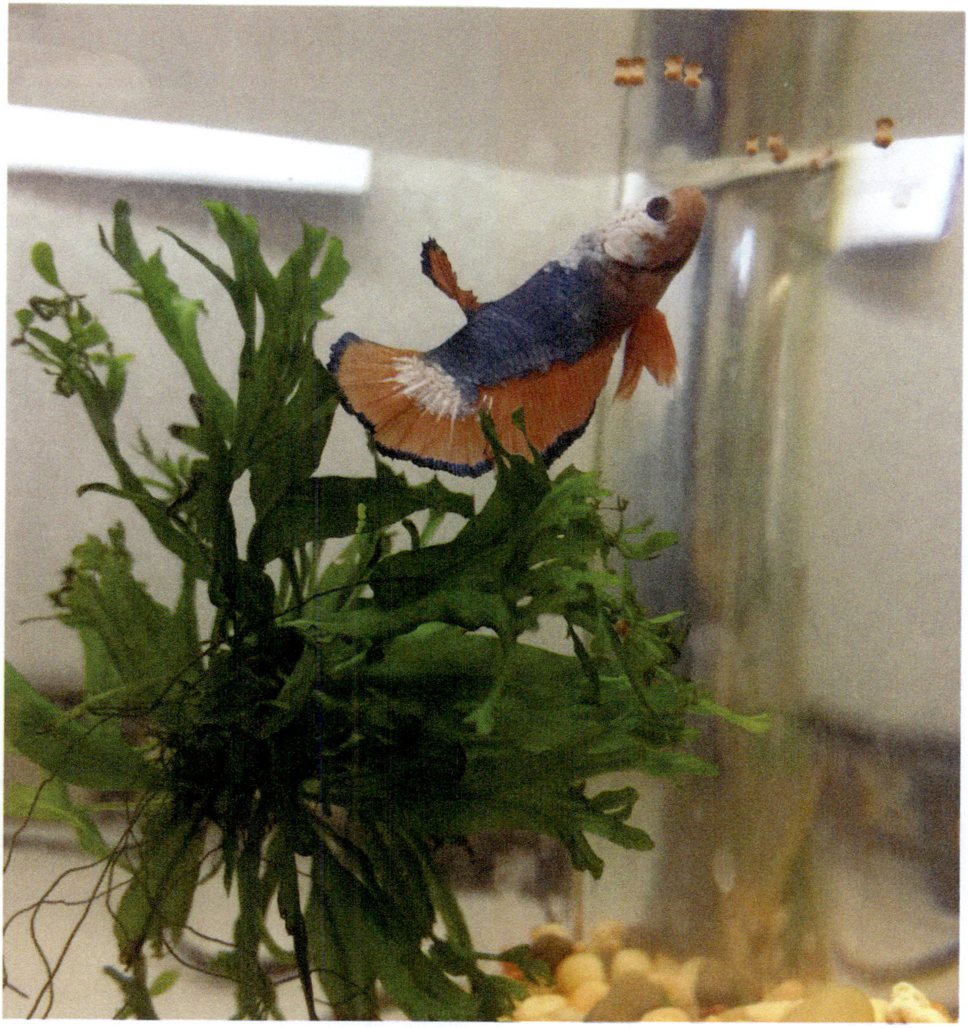

Fig. 8.3. Betta (*Betta splendens*) eating floating pellets. (Photograph by N. Saint-Erne.)

disease, and excess ammonia being released into the water. In many public aquariums, the fish are given foods designed for growing fish (trout chow or catfish pellets) that have a higher protein level than needed for adult fish and can lead to obesity in the fish. Fish are more efficient at using protein as an energy source than homeotherms, since ammonia synthesis does not require energy, as does the formation of uric acid in birds, or urea in mammals (Wright and Land, 1998).

The proteins in the diet are broken down into 20 different amino acids by enzymes in the digestive tract. These amino acids are then absorbed and resynthesized into new proteins in the fish's tissues. There are ten essential amino acids that must be supplied by the fish's protein consumption: arginine, histidine, isoleucine, leucine, lysine, methionine, phenylalanine, threonine, tryptophan, and valine. Tyrosine and cysteine are considered semi-essential because they can be synthesized from phenylalanine and methionine, respectively. Taurine is a necessary component of larval and juvenile diets of marine fish and comes from fish meal, but not vegetable proteins (Hardy, 2012). The rest of the amino acids can be synthesized by the fish from adequate dietary nitrogen (Hoopes and Koutsos, 2021). Deficiency of any of these essential amino acids, or an insufficient quantity of total protein will result in reduced growth and reproduction rates, and increased mortalities.

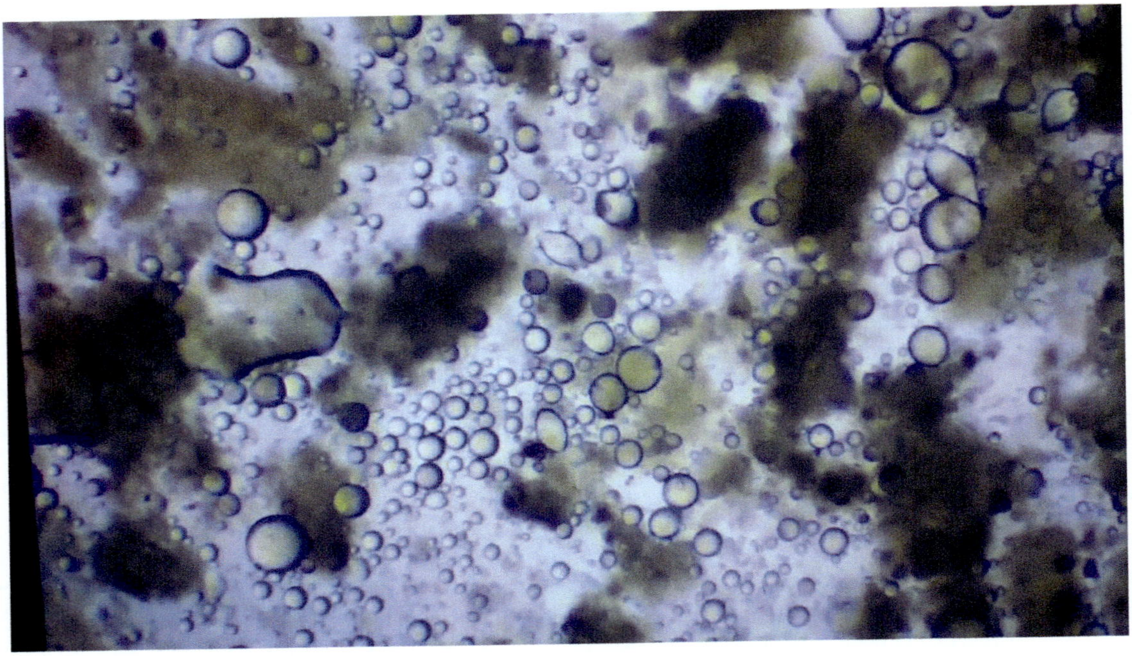

Fig. 8.4. Oil droplets in liver tissue of a Yaqui chub (*Gila purpurea*) with hepatic lipidosis. This was from an older fish living in an aquarium. (Microphotograph by N. Saint-Erne.)

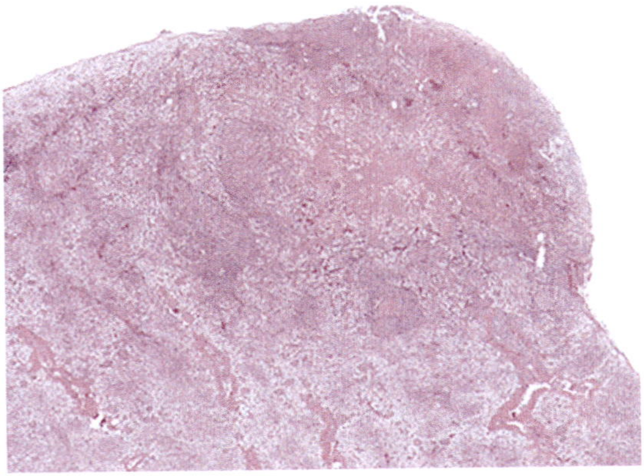

Fig. 8.5 Stained histopathology slide of a guineafowl pufferfish (*Arothron meleagris*) with hepatic lipidosis. This was from an 11-year-old fish living in an aquarium. (Microphotograph by Ethan Biswell, DVM MS Dipl ACVP.)

In nature, ingested protein is in the form of phytoplankton, zooplankton, algae, aquatic plants, bacteria, protozoa, crustacea, mollusks, worms, insects, and often other fish. In an aquarium or koi pond, the fish's nutritional needs are usually met by feeding a processed commercial flake or pelleted food. Prepared foods decrease in nutritional value over time, especially if exposed to air, sunlight, moisture, or high temperatures. Be sure to keep fish foods in closed airtight containers stored at refrigerated or room temperatures. All stored food should be used within three months to ensure freshness.

A good homemade protein supplement for feeding young fish can be made from eggs. Hen's eggs are 100% nutritious, contain all ten essential amino acids, and are high in lecithin and linoleic acid as well. They also contain 22 important minerals. Spinach or other dark green leafy vegetables can be added to the eggs as a source of vitamin A and other nutrients. The mixture is blended until it is homogenous and is then cooked until firm using a stove or microwave oven. Once cooked, it can be crumbled into bite-sized pieces and stored in airtight containers in the refrigerator or freezer. Use this to supplement other prepared fish foods if more protein in the diet is desired for breeding or rearing fry.

Excess proteins not needed for growth or reproduction are utilized as an energy source instead of fats or carbohydrates. However, because proteins average 16% nitrogen, the breakdown products of protein metabolism are ammonia (NH_3) and a small amount (less than 2%) of urea, $2(NH_2)CO$.

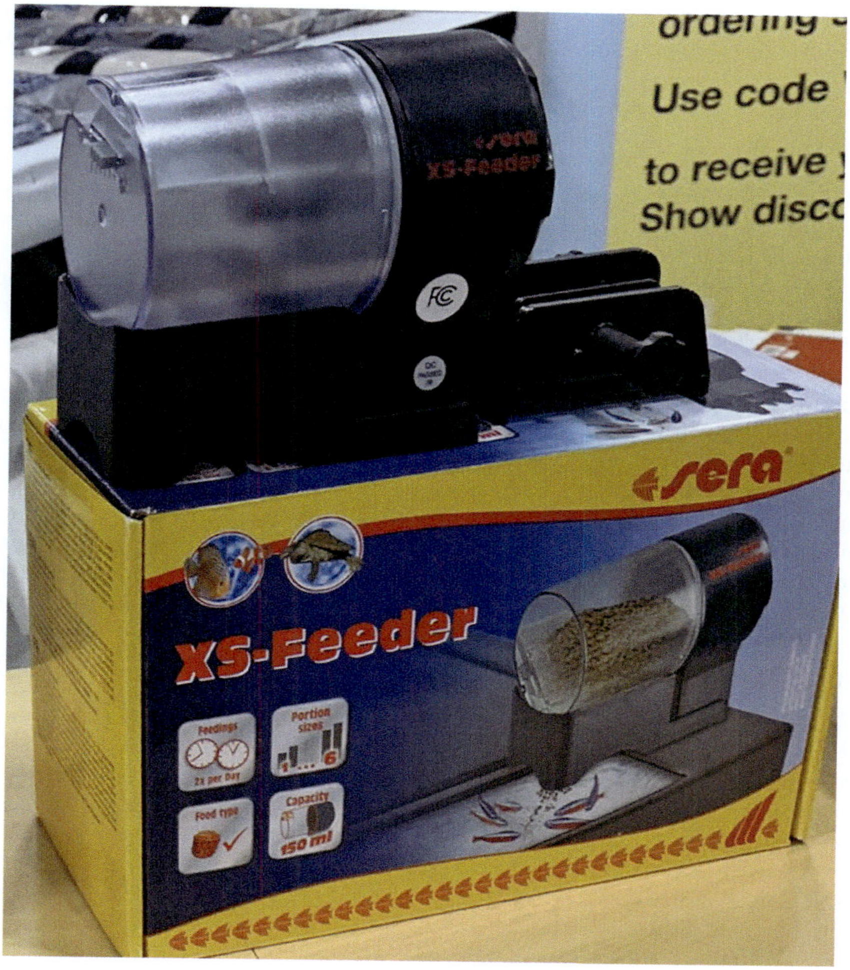

Fig. 8.6. Automatic fish feeder. (Photograph by N. Saint-Erne.)

The ammonia is passively released into the water through the fish's gills and can lead to toxicity if levels increase. Nonprotein energy metabolism does not cause ammonia production. Fats and simple carbohydrates added to the diet have a protein-sparing effect in that they can be used for energy instead of protein, without increasing ammonia production.

8.3 Fat

Fats (lipids) are another nutrient necessary in the fish's diet. Only low melting point unsaturated fats (oils) are readily digested and used by fish. Saturated (solid) fats are poorly digested and at water temperatures below 68°F/20°C can solidify and cause intestinal blockages. Rapidly growing fish utilize oils over carbohydrates or proteins as their primary source of energy. That is why young fish need higher fat in the diet than do mature fish. Fat metabolism produces CO_2 and H_2O as its by-products, which are non-toxic. Fats are an efficient energy source because they contain 9 kcal (or Cal.) per gram, while proteins and carbohydrates only produce 4 kcal/g.

In fish foods, 10–15% fat in the diet is optimal, although juvenile fish may need as much as 20% of the dry weight of the diet as fat (Hoopes and Koutsos, 2021). Excess fats can lead to hepatic lipidosis (fatty degeneration of the liver). Deficiency of fats, including essential fatty acids, causes fin erosions, slow growth, and neuromuscular shock.

The fat-soluble vitamins (A, D, E, and K) will not be absorbed without adequate fat in the diet.

Fats are used in the formation of cell structures and membranes, and in the formation of some steroids and other hormones. Two polyunsaturated fatty acids (PUFAs) are essential for growth: linolenic acid (18:3 Ω-3) [= 18 carbons, three double bonds, first double bond is on the 3rd carbon away from the end omega (Ω) carbon] and linoleic acid (18:2 Ω-6). These should be provided at 1% of the total diet on a dry matter basis for each of the omega-3 (Ω-3) and omega-6 (Ω-6) fatty acids.

Unsaturated fatty acids oxidize readily and will go rancid if exposed to oxygen, light, and heat. The oxidation metabolites can be toxic to fish. Sekoke disease in koi occurs when oxidized (rancid) fats destroy α-tocopherol in the food, resulting in vitamin E deficiency. Keep fish food in closed containers away from sunlight or heat. Do not use food that is moldy or has a rancid odor.

8.4 Carbohydrate

Carbohydrates (sugars, starches, and fiber) are not a major nutrient source in fishes, as they are poorly digested, but can be used as an energy source. Carbohydrates are less preferred for carnivores compared with omnivores and herbivores, especially in marine fish (Hoopes and Koutsos, 2021). Most fish cannot utilize complex starches (polysaccharides). Simple sugars (monosaccharides) are a readily digestible energy source, but they are not available in most of the natural diet of fish. Adding small amounts of monosaccharides or disaccharides to fish food will have a protein-sparing effect on energy production. Microflora (beneficial bacteria) in the intestines will break down some complex carbohydrates from plants, but it is the least digestible nutrient for fish. Carbohydrates are only about 34% digestible by fish, compared with 85–95% digestibility of proteins and fats. Carbohydrate digestion produces carbon dioxide, water, and energy.

Total carbohydrates in the diet of carnivores should be 5–25% (Hua and Bureau, 2009), while with omnivores and herbivores, it can be as high as 25–40% (Becker *et al.*, 2022), which includes indigestible fiber at no more than half the total amount of carbohydrates. Fiber consists of indigestible plant polysaccharides such as cellulose, hemicellulose, and lignin. Excess carbohydrates are stored in the liver as glycogen or converted into stored fat. Diets too high in carbohydrates can produce liver cell degeneration (hepatic lipidosis).

8.5 Vitamins

Both water-soluble and fat-soluble vitamins are necessary in the diet of fishes. Most water-soluble vitamins (B complex and C) are coenzymes used in cellular metabolism. A constant supply of these vitamins is required in the diet, as they are not stored in the body tissues. Fat-soluble vitamins (A, D, E, K) may be stored in the liver or other tissues after ingestion. Overdosage of fat-soluble vitamins can occur, since they are stored in the liver.

In several fish species, β-carotene, astaxanthin, and canthaxanthin can be converted to vitamin A (Moren *et al.*, 2002). Vitamin D functions in calcium homeostasis and in the development of skeletal tissues and cellular differentiation (NRC, 2011). Excess vitamin D can cause vertebral deformities in larval fish. Vitamin E serves as an antioxidant and protects PUFAs from becoming rancid. In koi that were fed a diet deficient in vitamin E consisting of oxidized silkworm pupae, the fish developed a condition called Sekoke disease, which caused loss of epaxial muscling on the dorsum of the fish. It was treated by adding α-tocopherol acetate (50 mg/kg food) to the diet (Saint-Erne, 2010).

One of the first signs of any vitamin deficiency is a decreased appetite, resulting in poor growth. More specific signs of a particular vitamin deficiency will develop after several weeks of feeding a vitamin-deficient diet. See Table 8.1 for specific vitamin deficiency signs.

Vitamin C deficiency is a common problem in fish. Vitamin C (L-ascorbic acid) is necessary for the metabolism of collagen for bones and joints. Deficiency causes poor bone and cartilage formation, resulting in scoliosis (curvature of the spine) and petechial hemorrhaging. It is usually due to the decay of vitamin C in processed fish food. Vitamin C can decay in food in as short a period as 3–6 months after processing. Excess heat and exposure to the air hastens the process. Always keep fish food in airtight containers and in dry, cool storage areas. Using a stabilized form of vitamin C, such as L-ascorbyl-2-polyphosphate, in the manufacture of commercial fish foods increases the shelf life of vitamin C in the food considerably. Additional vitamin C can be given to koi by floating orange slices

Table 8.1. Essential vitamin dosages and deficiency signs (Saint-Erne, 2010).

Vitamin	Daily requirement (mg/kg of diet)	Deficiency signs
Water-soluble vitamins:		
Thiamine (B_1)	1–11	Fin congestion, fading color, neurologic signs
Riboflavin (B_2)	4–25	Skin and fin hemorrhages, poor growth, cataracts
Niacin (nicotinic acid) (B_3)	10–150	Skin hemorrhages, muscle spasms, exophthalmia
Pantothenic acid (B_5)	10–50	Skin hemorrhages, anemia, exophthalmia, gill hyperplasia, and necrosis
Pyridoxine (B_6)	3–15	Neurological disorders, ascites, anemia
Biotin (B_7)	0.1–2.5	Poor growth, anemia, muscle atrophy, convulsions
Folacin (folic acid) (B_9)	1.0–4.0	Poor growth, anemia, lethargy
Cyanocobalamin (B_{12})	0.02–0.09	Hematological disorders, anemia
Choline	400–1500	Fatty liver, hemorrhagic kidneys, and intestines
Inositol	250–500	Skin lesions, poor digestion
L-Ascorbic acid (C)	60–500	Spinal deformities, hemorrhages
Fat-soluble vitamins:		
Vitamin A (retinol)	1–6	Hemorrhages, paleness, abnormal gill opercula, exophthalmia, poor vision, edema
Vitamin D_3 (cholecalciferol)	6–60	Poor growth, impaired bone calcification
Vitamin E (α-tocopherol)	25–200	Muscular dystrophy, anemia, hemosiderosis, death
Vitamin K (methyl-naphtho-quinone)	0.2–2	Skin hemorrhages, anemia

in the pond, which koi will nibble on, and for other fish, by soaking pelleted foods briefly in orange juice or vitamin C solution before feeding on an occasional basis.

8.6 Minerals

Fish have mineral requirements similar to other vertebrates. There are seven minerals that are needed in large amounts (calcium, chloride, magnesium, phosphorus, potassium, sodium, and sulfur) and 14 that are needed in only trace amounts (chromium, cobalt, copper, fluorine, iodine, iron, manganese, molybdenum, nickel, selenium, silicon, tin, vanadium, and zinc). Aluminum and arsenic may be required in even smaller amounts. Most minerals are obtained directly from the food, although some essential and nonessential compounds are absorbed from the water (Hoopes and Koutsos, 2021). Mineral ions capable of being diffused through the gill membranes include calcium, chloride, cobalt, copper, iron, magnesium, potassium, sodium, selenium, and zinc (Ca, Cl^-, Co, Cu, Fe, Mg, K, Na, Se, and Zn, respectively). The rest, especially phosphorus, must be provided in the food.

The minerals calcium, phosphorus, and magnesium function in the formation of bones, scales, skin, and muscle functions. Phosphorus is also used in phospholipid formation. Iron is necessary to form hemoglobin. Selenium is used to make glutathione peroxidase. Iodine is essential for thyroid function. Sodium and potassium create ionic balance in body fluids. Copper, manganese, and zinc are used as cofactors in enzyme activity (Hardy, 2001).

8.7 Water

Most prepared commercial fish foods contain about 9–10% moisture. Foods higher in water content will spoil more rapidly and may need to be kept refrigerated or even frozen. Freshwater fish do not drink water, as they are constantly trying to eliminate excess water from their bodies by producing copious urine. Their kidneys' primary function is water excretion, and nitrogenous waste excretion occurs through the gills. Saltwater fish take in seawater orally to keep the body hydrated and excrete the excess salt from their blood through specialized cells in the gills.

Water quality in an aquarium can be affected by the diet. Uneaten food will decay and promote bacterial and fungal growth, as well as increase the ammonia and phosphorus in the water, which can promote algae growth. Nitrogenous wastes can be reduced by decreasing the protein in the diet to the optimum level (McGoogan and Gatlin, 1999). Excess phosphorus can come from plant-based ingredients (phytate) in the diet, which are not readily digestible by fish. Regular water changes (with phosphate-free water) will help reduce phosphate accumulation.

8.8 Nutritional Deficiencies

Abnormalities in fish growth may be attributed to nutritional deficiencies, as can an increase in susceptibility to disease (Becker *et al.*, 2022). Changing foods may be beneficial when problems are seen, but nutritional deficiencies associated with improper food storage (high humidity and temperature, or exposure to air or sunlight) may cause feed degradation leading to diseases. Proteins are essential for growth, reproduction, cellular repair, and energy metabolism, especially in larval fish (Hardy, 2012). Fin erosion can occur due to a deficiency in the amino acid lysine. Tryptophan and histidine deficiencies have been associated with scoliosis and lordosis (Roberts, 2002). Lens cataracts (Fig. 8.7) can occur due to deficiencies in vitamin A, vitamin C, riboflavin (vitamin B_2), methionine, histidine, tryptophan, manganese, or zinc (Hadfield and Clayton, 2021).

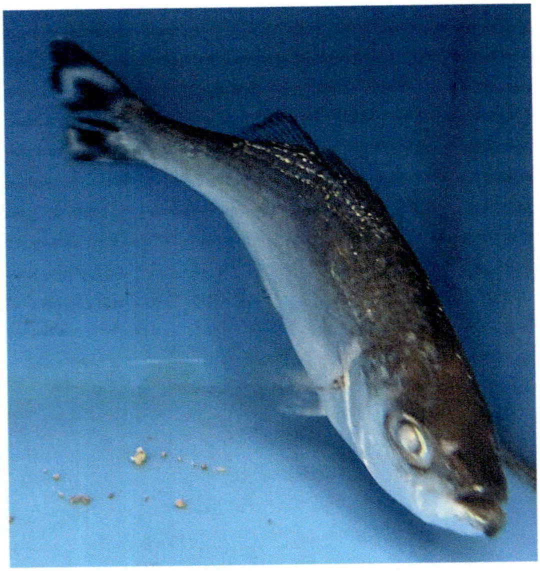

Fig. 8.7. Cataracts in fivebar flagtail fish (*Kuhlia mugil*). Deficiency of vitamins, minerals, or amino acids in the diet can cause cataracts in fish. (Photograph by N. Saint-Erne.)

Lipoid liver disease and anemia can occur in fish when fed diets containing rancid fats. The lack of essential fatty acids in the diet can result in slow growth rates and decreased absorption of fat-soluble vitamins (A, D, E, K). At least 1–2% of the diet formulation should be Ω-3 and Ω-6 fatty acids. Vitamin A deficiency can result in poor growth, keratomalacia, blindness, exophthalmia, hemorrhages at the base of fins, erosion of the caudal peduncle, and shortening of the operculum (Hardy, 2012). Vitamin E deficiency can cause muscle degeneration, steatitis, and anemia. Vitamin D is important in calcium metabolism. Vitamin K deficiency causes an increase in clotting time and decreases hematocrit values (Roberts, 2002).

Deficiencies of vitamins can result from omission of vitamins in preparation of commercial diets or from antagonistic interactions with other compounds in the diet (Hardy, 2001). The most commonly deficient vitamins in prepared diets include ascorbic acid (Fig. 8.8), α-tocopherol, pantothenic acid, pyridoxine, niacin, and thiamine. Vitamin deficiency commonly results in loss of appetite (anorexia), as well as other signs listed in Table 8.1. Using prepared diets within 3 months of purchasing best ensures the vitamins will still be active (Hardy, 2001).

Deficiencies of minerals cause a multitude of signs, including stunted growth, anorexia, anemia, cataracts, and increased mortalities, depending on the mineral that is lacking. Placing fish in deionized or distilled water would result in mineral imbalances, because of mineral loss from the fish into the water by osmosis. Diets high in plant rather than animal-derived ingredients may be deficient in phosphorus, as plant phosphorus is in the form of phytate, which is not digestible by fish. Phosphorus deficiency causes the fish to stop eating and growing, and the bones become flexible, especially seen as abnormalities in the jaw and operculum (Hardy, 2001). However, excess phosphorus results in excretion and eutrophication of the water, promoting algae growth. Phosphorus should be 1.0–1.4% in the diet.

Excess copper, especially the cupric ion (Cu_2^+), is toxic to fish and aquatic invertebrates. Copper sulfate has been used to treat protozoan parasites on fish. Chronic high copper exposure can cause damage to the gills, kidney, and spleen and can cause death (Becker *et al.*, 2022). Growth reduction and cataracts occur with manganese deficiency. Zinc deficiency causes poor growth, skin, and fin

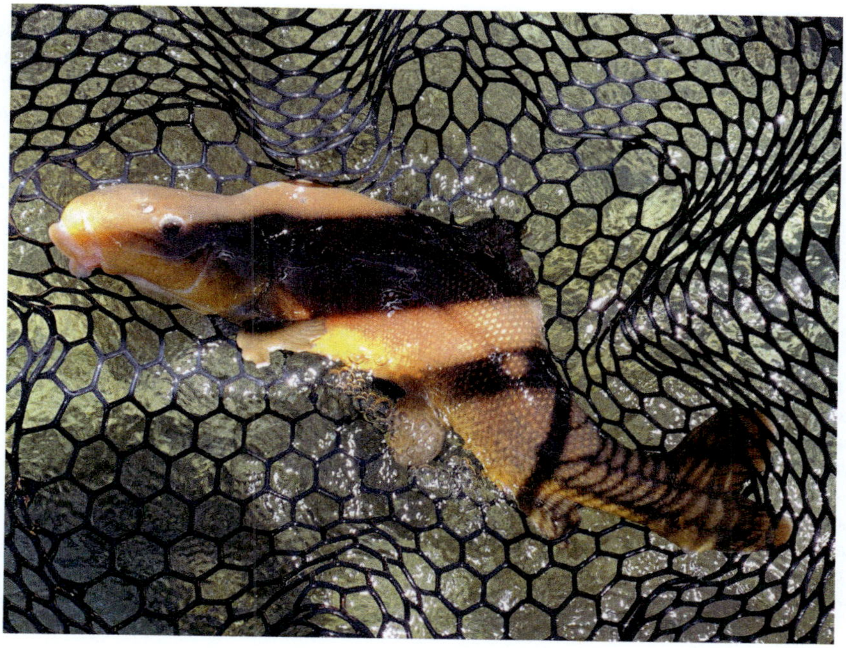

Fig. 8.8. Razorback Sucker (*Zyrauchen texanus*) with scoliosis of spine, believed to be secondary to vitamin C deficiency, which causes weakness in bone and cartilage. Muscular contractions during swimming can then compress the vertebrae and cause spinal deviation. (Photograph by N. Saint-Erne.)

erosion, and bilateral cataracts (Roberts, 2002; Becker *et al.*, 2022). Iodine deficiency causes thyroid hyperplasia (goiter) in fish (Hardy, 2001).

8.9 Food Storage

Protect fish foods from exposure to high temperatures, humidity, moisture, insects, rodents, and sunlight. Store the food for the least amount of time practical. Moist food should be used within 60 days of opening the package, and dry food should be used within 6 months. Refrigerating or freezing the food will allow a safer and longer storage. Keep the food in an airtight container to reduce oxidation and rancidity.

Calculating the average weight of the fish and counting or estimating the number of fish will help determine the approximate total BW of the fish in an aquarium or pond. Using the desired percentage of BW to be fed, the amount of food needed per day can be calculated. This will help ensure that the fish are not getting underfed or overfed. From this, it can also be determined how long a quantity of food should last for those fish at a set percentage of BW to be fed. Then the appropriate size food container can be purchased to feed the fish with the adequate amount of food that will be used within a specific period.

8.10 Conclusion

Deficiencies or excesses of any nutrients may affect the fish's growth, reproduction, immunity against disease, its welfare, and its survival. While commercial fish diets are produced to include the required nutrients for aquarium fish, they must be stored properly and used within a limited time, preferably 3 months, to ensure they are nutritionally complete. Store fish food in airtight, lightproof containers away from heat and moisture. Refrigerating or freezing food helps maintain its nourishment. Using several different foods to feed aquarium fish may reduce the risk of nutrient deficiency. If large numbers of fish from a population are showing similar signs of disease, nutritional deficiency should be investigated.

References

Becker, T., Adeyemo, O., Danyer, E. and Saint-Erne, N. (2022) Nutrition. In: Urdes, L., Walster, C. and Tepper, J. (eds) *Fundamentals of Aquatic Veterinary Medicine*. Wiley, Oxford, pp. 64–72.

Hadfield, C. and Clayton, L. (2021) *Clinical Guide to Fish Medicine*. Wiley, Hoboken, New Jersey.

Hardy, R.W. (2001) Nutritional deficiencies in commercial aquaculture: likelihood, onset, and identification. In: Lim, C. and Webster, C.D. (eds) *Nutrition and Fish Health*. Food Products Press, New York, pp. 131–147.

Hardy, R.W. (2012) The nutritional pathology of teleosts. In: Roberts, R.J. (ed.) *Fish Pathology*. 4th edn. Wiley, Oxford, pp. 402–424.

Hoopes, L.A. and Koutsos, E.A. (2021) Nutrition and nutritional support. In: Hadfield, C. and Clayton, L. (eds) *Clinical Guide to Fish Medicine*. Wiley, Oxford, pp. 67–96.

Hua, K. and Bureau, D. (2009) A mathematical model to explain variations in estimates of starch digestibility and predict digestible starch content of salmonid fish feeds. *Aquaculture* 294, 282–287.

McGoogan, B.B. and Gatlin, D.M. (1999) Dietary manipulations affecting growth and nitrogenous waste production of red drum, *Sciaenops ocellatus* I. Effects of dietary protein and energy levels. *Aquaculture* 178, 333–348.

Moren, M., Naess, T. and Hamre, K. (2002) Conversion of β-carotene, canthaxanthin and astaxanthin to vitamin A in Atlantic halibut (*Hippoglossus hippoglossus* L.) juveniles. *Fish Physiology and Biochemistry* 27, 71–80.

NRC (National Research Council) (2011) *Nutrient Requirements of Fish and Shrimp*. National Academies Press, Washington, DC.

Roberts, R.J. (2002) Nutritional pathology. In: Halver, J.E. and Hardy, R.W. (eds) *Fish Nutrition*. Academic Press, Washington, DC, pp. 453–504.

Saint-Erne, N. (2010) Koi nutrition. In: Saint-Erne, N. (ed.) *Advanced Koi Care*. 2nd edn. Erne Enterprises, Glendale, Arizona, pp. 89–93.

Wright, P.A. and Land, M.D. (1998) Urea production and transport in teleost fish. *Comparative Biochemistry and Physiology Part A* 119, 47–54.

9 Equipping the Veterinary Hospital to Treat Fish Patients

ROBERT MARTINEZ

Aquatic Veterinary Consulting, PLLC, Edmond, Oklahoma, USA

Abstract

Adding fish to the list of patients seen in a small animal veterinary clinic is not as hard as it might first seem. Most of the standard veterinary hospital equipment can also be used with fish patients. Here is information on additional items needed to practice fish medicine.

9.1 Equipment and Medications

The typical veterinary hospital is already well equipped to see fish patients, as the basic medical supplies are already available (Lewbart, 2009). Most veterinary equipment used for small animal medicine is also useful with fish patients. The additional equipment necessary for treating fish can be obtained inexpensively, excluding material necessary for specialized procedures. The basic equipment needed for fish diagnostics (Fig. 9.1) includes a high-quality microscope, latex gloves, simple surgical instruments (Fig. 9.2), microscope slides, coverslips, various-sized hypodermic needles, syringes, red rubber catheters, transport media for bacterial cultures, and other common laboratory supplies (Noga, 2010). The special items needed for treating fish patients include aquariums or tubs to hold the fish (Fig. 9.3), dechlorinator to make the tap water safe for fish, ammonia-neutralizing water treatment, air pumps with air tubing and air stones for aerating the water, a water pump and aquarium filter, water test kit, an aquarium water heater, and thermometer. For a more comprehensive list, please refer to Table 9.1.

The water quality test kits available can be as simple or advanced as preferred, depending on the fish caseload and finances. There are simple colorimetric kits to advanced electronic meters. There are test strips, which are fast and inexpensive but only provide a "ballpark" estimate of water quality, and spectrophotometers that are accurate to several decimal places. All have their uses, and the goal is to determine if the water is safe for the fish, or if any of the water parameters are at unhealthy levels.

The standard veterinary hospital medications are usually adequate. It is best to refer to an exotic veterinary formulary (Lewbart and Yanong, 2022) for the most up-to-date dosages of therapeutics. Most veterinary hospitals will need to purchase a fish anesthetic (such as MS 222) to use for sedation when performing physical exams, simple clinical procedures, diagnostics, and for anesthesia during surgery and euthanasia. Refer to Table 9.2 for a list of drugs and other common compounds used in aquatic veterinary medicine (Lewbart, 2009).

Other basic pieces of equipment that a veterinary hospital usually has readily available are an ophthalmoscope, ultrasound, radiography, and surgical instruments. Further details on their usage will be discussed in later chapters. Though some of these tools may not be routinely used, they can be useful for certain cases. Refer to Tables 9.3 and 9.4 for other recommended medical and diagnostic equipment (Lewbart, 2009).

9.2 House Calls Versus Hospitalization

Most fish patients can be treated as an out-patient at home by the owner, or with repeated home visits

Corresponding author: drrobmartinez@aquaticvetconsulting.com

© CAB International 2025. *The Handbook of Ornamental Fish Health and Welfare* (ed. N. Saint-Erne)
DOI: 10.1079/9781789246032.0009

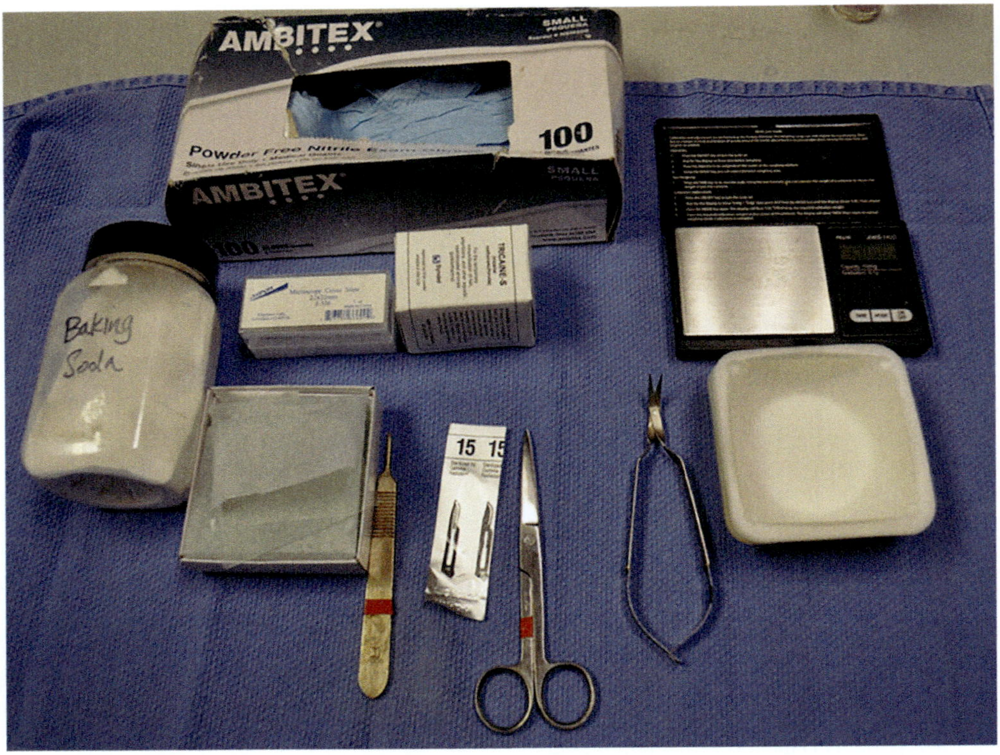

Fig. 9.1. Common supplies for treating fish include gloves, microscope slides, and coverslips, a gram scale, MS 222 fish anesthetic, and baking soda to buffer the anesthetic water. (Photograph by Azureen Erdman.)

by the veterinarian. If hospitalization of a fish patient is considered, this can be more labor-intensive. Typical reasons to consider hospitalization include cases that require intensive care, daily treatments, surgery, or postoperative recovery. Besides having appropriate equipment available, hospitalization of fish patients requires considering these factors:

- Space available in the clinic and equipment requirements (pumps, filters, tanks, tubs)
- Structural support due to the weight of the aquarium (water weighs 8 pounds per gallon)
- Biosecurity
- Staff training in biosecurity, monitoring patients, monitoring water quality, and maintaining equipment
- Cleaning and disinfection of the aquarium and equipment between patients
- Minimizing stress to the patient while in the hospital (lights, sounds, vibrations, motion)
- Placing lids, tops, or nets over the systems to prevent accidental jumping deaths or escapes
- Other considerations for the hospitalization tanks are to provide hiding places to reduce stress. Polyvinyl chloride (PVC) pipes of various sizes (Fig. 9.5) and plastic aquarium plants provide adequate places to hide and are easy to clean and disinfect (Roberts, 2010)

9.3 Conclusion

The Husbandry Equipment listed in Table 9.1 includes most of the equipment necessary to hospitalize a fish patient. The other equipment and medications used with fish are typically found in a small animal veterinary clinic. The specific fish-related materials can be purchased at local pet or fish stores or found at online retailers. There are several online companies that specialize in products for aquaculture and fish farming that carry the necessary medications and products required for setting up a fish hospital.

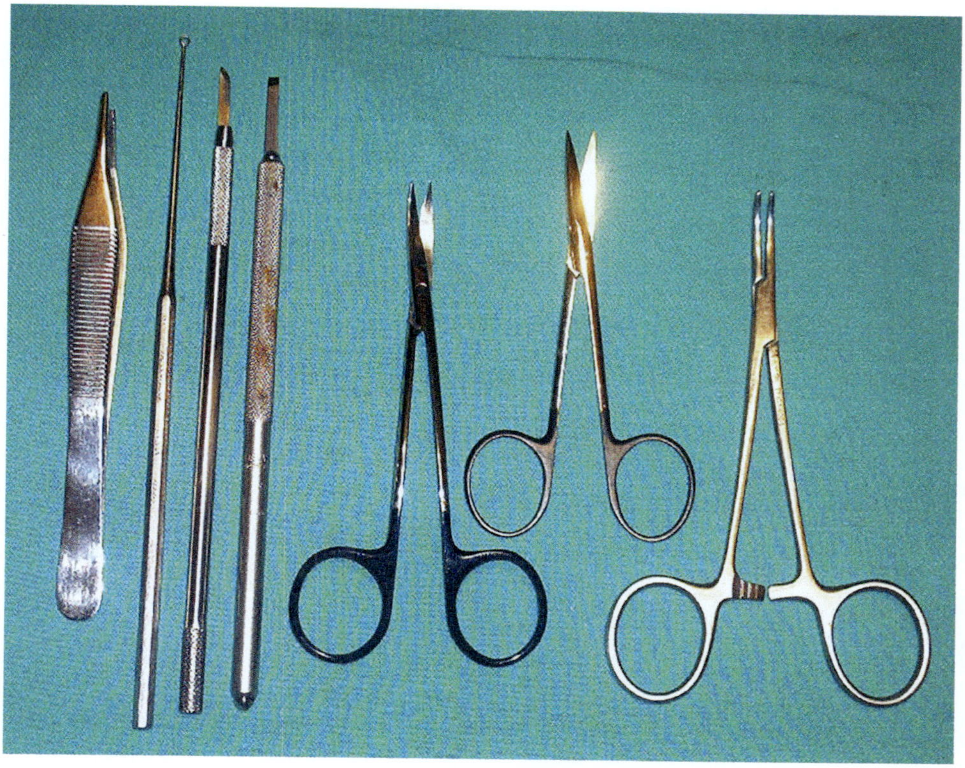

Fig. 9.2. Fine end forceps, scalpels with microblades, iris scissors, and mosquito hemostats are useful for biopsy and necropsy procedures on fish. (Photograph by N. Saint-Erne.)

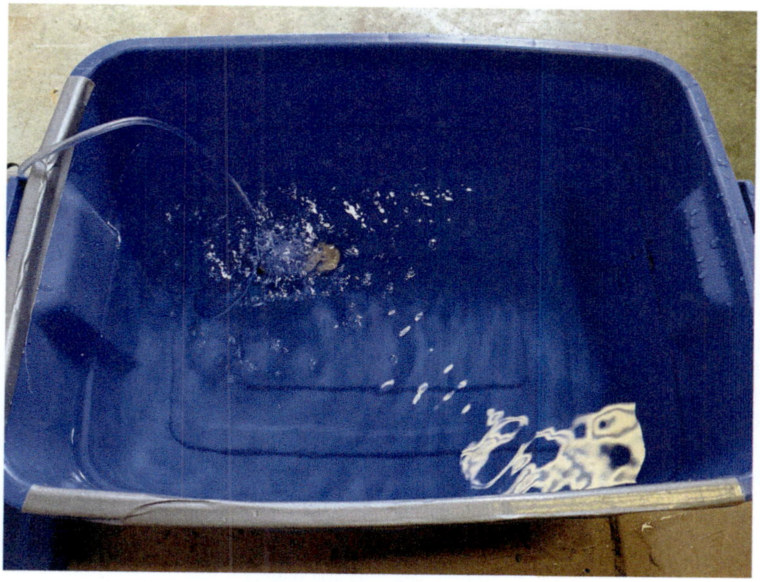

Fig. 9.3. Plastic tubs are more portable and sturdier than glass aquariums. The water should always be aerated using an air pump or water pump. Note the water level volume markings on the right side inside the tub. (Photograph by N. Saint-Erne.)

Table 9.1. Husbandry equipment. Author's own table.

Air pumps
Air tubing and air stone
Assorted glass aquariums
Assorted nets
Assorted plastic totes or boxes
Assorted sizes of plastic fish bags
Commercial dechlorinator and ammonia-neutralizing water conditioner
Rubber bands
Sea salt/non-iodized salt
Sponge filters
Submersible aquarium heaters
Thermometers
Water quality tests
Water sample bottles (plastic, 250 ml)
Water siphon for water changes
5-gallon buckets (Fig. 9.4)

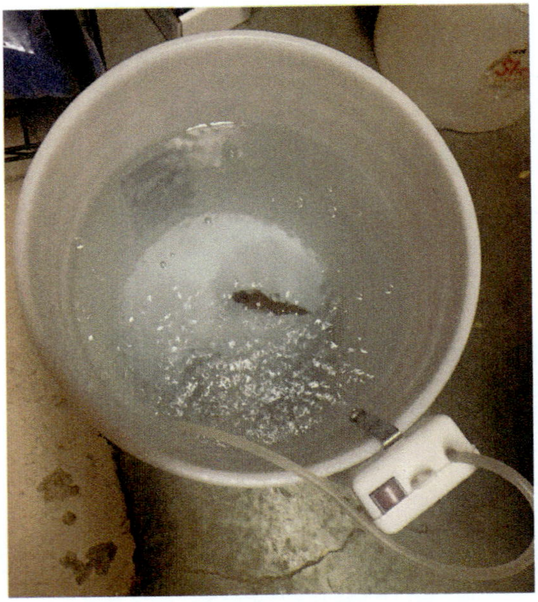

Fig. 9.4. Five-gallon buckets are useful for anesthesia administration prior to examinations. Battery-powered air pumps can aerate the water without needing electrical plugs, making them useful for transporting fish to and from the veterinary hospital as well. (Photograph by N. Saint-Erne.)

Table 9.2. Drugs and other compounds used in ornamental fish medicine. Author's own table.

Alfaxalone
Amikacin
Atropine
Betadine (Povidone iodine)
Calcium gluconate
Ceftazidime
Commercial water dechlorinator
Dexamethasone injectable
Diflubenzuron
EDTA
Enrofloxacin (22.7 mg/ml injectable and tablets)
Epinephrine
Eugenol (clove oil)
Fenbendazole
Florfenicol injectable
Furosemide
Heparin 1000 U
Hydrogen peroxide 3%
Isoflurane
Kanamycin
Lidocaine 2%
Lubricating jelly
Lufenuron
Metronidazole
MS 222 anesthetic, along with baking soda (sodium bicarbonate)
10% neutral buffered formalin
Nitrofurazone
Orabase gel (topical bandage for fish skin)
Ovaprim (injectable hormone to stimulate spawning)
Praziquantel (tablets, powder, and injectable)
Sea Salt/non-iodized salt (sodium chloride)
Silver sulfadiazine cream
Sterile water
Topical antibiotic/anti-inflammatory ointment
Trimethoprim/sulfamethoxazole tablets

Table 9.3. Medical equipment. Author's own table.

Centrifuge
Complete dissecting kit
Compound microscope
Fish anesthesia tub with recirculating setup
Gram scale (up to 1 kg)
Kilogram scale (up to 10 kg)
Ophthalmoscope/slit lamp/otoscope
Oxygen tank with regulator and hoses
Refractometer
Scalpel blades, especially microblades
Sterile surgical instrument pack
Suture removal scissors (useful for performing gill tip biopsies)

Table 9.4. Diagnostic materials. Author's own table.

Assorted hypodermic needle sizes (18 g, 20 g, 22 g, 25 g)
Assorted red rubber catheters (5–12 French)
Assorted suture material
Assorted syringes (1 cc, 3 cc, 6 cc, 12 cc, 35 cc, 60 cc) with Luer lock or catheter tip
Blood collection tubes: red top (clot tube), green (heparin), yellow (acid citrate dextrose)
Cover slips (glass or plastic)
Culturettes (minitip, portacult, regular, ARD bottle)
Fluorescein strips
Gauze pads (2 × 2 and 4 × 4)
Microcentrifuge
Microhematocrit tubes with putty to seal end
Microscope slides
Non-sterile gloves
Paper towels
Plastic pipettes
Tongue depressors
Wet wipes

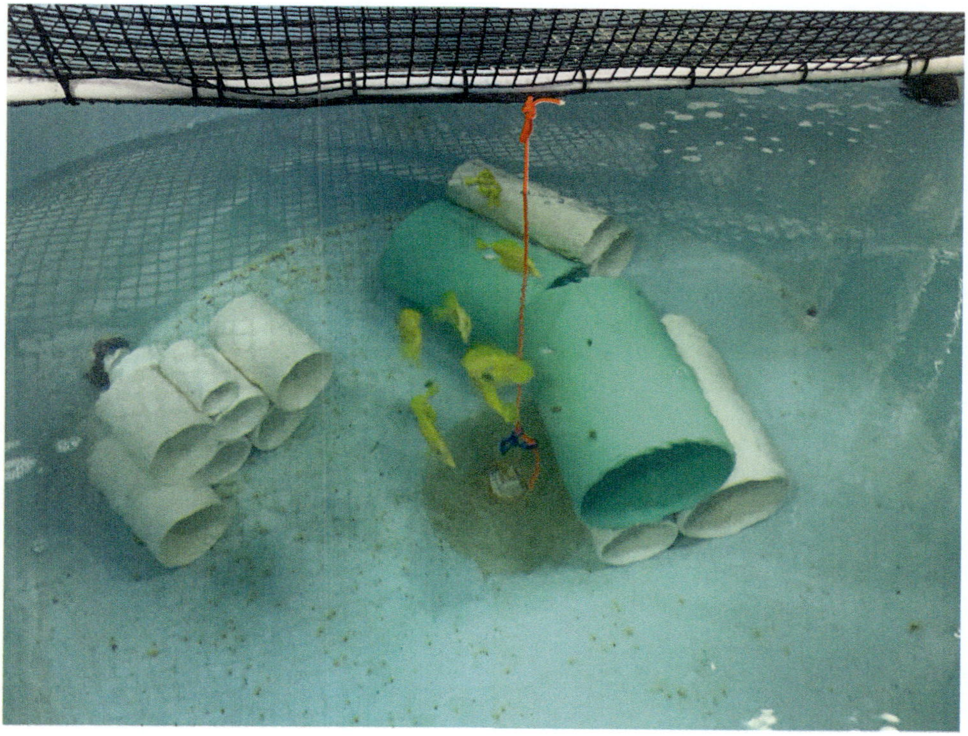

Fig. 9.5. Yellow tangs (*Zebrasoma flavescens*) in a bare quarantine tank with various sizes of PVC tubes for hiding shelters. Using PVC tubes is an easy way to give fish shelter but still keep the tank easy to treat and clean. Note the netting that can be closed over the top of the tank to prevent the fish from jumping out. (Photograph by N. Saint-Erne.)

References

Lewbart, G.A. (2009) Equipment and supplies. In: Lewbart, G.A. (ed.) *Fish Medicine Handbook*. Zoological Education Network, West Palm Beach, Florida, pp. 49–51.

Lewbart, G.A. and Yanong, R.P.E. (2022) Fish. In: Carpenter, J.W. and Harms, C. (eds) *Exotic Animal Formulary*. 6th edn. Elsevier, St. Louis, Missouri, pp. 16–52.

Noga, E.J. (2010) Equipping a fish disease diagnostic facility. In: Noga, E.J. (ed.) *Fish Disease Diagnosis and Treatment*. 2nd edn. Blackwell Publishing, Ames, Iowa, p. 13.

Roberts, H.E. (2010) Transport and hospitalization of the fish patient. In: Roberts, H.E. (ed.) *Fundamentals of Ornamental Fish Health*. Blackwell Publishing, Ames, Iowa, pp. 153–157.

10 Clinical Procedures

Robert Martinez

Aquatic Veterinary Consulting, PLLC, Salt Lake City, Utah, USA

Abstract

Collecting a history and then performing physical examinations and diagnostic tests are just as important with fish as with other animals. However, with fish in an aquatic environment, testing the water quality parameters must be done to ensure that the fish will recover with the administered medications. Treating the fish without correcting the water quality will not likely improve the health of the fish. Fish can be treated with medications like those used in other animal species, but in addition to injections and oral medications, they can be treated through the aquatic environment by adding medications to the water.

10.1 Practicing Veterinary Medicine on Ornamental Fish

Practicing veterinary medicine on fish is similar to the approach used in other companion animal species, the major difference being the environment that fish occupy, which can be a cause of added stress to some veterinarians on how to approach a fish case. Another challenge is the fish owner who most likely has done their own research and applied treatments prior to contacting a veterinarian. Regardless of these challenges, a systematic approach to working up a fish case is the same as in small and large animal medicine.

The clinical approach includes (but is not limited to) history, water quality testing, observation/physical exam, clinical procedures, diagnostic tests/interpretation, treatment, and post-mortem examination. What will be required of the veterinarian is a further understanding of basic husbandry and the environment of the species being examined. A thorough history is necessary to fully understand the issue that is occurring with an individual or group of fish (Table 10.1). Stoskopf (2010) elegantly stated, "It is usually easier to learn something by listening than by talking."

Learning how to obtain a proper history and ask appropriate questions takes experience and skill. One way to obtain an initial history is via a history form/template with stock questions regarding the husbandry (number of fish and species, size of aquarium or pond), water quality and filtration method, history of disease, treatment performed, feeding routine, additions of new fish, and other pertinent information. These forms can be created for the fish species with which you tend to work. The information obtained from the history will hopefully help determine acute or chronic disease processes and allow you to begin building a differential diagnosis list.

Water quality analysis is important in understanding the environment in which the patient is living. The results of water tests could explain certain behaviors noted or could indicate abnormal levels that cause the stress that allowed for the disease process to begin. Treating the fish without considering how to improve or correct the water quality issue is only addressing half of the issue. Proper water quality is often the best treatment. Evaluation of the filtration system is important in understanding the water quality of the aquarium or pond, and the reasons water quality test results may not be in the appropriate ranges.

Another consideration in fish medicine is in-clinic examination versus home visits. A home visit will provide information that may have been missed or possibly deemed unimportant by the owner. The ability to observe the patient in their environment and to examine the life support system is also

Corresponding author: drrobmartinez@aquaticvetconsulting.com

© CAB International 2025. *The Handbook of Ornamental Fish Health and Welfare* (ed. N. Saint-Erne)
DOI: 10.1079/9781789246032.0010

Table 10.1. Recording a thorough history. Author's own table.

- Species of affected fish, age, size, weight, gender, number affected
- How many fish and what species are in the habitat
- Disease signs—lesions or abnormal behavior
- Are the fish alive (moribund) or dead; if dead, when did they die, or were euthanized?
- What are the environmental conditions?
    - Aquarium or pond size
    - Substrate
    - Filtration system
    - Water quality
    - Recent water changes or treatments
- Diet, nutritional condition
- Reproductive status
- Previous history of diseases

advantageous. Another advantage is the decreased stress involved with transporting a fish patient to and from the clinic. Although home visits do require flexibility, time commitment, traveling, and, at times, a higher financial investment from the owner and the veterinarian, in-clinic examinations are still valuable, especially for certain diagnostic tests that cannot be performed tank/pond side, such as radiology or sonography. Also, based on the home visit examination, it may be determined that certain procedures are necessary that require transport to the veterinary clinic anyway (Butcher, 1996).

10.2 Handling and Examination

Examination of the fish patient is typically more involved when compared to other companion animals. The process of the exam is separated into three parts: environmental exam, indirect exam, and direct exam (Roberts, 2010). Depending on the case, these can be mutually exclusive, but a full exam should utilize all three parts.

The environmental aspects to be considered are the water quality and the life support systems (aeration and filtration). If possible, home visits to evaluate the fish in its aquarium can be invaluable. Water quality parameters—including temperature, pH, hardness, alkalinity, ammonia, nitrite, and nitrate—should be checked during the exam. If the owners have been monitoring water quality (Fig. 10.1), consider checking parameters that the owner did not evaluate, such as dissolved oxygen, alkalinity, salinity, or chlorine (Roberts, 2010). Check that their life support system is correctly arranged and adequately sized for the specific fish species and size of the aquarium, assess the condition of the filter system, and discuss the cleaning schedule and maintenance procedures. Educate the owners on the importance of maintenance of the filtration system, proper disinfecting and sterilization of equipment, and monitoring water quality parameters in the quarantine or treatment tanks. As mentioned before, home visits are not always feasible, so the client should be encouraged to provide photos of the aquarium and filtration system or provide a diagram of the life support system and ancillary equipment when coming into the clinic (Roberts, 2010). The owners can use their cell phones to take videos of specific behaviors and email them to the veterinarian.

An indirect exam of the fish or group of fish in their environment is the next step. It is important to examine the entire picture in front of you. Pay attention to the entire fish community in the aquarium and how they interact (Stoskopf, 2010). Observe their behavior in the aquarium. Are they congregating in a certain area of a pond? Are they swimming normally or abnormally? Where is their position in the water column? Are they utilizing the entire tank or staying to one side or aggregating at the top or bottom (Figs 10.2a and b)? Any flashing (Fig. 10.3) noticed? Any piping at the surface (Fig. 10.4)? Are there more than one fish affected? What is the location of the lesions? Do they still have an appetite (Lewbart, 2001; Roberts, 2010; Stoskopf, 2010)? These observations will provide further insight and hopefully explain the associations of the findings noted in the direct examination.

A direct physical exam can be performed once the fish is placed in an appropriately sized container. Some fish will be amenable to handling, though handling can be stressful. Sedation may be necessary to minimize stress during handling (Fig. 10.5) and minimize further injury (Roberts, 2010). Also,

Daily Water Quality Log

Week ending________________ Store #____________ Keep completed logs for six months.

All readings must be done manually. Do not use readings from Aquaguard or probes.
If water quality is outside normal limits, retest to ensure accuracy. After retesting, if results are still outside normal limits. contact the Pet Care or Store Manager immediately.

Main System	Normal Limits	Mon.	Tues.	Wed.	Thurs.	Fri.	Sat.	Sun.
		op.[x] / cl.[x]	op.[x] / cl.[x]	op.[x] / cl.[x]	op.[x] / cl.[x]	op.[x] / cl.[x]	op.[x] / cl.[x]	op.[x] / cl.[x]
Temperature	76–78 F (24–26 C)	/	/	/	/	/	/	/
Ammonia	0 – 0.25 mg/L	/	/	/	/	/	/	/
Chlorine	0 mg/L	/	/	/	/	/	/	/
Nitrate	0 – 40 mg/L	/	/	/	/	/	/	/
Nitrite	0 – 0.5 mg/L	/	/	/	/	/	/	/
Hardness	75–150 mg/L (ppm)	/	/	/	/	/	/	/
Alkalinity	80–180 mg/L (ppm)	/	/	/	/	/	/	/
pH	6.8 – 8.4	/	/	/	/	/	/	/
Salinity	0.2%	/	/	/	/	/	/	/
Number of Cups of Salt Added to Sump		/	/	/	/	/	/	/

Comet System	Normal Limits	Mon.	Tues.	Wed.	Thurs.	Fri.	Sat.	Sun.
		op.[x] / cl.[x]	op.[x] / cl.[x]	op.[x] / cl.[x]	op.[x] / cl.[x]	op.[x] / cl.[x]	op.[x] / cl.[x]	op.[x] / cl.[x]
Temperature	65–70 F (18–21 C)	/	/	/	/	/	/	/
Ammonia	0 – 0.25 mg/L	/	/	/	/	/	/	/
Chlorine	0 mg/L	/	/	/	/	/	/	/
Nitrate	0 – 40 mg/L	/	/	/	/	/	/	/
Nitrite	0 – 0.5 mg/L	/	/	/	/	/	/	/
Hardness	75–150 mg/L (ppm)	/	/	/	/	/	/	/
Alkalinity	80–180 mg/L (ppm)	/	/	/	/	/	/	/
pH	6.8 – 8.4	/	/	/	/	/	/	/
Salinity	0.2%	/	/	/	/	/	/	/
Number of Cups of Salt Added to Sump		/	/	/	/	/	/	/

Koi Pond	Normal Limits	Mon.	Tues.	Wed.	Thurs.	Fri.	Sat.	Sun.
(write N/A if not currently displayed)		op.[x] / cl.[x]	op.[x] / cl.[x]	op.[x] / cl.[x]	op.[x] / cl.[x]	op.[x] / cl.[x]	op.[x] / cl.[x]	op.[x] / cl.[x]
Temperature	65–70 F (18–21 C)	/	/	/	/	/	/	/
Ammonia	0 – 0.25 mg/L	/	/	/	/	/	/	/
Chlorine	0 mg/L	/	/	/	/	/	/	/
Nitrate	0 – 40 mg/L	/	/	/	/	/	/	/
Nitrite	0 – 0.5 mg/L	/	/	/	/	/	/	/
Hardness	75–150 mg/L (ppm)	/	/	/	/	/	/	/
Alkalinity	80–180 mg/L (ppm)	/	/	/	/	/	/	/
pH	6.8 – 8.4	/	/	/	/	/	/	/
Salinity	0.2%	/	/	/	/	/	/	/
Number of Cups of Salt Added		/	/	/	/	/	/	/
Opening and Closing Manager initial daily that the water tests are complete:		/	/	/	/	/	/	/

Notes Section:

File with Opening & Closing Checklists. * Test and record results at opening and closing.

Fig. 10.1. Water quality log used in a fish store. (Photograph by N. Saint-Erne.)

sedation should be considered with species of fish that have sharp spines, venomous barbs, sharp teeth, or are aggressive (Noga, 2010; Roberts, 2010). Tricaine methanesulfonate, MS-222, is the only US Food and Drug Administration-approved anesthetic for food fish (Roberts, 2010).

Once the patient is sedated, it is recommended to handle and palpate the patient with gloves to

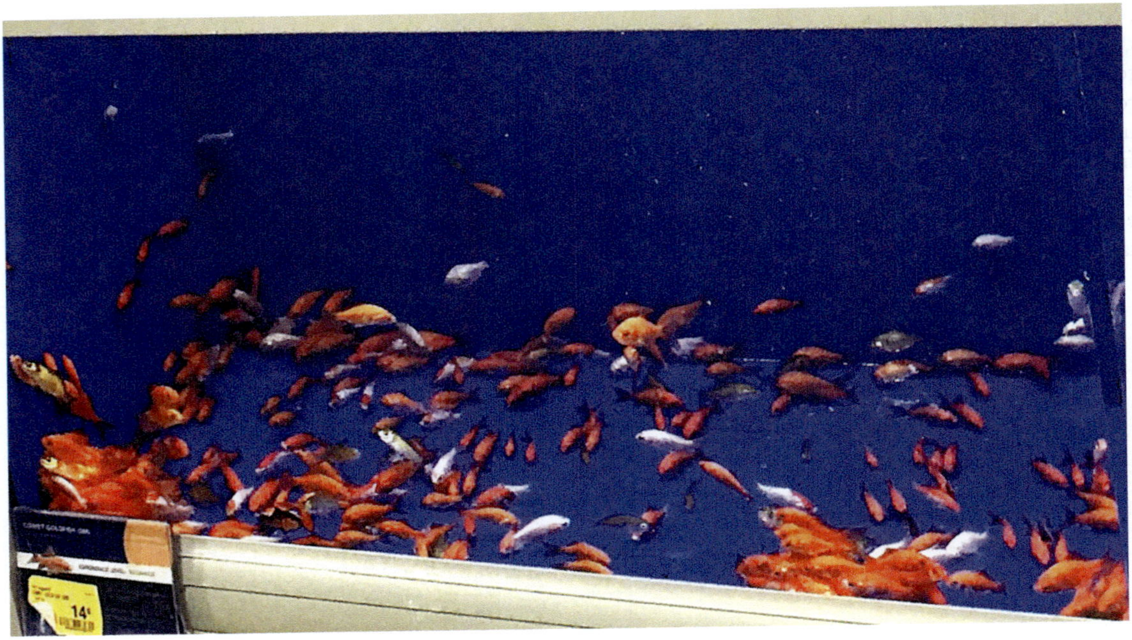

Fig. 10.2a. The abnormal position of goldfish (*Carassius auratus*) huddling near the bottom of the aquarium indicates a problem with the fish or water quality. (Photograph by N. Saint-Erne.)

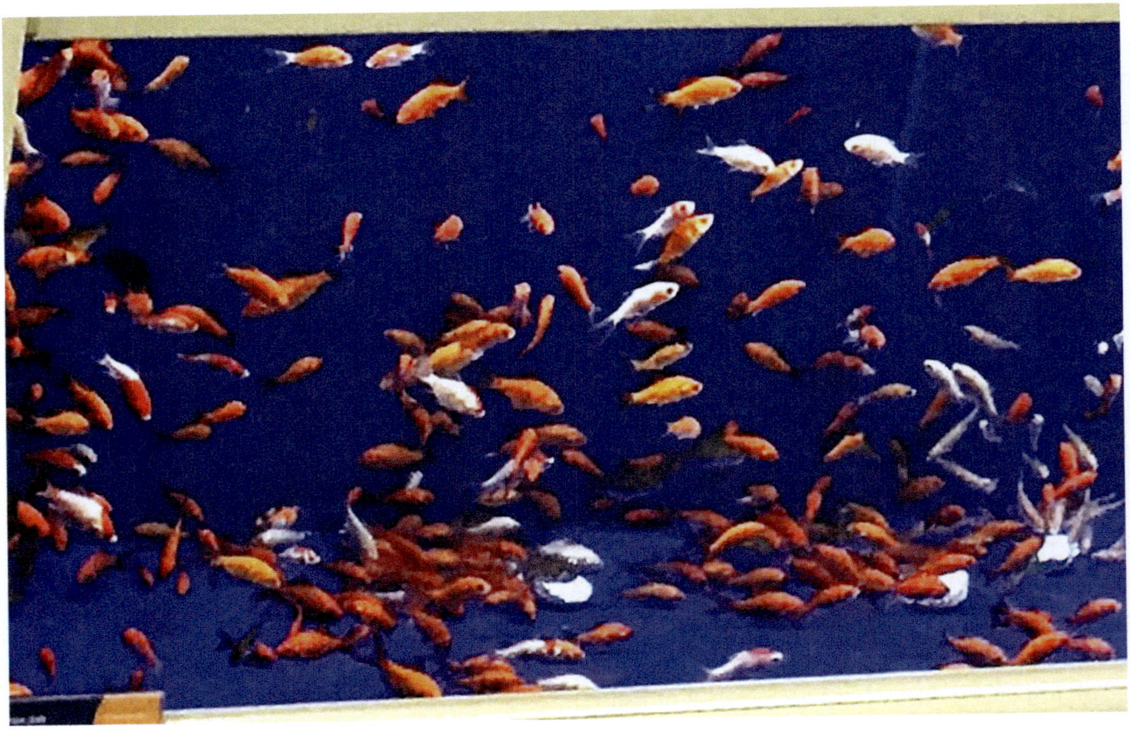

Fig. 10.2b. The same goldfish are swimming normally 9 min later, after adjusting the water flow to provide more surface aeration. (Photograph by N. Saint-Erne.)

protect the mucous layer or slime coat. Either keep the fish in the small water container or, if they need to be removed from the water, keep the skin moist to prevent desiccation. You can achieve this by using moist cloths or pouring tank water over the fish occasionally if they are out of the water for an extended period. Also, consider performing the exam over the container of water in case of accidental drop or fall. Dr Stoskopf says he holds his breath during the examination and will return the fish back to the water when he needs to breathe. This allows him to perform his examinations in 2–3 min, breaking at 45–60-s intervals to let the fish respire (Stoskopf, 2010).

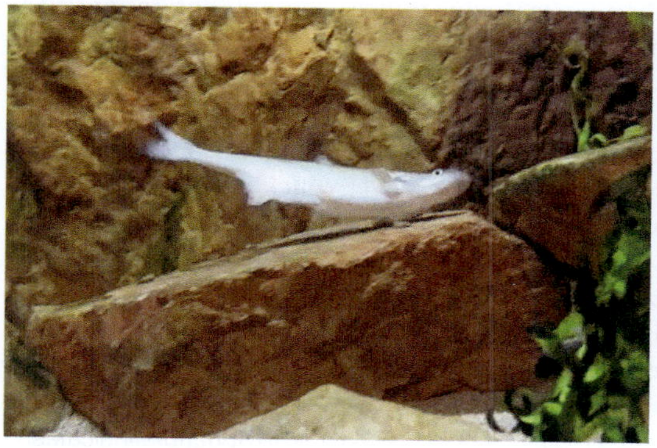

Fig. 10.3. Humpback chub (*Gila cypha*) flashing its light-colored belly, as it rubs its body against a rock in its aquarium. (Photograph by N. Saint-Erne.)

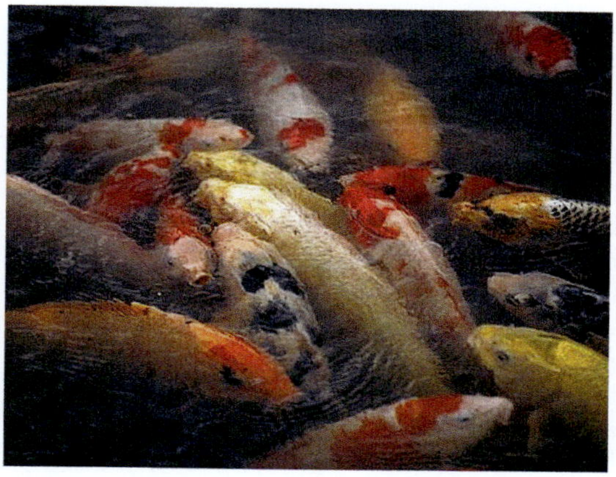

Fig. 10.4. Koi (*Cyprinus rubrofuscus*) piping, or gulping air at the surface of the water, especially if near a waterfall or water inlet, is a sign of low oxygen or other water quality problems that can affect respiration. (Photograph by N. Saint-Erne.)

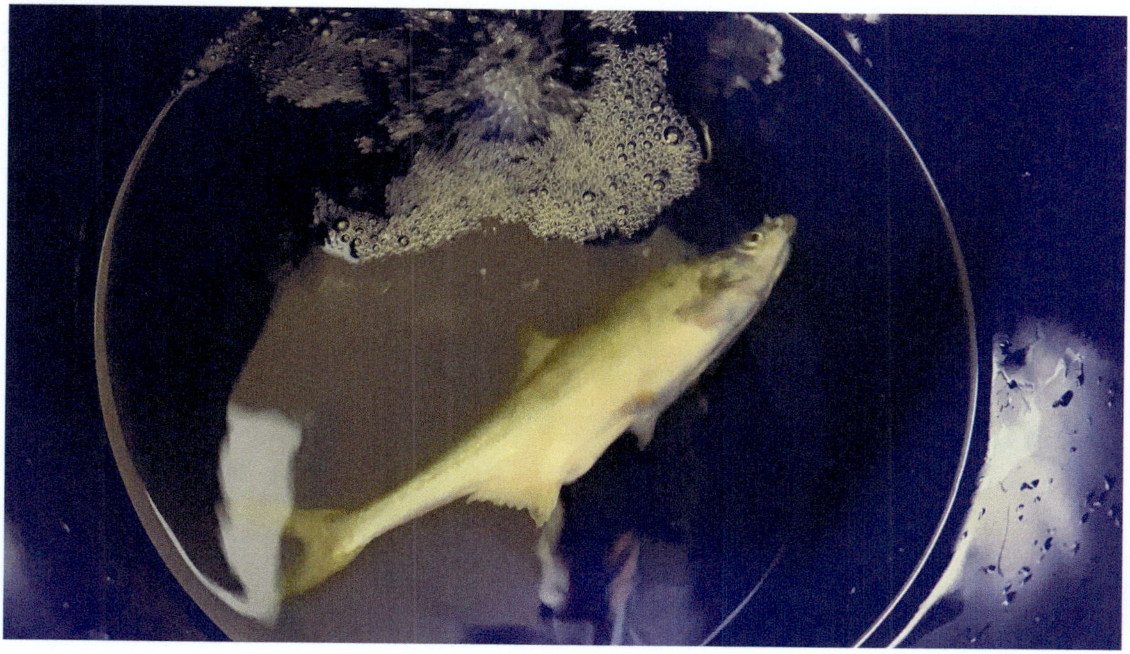

Fig. 10.5. Humpback chub (*G. cypha*) in an aerated, plastic five-gallon bucket being tranquilized using MS-222 anesthetic. (Photograph by N. Saint-Erne.)

A systematic and methodical approach should be used on all fish patients. Most veterinarians would advocate for the head-to-tail method of physical examination to be as thorough as possible (Lewbart, 2001; Roberts, 2010). Evaluate the fish's general body condition and appearance. While the patient is sedated, obtain its weight using an appropriate gram scale (Fig. 10.6) and measure its body length. Length can be measured as total length (snout to the tip of the tail in its normal position) or standard length (snout to the end of the body at the base of the caudal fin) to make up for the variation in caudal fin length in some species (Lewbart, 2001). Assess the body condition score to determine if the fish is normal, underweight, or overweight. Underweight fish have a triangular appearance in cross section due to decreased epaxial muscle mass with visible vertebral processes, and the head may appear too large for the body (Lewbart, 2001). Swollen or abnormally large abdomens in fish may be due to retained coelomic fluid, breeding season, air accumulation, abdominal fat, or a coelomic mass (Lewbart, 2001). While sedated, the body should be gently flexed and manipulated to assess for any rigidity or spinal deformities.

The skin is the largest organ on the fish (Lewbart, 2001). It is recommended to use powder-free latex gloves when handling fish during examination. Evaluate all skin surfaces (dorsal, ventral, and lateral) for external lesions, ectoparasites, discoloration, or abnormalities. Melanin pigmentation in a fish's skin is under neuroendocrine control and is affected by hormones (Noga, 2010). When a fish is sick or stressed, maintenance of normal pigmentation presumably takes less precedence compared to other vital body systems (Noga, 2010). Fish, when sick or stressed, can have either a paler or darker than normal appearance. These discolorations can also be localized based on focal tissue irritation and nerve damage. For example, ectoparasites can elicit thickening of the skin leading to a whitish or bluish color (Noga, 2010). Reddening of the body is usually due to hemorrhage, which can be a result of systemic bacterial or viral infections.

The fins consist of supportive bony spines and softer cartilage rays, connected by a thin layer of epithelial tissue. Lesions and parasites often are easier to notice on the fins. Therefore, a fin biopsy is recommended during clinical work-up (Lewbart, 2001). Also, many owners will first notice erosion or reddening of the fins before other clinical signs. Fins should be flared open, in a normal position, and the fish should be using them normally to

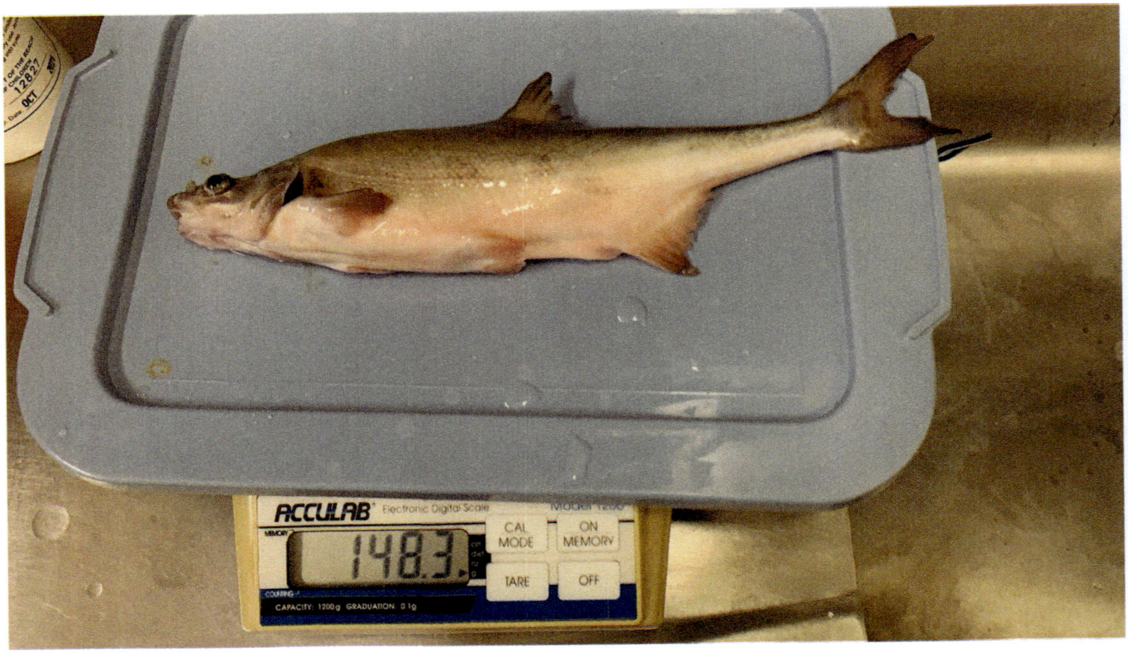

Fig. 10.6. Humpback chub (*G. cypha*) being weighed on a plastic lid being used for an examination tray. (Photograph by N. Saint-Erne.)

swim through the water. If the fins are clamped, held close to the body wall, or not being used normally, this can be an indication of systemic disease, stress, parasites, or even poor water quality (Roberts, 2010).

The mouth should be evaluated with a light/headlamp or an otoscope in smaller fish (Roberts, 2010). Also, using a tongue depressor or blunt spatula to aid in opening the oral cavity helps to visualize lesions or foreign bodies in the mouth (Lewbart, 2001). Care should be taken with fish that have sharp teeth. When opening the oral cavity, take note of any instability or fractures of the jaws caused by trauma. Foreign objects, such as pebbles or gravel, can get caught in the pharynx of fish and fish that are not eating or have difficulty breathing should have the oral cavity examined.

The eyes can be evaluated using an ophthalmoscope, penlight, or flashlight. The size and shape of the globes should be identical, unless enlarged eyes are specific to that breed of fish (Lewbart, 2001). Enophthalmos is associated with emaciation and exophthalmos (Fig. 10.7) can be associated with systemic disease or trauma (Noga, 2010). When either of these issues are noted, determine whether it is unilateral or bilateral. The corneas should be clear and symmetrical. Corneal lipidosis can occur in fish given feed containing high levels of cholesterol. An ophthalmoscope can be used to evaluate the intraocular structures and retina (Lewbart, 2001). The eye can be evaluated for abnormalities such as parasites, air/gas bubbles, hyphema, hypopyon, corneal edema, cataracts, or other lesions (Roberts, 2010). Fluorescein stain can be used on the eyes to check for corneal ulcers.

The gills can be evaluated by gently lifting the operculum with a thumb or forceps (Fig. 10.8). When lifting the operculum, evaluate for any lesions, masses, or abnormalities along the external or internal surface of the operculum. Most fish have four gill arches, and gill rakers are located at the base of each gill arch (Lewbart, 2001). The gill lamellae should appear dark red, with no mottling, masses, ragged edges, necrosis, or mucous covering (Roberts, 2010). A gill tip biopsy is recommended during clinical work-up.

The abdomen should be palpated and percussed, especially if there is any coelomic swelling (Lewbart, 2001). Palpation will allow you to detect fluid, masses, foreign bodies, swelling, or air/gas accumulation.

The vent is the one external opening for the elimination of fecal and urinary waste, as well as reproductive products (Lewbart, 2001). The vent should be evaluated for inflammation, swelling, protrusion, and the presence of endoparasites. Also, abnormal feces can be associated with gastrointestinal disease

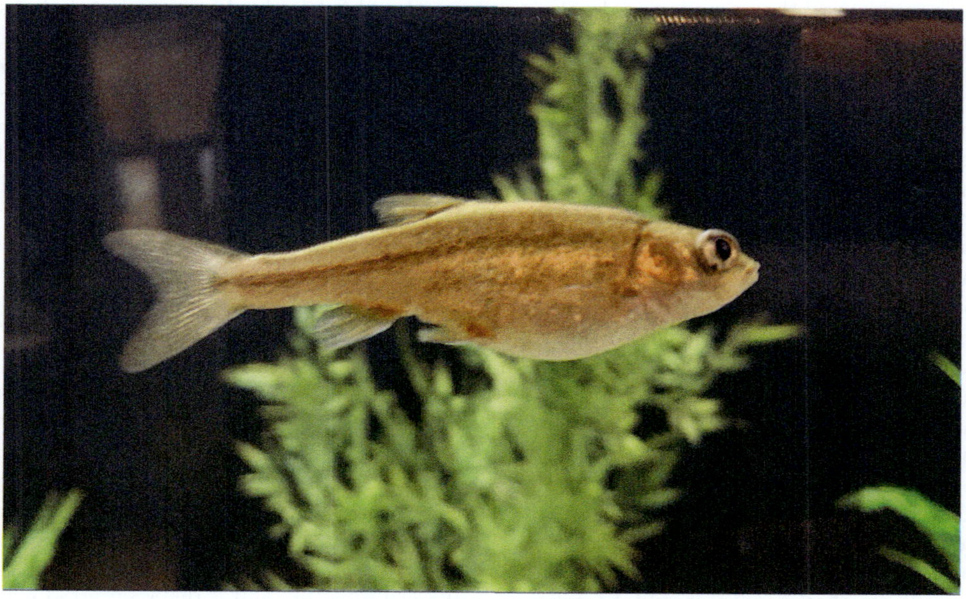

Fig. 10.7. A Sonora Chub (*Gila ditaenia*) with exophthalmos. (Photograph by N. Saint-Erne.)

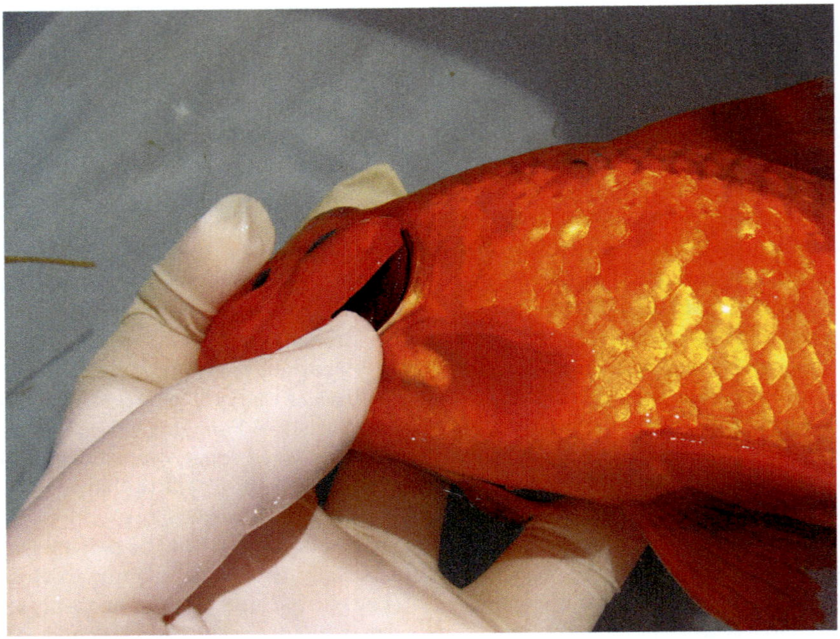

Fig. 10.8. Examination of a goldfish's (*C. auratus*) gills. (Photograph by N. Saint-Erne.)

(Lewbart, 2001). Feces should be collected during the examination, if possible, for microscopic analysis.

10.3 Diagnostic Tests

After the examination, the next step is deciding the diagnostic tests that will help further the investigation. Baseline procedures to consider as a part of the physical exam are a skin mucus scrape (Fig. 10.9), fin edge clip, and gill tip biopsy (Fig. 10.10). Further diagnostics beyond these have their advantages and disadvantages. Hematology and biochemistry, for example, will give you further insight, though depending on the species of fish, there may not be any reference ranges to compare to conspecifics. Imaging, such as radiographs (Fig. 10.11) and ultrasound, will give specific visualizations to help diagnose certain diseases. Also, if available advanced imaging, such as CT/MRI, can be pursued, though this modality is not always readily available or affordable by the client.

Necropsies should be performed on recently deceased fish (Fig. 10.12), and euthanasia of moribund fish can be considered in a community tank where there is a disease outbreak. Careful notes as well as photographs should be taken when performing a necropsy (Table 10.2). Necropsies can be performed tank side and samples saved to be submitted for cytology, histopathology, bacterial culture, or other diagnostic testing. Another consideration is sacrificing a moribund fish and submitting the whole fish to a lab for necropsy and further testing. Practicing veterinary medicine in ornamental fish is like treating our companion animal species. Of course, there are differences that need to be considered and understood to properly diagnose and treat fish patients. Many fish owners consider the fish to be pets and would not be willing to sacrifice a fish for diagnostic testing, as you might do in a herd-health situation, or with food fish species.

10.4 Treating Ornamental Fish

Treatment methods of the fish patient are similar to our domestic species. You can administer medications parenterally and orally. However, fish patients can also receive medications by immersion in medicated water, which can be either over a short, specific period (dip) or prolonged for days (bath). Considerations regarding the medications used are the water quality and if the medication will affect

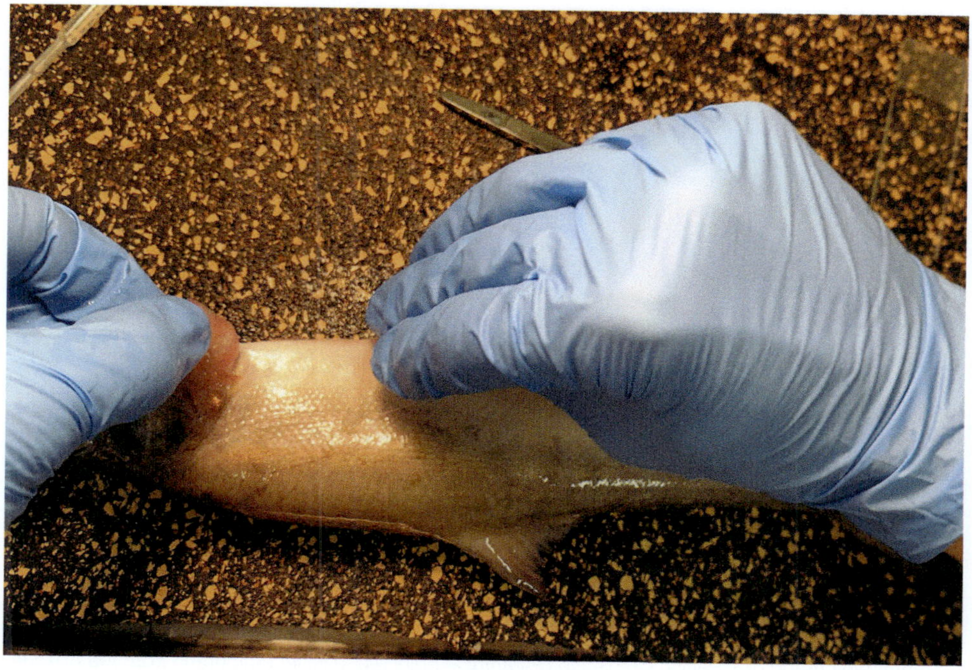

Fig. 10.9. Skin mucus biopsy on a humpback chub (*G. cypha*) using a glass cover slip (in the right hand) to collect the mucus sample. (Photograph by N. Saint-Erne.)

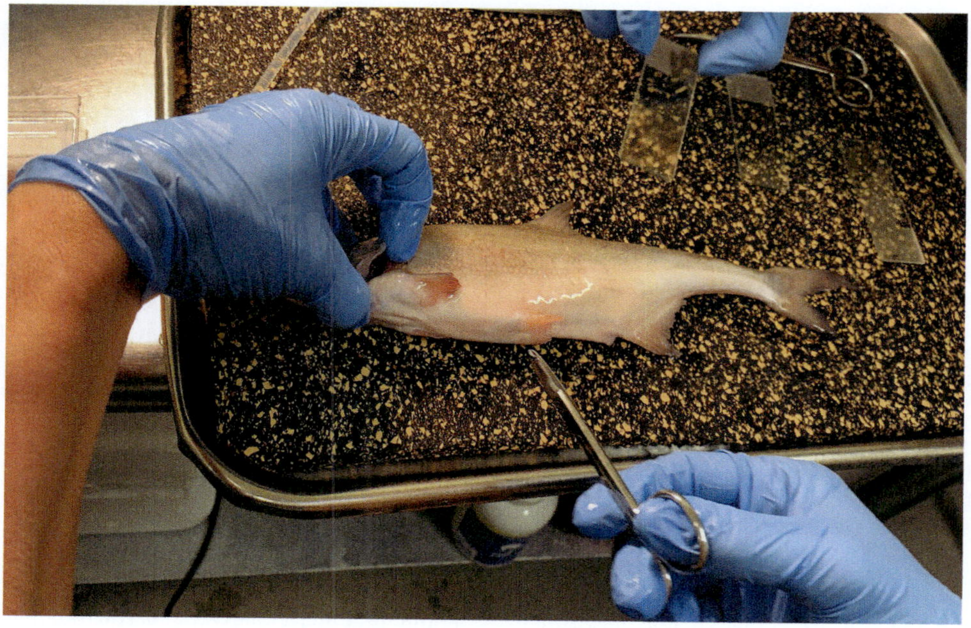

Fig. 10.10. Gill tip biopsy on a humpback chub (*G. cypha*). (Photograph by N. Saint-Erne.)

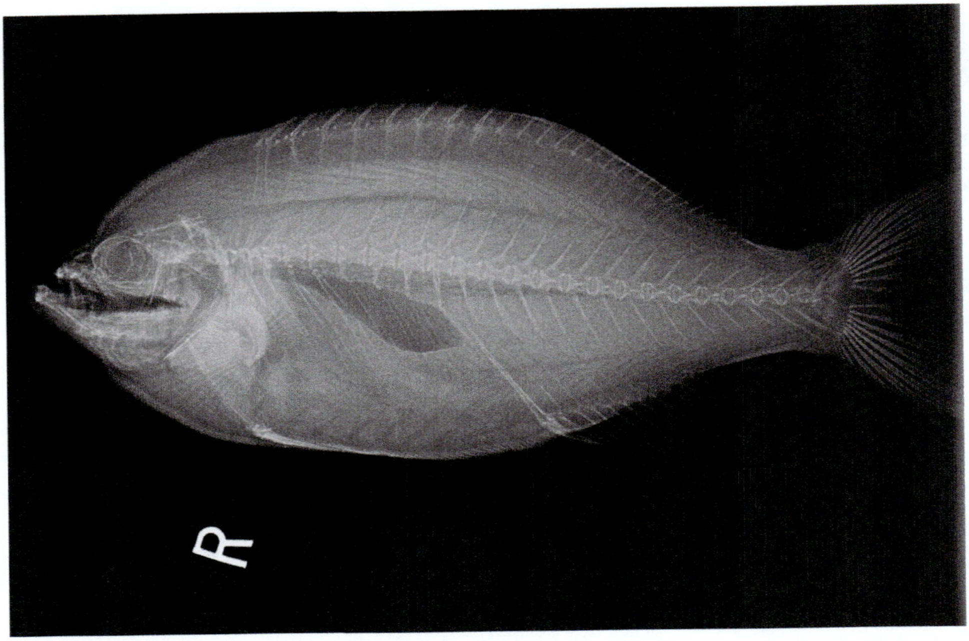

Fig. 10.11. Lateral radiograph of a Pacific Creolefish (*Paranthias colonus*). (Digital radiograph from the Arizona Sonora Desert Museum, Tucson, Arizona.)

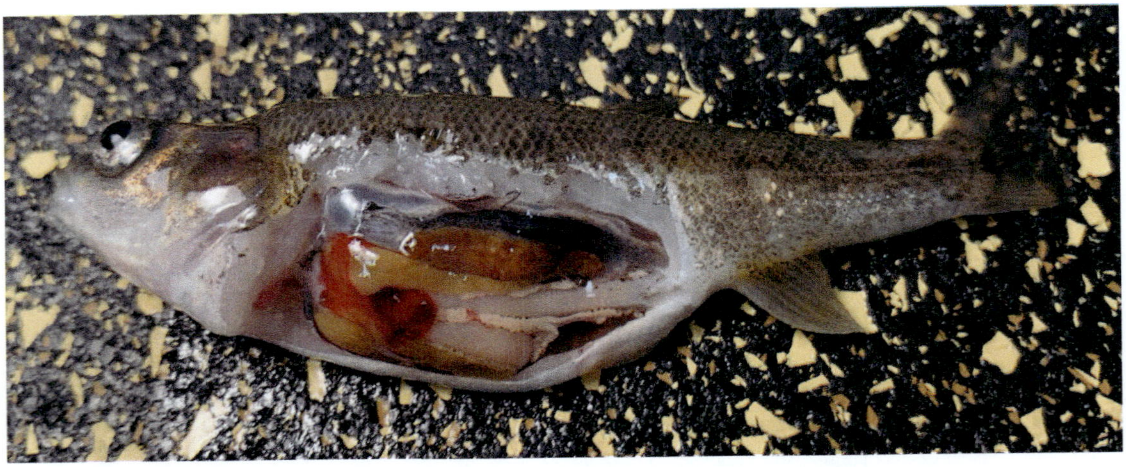

Fig. 10.12. The Sonora Chub (*G. ditaenia*) with exophthalmos and abdominal distension had 1.5 ml of serosanguinous fluid aspirated from its coelom. It was necropsied, and no parasites were seen on microscopic examination. The liver was pale yellow, and many oil droplets were seen on microscopic examination of an organ squash preparation. The diagnosis was fatty liver degeneration (hepatic lipidosis). (Photograph by N. Saint-Erne.)

any of those parameters (e.g. change pH or decrease oxygen), if the fish are eating (if not, medicated food will not be effective unless it is given by tube feeding) and how many fish are you treating. All these factors should be considered to determine what you may use to treat an individual fish, preferably in a quarantine tank, versus treating all the fish in a community aquarium.

In situations where it is not too stressful to handle the fish, topical medications can be used on external wounds (Saint-Erne, 2019). Gently debride open wounds and then swab with povidone-iodine solution and apply an antibiotic cream. This will remove necrotic tissue and reduce bacterial and fungal growth.

If the fish are still eating, medications such as antibiotics can be administered in the food. Aquaflor (Florfenicol) antibiotic is available as a Veterinary Feed Directive medication for adding to fish food and is approved by the FDA. Medicated food can be made with gelatin formulations, or by mixing the medication with the appropriate amount of fish food pellets, then add some egg whites or fish oil and stir together, then spread out in a pan and let dry. Store medicated food in an airtight container in the refrigerator.

Larger fish, such as cichlids, goldfish, and koi, can be injected with antibiotics or other medications. Intramuscular (IM) injections are given in the epaxial muscles along the back (Fig. 10.13),

Table 10.2. Necropsy observations. Author's own table.

- Take notes: small details are easily forgotten
- External Exam: record morphometrics (length and body weight), carcass condition, skin and fin defects/discoloration, lesions (acute or chronic condition)
- Collect sterile samples for bacteriology: tissues usually produce higher yield than effusion
- Make wet mounts for ectoparasite (protozoa, metazoa) examinations
- Collect feces and blood for testing
- Make impression smears of tissues for microscopic cytology
- Examine GI content: quantity and consistency; check for parasites
- Complete tissue set for examination/histopathology: regardless of if normal or not
- Multiple smaller sections are better than a few large sections of tissues
- Tissue sample thickness <1 cm; to be adequately preserved in formalin

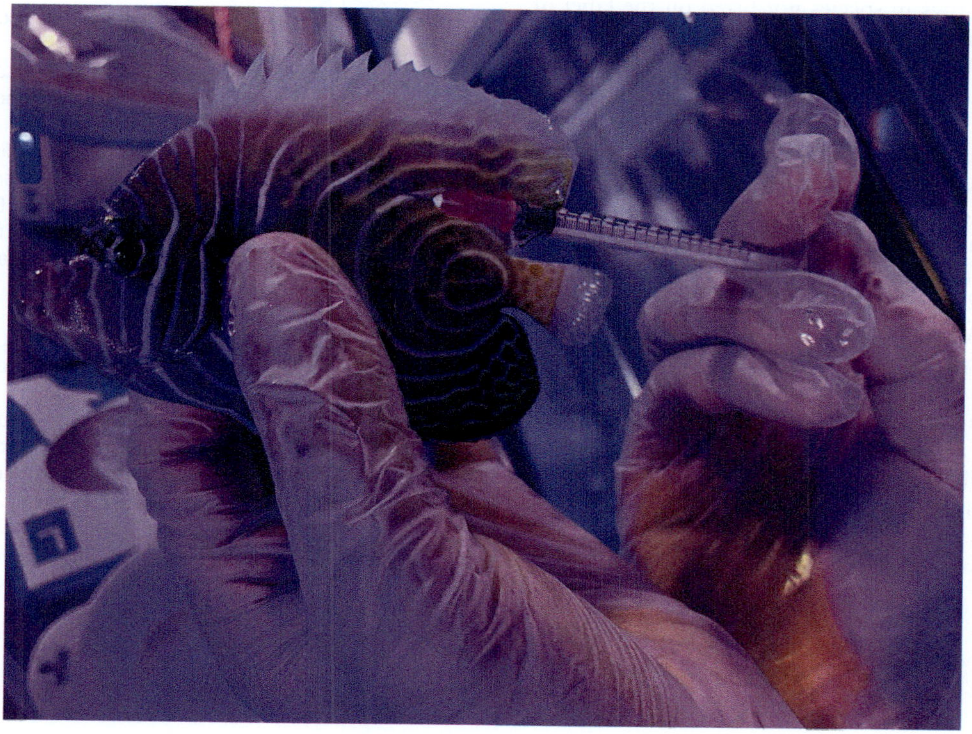

Fig. 10.13. Giving an intramuscular antibiotic injection to an emperor angelfish (*Pomacanthus imperator*). (Photograph by N. Saint-Erne.)

below or immediately behind the dorsal fin. Intracoelomic (ICoe) injections are given on the belly, above and behind the pelvic fin. Intravenous (IV) injections can be given in the caudal vein below the spine in the caudal peduncle. When injecting fish intramuscularly from behind the dorsal fin, direct the needle to the right or left into the epaxial muscle, not straight into the midline. Large volumes can be given by injecting half to the right side, then redirecting the needle and injecting half to the left side muscles. A butterfly catheter extension can be placed between the syringe and needle to prevent tissue trauma while injecting if the fish suddenly reacts, as the needle will move with the fish while the syringe is being held separately from the needle.

The veterinary drugs that are used in fish medicine are largely not approved for use in fish species. In the United States, chemical treatments (drugs) are approved by the US Food and Drug Administration (FDA, 2023), and biological treatments (vaccines) are approved for use by the US Department of Agriculture (USDA Approved Biologicals, 2023). Using approved human or animal drugs in species not listed on the label of the medication, or in a manner inconsistent with the label instructions, is considered Extra-Label Drug Use (ELDU). Extra-label drug use is permitted only by, or on the order of, a licensed veterinarian when a valid veterinarian-client-patient relationship exists. Be aware that examination of the patient and informing the owner that the medications being used are not approved for use in ornamental fish is important. There are many drugs available for use in ornamental fish that are not FDA approved for use in any species, so they do not qualify as ELDU. These drugs should not be used in fish produced for food. Follow label directions carefully on fish medications and be sure of accurate water volume measurement to ensure the medication is not being overdosed or underdosed.

10.5 Conclusion

Practicing fish medicine utilizes a combination of pet medicine and herd-health management practices. Some ornamental fish are very valuable individually and should be treated as any pet patient would be, while in other cases, the individual fish in an aquarium is less important than the whole collection of fish, and the owner may be willing to have a fish examined for diagnostic purposes to determine the best treatment for the other fish. Using all the equipment and medications available to a veterinary practice will help to better diagnose and treat our fish patients.

References

Butcher, R.L. (1996) General approach. In: Wildgoose, W.H. (ed.) *BSAVA Manual of Ornamental Fish*. 2nd edn. British Small Animal Veterinary Association, Quedgeley, UK, pp. 63–67.

FDA (2023) Approved aquaculture drugs. Available at: https://www.fda.gov/animal-veterinary/aquaculture/approved-aquaculture-drugs (accessed 5 March 2023).

Lewbart, G.A. (2001) Clinical examination. In: Wildgoose, W.H. (ed.) *BSAVA Manual of Ornamental Fish*. 2nd edn. British Small Animal Veterinary Association, Quedgeley, UK, pp. 85–89.

Noga, E.J. (2010) The physical exam. In: Noga, E.J. (ed.) *Fish Disease Diagnosis and Treatment*. 2nd edn. Blackwell, Ames, Iowa, pp. 17–20.

Roberts, H.E. (2010) Physical examination of fish. In: Roberts, H.E. (ed.) *Fundamentals of Ornamental Fish Health*. Blackwell, Ames, Iowa, pp. 161–165.

Saint-Erne, N. (2019) Therapeutics in ornamental fish. In: Smith, S.A. (ed.) *Fish Diseases and Medicine*. CRC Press, Boca Raton, Florida, pp. 344–347.

Stoskopf, M.K. (2010) Clinical examination and procedures. In: Stoskopf, M.K. (ed.) *Fish Medicine*. Vol. 1, 2nd edn. ART Sciences LLC, Apex, North Carolina, pp. 62–78.

USDA Approved Biologicals (2023) Veterinary biological products. Available at: https://www.aphis.usda.gov/animal_health/vet_biologics/publications/currentprodcodebook.pdf (accessed 5 March 2023).

11 Diagnostic Tests

AZUREEN ERDMAN

New River, Arizona

Abstract

Examining tissue samples taken from patients to obtain diagnostic information refers to the field of clinical pathology. Samples can be taken from the environment (water, substrate, biofilm), or from the fish's skin, fins, gills, feces, blood, and internal organs. Microscopic examination or other testing of these tissues will help determine the etiology of a disease.

11.1 Disease Diagnosis

Diseases found in aquatic animal species are not unlike those found in land-dwelling species. They can be classified in the same ways: viral, bacterial, fungal, parasitic, metabolic, neoplastic, genetic, degenerative, traumatic, and toxic. The goal of this chapter is to discuss sample collection from aquatic species for a minimum clinical database to facilitate the diagnosis of different disease processes. A minimum clinical database when working with an aquatic species includes a water quality test, physical exam, skin or mucus sampling, gill biopsy, fin edge biopsy, and fecal exam (Reavill and Roberts, 2007). It is recommended that these clinical tests be used in both screening for disease in newly acquired populations during quarantine, as well as in those individuals who are showing signs of clinical disease. Handling should be kept to a minimum and a physical exam should be performed at the same time as collection of clinical samples to facilitate fewer handling events. Latex, nitrile, or neoprene gloves should always be worn when handling aquatic species to prevent skin abrasions and minimize disruption of their mucous coating. The patient should be suspended within the water, just above the surface, or over a net when being examined. This allows for the patient to fall into a contained safe area with minimal trauma if wriggling out of the handler's grasp during the exam (Noga, 2010).

The equipment needed to perform a minimum clinical database does not require a large financial investment. The equipment is often already present in most veterinary clinics and includes smooth gloves, microscope slides, coverslips, iris scissors or suture removal scissors, a gram scale, a microscope, and a high-quality water testing kit. Sedation should be used based on the patient's status and the clinician's comfort level. Sedation in an MS-222 bath is commonly used in smaller species but is not recommended for very large species, such as sharks, where team members would be submerged in the anesthetic water handling larger species (Wildgoose, 2001). In cases with larger species, a 2-Phenoxyethanol bath or injectable protocols have been recommended. Sedation should always be used if the patient is venomous, poisonous, or a health risk to the handlers. It has been the author's experience that sedation be used with most patients to decrease the stress of handling and decrease the risk of artifact in sample collection. A bath using MS-222 at a concentration of 30–50 mg/l, buffered 1:1 with baking soda (Fig. 11.1), is often adequate to reach a desired plane of sedation for simple diagnostics. This concentration can be titrated up or down based on the clinical status of a patient.

11.2 Water Quality

Perhaps the most important point to remember is that when clinically diagnosing an animal that lives in an aquatic environment you must analyze the environment it lives in. In the private practice set-

Corresponding author: az.erdman@gmail.com

© CAB International 2025. *The Handbook of Ornamental Fish Health and Welfare* (ed. N. Saint-Erne)
DOI: 10.1079/9781789246032.0011

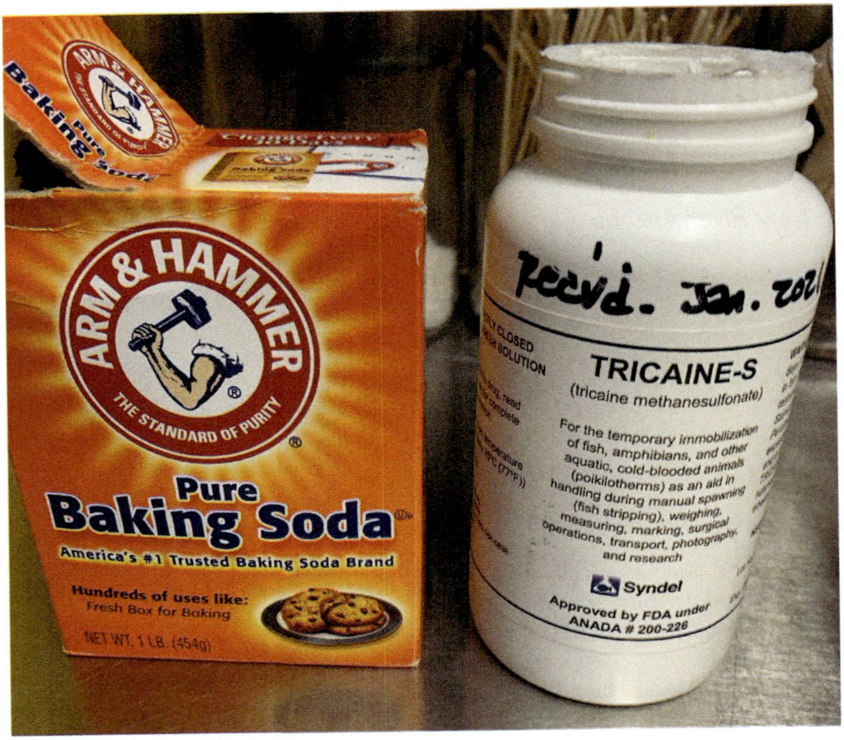

Fig. 11.1. Baking soda is mixed with equal portions of MS-222 powder to buffer the anesthetic solution to prevent it from becoming acidic. (Photograph by N. Saint-Erne.)

ting, it has been the author's experience that a majority of cases present medical problems stemming from issues with water quality. Due to the importance and breadth of information involving water quality, this topic is discussed in Chapter 5. Water quality testing should be performed in the hospital with every aquatic animal exam. Owners and aquarists should be testing water quality at home weekly (Andrews *et al.*, 2010). Temperature should be monitored daily. The hospital water testing kit (Fig. 11.2) should include the following parameters: ammonia, nitrite, nitrate, pH, temperature, hardness, alkalinity, salinity or specific gravity, dissolved oxygen, iron, copper, and phosphate (Brightwell, 2007). When working with elasmobranchs and marine mammals, coliform bacteria levels should also be tested.

11.3 Skin Scrape

A skin scrape, also known as a mucus sample, is indicated for patients showing signs of dermatological disease. Behaviorally, patients may be flashing, swim erratically, or have changes in appetite and energy. Physically a patient could present with ulcerations, discharge, growths, skin or scale color changes, and excess mucus on the skin and the fins.

To collect a mucus sample, use the back side of a scalpel, a microscope coverslip, or a spatula, and scrape the skin in a head-to-tail direction to avoid dislodging scales (Fig. 11.3). Collect two to three samples from along the dorsum, behind the pectoral fin, or along the abdomen. While scraping, perform a superficial scrape to collect a mucus sample without dislodging scales or epithelium. It is not like scraping for *Demodex* on a dog but rather for superficial parasites and bacterial infections. Light pressure is often sufficient to attain a sample (Fig. 11.4). Focus your sampling technique on areas behind fins and the operculum, as these areas are protected from currents while a fish is swimming and will likely yield better samples.

Place the mucus sample on a slide, add a drop of tank water, gently use the coverslip to spread out the mucus by tapping, and then place a coverslip

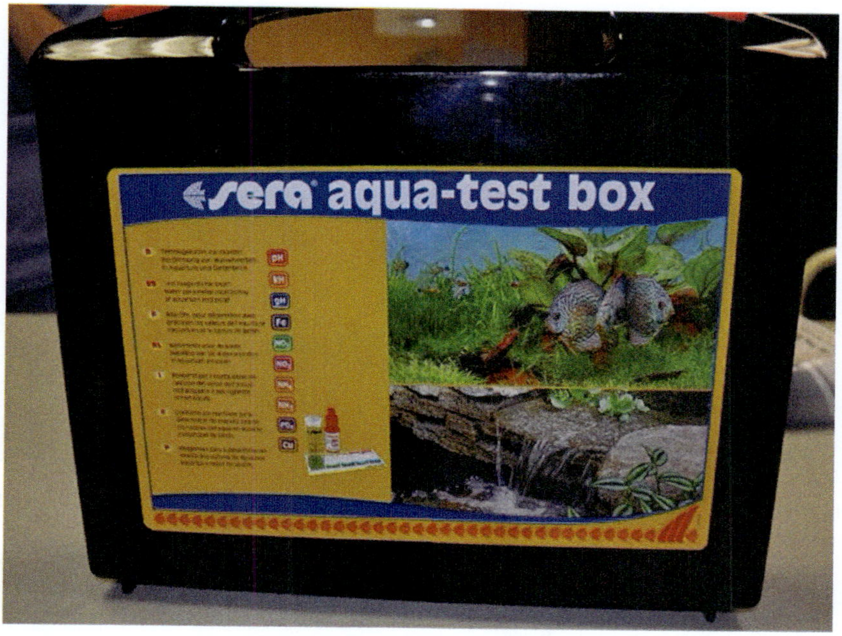

Fig. 11.2. An example of a water quality testing kit. (Photograph by Azureen Erdman.)

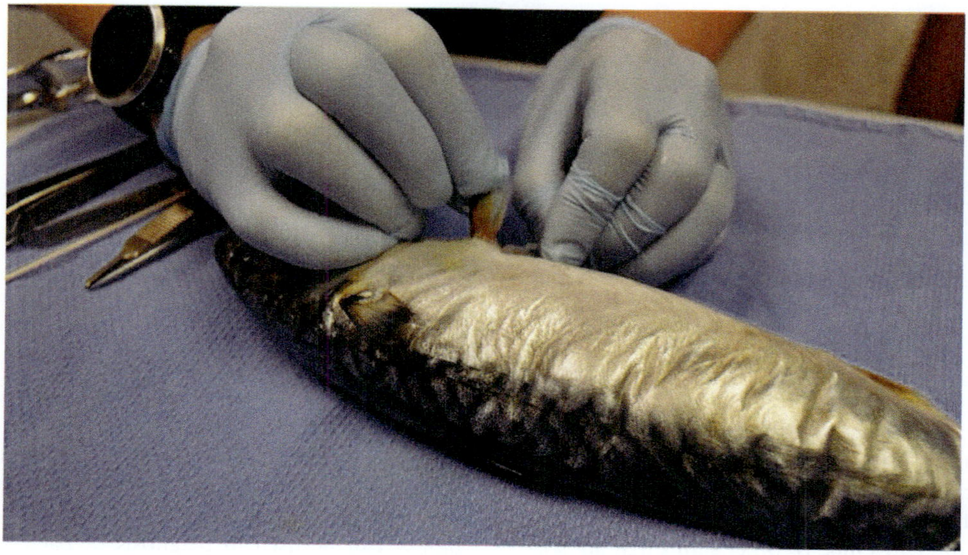

Fig. 11.3. Using the back of a #15 scalpel blade to scrape behind the pelvic fin of a mackerel. (Photograph by Azureen Erdman.)

over the sample (Fig. 11.5). Examine the sample under the microscope looking for motile parasites and bacteria. When creating a wet mount, it is easiest to use a drop of water from the fish's tank to ensure the same salinity between the slide and the fish's environment. Using normotonic saline on a marine fish sample can affect your results by slowing down or killing the motile organisms. The same can be said for using a higher salinity water sample on a freshwater fish mucus sample. Wet mounts

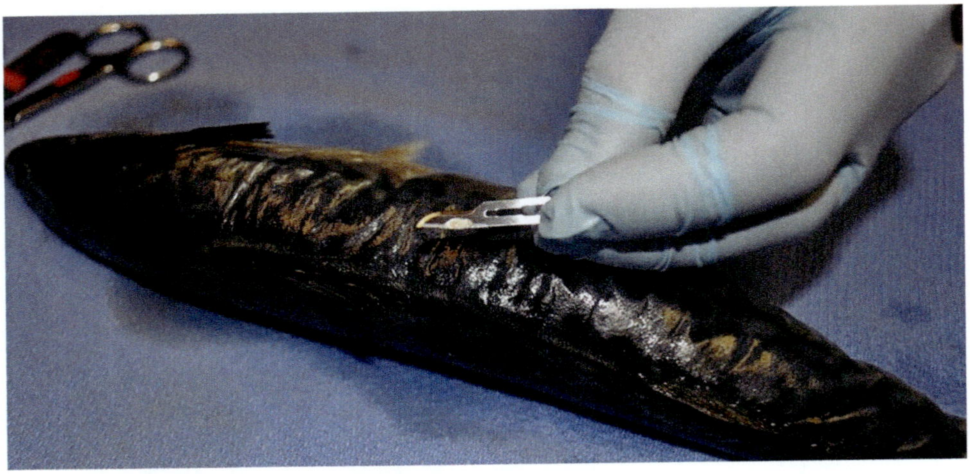

Fig. 11.4. Showing the mucus sample collected on the back of a scalpel blade. (Photograph by Azureen Erdman.)

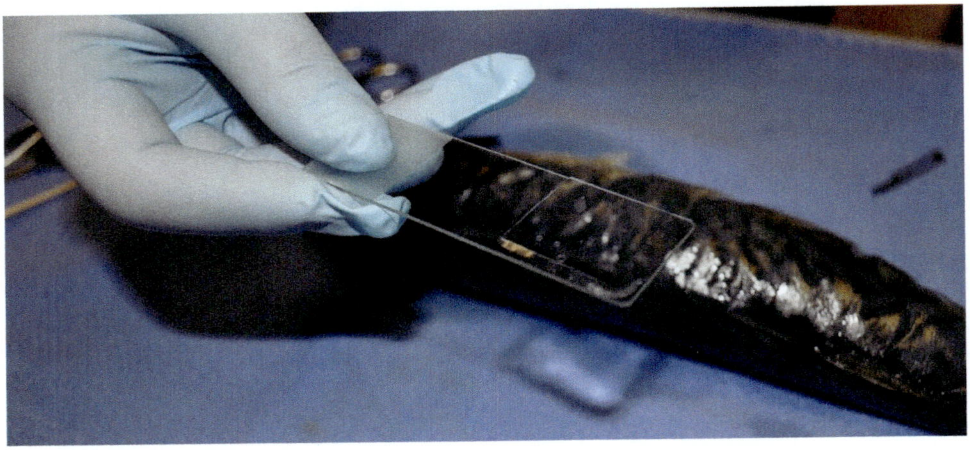

Fig. 11.5. The mucus sample is made into a wet mount slide. (Photograph by Azureen Erdman.)

must be examined right away, as motility will decrease or stop as a sample becomes desiccated.

This mucus sampling technique can be repeated to collect another sample that can be allowed to dry for future staining. Slides can be stained with Gram stain, Diff-Quik, or other stains that are specific to pathogens like *Mycobacterium* and fungal entities.

11.4 Gill Biopsy

A gill biopsy is one of the more important clinical diagnostic tests. As gills are exposed to environmental irritants, toxins, and pathogens, the tissue will undergo hyperplasia with an increase in epithelial cells, white blood cells, and mucus production. Microscopically, this change is known as gill "clubbing" because the gill lamellae turn from individual layers to one cohesive piece of tissue due to the hyperplasia (Nowak and Lucas, 1997). A gill biopsy can be used in diagnosis of bacterial and parasitic diseases, as well as a screening tool for environmental irritants. Often, the degree of hyperplasia can also help a clinician identify the chronicity of a disease process (Strzyzewska *et al.*, 2016).

The gills are composed of gill arches, gill filaments, and lamellae. The gill arches are the bony structures in the pharynx from which the gill filaments are suspended. The gill filaments are composed of a cartilaginous support that runs centrally with larger blood vessels. From the gill filaments branch the pairs of leaf-like tissues known as lamellae. Each lamella has a loop of capillaries through which blood flows. It is within the lamellae that gas exchange occurs between the blood and the water.

Grossly, upon lifting the operculum, you can visualize the gill arches and filaments. Observe the tissues and look for obvious lesions, areas of discoloration, or general changes in color. The lamellae are visualized and examined through a microscope after biopsy. To perform a gill biopsy, lift the operculum and using small scissors remove the distal tips of four to six gill filaments and place them on a clean microscope slide (Fig. 11.6). Add a drop of tank water and, using the edge of the coverslip, gently tap the gill tissue to spread the lamellae to get them on a flatter plane (Fig. 11.7). Place the coverslip over the surface and ensure that the drop of water covers all the tissue under the coverslip. Add more water to the edge of the coverslip if necessary. Examine the tissue under the microscope, looking for signs of motile organisms, hyperplasia of the lamellae tissue, blood clots and capillary widening (telangiectasia), increased white blood cells, and increased mucus production within the gill tissues (Fig. 11.8). Small numbers of protozoa can often be seen in most species without causing pathological lesions. Heavy infestations are more likely to be pathogenic.

It is important to note some differences in biopsy techniques that occur among species, specifically with elasmobranchs and syngnathids. The above technique should be used carefully with elasmobranchs. Due to the larger and more vascular nature of the gill filaments in elasmobranchs, they have a much higher likelihood of hemorrhage complications. Multiple resources note that it is better to use the back of a scalpel and scrape the gills as if performing a mucus sampling rather than biopsy of the tissue. Many syngnathids have a thick gill plate that acts as the operculum. This thickened tissue, as well as the general size of the patients, makes it difficult to perform a biopsy of the underlying gills. In the case of these patients, a brachial flush can be performed. This procedure involves flushing a small amount of seawater over the gills with a catheter tip syringe placed under the gill plate (Koldewey, 2005). The water runoff can be collected and examined microscopically for pathogens.

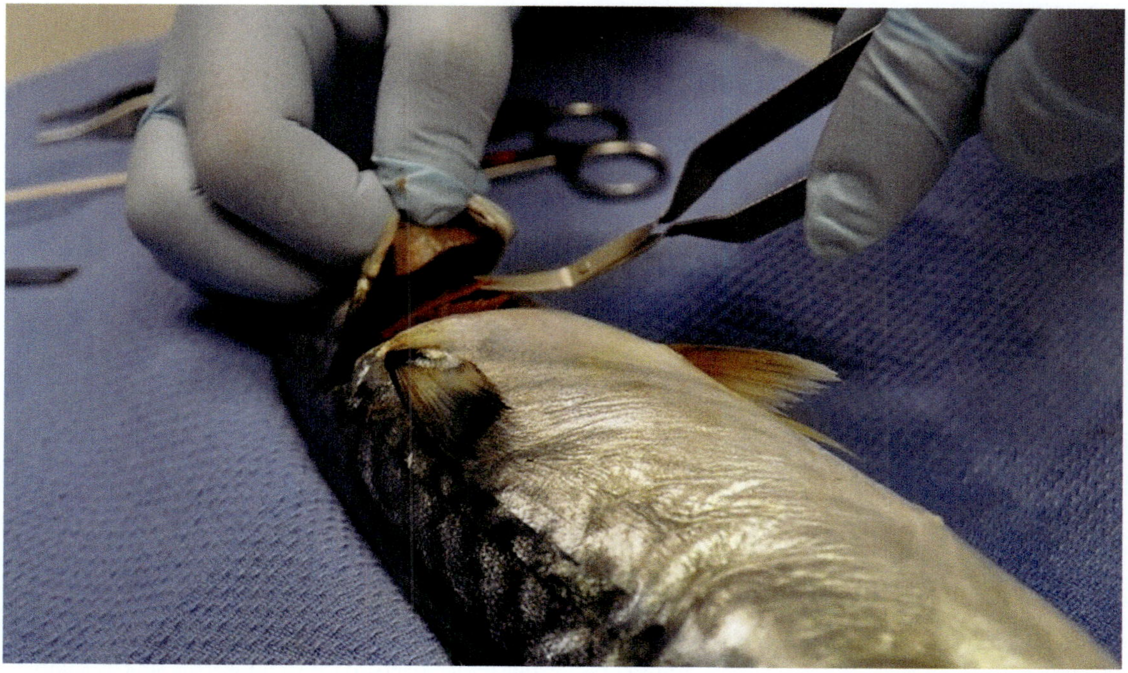

Fig. 11.6. Lifting the operculum to remove a small portion of the gill tips for microscopic examination. (Photograph by Azureen Erdman.)

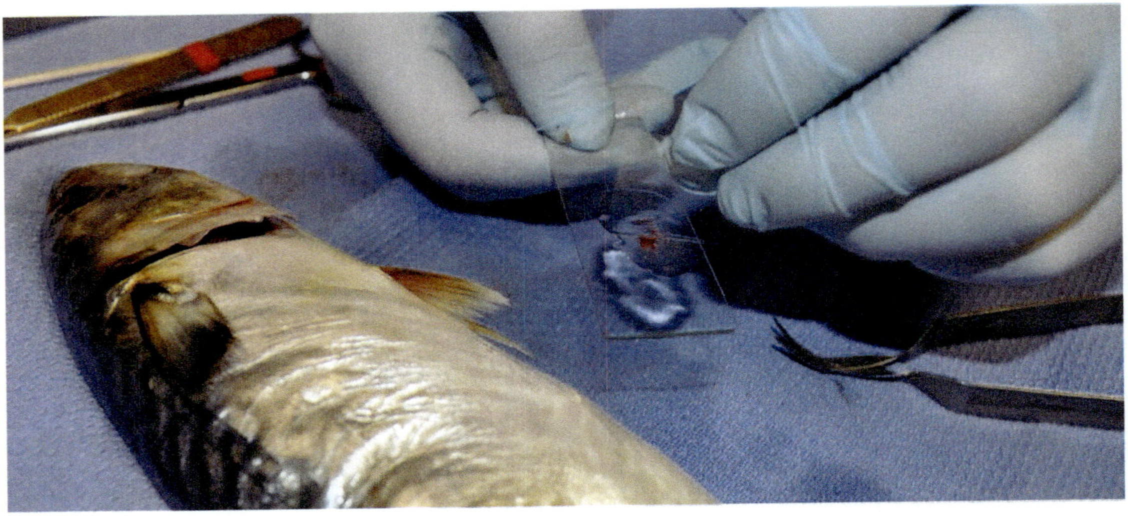

Fig. 11.7. Spreading the gill tip biopsy sample in the drop of water on the microscope slide using the coverslip. (Photograph by Azureen Erdman.)

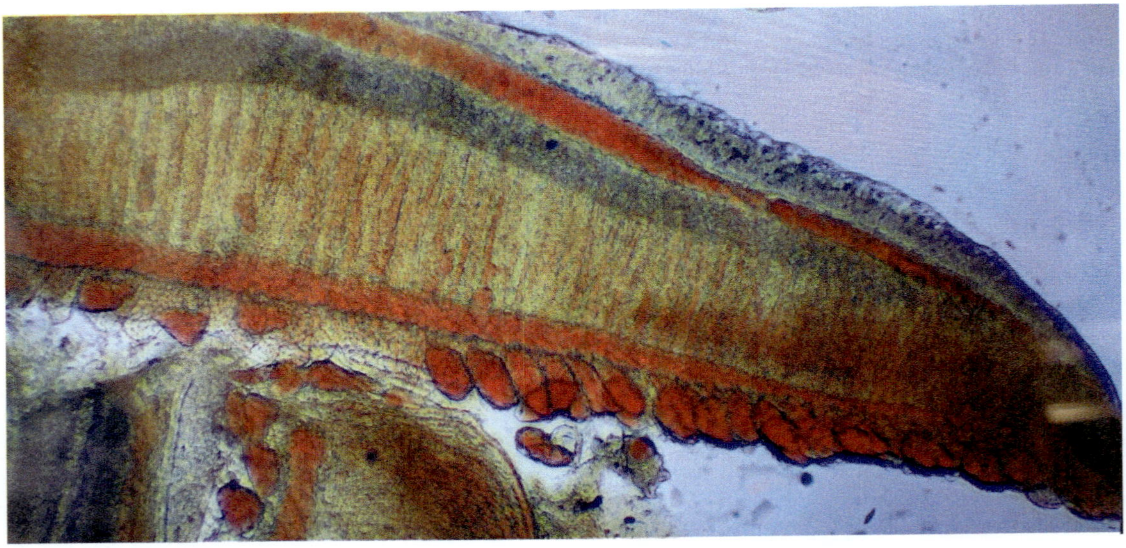

Fig. 11.8. Gill filament with hyperplasia along upper side of filament and telangiectasia on the lower lamellae. (Microphotograph by N. Saint-Erne.)

11.5 Fin Clip Biopsy

A fin clip biopsy is a diagnostic test that can be used to identify pathogens on the fin edges. To take a sample, fan the fin out and using sharp scissors cut a small portion from the fin edge (Figs 11.9a and b). Place the fin tissue on a microscope slide and add a drop of tank or tap water (Fig. 11.10). Then use the coverslip to spread the fin tissue out normally and place the coverslip on top. Like the mucus sample, this must be evaluated right away for parasites and other motile organisms.

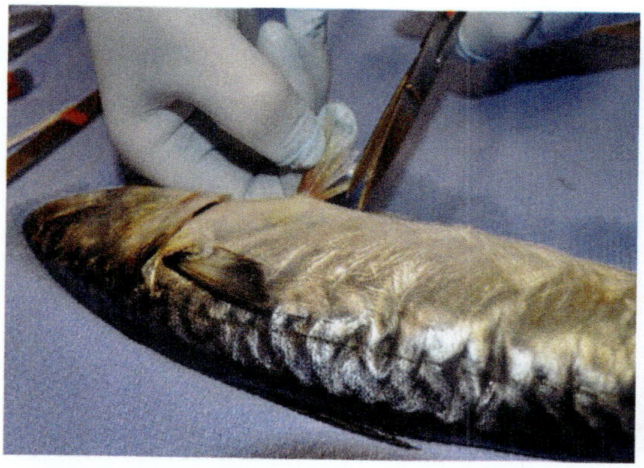

Fig. 11.9a. Cutting the edge of a pelvic fin for a biopsy sample. (Photograph by Azureen Erdman.)

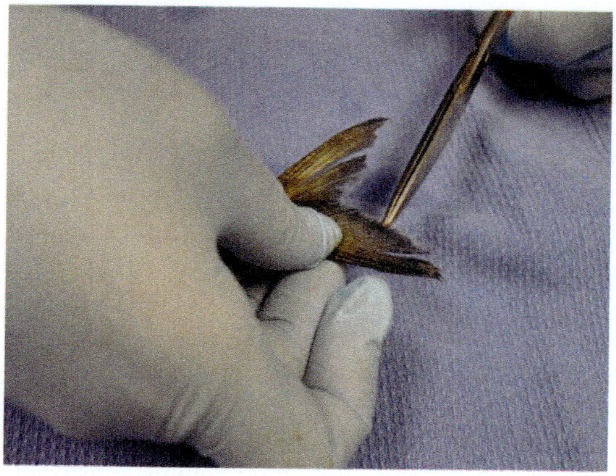

Fig. 11.9b. Cutting the edge of the caudal fin for a biopsy sample. (Photograph by Azureen Erdman.)

11.6 Fecal Examination

Fecal sample examinations should be performed regularly on patients in quarantine or those entering a new collection. Regular fecal screenings should be considered in populations living outdoors. A fecal sample can be used to identify intestinal parasites. Samples can be collected by skimming the bottom of the tank and collecting the sediment. This is less stressful for a patient, but often the patient is co-housed with other fish, and this does not allow for ease of separation of samples from one animal to another. If possible, separate the patient of interest and collect the fresh feces from the bottom of the separate tank. If the fecal samples are not fresh, they will contain microorganisms from the aquarium substrate that are not actually pathogens found in the fish.

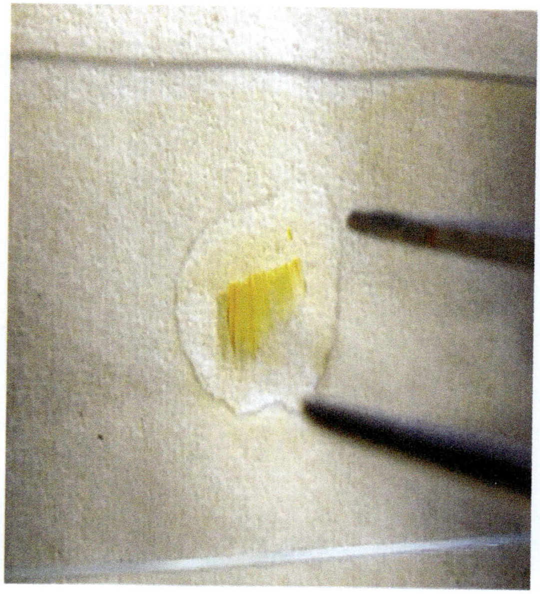

Fig. 11.10. Caudal fin biopsy from a guppy (*Poecilia reticulata*). (Photograph by N. Saint-Erne.)

Fish often pass feces in transport containers, and these should be collected and examined when fish are brought into the clinic. Fish may also pass feces while being anesthetized, and the feces should be collected and examined (Fig. 11.11). In larger fish species, feces can be collected by an anal wash. Using a small amount of saline, infuse the saline rectally and collect the fecal fluid that is expelled.

Fecal material is examined microscopically under a wet mount using water from the tank. Evaluate the wet mount sample promptly. Some parasites can be found on a fecal float using the sodium nitrate suspension technique, though often the fecal wet mount is more likely to yield results as piscine parasites can be delicate and easily destroyed in the floatation process.

11.7 Blood Collection

Blood collection in fish historically has not often been used routinely in the clinical setting. Perhaps it is gaining more use in collections where serial samples can be compared and monitored throughout a patient's life. As more databases are created with comparatively "normal" values among certain species of fish, this clinical technique may become more popular. Artifacts and changes to biochemistry and complete blood counts can be seen associated

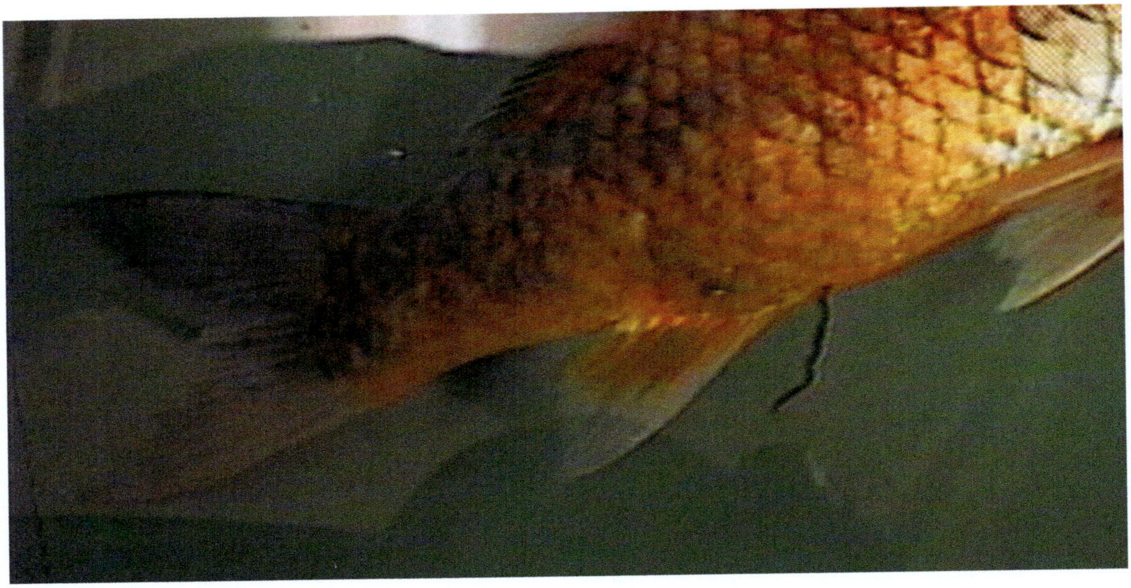

Fig. 11.11. Koi (*Cyprinus rubrofuscus*) passing feces while being anesthetized. (Photograph by N. Saint-Erne.)

with hemodilution with lymphatic fluid, stress from handling, sedation protocol, location of blood draw, and use of certain anticoagulants (Campbell, 2015). Sedatives like MS-222 can cause hemolysis, especially once the blood of a sedated fish is added to EDTA. In general, cooling fish blood can also cause hemolysis creating further artifacts. For this reason, it is best to create blood smears directly after a blood draw. Due to the biochemical artifacts associated with hemolysis, blood should be spun in a serum separator tube before cooling the sample (Duman *et al.*, 2019).

Lithium heparin and EDTA have been used as anticoagulants in fish blood samples. Fish have an alternate pathway for clot formation that is not stopped when heparin is used. The use of EDTA prevents the formation of blood clots, important when running whole blood samples and creating blood smears. However, EDTA can acidify the blood and lower serum calcium level readings. Due to this, EDTA should not be used for the purpose of running blood-gas analysis. Lithium heparin should be used for acid-base testing, and in smaller species where the syringe needs to be primed with an anticoagulant to help prevent clot formation. However, micro-clots can still form, and it is important to process the blood smears quickly if using heparin. Heparin allows for red blood cell clumping, and it can cause a blue-tinged discoloration of the cells on a blood smear. For those working with elasmobranchs, the anticoagulants will need to be balanced to match the osmolarity of the patient to prevent hemolysis of the cells. Multiple recipes of modified heparin-EDTA and modified phosphate-buffered saline can be found (Smith, 2004).

A fish carries a blood volume that is 5% of its body weight. Of this total blood volume, a fish can lose up to 30–40% before succumbing to blood loss. Blood can be collected from multiple locations depending on the species and size of the patient. The easiest and most widely used location in teleosts and elasmobranchs is the caudal tail vein. This vein runs ventral to the vertebral column and can be approached from the ventral midline region on the caudal peduncle by inserting the needle straight upward until hitting the vertebrae, then backing out slightly to collect blood (Fig. 11.12). A lateral approach (Fig. 11.13) on the caudal peduncle, aiming the needle at a 45° angle forward and inserting it 1–2 mm ventral to the lateral line organ and ventral to the vertebrae can also be used (Zang *et al.*, 2013).

It is important to note that in elasmobranchs this vessel is surrounded by a cartilaginous ring and, while entering the vascular space, you may feel a "popping" sensation as you move through the cartilage. In larger elasmobranch species, a vascular sinus can be utilized. The sinus is located caudal

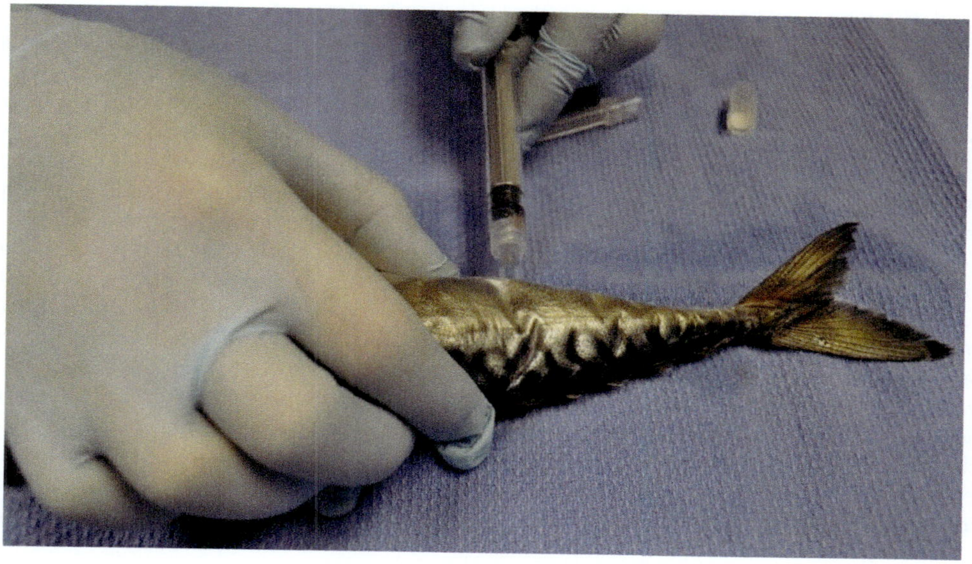

Fig. 11.12. Ventral approach for collecting a blood sample. (Photograph by Azureen Erdman.)

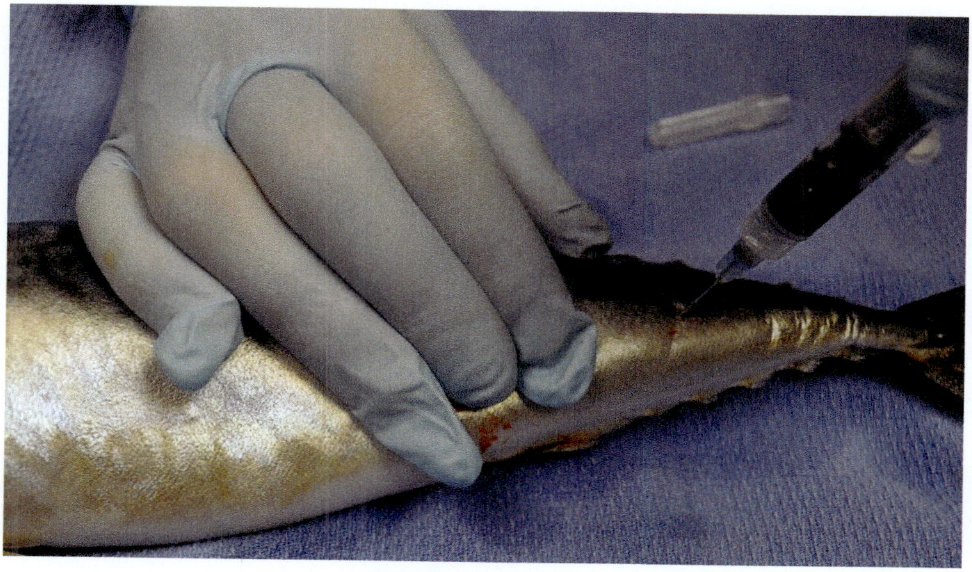

Fig. 11.13. Lateral approach for collecting a blood sample. (Photograph by Azureen Erdman.)

and ventral to the dorsal fin and can be approached by inserting the needle almost parallel to the fin base entering through the softer area of skin in the region. It is possible to obtain a blood sample through cardiocentesis. This must be performed under full anesthesia. Using this technique, up to a 25% rise in the packed cell volume has been reported.

11.8 Necropsy

Necropsy (or post-mortem examination) is an important diagnostic tool in veterinary medicine. Examining freshly dead fish, or fish that have been recently euthanized, may be helpful in determining the cause of disease or death. Necropsies are not performed on all deceased fish but may be useful in determining the cause of death if it has not already been identified. Necropsy is useful in aquatic veterinary medicine when the patients are part of a large population. It is beneficial to euthanize and perform necropsies on some fish that are sick to identify pathogens and treat the larger population involved. Sometimes euthanasia and necropsy are used merely because of the small size of the patient and lack of ability to perform antemortem diagnostics without harming the fish. Aquatic species undergo autolysis very quickly, within hours, causing contamination of tissue with bacteria as well as causing artifacts that can impede histopathologic diagnosis. It is best to choose a moribund patient and euthanize it just prior to necropsy. If this cannot be done, the remains should be stored in a refrigerator, wrapped in a wet towel or paper, and placed in a plastic bag without water. The necropsy should be performed preferably within 8 h (Wolf *et al*., 2014).

Larger fish can be necropsied using the following technique: make an incision on the ventral midline from vent to just caudal to the operculum (Fig. 11.14). It may be necessary to use bandage scissors or bone cutters to cut through the pelvic fin bones. Be careful not to cut the organs or intestines. Make two perpendicular incisions from the ventral midline extending as far dorsally as possible, one at each end of the coelomic cavity (Fig. 11.15). These cuts will form a flap that can be lifted dorsally. Elevate the flap of the body wall to examine and attain samples for pathology (Fig. 11.16). The lifted flap will contain the rib bones and can be cut out using large bandage scissors. Look at the color, size, and position of each of the coelomic organs.

Bacteriology samples are best taken by sampling the kidney in a sterile manner. Due to autolysis and the risk of bacterial contamination from the

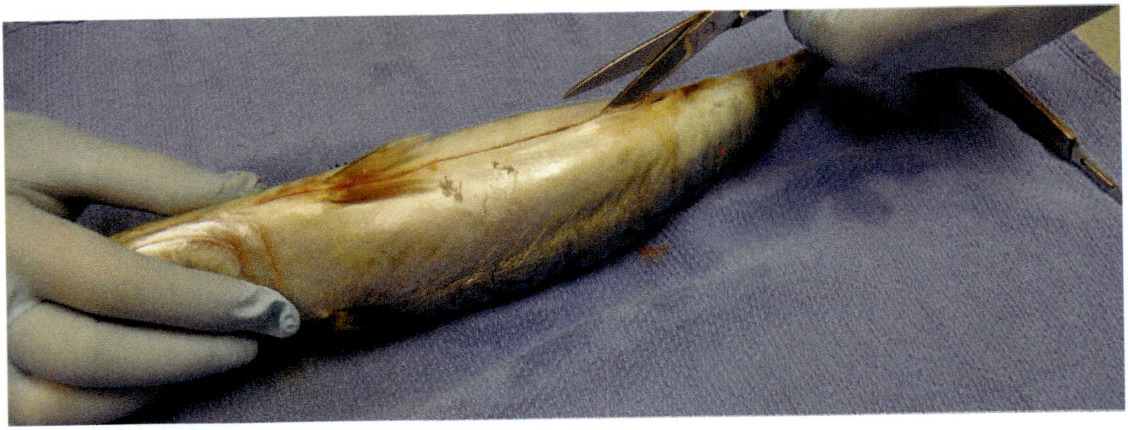

Fig. 11.14. Midline incision for ventral approach for necropsy. (Photograph by Azureen Erdman.)

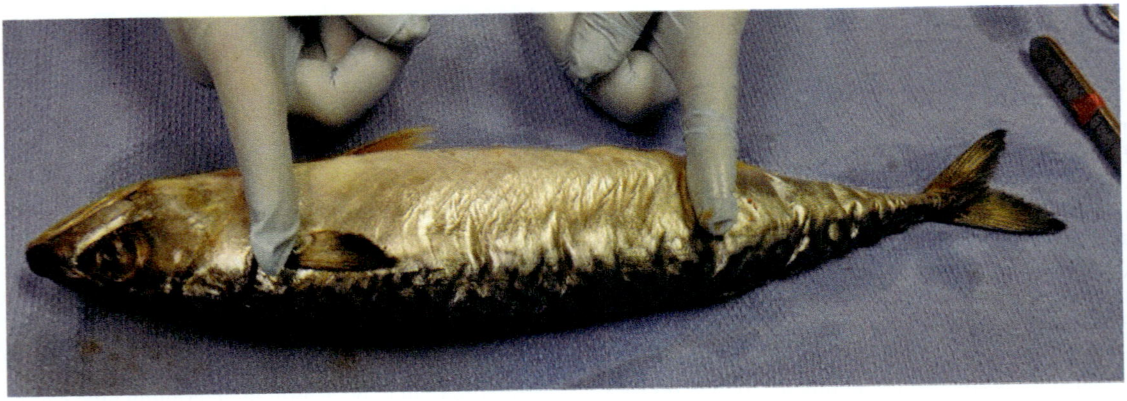

Fig. 11.15. Indicating where sides are cut to raise body wall for necropsy. (Photograph by Azureen Erdman.)

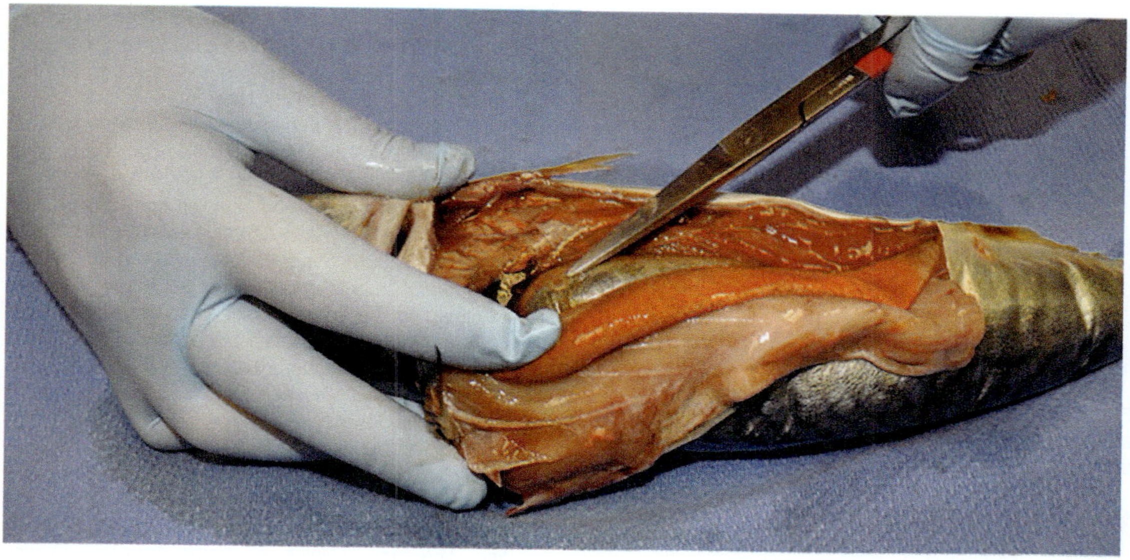

Fig. 11.16. The body wall has been raised dorsally to examine internal organs. (Photograph by Azureen Erdman.)

gastrointestinal tract within the coelom, it is necessary to sear the surface of the kidney with a hot sterile scalpel blade prior to taking a swab sample from inside the kidney tissue. Using the sterile bacterial swab enter the kidney through the recently sterilized area (Fig. 11.17). An alternative method of collecting a swab from the kidney is through a dorsal approach. Use a disinfectant on the surface of the fish, and use sterile scissors to incise into the body cavity anterior to the dorsal fin (Figs 11.18a and b). This will allow for a sterile bacterial culture swab to be used to swab directly from the dorsal aspect of the kidney. Bacterial samples from fish should be cultured at 25°C. An additional culture can be grown at 37°C if there is a concern about the bacteria having zoonotic potential, such as with *Mycobacterium*.

Tissue samples for pathology should be saved in 10% buffered neutral formalin. Formalin will only penetrate and fix through one cubic centimeter (1 cm^3) of tissue, so any samples should be smaller than that. It is better to take multiple samples of a tissue and have them fully fixed rather than a half-fixed larger piece. If sending a larger piece of tissue, you can facilitate formalin penetration by making linear cuts through the tissue. Whole fish placed into fixative should have the coelom incised so the internal organs will be in contact with the formalin. The fish can be bent gently to open the region of the cut to facilitate entrance of formalin into the coelomic cavity, allowing for fixation of the entire body. In these cases, the pathologist will be looking at whole-body slices.

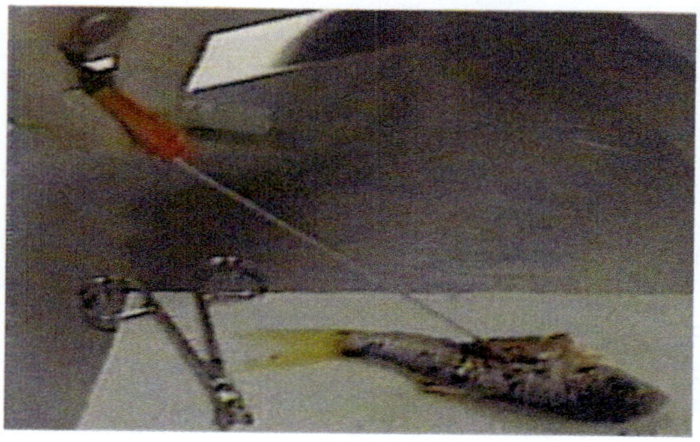

Fig. 11.17. Ventral approach for collecting a bacterial culture sample from the kidney. (Photograph by N. Saint-Erne.)

11.9 Conclusion

The use of clinical diagnostic tests will help determine the cause of diseases in fish. In some cases, more than one etiology may be present, so finding one positive test that leads to a diagnosis does not rule out other options occurring as well. The results of water quality testing, physical exams, and diagnostic tests are all important in discovering the cause of a disease. That will result in a better-informed course of action in treating the fish, rather than using empirical medical treatments.

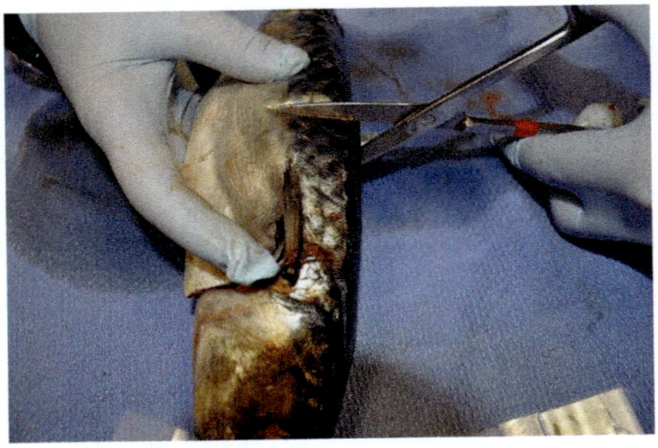

Fig. 11.18a. Cutting through the spine for a dorsal approach to the kidney for collecting a bacterial culture sample. (Photograph by Azureen Erdman.)

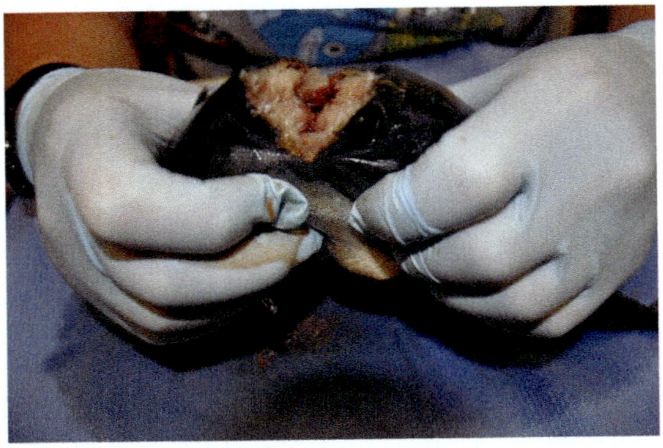

Fig. 11.18b. Dorsal approach for collecting a bacterial culture sample from the kidney. (Photograph by Azureen Erdman.)

References

Andrews, C., Carrington, N. and Exell, A. (2010) *Manual of Fish Health: Everything You Need to Know about Aquarium Fish, Their Environment and Disease Prevention*. Firefly Books, Richmond Hill, Ontario, Canada.

Brightwell, C. (2007) *Marine Chemistry*. T.F.H. Publications, Neptune City, New Jersey.

Campbell, T.W. (2015) *Exotic Animal Hematology and Cytology*. Wiley, Ames, Iowa.

Duman, M., Saticioglu, I.B., Suzer, B. and Altun, S. (2019) Practices for drawing blood samples from teleost fish. *North American Journal of Aquaculture* 81(2), 119–125.

Koldewey, H. (2005) *Syngnathid Husbandry in Public Aquariums, 2005 Manual*. Project Seahorse, London. Available at: https://projectseahorse.org/wp-content/uploads/2021/06/Syngnathid_Husbandry_Manual2005.pdf (accessed 6 October 2020).

Noga, E.J. (2010) *Fish Disease: Diagnosis and Treatment*. Wiley, Ames, Iowa.

Nowak, B.F. and Lucas, C.T. (1997) Diagnosis of structural changes in fish gills—can biopsy replace necropsy? *Aquaculture* 159(1–2), 1–10.

Reavill, D. and Roberts, H. (2007) Diagnostic cytology of fish. *Veterinary Clinics of North America: Exotic Animal Practice* 10(1), 207–234.

Smith, M. (2004) *The Elasmobranch Husbandry Manual: Captive Care of Sharks, Rays and Their Relatives*. Ohio Biological Survey, Columbus, Ohio.

Strzyzewska, E., Szarek, J. and Babinska, I. (2016). Morphologic evaluation of the gills as a tool in the diagnostics of pathological conditions in fish and pollution in the aquatic environment: a review. *Veterinární Medicína* 61(3), 123–132.

Wildgoose, W.H. (2001). *BSAVA Manual of Ornamental Fish*. British Small Animal Veterinary Association, Gloucester, UK.

Wolf, J.C., Baumgartner, W.A., Blazer, V.S., Camus, A.C., Engelhardt, J.A. *et al*. (2014). Nonlesions, misdiagnoses, missed diagnoses, and other interpretive challenges in fish histopathology studies. *Toxicologic Pathology* 43(3), 297–325.

Zang, L., Shimada, Y., Nishimura, Y., Tanaka, T. and Nishimura, N. (2013). A novel, reliable method for repeated blood collection from aquarium fish. *Zebrafish* 10(3), 425–432.

12 Fish Hematology and Biochemistry

LILY PARKINSON

Brookfield Zoo, Brookfield, Illinois

Abstract

Blood collection and evaluation can be a useful tool in determining fish health. However, risks of injury from blood collection due to handling and the stress on the fish, especially the smaller tropical fish species, must be considered. The practitioner must be experienced in the collection and evaluation of the blood for the species of fish being diagnosed, and a consistent protocol for all blood collection and analysis is necessary to obtain the best information from any blood analysis performed.

12.1 Considerations Prior to Blood Analysis

Blood analysis has not traditionally been a mainstay diagnostic test in fish medicine (Noga, 2010; Campbell, 2012b). For freshwater aquarium fish, limitations due to size and blood volume that can be safely obtained are frequently encountered. Traditionally, the risk of mortality due to a blood draw in fish less than 8 cm (3 inches) body length made this diagnostic not recommended for most aquarium species (Noga, 2010). It has also been historically recommended to only obtain a blood sample if the fish appeared anemic based on gill evaluation (Noga, 2010). Care for aquarium fish continues to expand, however, and utilizing blood analysis can help provide a more complete picture of health, so this diagnostic tool is being utilized more commonly (Clauss *et al.*, 2008; Grant, 2015). Rather than obtaining a blood sample and considering it a portion of a "minimum clinical database," as it might be in other species, it is strongly recommended that blood sampling in fish patients be carefully considered with definitive goals for analysis formulated prior to obtaining the sample.

Extreme variability has been found in fish hematology and clinical chemistry results, with everything from temperature, stocking density, age, water quality, season, and handling variables altering results (Pickering and Pottinger, 1987; Hrubec *et al.*, 2001; Clauss *et al.*, 2008; Gholipourkanani and Ahadizadeh, 2013; Eslamloo *et al.*, 2015). The clinician should research if a clinical reference interval will be available for the fish species to help interpret any results obtained. Many fish species do not have normal blood values available. Even with a published reference interval, the clinician should also recognize that any outlier results obtained may not represent a disease state but rather a normal physiologic adaptation to a different living environment, stressful handling event, or due to drug administration.

Blood analysis can provide different information to the clinician. Hematology, the study of the blood cells, can reveal anemia or polycythemia, white blood cell responses to stress, infection, neoplasia, or the presence of blood parasites. Biochemical analysis of the blood can evaluate electrolytes (which can be altered a great deal in an ill fish living surrounded in an aquatic environment) and evaluate specific metabolic processes or enzyme presence or activity, which may reflect organ function. Each of these elements can provide a great deal of information, but each requires a specific volume of blood to obtain results. In small species of fish, only small volumes of blood can be obtained, so only a small amount of blood analysis can be performed. The clinician may need to choose which results are most important to the evaluation of the case. This decision should be made based upon a holistic evaluation of

Corresponding author: lilyparkinson@gmail.com

© CAB International 2025. *The Handbook of Ornamental Fish Health and Welfare* (ed. N. Saint-Erne)
DOI: 10.1079/9781789246032.0012

the case; a fish that appears quite anemic might benefit from evaluation of its red blood cells, whereas a fish with a great deal of skin ulcerations present, should likely have its electrolyte status evaluated to determine if it is compensating adequately for its compromised state.

Obtaining blood for analysis is not without risk. This risk should be carefully considered and should be discussed with all stakeholders in the case (owner, breeder, purchasers). The most dramatic risk that can occur from a blood draw is death. This can occur from exsanguination, whether due to too much blood being taken during the blood draw, or continued bleeding from the blood draw site after the collection has been completed. The stress involved in the blood draw procedure in a severely compromised fish patient can also lead to clinical decompensation and death. Other potential complications include damage to internal organs, including spinal nerves, which are often near blood collection sites. Spinal nerve damage can lead to a fish's inability to swim and/or hypopigmentation of the fish caudal to the site of damage, since these nerves often control the chromatophores that give each fish its coloration (Noga, 2010).

12.2 Obtaining Blood

There are numerous techniques described for obtaining blood from fish. Many of these sampling techniques are meant to be performed as a terminal procedure (Duman *et al.*, 2019). This may need to be explored in large populations or with serious disease outbreaks to obtain as much information as possible. If this is pursued, histopathology of the fish for full evaluation is also strongly recommended. For most aquarium fish, the survival of the fish is desired to improve its health based on the results of the blood analysis. When obtaining blood samples, use a needle with length sufficiently long to pass through the muscles to reach the blood vessel. It is helpful for working with large fish to use a butterfly catheter attachment between the needle and syringe to make inserting the needle easier. Two people can work together to draw blood in this way, one holding the syringe and the other positioning the needle.

The most common location for blood collection in fish is the ventral caudal vasculature, referred to as such, since the artery and vein run together very closely, and it is impossible to determine if venous or arterial blood is being obtained (Noga, 2010; Campbell, 2012b; Lawrence *et al.*, 2020). While all non-terminal blood collection techniques in fish are generally nonvisual, this technique allows palpation or visualization of the lateral processes of the spine, and the needle being utilized to obtain the blood can be "walked off" the spine to help find the correct location (Campbell, 2012b; Grant, 2015; Duman *et al.*, 2019). This can be particularly useful due to the extremely wide variety of sizes and shapes present within fish. Being able to visualize where the spine and the ventral hemal arch are within each unique body type can allow the practitioner to adapt this technique to each new fish species that is encountered (Lawrence *et al.*, 2020).

While this location can lead to complications (exsanguination, damage to spinal nerves), they are generally considered less severe than those that may occur in other blood draw sites. This location has even been described for nonlethal blood collection in extremely small zebra fish with small volumes (1–25 μl) being obtained (Zang *et al.*, 2013). While this small volume would necessitate very judicious use of the blood obtained, it could provide valuable insight for a clinician with a pointed clinical question, and this technique had a low mortality rate of 2.3% (Zang *et al.*, 2013).

The heart, dorsal aorta, and bulbus arteriosus can also be utilized for blood collection (Campbell, 2012b; Duman *et al.*, 2019). This is another blind stick that has the potential to lead to damage to nearby internal organs (head kidney, gills, heart), and due to the higher pressure and larger volume of blood present in these locations, the possibility of blood loss after the blood sampling is much higher (Campbell, 2012b; Grant, 2015; Duman *et al.*, 2019). Blood can be collected from sharks by caudal venipuncture or by using the vascular sinus located caudal and slightly ventral to the dorsal fins. The advantage of using the vascular sinus as a site for blood collection instead of venipuncture of the caudal vertebral vessels in large elasmobranch fish is the relative ease of access to the sinus with proper restraint (Campbell, 2015). Blood samples can be taken from rays either by caudal puncture or from the vasculature in the pectoral fins (Fig. 12.1).

In general, blood collection can be accomplished with a needle and syringe that have been pre-coated with an anticoagulant (Campbell, 2012b; Zang *et al.*, 2013; Grant, 2015; Duman *et al.*, 2019; Lawrence *et al.*, 2020). Each anticoagulant has several advantages and disadvantages associated with it (Campbell, 2012b; Duman *et al.*, 2019). The most

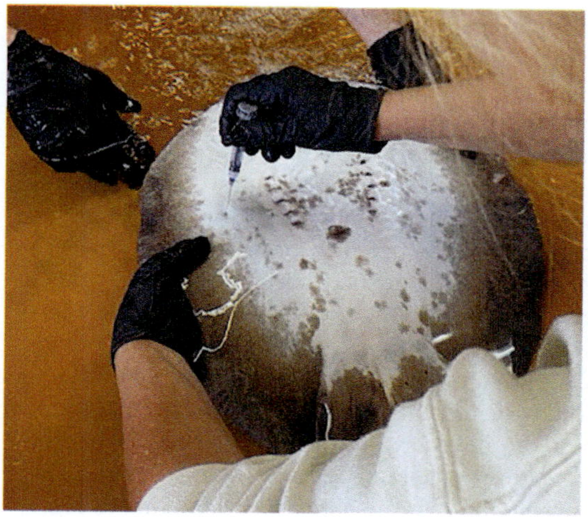

Fig. 12.1. Dr. Sharmie Johnson obtaining a blood sample from an anesthetized freshwater stingray (*Potamotrygon motoro*) from the blood vessels in the ventral surface of the pectoral fin. (Photograph by Marie Dillon, B.S., CVT.)

commonly utilized anticoagulant in clinical fish veterinary practice appears to be lithium heparin (Grant, 2015). While heparin can lead to changes in the visualization of blood cells and allow continuation of blood clotting if it has already begun, it minimally affects biochemical results (Campbell, 2012b; Duman *et al.*, 2019). Another commonly available veterinary anticoagulant, ethylenediaminetetraacetic acid (EDTA), can lead to hemolysis in certain fish species (Campbell, 2012b). Due to the small volumes that might be obtained from many species, and the low likelihood of being able to perform a repeat blood collection in the species evaluated in freshwater aquariums, it is recommended to avoid the potential for valuable sample loss via hemolysis, especially when the hemolysis risk for each species' blood in EDTA is largely unknown.

Blood collection is generally difficult in fish due to the necessity of performing blind blood collection, the small volumes that can be obtained, and their rapid clotting times. Perhaps even more difficult than this, however, is the speed with which blood collection needs to be accomplished, or the requirement for sedation or anesthesia to obtain the blood. Several factors need to be considered when determining if blood sampling will be performed with an awake or a sedated/anesthetized fish (Lawrence *et al.*, 2020). If other diagnostics that require time (e.g. radiographs, ultrasound) are desired, then sedation or anesthesia will likely be required, and blood collection should be planned concurrently. If only blood sampling, skin scraping, and/or gill clipping is planned, then awake sampling may be acceptable and advantageous.

While no definitive time limit can be given for the collection of blood and other samples in order to be the safest and least stressful procedure for the fish, many sources recommend obtaining all samples in 30 s or less if the fish will have its gills out of water (Campbell, 2012b; Chen *et al.*, 2014; Lawrence *et al.*, 2020). As this will often not be feasible, designing a trough to help place the fish in an optimal position for blood draw and to allow for bathing of the gills in water during collection procedures is likely ideal (Lawrence *et al.*, 2020). Preplanning prior to the collection procedure will help provide the most rapid procedure so that it may be safest for the fish patient.

Finally, once the sampling is occurring, the clinician should be mindful that an appropriate amount of blood is obtained—carefully balancing maximizing the information obtained from the blood sample and allowing the fish being sampled to maintain an appropriate remaining blood volume. There is no definitive parameter for determining a safe amount of blood to obtain from a fish, and very wide ranges have been published: from 30 to 50% of blood volume in some locations, or much lower recommendations of 0.1 to 10% of blood volume (Grant, 2015; Lawrence *et al.*, 2020). The total blood volume in a fish may be 5% of its body weight (Saint-Erne, 2010). When obtaining blood volumes from zebra fish, a maximum of 2% of body weight could be obtained (Zang *et al.*, 2013).

Many of these recommendations and amounts are determined by a fish's body weight. It is recommended that a fish clinician work on learning the general weights of many aquarium fishes that are generally worked with. Body weights obtained during anesthetized examinations or during recovery periods when a fish is in a small recovery tank are recommended, and the clinician is encouraged to maintain a list of these weights along with the age, size, and gender (if known) of the species that provided the weight, to help the clinician to better estimate how much blood can be obtained from a new patient that is presented prior to any diagnostics or body weights being performed. In general, it is recommended that the clinician obtain 1% of body weight or less in blood samples.

12.3 Blood Analysis

12.3.1 Hematology

Only a single drop of blood is required for a hematologic assessment. Even very small patients can provide this sample. The best preparation for assessing blood morphology is to make a blood smear immediately from a sample obtained with no anticoagulant (Grant, 2015). If a very small patient is being sampled, this is the recommended method; however, in larger patients where additional analyses will be performed, then an anticoagulant will need to be utilized, as multiple blood draws are not recommended due to the time constraints of sample procurement and the increased risk for complications. The practitioner should become very comfortable creating blood smears in order to make the most of any sample obtained (Allison and Meinkoth, 2007). Practicing with larger volumes of blood when available until proficient is recommended. If only a blood smear is obtained, the hemogram (red blood cells), leukogram (white blood cells) and thrombogram (clotting cells—thrombocytes) can be qualitatively evaluated.

Due to the extreme variability that can be seen in hematology results in fish due to many different factors, it is recommended that a fish practitioner choose one method for evaluating fish blood with no deviations. This will give the best chance for accurate assessment of results and comparison between samples. Results will usually be more accurate if analyzed almost immediately (Noga, 2010; Campbell, 2012b; Lawrence *et al.*, 2020), so learning to perform blood smear evaluation and even a manual complete blood count with a hemocytometer is recommended, but if this is not possible, then blood can be sent to an outside laboratory familiar with fish specimens for analysis. The blood should be handled and shipped in the exact same manner every time. A method for preserving whole blood samples from fish in 10% formalin has been described to allow for later analysis, which may be useful for a practitioner with a busy schedule or multiple fish samples being collected (Arnold *et al.*, 2014). Again, the practitioner is urged to maintain consistency in how blood samples are collected, preserved, and analyzed, especially within the same patient and case.

The hemogram (red blood cells) of a fish patient can be evaluated on a blood smear. The red blood cells of fish are ovoid and contain a nucleus, with rare exceptions (Grant, 2015). Immature red blood cells are more circular and are usually more basophilic in color. These cells are generally smaller than mature red blood cells, in contrast to mammals where immature red blood cells are generally larger. If blood for more than just a blood smear is obtained, a packed cell volume (PCV) and total solids (TS) evaluation should be obtained to help best assess the patient's health and evaluate the hemogram in context (Clauss *et al.*, 2008). In general, most fish have a PCV between 20% and 40% (Clauss *et al.*, 2008; Grant, 2015; Lawrence *et al.*, 2020). If a patient appears to have a low PCV, then it may be anemic. This can be assessed in the context of gill color and the hemogram. If numerous immature red blood cells exist, this may indicate anemia and that the patient is attempting to regenerate a normal amount of red blood cells. It should be noted, however, that very minimal red blood cell regeneration is likely to occur in the peripheral blood and is, instead, likely occurring in the erythropoietic organ, the head kidney (Clauss *et al.*, 2008; Grant, 2015). Alternatively, if the fish appears to have a relatively high PCV (especially in an ill or slow-moving species—high PCVs typically exist in athletic and fast swimming species), this may be an indication of dehydration and should be interpreted with biochemical parameters, if available (Clauss *et al.*, 2008). Hypoxia, stress, splenic contraction, and erythrocyte swelling can also be responsible for an elevated PCV (Grant, 2015). If even more blood has been obtained and a manual cell count is going to be performed, a red blood cell count can be obtained as well (Grant, 2015).

The leukogram should next be evaluated on a blood smear. White blood cell evaluation of fish is a highly specialized skill (Clauss *et al.*, 2008; Campbell, 2012b; Grant, 2015). A consensus on what terminology to utilize when referring to white blood cells has not even been reached (Tripathi *et al.*, 2004; Campbell, 2012b; Grant, 2015). With a consistent approach, however, a practitioner will be able to pick out general trends or changes in patients. The most numerous white blood cells seen when evaluating a fish blood smear are generally either lymphocytes, neutrophils, or heterophils. The lymphocyte (an agranulocyte) and the neutrophil or heterophil (a granulocyte) should be easily distinguished from one another. The morphology of the cells and a qualitative assessment of white blood cell numbers can be made from a well-made blood smear.

A quantitative assessment of white blood cells can be made by performing a manual complete blood cell count (CBC). Natt and Herrick's procedure and solution for the complete blood count is the preferred method in fish (Noga, 2010; Campbell, 2012b). Very little blood (around 20 μl) is required to perform a manual complete blood count. Those who are familiar with this procedure in other species should be warned that thrombocytes are also stained with Natt and Herrick's solution in fish, so it may be difficult to differentiate these from the white blood cells present (Campbell, 2012b). Care should be taken to ascertain that an accurate white blood cell count is obtained.

A differential count of the white blood cells should be performed on the blood smear, with or without a manual complete blood count. The morphology of the white blood cells should also be evaluated. Increases or decreases in white blood cell lineages and markers of toxicity, or a left shift, have been documented to occur in reaction to disease processes, and can often be interpreted similarly to how they are in mammalian patients (Clauss *et al.*, 2008; Campbell, 2012b). A low white blood cell count could indicate a fish is healthy and has no need for a stress or inflammatory response or that the fish is experiencing a severely septic process; evaluation of the morphology of the white blood cells present in the blood smear would be essential to determine which situation is present.

Finally, the thrombocytes in the blood smear should be evaluated. They are generally elliptical with a central nucleus, although their morphology varies a great deal among species (Grant, 2015). As multifocal hemorrhage is often a manifestation of disease in fish, an assessment of whether the thrombocytes are being fully consumed and are no longer present in the peripheral blood can help a clinician determine how afflicted the evaluated fish truly is. An extremely low thrombocyte count should prompt the clinician to evaluate the sample for a blood clot or clumped thrombocytes in the feathered edge of the blood smear. If neither of these situations is present, careful observation of the sampled fish should be undertaken to ascertain that evidence of ongoing hemorrhage is not present.

12.3.2 Biochemistry

As previously discussed, reference intervals for most aquarium fish are lacking, which can make it very difficult to best interpret any results obtained. In addition, what might be considered a normal or baseline value for any sampled fish could vary widely based upon the environment it came from or the handling it experienced for the blood sample collection (de Souza Neves *et al.*, 2018). Nevertheless, with continued sampling and targeted clinical questioning, a practitioner can begin to elucidate the health status of a fish patient via biochemical analysis. While biochemical analysis can be performed on serum or plasma, due to the small amount of blood that can often be obtained from the species dealt with in freshwater aquarium medicine, plasma is recommended to maximize the sample available for analysis and to maintain consistency in results (Hrubec and Smith, 1999). Again, the clinician is urged to perform all collection and analysis in a similar manner to allow for the maximum ability to compare results between samples. With this in mind, the separation of plasma from the red blood cell pellet should be performed as soon as possible to minimize changes occurring due to metabolism in the red blood cells (Noga, 2010; Campbell, 2012b). This may necessitate having a traveling centrifuge. If this is not possible, the amount of time that has elapsed between blood collection and separation should be recorded to help the clinician remain cognizant of any artifacts that may have been introduced due to the delay in separation.

There are now several portable analyzers available that can be utilized to evaluate electrolyte levels in fish. While there may be variation present between species, in general, all fish need to maintain a tight electrolyte homeostasis for normal electrochemical functioning (Sakamoto *et al.*, 2001). In freshwater fish, a decrease in sodium below 140 mmol/l (with chloride generally being around 10–20 mmol/l lower than sodium) indicates that the fish is very ill and has not been able to maintain its normal osmoregulation (Campbell, 2012a). This can be due to severe ulcerations in the integument leading to fluid entering across the compromised barrier, or it could be due to decreased appropriate ionic movement in the intestines, kidney, urinary bladder, or across the gills. Rapid intervention should be undertaken, usually in the form of increasing the salinity in the fish's environment.

With very minimal blood, a practitioner can evaluate the blood glucose concentration of a fish (Zang *et al.*, 2013). Glucose levels in fish are generally lower than values obtained in mammals (Snellgrove and Alexander, 2011). Glucose can increase with a stress response and may be an indicator to the practitioner that the sampling method was not as stress-free for the fish as was hoped (Snellgrove and Alexander, 2011). Lactate evaluation, which is also often available for analysis on small handheld analyzers, can also help the practitioner assess the degree of stress or the degree of derangement in cellular metabolism that is present (Campbell, 2012a). Low glucose would be presumed also to reflect a potential bacteremia or severe malnutrition, as can be seen in mammals, but with the lower normal values present in fish and delays in analysis that may allow glucose consumption by erythrocytes, it may be difficult to determine if an obtained glucose value is truly pathologically low.

Any further biochemistry analysis in fish remains largely untapped. Renal and liver function have been evaluated (Sakamoto *et al.*, 2001; Campbell, 2012a), as have metabolic processes and thyroid function (Campbell, 2012a; Zang *et al.*, 2013). No generalizations can be made, however, for the majority of fish species. The practitioner is encouraged to create their own internal reference intervals when dealing with a great number of certain species to help with the assessment of those animals if the animals become ill. Discussing the creation of an internal reference interval when animals are healthy with owners as a recommendation to aid when patients have aged or become ill can greatly aid in the interpretation of any biochemistry analysis performed in the future during ill health.

12.4 Conclusions

Overall, blood analysis in freshwater aquarium fish remains an area requiring further research and knowledge. This should not prevent a clinician from utilizing this diagnostic tool in clinical cases when it is carefully considered and planned. The practitioner is urged to have a consistent protocol for all blood collection and analysis to aid in obtaining the best information from any blood analysis performed.

References

Allison, R.W. and Meinkoth, J.H. (2007) Hematology without the numbers: in-clinic blood film evaluation. *Veterinary Clinics of North America: Small Animal Practice* 37, 245–266, vi.

Arnold, J.E., Matsche, M.A. and Rosemary, K. (2014) Preserving whole blood in formalin extends the specimen stability period for manual cell counts for fish. *Veterinary Clinical Pathology* 43, 613–620.

Campbell, T. (2012a) Clinical chemistry of fish and amphibians. In: Thrall, M.A., Weiser, G., Allison, R.W. and Campbell, T. (eds) *Veterinary Hematology and Clinical Chemistry*. 2nd edn. Wiley, Ames, Iowa, pp. 607–614.

Campbell, T. (2012b) Hematology of fish. In: Thrall, M.A., Weiser, G., Allison, R.W. and Campbell, T. (eds) *Veterinary Hematology and Clinical Chemistry*. 2nd edn. Wiley, Ames, Iowa, pp. 298–312.

Campbell, T. (2015) Blood sample collection and preparation in fish. In: Campbell, T.W. (ed.) *Exotic Animal Hematology and Cytology*. Wiley, Ames, Iowa, pp. 183–186.

Chen, Y.-H., Chen, H.-H. and Jeng, S.-S. (2014) Rapid renewal of red blood cells in the common carp following prolonged exposure to air. *Fisheries Science* 81, 255–265.

Clauss, T.M., Dove, A.D. and Arnold, J.E. (2008) Hematologic disorders of fish. *Veterinary Clinics of North America: Exotic Animal Practice* 11, 445–462, v.

de Souza Neves, M., Barbas, L., do Couto, M., Lopes, J., Tavares-Dias, M. and Fujimoto, R. (2018) Hematological assessment of four amazonian ornamental armoured catfish (Teleostei, Loricariidae). *Acta Scientiarum* 40. doi:10.4025/actascibiolsci.v40i1.39554.

Duman, M., Saticioglu, I.B., Suzer, B. and Altun, S. (2019) Practices for drawing blood samples from teleost fish. *North American Journal of Aquaculture* 81, 119–125.

Eslamloo, K., Akhavan, S., Eslamifar, A. and Henry, M. (2015) Effects of background colour on growth performance, skin pigmentation, physiological condition and innate immune responses of goldfish, *Carassius auratus*. *Aquaculture Research* 46, 202–215.

Gholipourkanani, H. and Ahadizadeh, S. (2013) Use of propofol as an anesthetic and its efficacy on some hematological values of ornamental fish *Carassius auratus*. *SpringerPlus* 2, 1–5.

Grant, K.R. (2015) Fish hematology and associated disorders. *Veterinary Clinics of North America. Exotic Animal Practice* 18, 83–103.

Hrubec, T. and Smith, S. (1999) Differences between plasma and serum samples for the evaluation of blood chemistry values in rainbow trout, channel catfish, hybrid tilapias, and hybrid striped bass. *Journal of Aquatic Animal Health* 11, 116–122.

Hrubec, T., Smith, S. and Robertson, J. (2001) Age-related changes in hematology and plasma chemistry values of hybrid striped bass (*Morone chrysops x Morone saxatilis*). *Veterinary Clinical Pathology* 30, 8–15.

Lawrence, M.J., Raby, G.D., Teffer, A.K., Jeffries, K.M., Danylchuk, A.J. *et al.* (2020) Best practices for non-lethal blood sampling of fish via the caudal vasculature. *Journal of Fish Biology* 97, 4–15.

Noga, E. (2010) The clinical workup. In: Noga, E. (ed.) *Fish Disease: Diagnosis and Treatment*. 2nd edn. Wiley, Ames, Iowa, pp. 13–48.

Pickering, A. and Pottinger, T. (1987) Crowding causes prolonged leucopenia in salmonid fish, despite interrenal acclimation. *Journal of Fish Biology* 30, 701–712.
Saint-Erne, N. (2010) Hematology. In: Saint-Erne, N. (ed.) *Advanced Koi Care*, 2nd edn. Erne Enterprises, Glendale, Arizona, p. 45.
Sakamoto, K., Lewbart, G. and Smith, T. (2001) Blood chemistry values of juvenile red pacu (*Piaractus brachypomus*). *Veterinary Clinical Pathology* 30, 50–52.
Snellgrove, D.L. and Alexander, L.G. (2011) Haematology and plasma chemistry of the red top ice blue mbuna cichlid (*Metriaclima greshakei*). *British Journal of Nutrition* 106(Suppl. 1), S154–S157.
Tripathi, N., Latimer, K. and Burnley, V. (2004) Hematologic reference intervals for koi (*Cyprinus carpio*), including blood cell morphology, cytochemistry, and ultrastructure. *Veterinary Clinical Pathology* 33, 74–83.
Zang, L., Shimada, Y., Nishimura, Y., Tanaka, T. and Nishimura, N. (2013) A novel, reliable method for repeated blood collection from aquarium fish. *Zebrafish* 10, 425–432.

13 Transporting Samples for Laboratory Analysis

Lily Parkinson

Brookfield Zoo, Brookfield, Illinois

Abstract

Blood and tissue samples can be submitted to commercial or university diagnostic laboratories for specialized testing. Microbial cultures and other specimens that need to be received in a viable condition require specific packaging. It is important that the correct samples are submitted and that they are handled and shipped to the laboratory by the appropriate method for accurate diagnostic test results.

13.1 Sample Types

Caring for freshwater fish may necessitate analysis of multiple sample types after collection. While many samples may be collected and analyzed on-site by a veterinarian or fish owner, some samples will require laboratory analysis for more specialized testing. Blood samples, cytology slides, bacterial culture swabs, and tissues for histopathology will make up most samples collected and sent for laboratory analysis. Following excellent and consistent protocols in obtaining, handling, securing, and shipping samples will allow the best results to be obtained. No matter how excellent a laboratory is, they will be unable to overcome damage to samples during collection, handling, or shipping (Weiser, 2012). Receiving test results that are incorrect due to inappropriate sample handling can cause erroneous interpretation of results (and thus a waste of the sample and money) or a misdiagnosis and inappropriate treatment (Meinkoth and Allison, 2007). Most general guidelines for handling animal samples and shipping can be followed for fish samples, although a few specific additional rules or caveats should be considered. Advance communication with the laboratory that is receiving the samples to discuss their comfort level with fish diagnostics, their success rate with your desired testing, and their recommended sample preparation techniques will lead to the best results.

13.2 Blood and Cytology Samples

Choosing the correct tube for the blood analytes desired is the first important step in correctly transporting a sample to a laboratory. In general, blood tubes will either be meant to preserve whole blood that will be sent for analysis (lithium heparin tubes are utilized for complete blood counts, and occasionally sodium citrate tubes), serum (red top tubes that have no additive, or serum separator tubes), or plasma (typically lithium heparin tubes and occasionally sodium citrate tubes). For fish, in order to maximize sample volume and minimize alterations from clotting, plasma is typically recommended over serum (Hrubec and Smith, 1999). In addition to traditional blood tubes, a method has been described for better preserving whole blood in fish to allow evaluation of their cell morphology after a more prolonged period of time by utilizing 10% formalin (Arnold *et al.*, 2014).

In small fish patients, a method for obtaining plasma utilizing heparinized hematocrit capillary tubes, originally described for avian patients, should be considered to maximize the volume of

Corresponding author: lilyparkinson@gmail.com

 © CAB International 2025. *The Handbook of Ornamental Fish Health and Welfare* (ed. N. Saint-Erne)
DOI: 10.1079/9781789246032.0013

plasma obtained (Fudge, 1990). It should be noted, however, if this method is utilized, that an anticoagulated needle and syringe should not be used for collection, and the blood should be placed into the capillary tubes as quickly as possible. In very small patients, making a blood smear with one drop of blood for a manual complete blood cell count, and then utilizing the remainder in the hematocrit capillary tubes could provide a full complement of blood analytes with as little as 100–200 µl of blood.

Once the blood has been placed in the correct tube or collection container, it must be appropriately processed prior to shipping. When whole blood is being submitted, the sample should generally be kept refrigerated (although some samples should be kept at room temperature—always contact the lab receiving the submission for exact guidelines) prior to shipment. If the sample is being sent for a complete blood count, it is recommended that fresh slides are made and sent along with the tube to minimize artifactual changes in the blood and allow for the best analysis of cell morphology (Allison and Meinkoth, 2007). The exact same shipping and handling recommendations should be utilized when cytology samples are submitted. If cytologic analysis of an unknown fluid is desired (e.g. a fluid obtained when aspirating the coelom), it is recommended that slides of the sample are created and then a tube of the whole fluid sample is submitted as well.

In mammals, complete blood counts and cytologic fluid analysis are typically performed on samples in EDTA tubes, but EDTA can lead to hemolysis in many species of fish (and this may be compounded with MS-222 sedative that may have been used to obtain samples). Therefore, lithium heparin is generally recommended for blood and cytologic samples obtained for analysis in fish (Noga, 2010; Campbell, 2012). If an aspirated cytology sample or impression smear has been created, then the slides should be submitted as described below. Slides from highly cellular fluids (usually the sample will appear turbid) can be created just as blood smears (Allison and Meinkoth, 2007). If the sample does not appear highly cellular, then the sample can have a portion centrifuged to concentrate the cells and then have a slide made similar to a blood smear with the cellular pellet (Meinkoth and Allison, 2007). Alternatively, a relatively low cellularity sample could be prepared similar to a blood smear, but when the slide is "pushing" the sample along the other slide, the "pusher" slide can be abruptly lifted from the base slide resulting in an abrupt termination line of the fluid. This fluid line can then be allowed to dry. A greater concentration of cells should be present within this line, due to the drag the slide created, and will allow better analysis of what limited cells are present in the sample.

When blood or cytology samples are being shipped, the blood should be kept refrigerated, but should not be allowed to become frozen. This requires that the blood be within a cooler that contains an ice pack, but the tube must be physically separated from the ice to prevent freezing. This can be accomplished via cardboard physically separating the ice pack and the blood sample. Sufficient absorbent material is wrapped around the blood tube to absorb the liquid contents of the tube if the tube were to leak (Meinkoth and Allison, 2007). Surrounding the tube with absorbent material is a requirement for most shipping couriers. Additionally, the slides being sent along should be placed in specialized rigid plastic or foam containers—cardboard holders are inadequate for protecting glass slides (Meinkoth and Allison, 2007). In addition, any slides shipped and submitted to an outside laboratory should not be fixed by heat or chemical prior to shipment, nor should they be shipped in the same box as a formalin container, even if it is stored in an airtight manner, as all of these may prevent appropriate staining of the slide when it arrives at the laboratory (Meinkoth and Allison, 2007). Be sure to work with your courier service to determine their requirements for shipping biological specimens. Many veterinary laboratories will provide pickup services for blood samples, but samples should still be packaged as though they are being shipped, as transport is often prolonged (Weiser, 2012).

If plasma is being submitted, the blood tube should be immediately centrifuged, and then the plasma should be separated and placed in a new additive-free container to minimize changes due to metabolism by the red blood cells occurring in the sample (Meinkoth and Allison, 2007). If serum is required, the tube should be allowed to sit for only 15–20 min prior to centrifugation and then serum removal, where it will then be placed in an additive-free tube (Weiser, 2012). In general, plasma and serum can be refrigerated until shipment and can be shipped on ice packs as described above for whole blood samples (Meinkoth and Allison, 2007), but certain circumstances may require frozen samples and shipment with dry ice (frozen CO_2). Consultation with the receiving laboratory is recommended, and following the courier instructions for dry ice shipment is required to ascertain that the samples are shipped in an appropriate and timely manner.

13.3 Culture Samples

Culture samples are frequently taken from fish during a clinical workup. Swabs, whole tissue, and liquid culture samples all might be obtained. Once again, contacting and discussing with the receiving laboratory is critical to ensuring that the best results are obtained for each clinical case. When swabs are taken, the swab should be placed in transport media (Amies transport media and not Stuart media is recommended for fish), refrigerated, and then shipped with ice packs to keep the samples cool (Buller, 2004).

Culturing entire tissues is a more variable process that will depend on the length of time that will elapse between obtaining the sample and arrival at the laboratory. Sterile instruments should be utilized to handle the tissue, and the surface of the tissue itself should also be sterilized. This can be accomplished by washing the surface of the tissue with sterile saline 3–4 times or heat sterilizing the surface of the tissue with 70% ethanol and a flame (Buller, 2004). A sample of tissue can then be taken from the sterilized region using sterilized scissors and forceps. This tissue can then be placed into sterile saline, transport media, or it can be macerated. A swab can then be utilized to take a sample from the macerated tissue, and the swab can be placed in transport media. Consultation with your laboratory, when an estimate of transport time has been calculated, is recommended to determine which method is recommended for individual situations. Ideally, the laboratory receiving your samples will be familiar with the culture of fish pathogens and recognize that parallel incubations at multiple temperatures, or specific culture media or salinities, may be required for specific pathogens (Noga, 2010).

A particularly difficult pathogen to culture that may be a causative agent to consider in many disease processes in fish is mycobacterial organisms. Alerting the receiving laboratory that mycobacteria may be a differential and a separate culture request for mycobacterial organisms is often necessary in fish cases. It may take many weeks to months to receive a positive mycobacterial result, and exploring other diagnostic options in the meantime, such as PCR testing, may be advisable. Regardless, a positive culture is still considered the gold standard for mycobacterial diagnosis. Discussion with the lab prior to sample collection may indicate that any liquids you desire to culture for mycobacteria need to be mixed with a culture broth nearly immediately, and other procedures may need to be undertaken if contamination with other bacteria is suspected (Kent and Kubica, 1985).

13.4 Samples for Histopathology

Samples obtained via biopsy or even whole fish may need to be shipped for histopathologic examination. Formalin fixation solution (10% buffered neutral formalin) is most often utilized (Fig. 13.1). Formalin is a carcinogen, however, so careful attention to safety must be maintained when handling and shipping this solution. Any tissues or whole animals that are being sent should be fixed in formalin in a ratio of 10:1 (i.e. 10 ml formalin for every 1 cm^3 tissue), and if a whole fish is being submitted, the coelom should be opened to allow contact between the internal organs and the formalin fixative to ensure that the fixative is able to reach the organs and prevent autolysis (Noga, 2010). If achieving this ratio will result in an unmanageable amount of formalin for shipment, then the tissues can be allowed to fix for 3–7 days, and then can be removed from the fixative solution and wrapped in formalin-soaked gauze or paper towels and then placed in tightly sealed plastic bags (APHIS, USDA, 2020). If liquid formalin will be shipped, then it must be shipped in tightly sealed plastic containers, ideally secondarily sealed with Parafilm™ around the lid, and then placed in a tightly sealed plastic bag. Placing absorbent material around the container to absorb any potential leaks is also advisable (APHIS, USDA, 2020).

As previously discussed, in general, formalin-containing shipments should be shipped alone with no other types of specimens. Formalin can severely damage cytology samples preventing appropriate staining (Meinkoth and Allison, 2007) and can also kill biological samples that a clinician is trying to culture (Chua *et al.*, 2019). In addition, formalin should not be shipped with ice packs or dry ice; and, since this is often required for shipping other sample types, this provides another reason to separate shipment of differing sample types (APHIS, USDA, 2020).

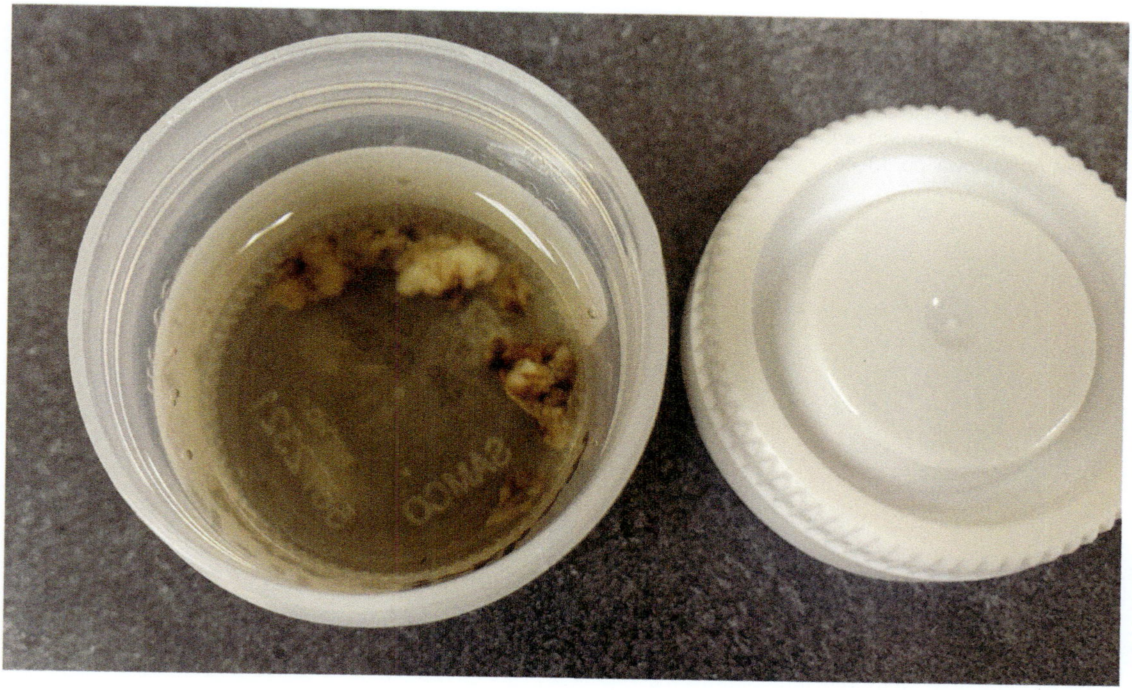

Fig. 13.1. Tissue samples submitted for histopathology in formalin should be less than 1 cm in thickness. (Photograph by N. Saint-Erne.)

13.5 Conclusions

Prior planning and communication with the personnel at the laboratory being utilized who have experience with fish-specific diagnostics will produce the most clinically useful results. Appropriate packaging of the samples will help preserve them and will be safest for all personnel involved.

References

Allison, R.W. and Meinkoth, J.H. (2007) Hematology without the numbers: in-clinic blood film evaluation. *Veterinary Clinics of North America: Small Animal Practice* 37, 245–266, vi.

APHIS, USDA (2020) Packaging and labeling submissions to the NVSL. 20 June 2020. Available: at: https://www.aphis.usda.gov/aphis/ourfocus/animalhealth/lab-info-services/SA_Diagnostic_Tests/CT_Packaging_labeling (accessed 24 November 2020).

Arnold, J.E., Matsche, M.A. and Rosemary, K. (2014) Preserving whole blood in formalin extends the specimen stability period for manual cell counts for fish. *Veterinary Clinical Pathology* 43, 613–620.

Buller, N. (2004) Bacteriological culture techniques: microscopy, culture and identification. In: Buller, N. (ed.) *Bacteria from Fish and Other Aquatic Animals: A Practical Identification Manual*. CAB International, Wallingford, UK.

Campbell, T. (2012) Hematology of fish. In: Thrall, M.A., Weiser, G., Allison, R.W. and Campbell, T. (eds) *Veterinary Hematology and Clinical Chemistry*. 2nd edn. Wiley, Ames, Iowa, pp. 298–312.

Chua, J., Bozue, J.A., Klimko, C.P., Shoe, J.L., Ruiz, S.I. *et al*. (2019) Formaldehyde and glutaraldehyde inactivation of bacterial tier 1 select agents in tissues. *Emerging Infectious Diseases* 25, 919–926.

Fudge, A. (1990) How to get the most from your avian diagnostic laboratory. *Journal of the Association of Avian Veterinarians* 4, 208–211.

Hrubec, T. and Smith, S. (1999) Differences between plasma and serum samples for the evaluation of blood chemistry values in rainbow trout, channel catfish, hybrid tilapias, and hybrid striped bass. *Journal of Aquatic Animal Health* 11, 116–122.

Kent, P. and Kubica, G. (1985) *Public Health Mycobacteriology: A Guide for the Level III Laboratory*. US Department of Health and Human Services, Atlanta, Georgia.

Meinkoth, J.H. and Allison, R.W. (2007) Sample collection and handling: getting accurate results. *Veterinary Clinics of North America: Small Animal Practice* 37, 203–219, v.

Noga, E. (2010) The clinical workup. In: Noga, E. (ed.) *Fish Disease: Diagnosis and Treatment*. 2nd edn. Wiley, Ames, Iowa, pp. 13–48.

Weiser, G. (2012) Sample collection, processing, and analysis of laboratory service options. In: Thrall, M.A., Weiser, G., Allison, R.W. and Campbell, T. (eds) *Veterinary Hematology and Clinical Chemistry*. 2nd edn. Wiley, Ames, Iowa, pp. 34–39.

14 Advanced Diagnostic Techniques

NICHOLAS SAINT-ERNE

Dr. Saint-Erne Consulting, PLLC, Phoenix, Arizona

Abstract

Diagnosing diseases in fish starts with a physical examination and testing the water quality. From there, the diagnostic tests can include biopsies, blood tests, and more advanced techniques, such as radiology, sonography, endoscopy, and other medical procedures. Diagnostic equipment used in a small animal medical clinic can be used on fish patients as well.

14.1 Further Diagnostic Tests

What are the next steps in diagnosing fish diseases after having completed skin and gill biopsy examinations and bacterial cultures? How about blood tests, radiographs, endoscopy, sonography, or even computed tomography (CT) and magnetic resonance imaging (MRI)? With some accommodations for handling fish, the same diagnostic tools that are frequently used for other animals can be applied to fish (Eshar *et al.*, 2009). Diagnosing diseases in fish, especially internal problems, can be made easier with the use of radiology, ultrasound, and endoscopy equipment already present in the veterinary clinic. Techniques such as CT and MRI, when available through specialty practices or veterinary colleges, can also be of great assistance in diagnosing abnormalities of the cardiovascular system, intestinal tract, gas bladder, and abdominal organs in larger fish, such as a koi with abdominal distension. These techniques, along with microscopic analysis of fluid and tissue biopsies, are very helpful in the diagnosis of fish diseases.

14.2 Hematology

Collecting blood for hematology can provide information about the fish's health. Drawing blood samples from larger fish, especially koi, can be done from the caudal vein below the spine in the caudal peduncle. Use a 1-ml tuberculin syringe with a 22- or 23-gauge needle of appropriate length. A butterfly catheter can be attached to the syringe to facilitate handling of the needle separately from the syringe. Fill the hub of the needle with a drop of lithium heparin to prevent the blood from clotting. This is preferable to ammonium heparin or sodium heparin, but they can also be used for hematology testing. The ammonium and sodium heparins will affect the ammonia and sodium blood values if used in samples for serology or electrolyte testing. Ethylenediamine tetraacetic acid (EDTA) is not recommended to be used to prevent blood clotting in fish blood samples, as it may cause erythrocyte lysis.

To collect a blood sample from an anesthetized fish, the needle is inserted at an angle pointing craniodorsally from the ventral midline of the caudal peduncle until it hits the vertebrae (Fig. 14.1). Withdraw the needle slightly and it should be in the caudal vein. Light aspiration on the syringe plunger should be applied to collect the blood. The total volume of blood in most fish makes up about 5% of its body weight (50 ml/kg). Up to 20% of the total blood volume can safely be removed in fish that are not excessively ill. This allows for 0.1 ml of blood to be removed from a 10-g fish (20% × 50 ml/kg × 10 g = 0.1 ml), 0.5 ml of blood removed from a 50-g fish, or 1 ml from a 100-g fish. Larger blood samples are usually not necessary, even though more blood could be drawn from a larger fish such as a koi (Saint-Erne, 2010a).

Corresponding author: DrSaintErne@gmail.com

© CAB International 2025. *The Handbook of Ornamental Fish Health and Welfare* (ed. N. Saint-Erne)
DOI: 10.1079/9781789246032.0014

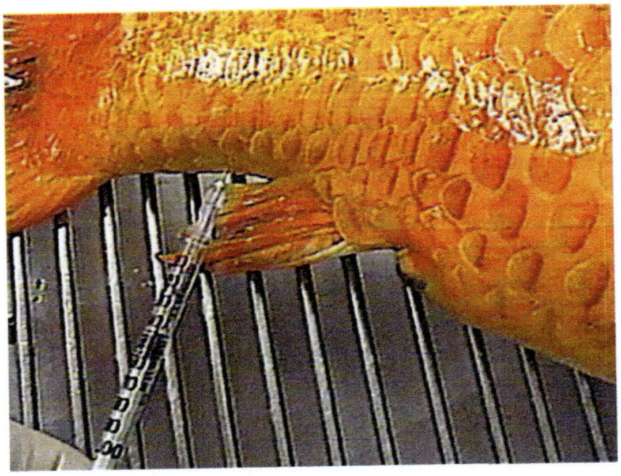

Fig. 14.1. Ventral approach to collect blood from the caudal vein of a koi (*Cyprinus rubrofuscus*). (Photograph by N. Saint-Erne.)

14.3 Radiology

Standard veterinary radiology equipment can be used to take radiographs of fish. The fish can be anesthetized and removed from the water for taking the radiographs, or it can be restrained in a plastic bag with a small volume of water taped to the table to keep the fish from moving. Many times, the fish will lie still without jumping even without restraint, but each case must be evaluated individually to determine the restraint needed (Fig. 14.2). Fish can also be anesthetized and then taken out of the water and positioned for radiographs.

Radiographs are good for examining the gas bladder (Fig. 14.3), bone structures, spinal deformities (Figs 14.4a and b), or abdominal swellings, and occasionally ingested foreign objects can be evaluated using radiology. Internal organs are not easily distinguishable in a radiograph without a contrast medium. A flexible rubber catheter can be inserted orally passing through the esophagus to place barium or iodinated contrast solution into the stomach or intestines to perform contrast studies on the intestinal tract (Figs 14.5a and b). The dosage for barium is 5–10 ml/kg body weight and the iodinated medium is dosed at 1–2 ml/kg. Be careful not to leak barium into the oral cavity and onto the gills, which could impair oxygen diffusion through the gills. Contrast radiology can be helpful in visualizing an intestinal obstruction or displacement of the intestines due to an abdominal mass. Ovaries filled with roe in females can sometimes be visualized on radiographs to help determine the sex of young koi.

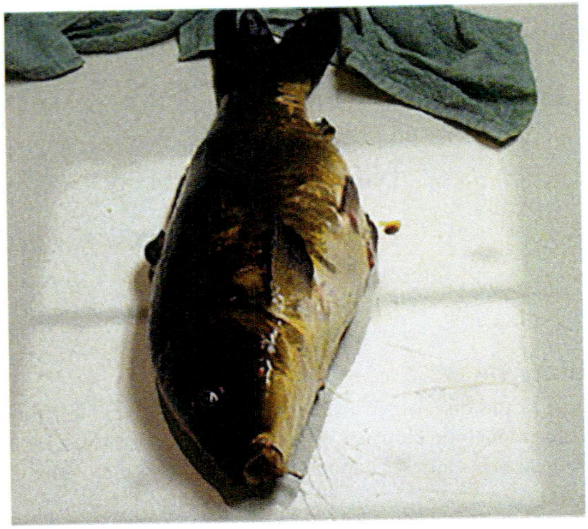

Fig. 14.2. An anesthetized Karasu koi (*C. rubrofuscus*) with a buoyancy problem is positioned for taking a lateral radiograph to evaluate the gas bladder. Note the wet towel used to carry the fish to the radiography table. (Photograph by N. Saint-Erne.)

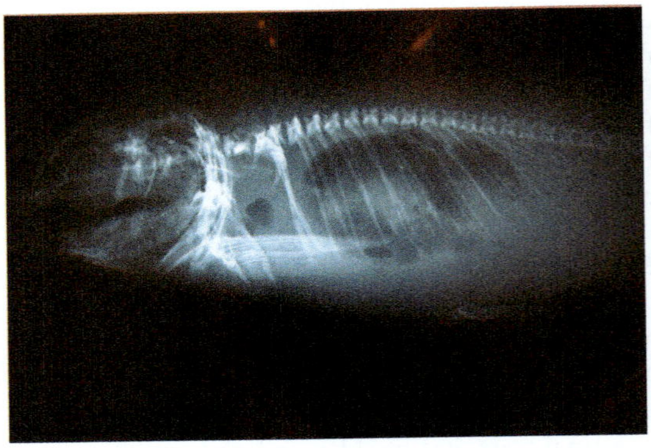

Fig. 14.3. The Karasu koi (*C. rubrofuscus*) has an abnormal accumulation of gas and fluid in its swim bladder. (Photograph by N. Saint-Erne.)

14.4 Sonography

Ultrasound imaging uses high-frequency (3–10 MHz) sound waves to produce a computer-generated cross-section (sonogram) of the area of the body being examined. Real-time computer sampling will produce a moving picture that can show the beating of the heart or peristalsis waves of the intestines. Different tissues propagate or reflect sound waves at varying quantities. Sound waves propagate in soft tissues, and they will appear in shades of gray, and fluids appear black. Sound is reflected by

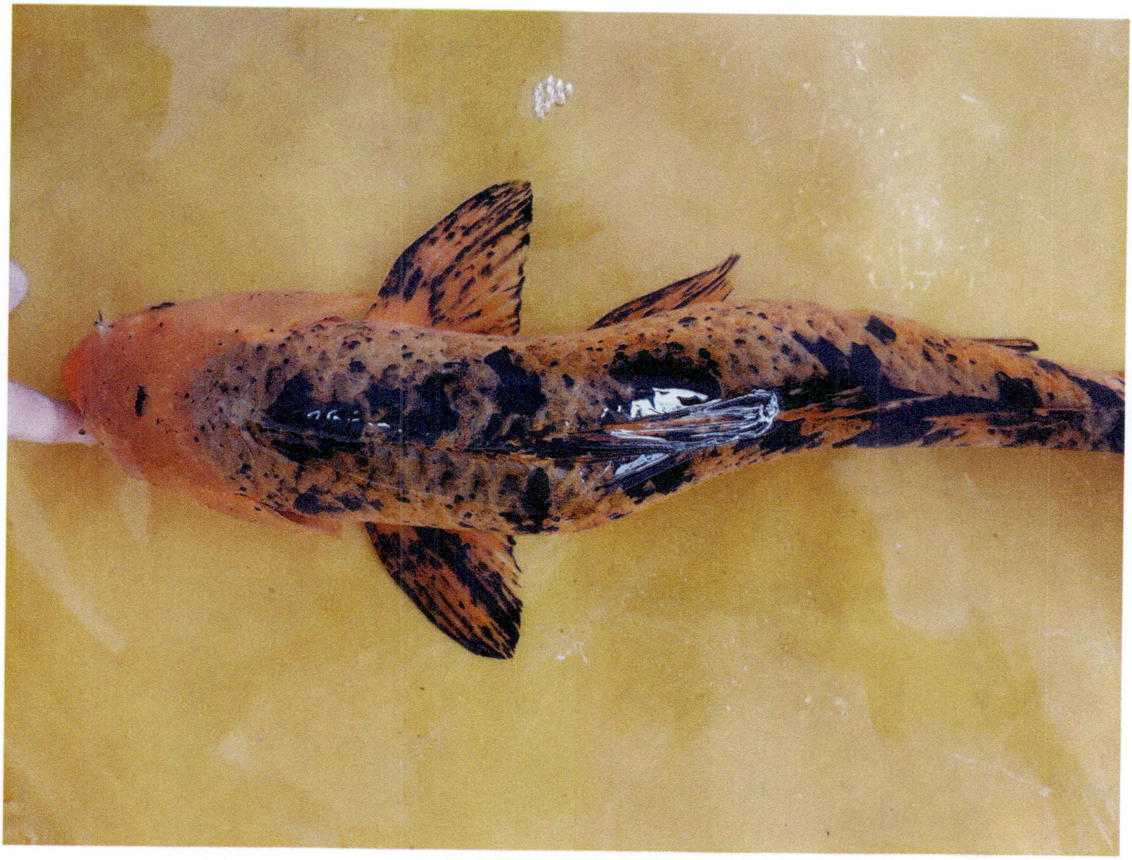

Fig. 14.4a. An adult Ki Utsuri koi with scoliosis associated with damaged vertebrae. (Photograph by S. Johnson.)

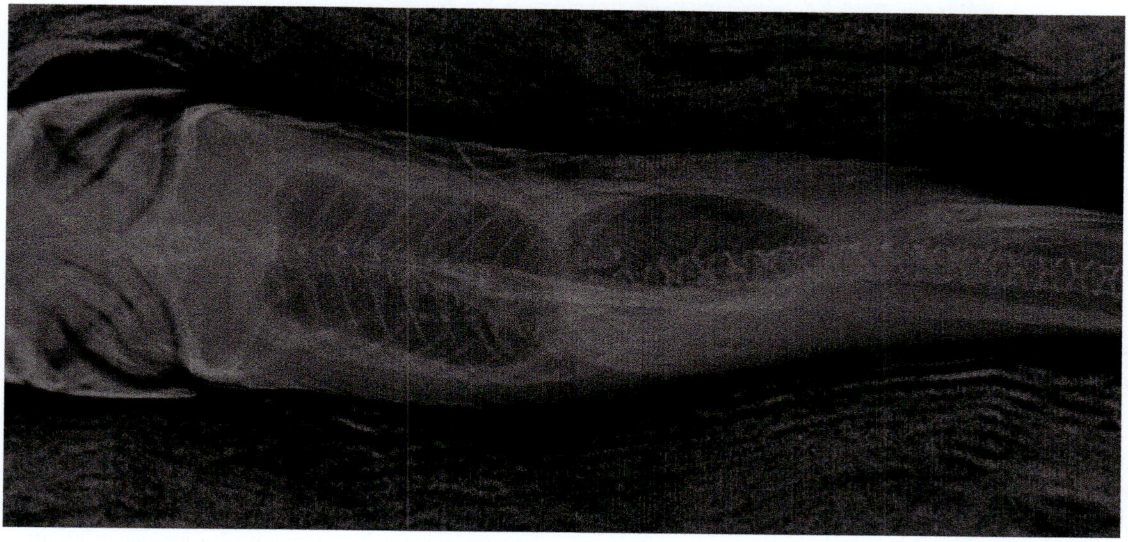

Fig. 14.4b. Radiograph of the Ki Utsuri koi with scoliosis. (Photograph by S. Johnson.)

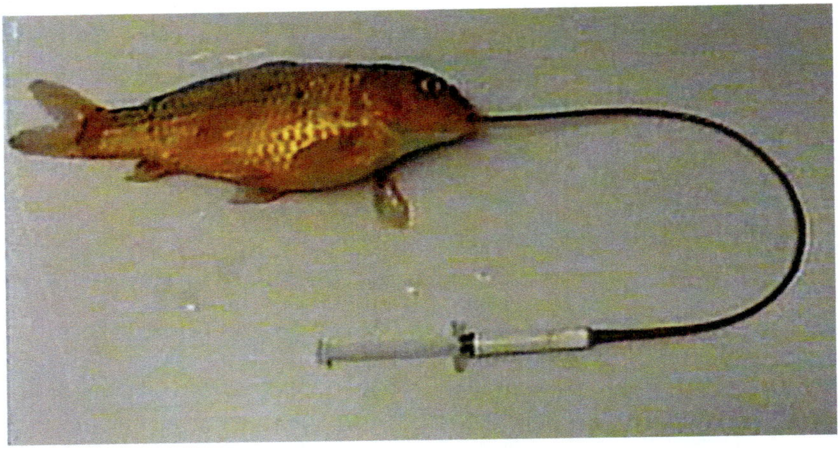

Fig. 14.5a. Barium is inserted into the intestines of an anesthetized koi using a rubber catheter down its pharynx. (Photograph by N. Saint-Erne.)

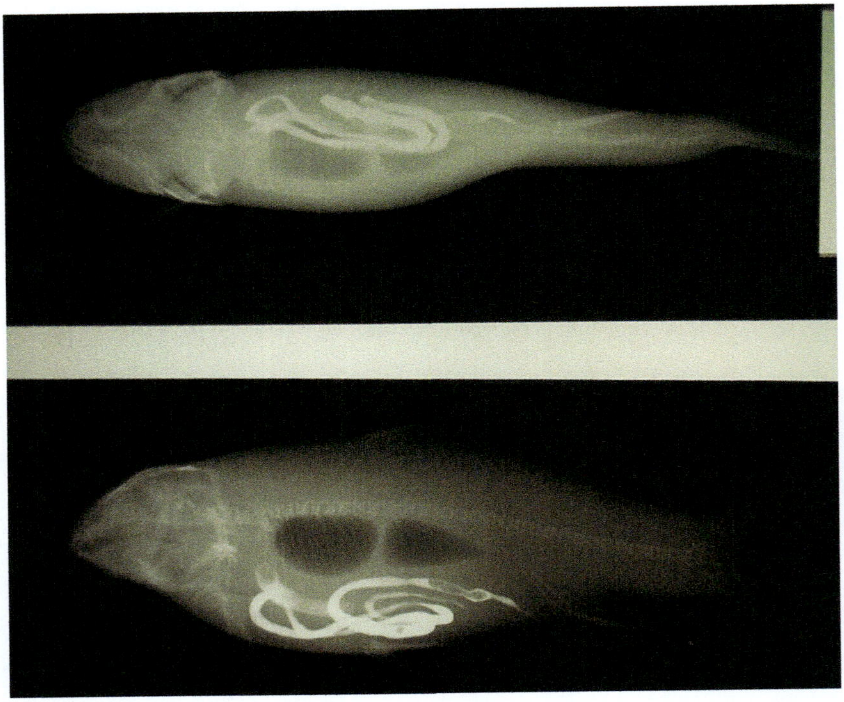

Fig. 14.5b. Dorsal ventral (DV) and lateral views of the koi with barium. The barium has reached the koi's distal intestines by three hours post administration. (Photograph by N. Saint-Erne.)

bones and air, which send echoes back and appear white. Ultrasound is a safe, rapid, and non-invasive diagnostic tool that usually does not require sedation of the patient. The fish is kept in the water, which aids in handling the fish and increases sound propagation. An ultrasound transducer of 5–10 MHz works well for visualization of internal organs at depths up to 20 cm into the body, with lower frequency transducers producing images at greater depths of tissue penetration (Stetter, 1999).

The transducer, if not waterproof, is wrapped in a waterproof cover (plastic bag, exam glove, condom) and is placed against the side of the fish while it is still in a shallow container of water (Fig. 14.6). Coupling gel is not necessary for fish in the water, and the transducer can be held several centimeters away from the skin surface while underwater. The transducer is repositioned until the desired image is obtained. Echocardiogram refers to an ultrasound that is used to monitor the beating of the heart (Fig. 14.7). The image can be in motion or frozen into a still picture. Most ultrasound units will save the images, so they can be replayed or printed. A motion image can be used to guide a biopsy needle into a specific organ or mass for a biopsy sample collection, abdominocentesis (coelocentesis), or pneumocystocentesis (Fig. 14.8). Anesthesia may be needed for biopsies, however.

14.5 Endoscopy

Endoscopic examination of the oral cavity, gill arches, and pharynx can be performed by passing the endoscope into the mouth (Fig. 14.9) or through the gill operculum (Fig. 14.10) of an anesthetized fish. Traditional biopsies of gill filament tips may miss lesions at the base of gill filaments that may be found using an endoscope. Flexible endoscopes can be passed through the esophagus into the stomach or intestines and have application in foreign body removal in larger fish (Sladakovic and Divers, 2021). Cyprinid fish such as koi and goldfish have no stomach, but the proximal intestine is elastic and can distend to hold ingesta.

Laparoscopy (coelioscopy) can be performed in larger fish to visualize internal organs or take biopsy samples. A few scales can be removed to access the dermis. A stab incision is made through an anesthetized fish's body wall and hemostats are

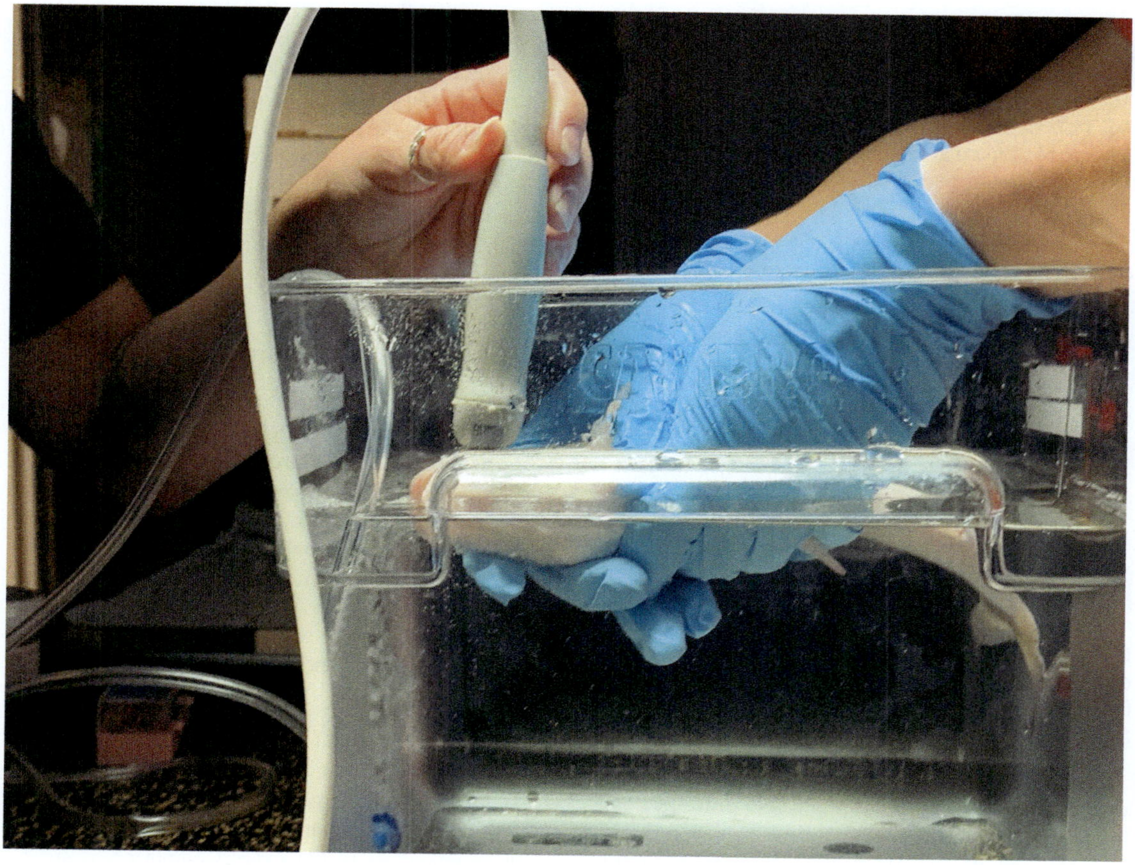

Fig. 14.6. Ultrasound imaging of the eye of a humpback chub. (Photograph by N. Saint-Erne.)

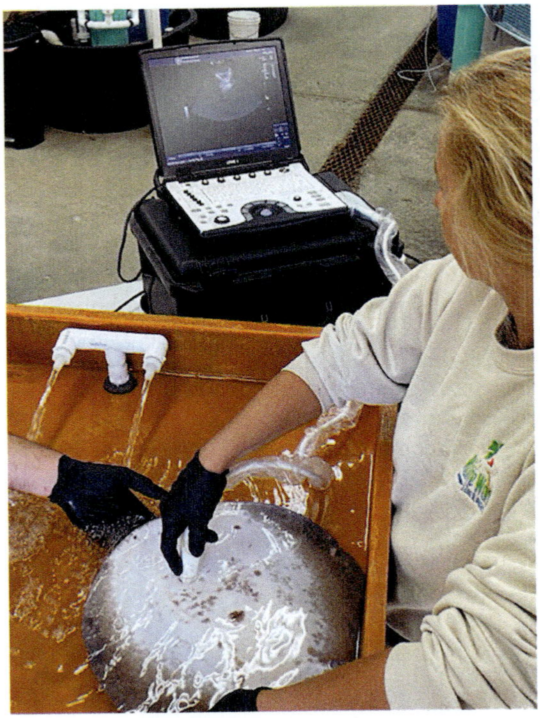

Fig. 14.7. Dr. Sharmie Johnson performing an echocardiogram on an anesthetized freshwater stingray. (Photograph by Marie Dillon, CVT.)

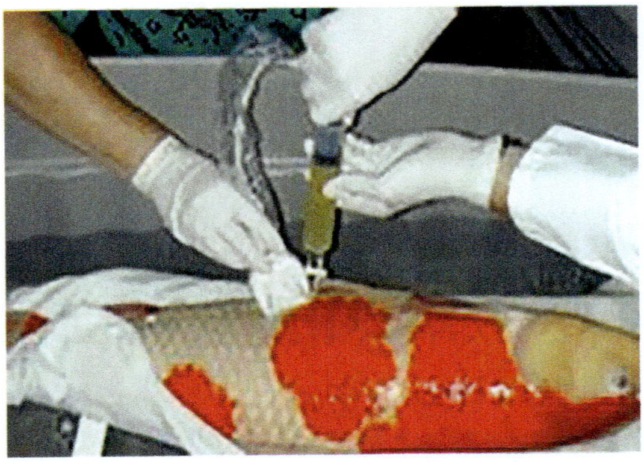

Fig. 14.8. Using ultrasonography to guide the needle during a pneumocystocentesis on a Kohaku koi's fluid-filled gas bladder. (Photo courtesy of Gregory A. Lewbart, MS, VMD, Dipl. ACZM.)

used to open the skin and muscle layer into the coelomic cavity, just large enough to insert an endoscope. Coelomic cavity visualization is used to evaluate the liver (hepatopancreas), the gonads to determine

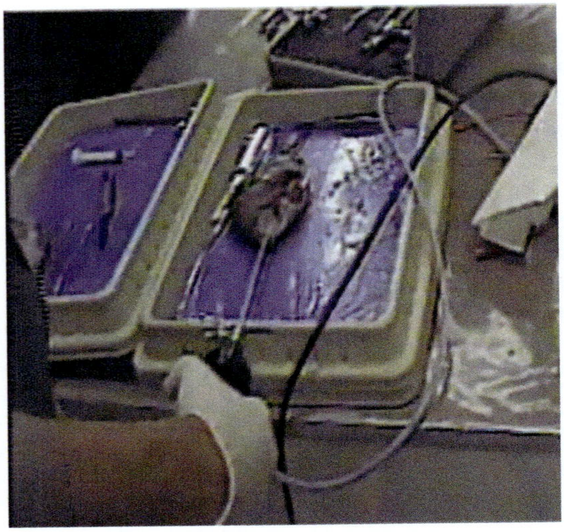

Fig. 14.9. Endoscopic exam of a fish's oral cavity and gills. (Photograph by N. Saint-Erne.)

gender or reproductive organ development, the presence of adhesions or inflammation, the gas bladder position and status (inflamed, deflated, or fluid infused), or to collect an abdominal swab for bacterial culture. If the coelomic cavity has been insufflated with air during the procedure, the air must be removed to prevent buoyancy problems immediately after the procedure. The small laparoscopy incision can be closed with a simple interrupted absorbable suture, which is preferably removed after the incision heals to minimize inflammation from the suture material.

14.6 Fluoroscopy

Fluoroscopy is an imaging technique used to obtain real-time moving images of the internal structures of a patient using a fluoroscope, which consists of an X-ray source that projects through the patient onto a fluorescent screen (Fig. 14.11). These images are useful when looking at the heart to assess its beating and blood flow.

14.7 Computed Tomography Scans

CT scans can be performed on fish, while they are in a small container of oxygenated water. The water does not affect the image in a CT scan (Saint-Erne, 2010b). The CT images are narrow slices through the body that are examined sequentially to diagnose abnormalities (Figs 14.12a and b). Computer reconstruction of the images can provide a three-dimensional

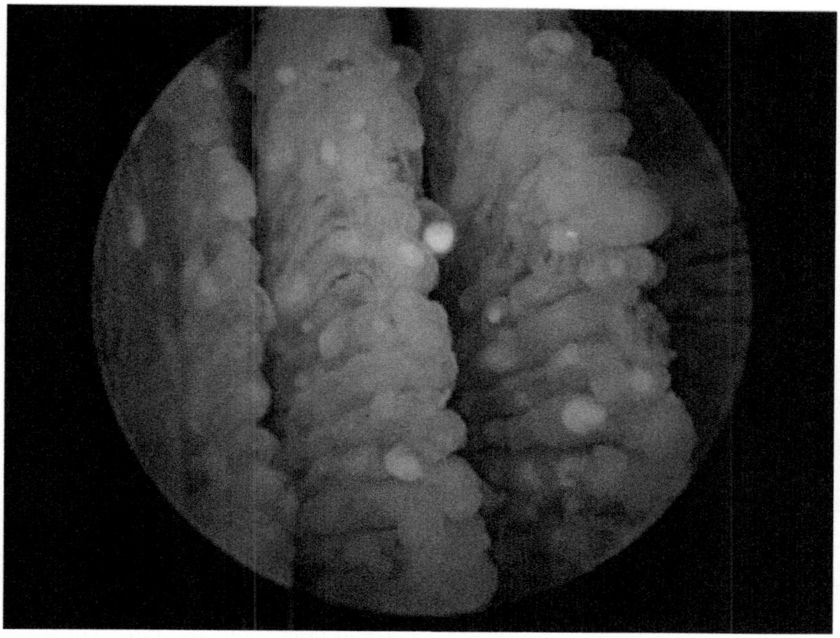

Fig. 14.10. Rigid endoscopic exam of *Acanthurus mata* gills infested with *Cryptocaryon* protozoa. (Photograph courtesy of Shane Boylan, DVM.)

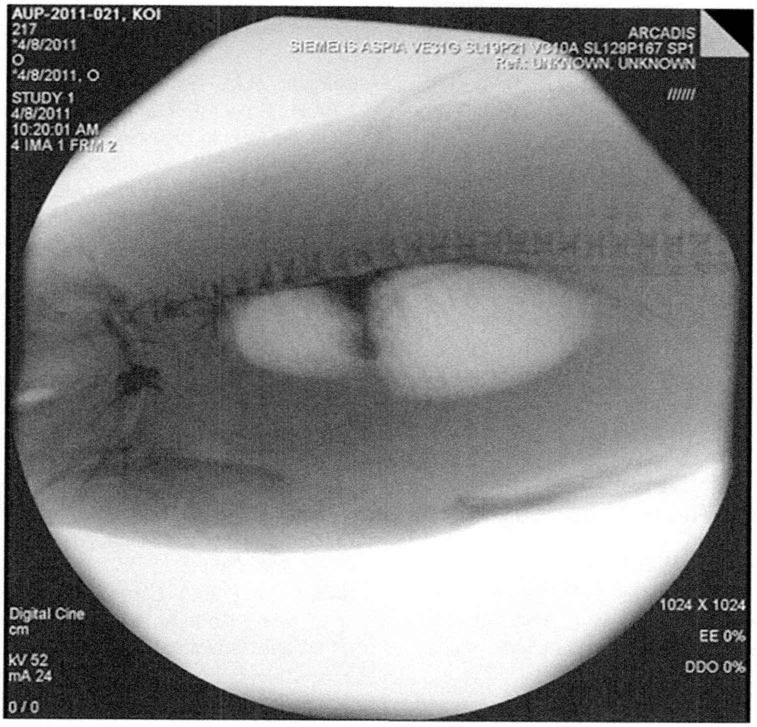

Fig. 14.11. Still image from a fluoroscopy video of a koi. (Photograph courtesy of Zoe Browning, DVM.)

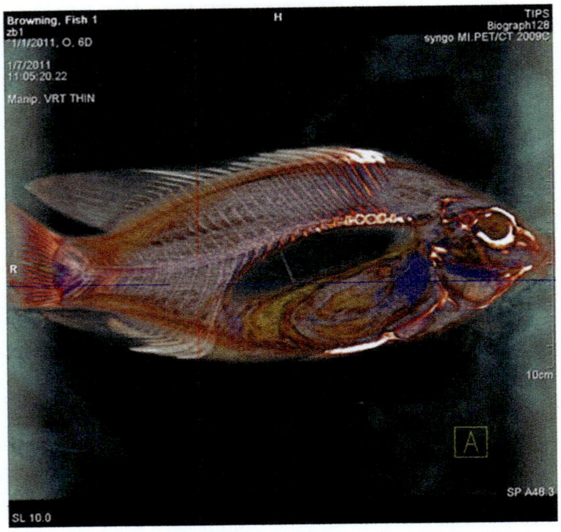

Fig. 14.12a. CT scan image of a tilapia cichlid. (Photograph courtesy of Zoe Browning, DVM.)

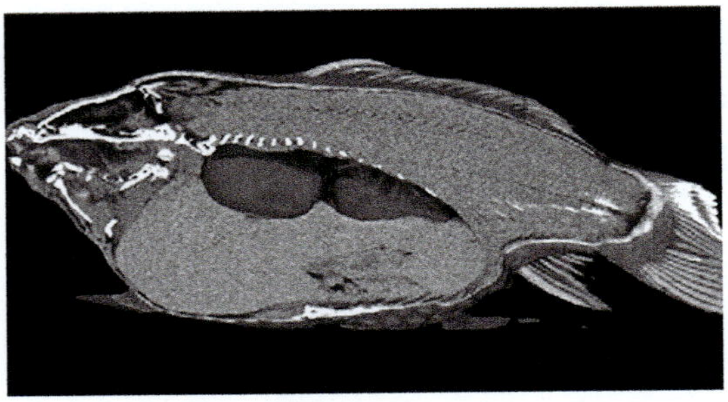

Fig. 14.12b. CT image of a gravid female koi, sagittal section. The large egg mass (roe) is visible below the two chambers of the gas bladder. (Photograph courtesy of Gregory A. Lewbart, MS, VMD, Dipl. ACZM.)

radiographic image of skin, muscles, skeleton, and other internal structures or two-dimensional views of sequential planes through the body.

14.8 Magnetic Resonance Imaging

MRI, which uses nuclear magnetic resonance instead of X-rays to generate an image, can produce very detailed images of the soft tissue and internal anatomy, and is useful in diagnosing neoplasia. Because the patient needs to remain motionless during the MRI procedure, anesthesia is required during imaging. MRI of preserved museum specimens has allowed them to be examined in detail without damage to the original fish (Berquist *et al.*, 2012). The Digital Fish Library (DFL, http://www.digitalfishlibrary.org) is an online digital archive of high-resolution, high-contrast MRI scans of the soft tissue anatomy of an array of fishes preserved in the Marine Vertebrate Collection of Scripps Institution of Oceanography. Examining the MRI of fishes in this collection can help understand the anatomy of each species.

14.9 Conclusion

Veterinarians have many diagnostic options available, and most of these can successfully be used with fish patients. Making the correct diagnosis of diseases in fish is as important as with any other patient. While most fish illnesses do not require these advanced diagnostic techniques, it is important to know that they can be effectively used with fish patients as well as with humans and other animals.

References

Berquist, R.M., Gledhill, K.M., Peterson, M.W., Doan, A.H., Baxter, G.T. *et al.* (2012) The digital fish library: using MRI to digitize, database, and document the morphological diversity of fish. *PLoS ONE* 7(4): e34499. doi:10.1371/journal.pone.0034499.

Eshar, D., Latney, L. and Wyre, N. (2009) Diagnostic contrast radiography in fish. *Lab Animal* 38, 323–324. doi:10.1038/laban1009-323.

Saint-Erne, N. (2010a) Diagnostic methods. In: Saint-Erne, N. (ed.) *Advanced Koi Care*. 2nd edn. Erne Enterprises, Glendale, Arizona, pp. 40–49.

Saint-Erne, N. (2010b) Diagnostic techniques and treatments for internal disorders of Koi. *Veterinary Clinics of North America Exotic Animal Practice* 13(3), 333–347.

Sladakovic, I. and Divers, S. (2021) Surgery and endoscopy. In: Hadfield, C. and Clayton, L. (eds) *Clinical Guide to Fish Medicine*. Wiley, Hoboken, New Jersey, pp. 213–223.

Stetter, M. (1999) *Ultrasonography of Non-domestic Species*. North American Veterinary Conference Fish Wetlab, Orlando, Florida.

15 Sedation, Anesthesia, and Euthanasia

NICHOLAS SAINT-ERNE

Dr. Saint-Erne Consulting, PLLC, Phoenix, Arizona

Abstract

Fish react to painful stimuli and should be given sedation or anesthesia prior to any handling that would cause stress or discomfort. There are many commonly used anesthetic drugs in small animal veterinary medicine that are effective for fish. Anesthetics are also effectively used for performing euthanasia in fish.

15.1 Fish Anesthesia

15.1.1 Anesthetics and equipment

When handling fish for examination, diagnostic testing, or disease treatment, it is often desirable to use an anesthetic agent to calm the fish to reduce stress and trauma. Surgery can also be performed on anesthetized fish to repair wounds, remove skin and fin tumors, or remove abdominal masses. Many chemicals have been used to induce sedation and anesthesia in fish (Table 15.1). All have some element of risk, but when used carefully they have successfully induced sedation or anesthesia in fish (Saint-Erne, 2010; Yanong and Lewbart, 2024).

The anesthetic dose is added to clean, well-oxygenated water in a suitable glass or plastic container (Fig. 15.1). The water is thoroughly mixed to ensure all the anesthetic chemical is dissolved and dispersed evenly. Using a syringe with a needle attached to inject liquid anesthetic under the water in the anesthesia chamber will help mix the anesthetic solution into the water. The anesthetic solution should be the same temperature, salinity, and pH as the aquarium or pond water. Use a thermometer to monitor the water temperature during anesthesia and monitor the dissolved oxygen concentration if an oxygen meter is available. The anesthetic solution should be aerated during the procedure. Ventilating the fish by having water pumped through the mouth and across the gills will ensure smoother anesthesia and reduce the risk of the fish becoming hypoxic.

Never leave a fish unattended while it is under anesthesia. Cover the anesthesia chamber to prevent the fish from jumping out. Monitor the respiration rate (opercular movements) to assess the depth of anesthesia. The fish will lie on its side, and the respiratory rate will slow as the chemical induces anesthesia (Fig. 15.2). The concentration of immersion anesthetic should be decreased by diluting the anesthetic solution with water after induction (Neiffer, 2021). Maintaining a fish for a prolonged period at the induction concentration will result in excessive anesthetic depth and can lead to prolonged recovery times and even death. After the examination, diagnostic procedure, or surgery is completed, the fish is placed into clean, aerated water without any anesthetic to recover safely, before being returned to the aquarium or pond (Fig. 15.3).

15.1.2 Anesthesia induction

Anesthesia is usually performed using two containers of good-quality water, with aeration. Aeration can be provided by an electric aquarium air pump or using a battery-operated air pump available at fishing supply stores for use with bait fish. A water pump, such as an aquarium filter power head, can

Corresponding author: DrSaintErne@gmail.com

© CAB International 2025. *The Handbook of Ornamental Fish Health and Welfare* (ed. N. Saint-Erne)
DOI: 10.1079/9781789246032.0015

Table 15.1. Anesthetic drugs and dosages used with fishes. Author's own table.

Alfaxalone (3-alpha-hydroxy-5-alpha-pregnane 11,20-dione)—Dose at 1–2 mg/l for sedation, 2–10 mg/l will achieve anesthesia. Induction time is 5 min with recovery in 3–10 min.

Benzocaine (ethyl p-aminobenzoate)—Dose at 15–40 mg/l for sedation during transportation. Dose at 50–500 mg (may need to dissolve in ethanol first)/l of water for anesthesia. Induction time in 1 min, recovery in fresh water in 3–15 min.

Butorphanol—0.1–0.2 mg/kg IV or 0.4 mg/kg IM for post-operative analgesia.

Carbon dioxide (CO_2)—A dose of 100–400 mg/l will cause unconsciousness; excessive exposure will cause death. Use it with caution, under constant observation! Can be used for euthanasia.

Induction is in 1–2 min and recovery in 5–10 min in fresh water.

Diazepam (Valium)—A sedative and muscle relaxant, used as a preanesthetic agent.

Can be injected intramuscularly at 0.1–0.5 mg/kg or mixed in food and given orally.

Ethanol (ethyl alcohol)—1% added to the water will produce sedation, 3% or more will result in euthanasia. Using 20 ml of 100-proof (50%) grain alcohol or vodka in 1 l of water will produce a 1% solution.

Etomidate—0.5–3.6 mg/l bath used for anesthesia.

Eugenol (85% clove oil)—Use 40–120 mg/l (1–3 drops/l of water). Mix vigorously.

Induction occurs in 2–5 min and recovery in 5 min in fresh water.

Can be made more water-soluble by mixing with ethanol.

Isoflurane (1-chloro-2,2,2-trifluoroethyl difluoromethyl ether)—Dose at 0.5–1 ml/l water. Spray the required dose through a 25-gauge needle under the water while mixing. Induction in 2–8 min, recovery in clean water in 3–30 min.

Ketamine hydrochloride—Dose at 1 g/l water, or 66–88 mg/kg injected intramuscularly.

Provides sedation and immobilization for handling or transportation.

Lidocaine—1–2 mg/kg IM for topical anesthesia.

Metomidate—Sedation concentration: 0.1–1.0 mg/l of water. Dosages for tranquilization used in transporting tropical fish vary from 1 to 5 mg/l. Anesthesia: 1.0–10.0 mg/l of water. The dosage should be individualized, depending upon the fish species and the degree of anesthesia required. May need buffering if water is at a low pH. Not recommended for long procedures.

Pentobarbital—20–40 mg/kg IM or ICoe. 60–100 mg/kg ICoe for euthanasia.

Induces long anesthesia time and may cause cardiac and respiratory depression.

Propofol (2,6-diisopropylphenol)—Anesthesia induction dose is 1.5–2.5 mg/kg intravenously. Use parenterally only. Can be used as an immersion anesthetic at 2.5–10 mg/l. Induction time is 5 min; recovery in 60–75 min.

Quinaldine sulfate (2-methylquinoline sulfate)—Dose at 5–10 mg/l for sedation, and 25–100 mg/l for anesthesia. Induction in 2–6 min, recovery in fresh water in 5–20 min.

Acidifies low alkaline water. Use buffer in water as necessary.

Sevoflurane—similar to isoflurane use.

Tricaine methane sulfonate, MS-222 (3-Aminobenzoic acid ethyl ester)—Dose at 10–40 mg/l for sedation (handling/shipping). Dose at 50–120 mg/l for anesthesia induction.

Induction in 1–5 min; recovery in 3–15 min in clean water.

Acidifies water—add sodium bicarbonate in a volume equal to measured MS-222 as buffer.

Add more sodium bicarbonate (baking soda) as needed to maintain pH of the solution equal to the aquarium water. Sodium carbonate (Na_2CO_3) also known as washing soda, or soda ash, is a stronger buffer than sodium bicarbonate and may be more useful in salt water to maintain the proper pH of the anesthetic solution.

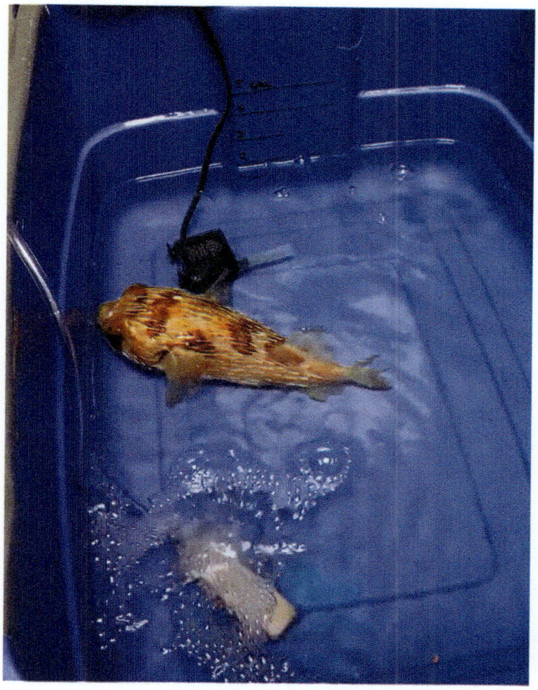

Fig. 15.1. Anesthesia induction container with a submersible water pump and an air stone for aeration being used to anesthetize a spiny pufferfish (*Diodon holocanthus*). (Photograph by N. Saint-Erne.)

also be used to create water surface agitation to provide aeration. In a veterinary clinic, using an oxygen canister with tubing that bubbles O_2 through the water can also be used. One of the water containers is used for induction with the anesthetic solution. Place the fish into the container and monitor it to determine the stages of anesthesia (Table 15.2). When the fish has reached the desired level of sedation or anesthesia, remove the fish for treatment, biopsy or other diagnostic tests, or surgery (Saint-Erne, 2019).

Use wet, powderless gloves for handling fish to prevent damage to the mucous layer of the skin. Keep the skin and gills wet if the fish is kept out of the water. Lubricate its eyes using sterile ophthalmic ointment. Place the fish on a wet, plastic drape, or cloth towel to keep its skin moist (Fig. 15.4). Pump lower dose anesthesia solution over gills to maintain anesthesia. This can be done by hand using a large syringe, by gravity using an IV bag filled with anesthetic solution and a drip line placed into the fish's mouth, or by using a small water pump/aquarium power head. Make sure there is an even flow of the anesthetic solution out of both opercula and that the solution is not going down the esophagus. Have oxygenated fresh water on hand to syringe across the gills if the plane of anesthesia becomes too deep.

15.1.3 Anesthetic monitoring

To determine the depth of anesthesia, monitor the fish's response to touch and righting reflex. Observe the opercular movement, as the respiratory rate will decrease with the anesthetic depth (Loh *et al.*, 2022). It is important to record the respiratory rate prior to anesthesia and keep track of the rate during the procedure. The anesthesia concentration in the water may need to be diluted if the respiratory rate is slowing.

An electrocardiogram (ECG) can be connected to larger fish by inserting hypodermic needles into the muscles at the base of the pectoral fins. A third needle can be inserted into the muscles anterior to the anal fin. Clamp the ECG leads onto the needles to monitor the heart rate (Fig. 15.5). Be aware that in fish the heart can continue to beat even after death, so the rate of change is important. Get an early heart rate reading when the fish is first under anesthesia and reduce the anesthetic level if the heart rate is slowing. An ultrasound machine can also be used to monitor the fish's heart rate. Using pulse oximetry on the fish's caudal fin can provide a pulse rate and blood oxygen saturation percentage (Fig. 15.6). If the oxygen saturation is decreasing, increase the aeration in the anesthetic solution by bubbling oxygen from an O_2 canister through the anesthetic solution. Monitor the water temperature and quality during anesthetic procedures.

15.1.4 Anesthesia recovery

Lower the anesthetic dose in the water by diluting the anesthesia container with fresh water when nearing the end of the procedure, or if the respiration or heart rate slows. Recuperation after anesthesia is accomplished by transferring the fish into a container of fresh well-aerated water. The longer the fish has been under anesthesia, the longer the fish will take to recover. Use dim lighting above the recovery tank and keep the recovery area quiet.

Moving larger fish gently in a forward direction will aid the flow of fresh water across the gills, hastening anesthesia release from the gills. Do not slosh the fish back and forth in the water. A small water pump can also be used to flow water into the

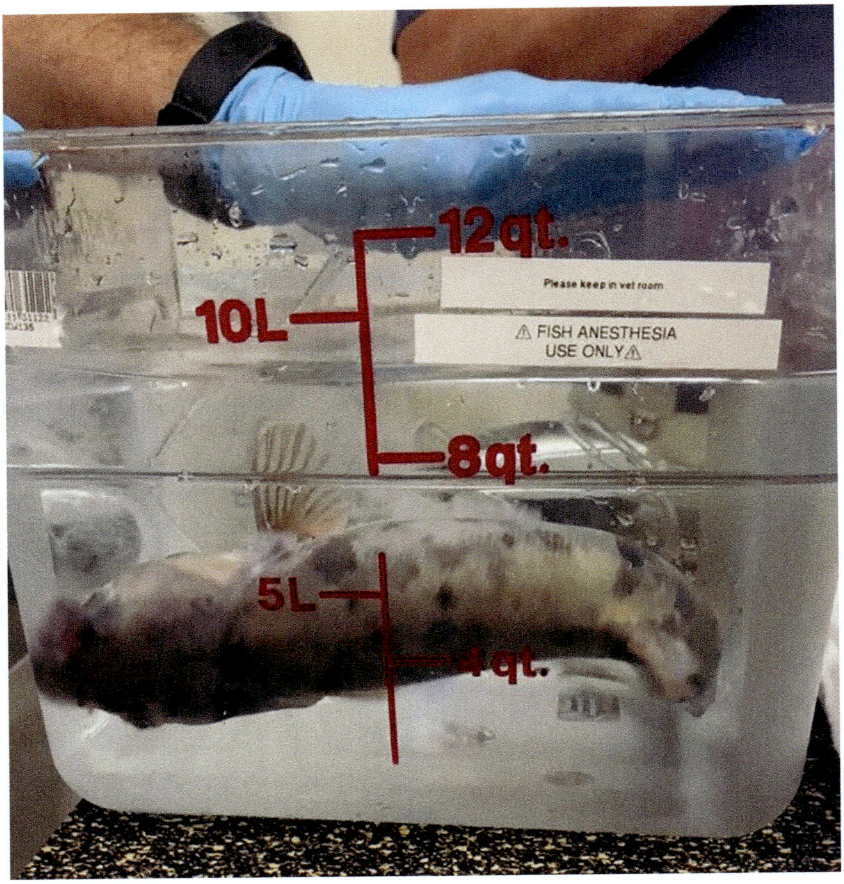

Fig. 15.2. A roundtail chub (*Gila robusta*) turns onto its side as it becomes anesthetized. (Photograph by N. Saint-Erne.)

fish's mouth and out its gills. Once there are steady opercular movements, let the fish rest and gradually recover in a quiet, dim environment. Cover the tank to prevent the fish from jumping out as it recovers, as the fish may become reactive when awakening from anesthesia (Loh *et al.*, 2022). Monitor it until it is swimming normally and can be transferred back into the aquarium or pond.

15.2 Sedation and Tranquilization

Sedation is inducing depression of consciousness, with the reduction of irritability or agitation, by administration of sedative drugs, generally to facilitate a diagnostic procedure. Sedation can be administered in varying dosages, from a smaller dose to relax a patient or at a higher dose to make the patient unconscious before a medical procedure that can cause pain or discomfort. Fish are often sedated to reduce the fish from squirming and possibly being injured during a physical examination, or when gill, fin, and skin mucus biopsies are taken for diagnostic purposes. They may be sedated before being given an injection or implanting a microchip transponder. The dose of anesthetic drug used to induce sedation is often the lower end of the range that would be used for general anesthesia for a more invasive or prolonged procedure, such as surgery. The length of time a fish is sedated is a shorter duration than for anesthesia.

Tranquilization is inducing a peaceful calmness in an animal by using a drug at a dose that does not induce total unconsciousness but just relaxation. The tranquilizer drug relieves anxiety and depresses physiological activity. Tranquilizers are sometimes added to the shipping water when fish are being transported for a considerable time. They can be administered prior to short-duration handling of fish

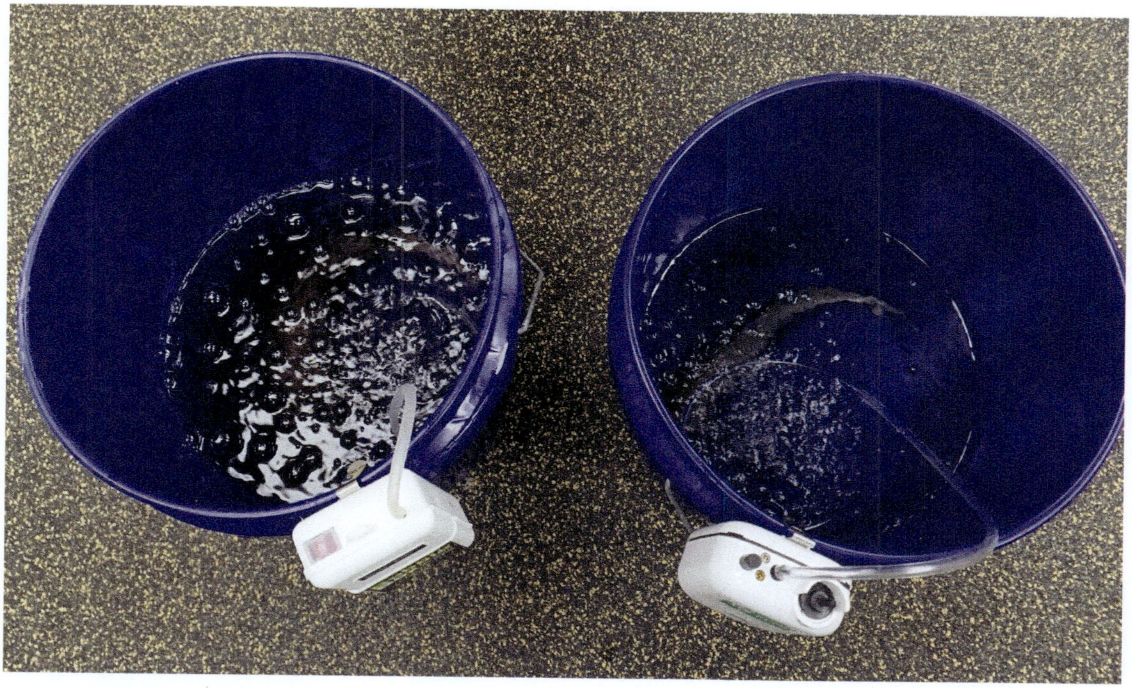

Fig. 15.3. Two containers with battery-operated air pumps can be used, one with anesthetic solution and a second with fresh water to be used for recovery of the fish from anesthesia. (Photograph by N. Saint-Erne.)

Table 15.2. Stages of anesthesia in fishes (Saint-Erne, 2019).

Stage	Plane	Description	Signs
0	0	Normal	Swimming actively, equilibrium normal
I	1	Light sedation	Reduced motion, ventilation decreased
I	2	Deeper sedation	Motionless unless stimulated
II	1	Light anesthesia	Partial loss of equilibrium
II	2	Deep anesthesia	Loss of equilibrium and righting reflex
III	1	Surgical anesthesia	Total loss of reactivity when stimulated
III	2	Deep surgical anesthesia	Decrease in respiratory and heart rates
IV	1	Medullary collapse	Cessation of respiratory movements
IV	2	Cardiac arrest	Death

for physical manipulation, such as stripping roe or milt when breeding fish. Suggested anesthetic drugs useful for tranquilization include benzocaine, ketamine, eugenol, quinaldine, and MS-222. Start with a lower dose and increase it, if necessary, especially if using an unfamiliar drug or on a new fish species.

15.3 Analgesia

Analgesia reduces the sensation of pain without the loss of consciousness. For the optimum health and welfare of fish patients that are suffering from traumatic wounds, or during post-surgical recovery periods, they can be provided with analgesic medications (Table 15.3). Fish have been shown to have a reduced response to noxious stimuli when given morphine, tramadol, buprenorphine, and dermorphine (Neiffer, 2021). Analgesic drugs are administered primarily by injection.

15.4 Euthanasia

Euthanasia is derived from the Greek terms *eu* meaning good and *thanatos* meaning death. The

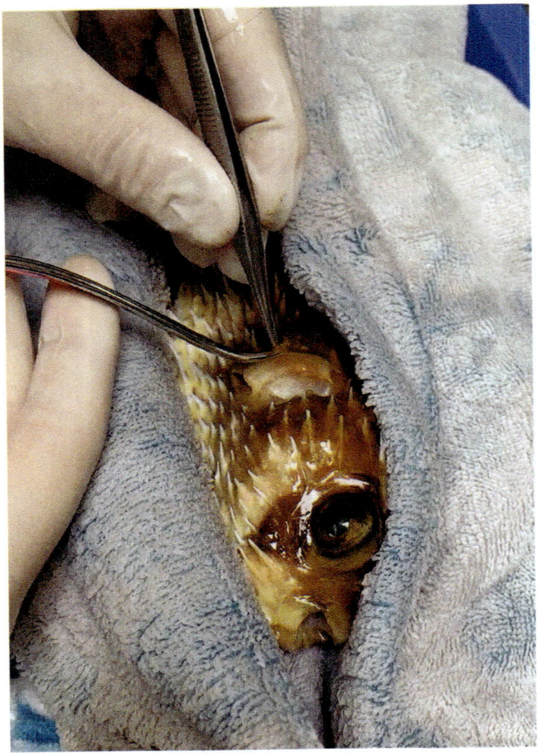

Fig. 15.4. Anesthetized spiny pufferfish (*D. holocanthus*) is wrapped in a wet towel during a procedure. (Photograph by N. Saint-Erne.)

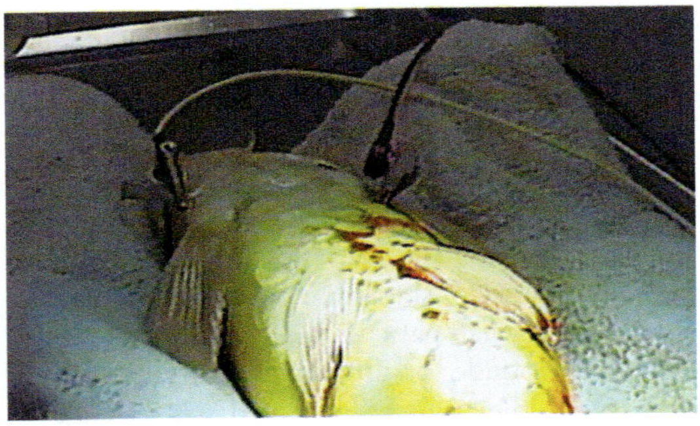

Fig. 15.5. ECG leads attached to hypodermic needles in the pectoral fin muscles of a koi (*Cyprinus rubrofuscus*). (Photograph by N. Saint-Erne.)

term is usually used to describe ending the life of an individual animal in a way that minimizes or eliminates pain and distress. Sometimes, severely sick or injured fish may need to be humanely euthanized. However, freezing is not an acceptable method of euthanasia by the American Veterinary Medical

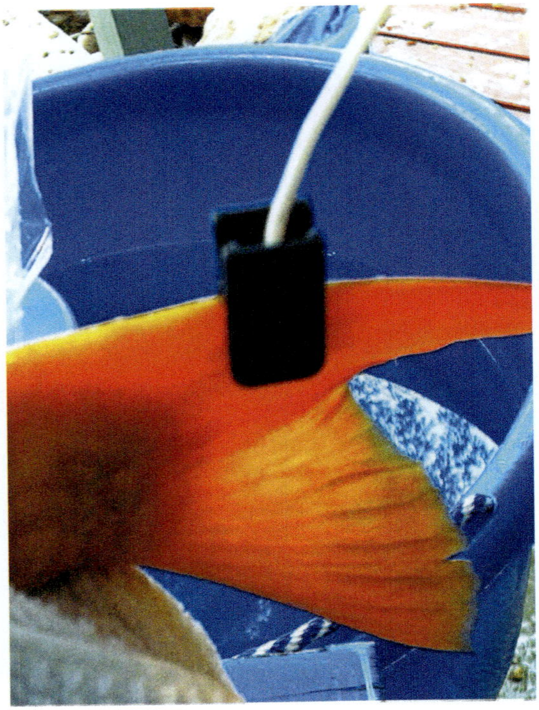

Fig. 15.6. A pulse oximeter clip is attached to the caudal fin of a koi (*C. rubrofuscus*) during surgery to monitor the heart rate and oxygen saturation of the blood. (Photograph by N. Saint-Erne.)

Table 15.3. Fish analgesia and anti-inflammatory drugs (Saint-Erne, 2019).

Analgesics:
Butorphanol—0.1–0.4 mg/kg body weight (BW) Intramuscular (IM) or Intracoelomic (ICoe)
Lidocaine—0.1–2.0 mg/kg IM around skin lesions
Steroids:
Dexamethasone—1–2 mg/kg IM or ICoe
Hydrocortisone—1–4 mg/kg IM or ICoe
Non-steroidal anti-inflammatory drugs:
Aspirin—325 mg/gallon (3.8 l) of water
Carprofen—1.0–5.0 mg/kg IM
Ketoprofen—0.5–2.0 mg/kg IM
Meloxicam—0.2–1.5 mg/kg IM

Association (AVMA, 2020) standards. It is preferable and more humane to use an overdose of anesthesia, which will render the fish unconscious quickly, and cause its respiration to cease. Use up to 10 times the recommended anesthetic dose and leave the fish in the solution for an hour or more after it has stopped opercular movements.

15.4.1 Methods of euthanasia

Common methods used to euthanize fish include immersion, injection, and physical intervention. The use of anesthetics in the water is considered immersion and is the most commonly used method of euthanasia by veterinarians. Fish rapidly absorb many chemicals through the gill membranes into the bloodstream. With immersion euthanasia, it is important to accurately measure the volume of water that is being medicated so that the correct dosage of anesthetic can be used. In some fish species that are tolerant of hypoxic conditions, death may not quickly occur after anesthesia, and a secondary physical method of euthanasia is also used: step 1, immersion to render the fish unconscious; step 2, a secondary adjunctive method to complete euthanasia (such as decapitation, cervical transection, pithing, or rapid freezing).

15.4.2 Confirmation of death

Death must be confirmed before disposal of any animal remains. A combination of criteria is most reliable in confirming death, including lack of heartbeat, lack of breathing (operculum movements), lack of response to painful stimuli, gills becoming pale, and rigor mortis. None of these signs alone, except rigor mortis, confirms death. A Doppler or ultrasound unit, or electrocardiogram can be used to monitor the fish's heartbeat to confirm cardiac arrest. After the heart stops beating, the gills should become pale colored. Some fish species (anabantids, catfish, lungfish) are highly tolerant to anoxic conditions and may need longer times in anesthetic solutions for euthanasia or may need secondary methods of euthanasia once anesthetized. Death can be ensured by physical intervention (pithing, decapitation) after anesthesia.

15.4.3 Euthanasia in veterinary clinics

The container used for euthanasia is best if it is dark colored, and the euthanasia is performed under reduced lighting in a quiet area. The water to which the euthanasia solution is added should be the same temperature, salinity, and pH as the aquarium or pond water. The fish should be maintained in the euthanasia solution for an hour or more after respiration (opercular movements) has stopped.

The following methods are acceptable for use in this environment (AVMA, 2020):

1. Immersion in a solution of buffered tricaine methanesulfonate (MS-222), buffered benzocaine, isoflurane, sevoflurane, quinaldine sulfate, eugenol, or clove oil.
2. Injections of pentobarbital; ketamine followed by pentobarbital; a combination of ketamine and medetomidine followed by pentobarbital; or propofol followed by pentobarbital. Owners should be advised about the possibility of ketamine-induced muscle spasms during induction when using that agent.

The following methods are not recommended for use in this environment:

1. Immersion in CO_2-saturated water is not recommended because some fish exposed to this method may become hyperactive, which can be disconcerting for staff and owners. However, in some cases, other appropriate anesthesia is not available for humane euthanasia. Using carbon dioxide for euthanasia is approved by the AVMA.
2. Manually applied blunt force trauma to the head, decapitation, and pithing are not recommended because their application can be distressing for owners and staff.

References

AVMA (2020) *AVMA Guidelines for the Euthanasia of Animals*. American Veterinary Medical Association, Schaumburg, Illinois. Available at: https://www.avma.org/sites/default/files/2020-02/Guidelines-on-Euthanasia-2020.pdf (accessed 1 August 2024).

Loh, R., Bogan, J., El-Matbouli, M., Hatem, S., Kottwitz, J. *et al.* (2022) Anesthetics and analgesics. In: Urdes, L., Walster, C. and Tepper, J. (eds) *Fundamentals of Aquatic Veterinary Medicine*. Wiley, Hoboken, New Jersey, pp. 164–169.

Neiffer, D.L. (2021) Anesthesia and analgesia. In: Hadfield, C. and Clayton, L. (eds) *Clinical Guide to Fish Medicine*. Wiley, Hoboken, New Jersey, pp. 198–212.

Saint-Erne, N. (2010) Anesthesia. In: Saint-Erne, N. (ed.) *Advanced Koi Care*. 2nd edn. Erne Enterprises, Glendale, Arizona, pp. 50–52.

Saint-Erne, N. (2019) Anesthesia and euthanasia in ornamental fish. *The Aquatic Veterinarian* 13(1), 28–33.

Yanong, R.P.E. and Lewbart G.A. (2024) *The Aquarium Fish Medicine Handbook*. CRC Press, Boca Raton, Florida.

16 Surgery

NICHOLAS SAINT-ERNE

Dr. Saint-Erne Consulting, PLLC, Phoenix, Arizona

Abstract

Surgery on fish can be performed using standard veterinary surgical equipment, including electrocardiogram and pulse oximeter machines for monitoring heartbeats and pulse. The anesthesia delivery method is usually by mixing the anesthetic into the water. Once anesthetized, fish can be removed from the water for many surgical procedures. Recovery from anesthesia occurs when the fish are placed back into untreated water.

16.1 Surgical Preparation

Surgical procedures have been successfully performed on fish. A variety of surgeries are described in the literature, including skin and fin wound repair, excision of skin masses, orthopedic procedures for repair of spinal fractures, resection of prolapsed cloacal tissues, and exploratory surgeries to remove coelomic masses (Harms and Lewbart, 2000). General surgical knowledge and experience will facilitate successful fish surgery, as will familiarity with normal fish anatomy (Saint-Erne, 2010a). Aseptic surgical technique should be maintained as best as possible, but post-surgery the fish will be placed back into water that contains myriad bacteria, so antibiotics are recommended if there is a risk of infection. Prepare the fish for surgery by placing it in a container of clean water that is the same temperature, pH, and salinity as the original tank or pond water, with additional aeration (Fig. 16.1). The anesthetic agent can be administered, usually by immersion, to the fish when the surgery is ready to be performed.

After the fish is in an adequate plane of anesthesia, it is removed from the induction container and placed on a wet cloth or foam in the appropriate position for surgery. For larger fish, rolled-up towels can be placed on either side of the body to maintain the fish in dorsal recumbency (Figs 16.2a and b). Exposed tissues not in the surgical field are covered with wet gauze or cloth to prevent desiccation (Fig. 16.3). The skin should be kept moist throughout the surgical procedures; a red rubber catheter attached to a large syringe can be used to carefully moisten the patient without splashing water into the incision site (Lewbart, 2006). An ophthalmic ointment should be placed on the eyes to keep them moist.

Fish have a mucous layer covering the epidermis that protects the fish from the environment. Aseptic presurgical skin disinfection used in terrestrial animals is not applied to fish, as it can remove the mucous layer (Sladakovic and Divers, 2021). The surgical site is flushed with sterile saline to remove surface debris prior to starting surgery. The surgical site can be gently cleaned or sprayed with 1% povidone-iodine (Betadine®) solution. A clear plastic surgical drape can be placed over the surgery site; small dabs of Vaseline will help adhere it to the skin (Fig. 16.4). The plastic drape retains moisture on the fish and allows a sterile surgical field (Lewbart, 2006).

16.2 Maintaining Anesthesia During Surgery

Several fish anesthetic "machines" have been described that are designed around a submersible pump, such as an aquarium powerhead, to create a constant and steady water flow (Lewbart, 2006). The aerated

Corresponding author: DrSaintErne@gmail.com

© CAB International 2025. *The Handbook of Ornamental Fish Health and Welfare* (ed. N. Saint-Erne)
DOI: 10.1079/9781789246032.0016

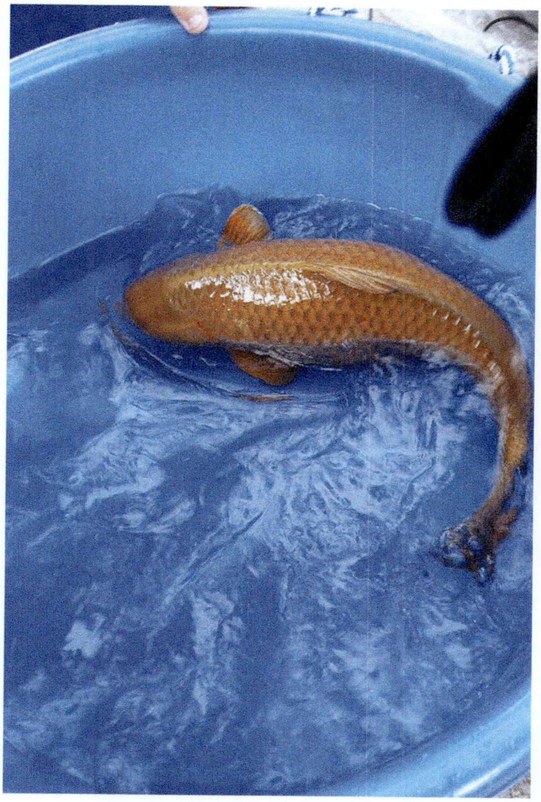

Fig. 16.1. Chagoi koi (*Cyprinus rubrofuscus*) is placed in a container of water containing anesthetic solution. (Photograph by N. Saint-Erne.)

anesthetic solution is dripped over the gills to maintain anesthesia, or plastic tubing can be placed into the fish's mouth and the solution slowly pumped in and across the gills (Figs 16.5a–c). The fish is placed onto a surgical platform so that a tube delivers the anesthetic-laden water through the patient's mouth and over its gills. The water flows through a foam or perforated platform back into a tank under the surgical table for recirculation. Anesthetized fish can be maintained on such systems for several hours (Harms and Lewbart, 2000).

The anesthetic solution flow can also be maintained by gravity using an IV bag filled with anesthetic solution and a drip set, or by hand with a syringe attached to IV tubing or aquarium air tubing (Saint-Erne, 2010a). Having the fish on a perforated platform, towel, or sponge will allow the anesthetic solution to run out from under the fish and into a catch basin. Recirculation of the water will allow it to continue to be pumped into the fish's mouth and out the gills. The anesthetic water should be aerated during the surgery to ensure adequate dissolved oxygen concentration. The anesthetic concentration can be diluted with premeasured water to adjust the depth of anesthesia during surgery.

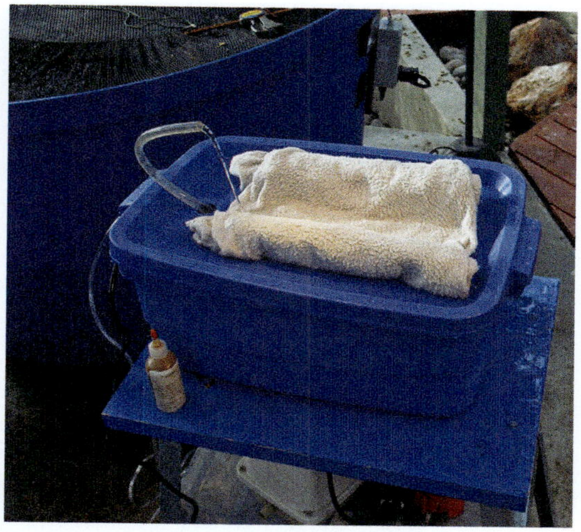

Fig. 16.2a. The portable surgery table is prepared with anesthetic solution in the base, an air pump attached to an air stone in the water providing aeration, a water pump flowing anesthetic solution to where the fish will be positioned on the wet towel, rolled to hold the fish in dorsal recumbency for coelomic surgery. (Photograph by N. Saint-Erne.)

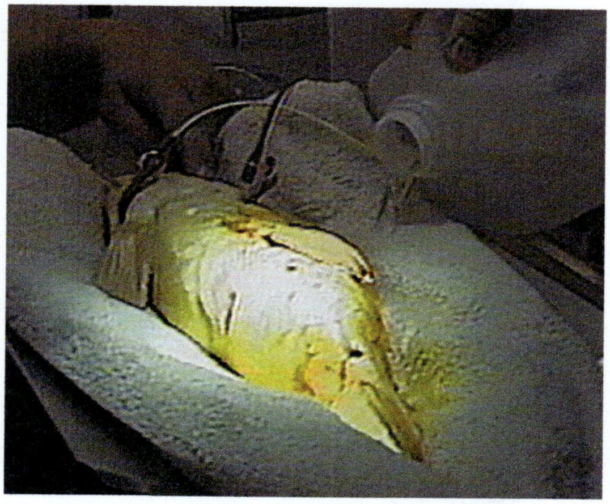

Fig. 16.2b. A wet towel is being used over a V-tray to maintain dorsal recumbency of a koi (*C. rubrofuscus*) for coelomic surgery to remove a gonadal tumor. Water is added to the towel to maintain moisture in the skin. (Photograph by N. Saint-Erne.)

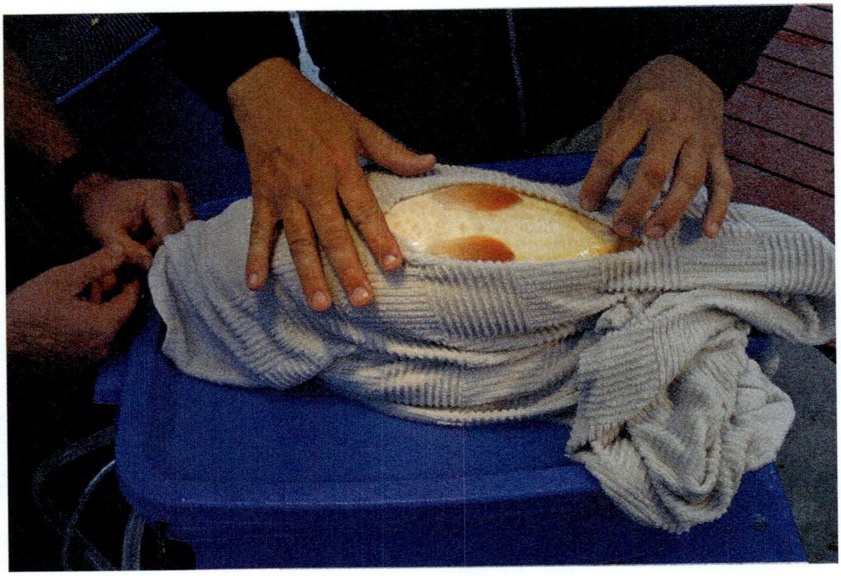

Fig. 16.3. Water is being pumped into the koi's mouth and out the operculum. The body is covered with a wet towel to maintain hydration of the skin. (Photograph by N. Saint-Erne.)

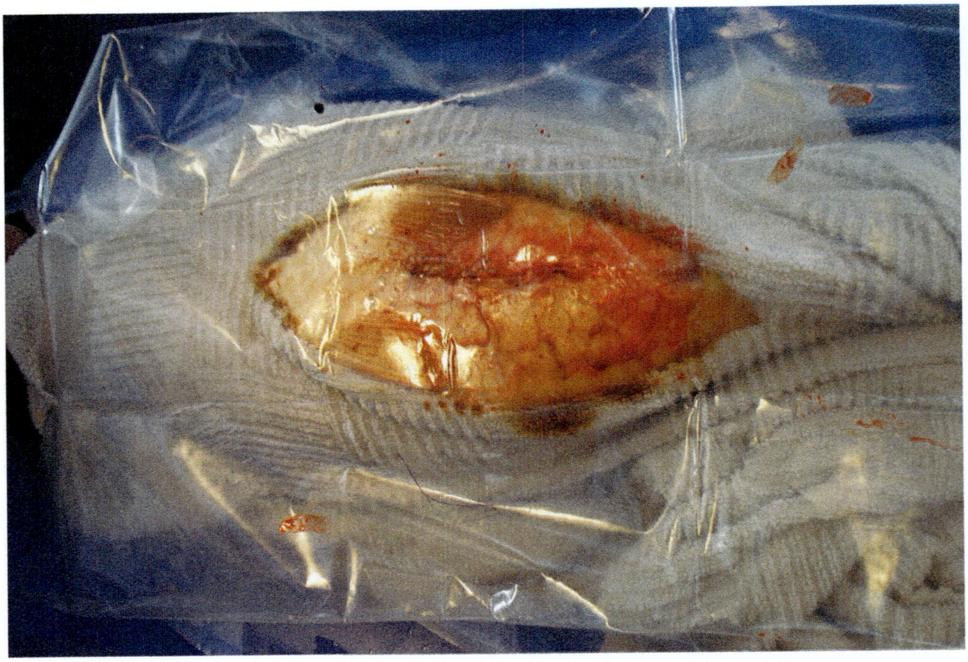

Fig. 16.4. Clear, sterile drapes are used over the body to help maintain a sterile surgical field. (Photograph by N. Saint-Erne.)

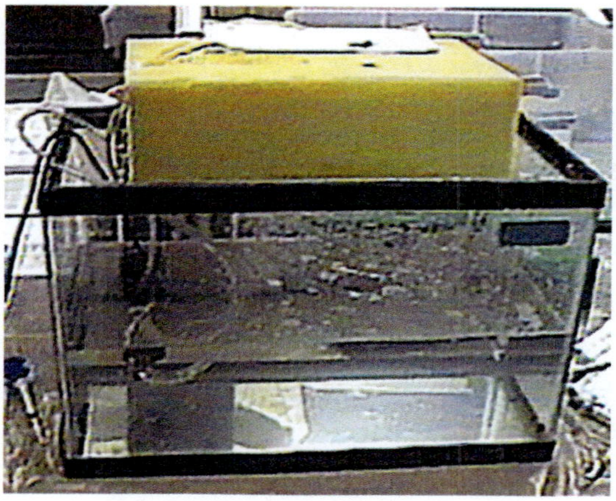

Fig. 16.5a. Glass aquarium used for anesthesia chamber, as described by Harms and Lewbart, with the water pumped through tubing into the fish's mouth, across the gills, and out the operculum. The water flows through the foam pad back into the anesthetic chamber. (Photograph by N. Saint-Erne.)

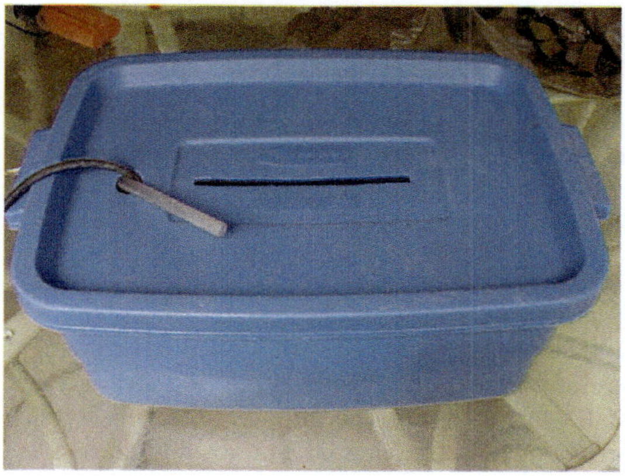

Fig. 16.5b. Anesthetic chamber made from a plastic bin so that it is lighter weight, sturdier, and more portable than a glass aquarium. The water is pumped from inside the bin through the tube into the fish's mouth, and then it is collected in the top tray of the lid and flows back down through the center slit into the bin. (Photograph by N. Saint-Erne.)

16.3 Surgical Equipment

16.3.1 Veterinary supplies

Most small and exotic animal hospitals will already possess the necessary surgical instruments and other supplies (Table 16.1) necessary to perform surgery on fish (Lewbart, 2006). The best surgical instruments to use with fish are ophthalmic or microsurgery instruments because of their small size; but many surgeries can be performed with a scalpel handle and a #11 or #15 blade, iris scissors, Metzenbaum scissors, mosquito hemostats, and a pair of fine forceps. A magnifying loupe or other magnifying lens is very helpful.

16.3.2 Electrocardiogram

During a surgical procedure, an electrocardiogram (ECG) reading can be taken to monitor the heart rate and rhythm. Three ECG lead clips can each be attached to the metal part of 22-gauge hypodermic needles. These needles are then placed through the skin and just into the muscle tissue at the base of the right pectoral fin (RA lead), the left pectoral fin (LA lead), and the cranial to the vent opening (LL lead). The P-QRS-T waves produced are of low amplitude (1 mV QRS complex) but similar to those in other animals (Fig. 16.6). Heart rates are temperature dependent, as well as being affected by anesthesia. Normal heart rates are 30–40 beats per min but can range from 15 to 100 beats per min. It is important to get a heart rate early during anesthesia and monitor for bradycardia. If the heart rate decreases excessively, reducing the anesthesia concentration in the water is necessary to increase the heart rate.

16.3.3 Pulse oximeter

Any time a fish is anesthetized, a pulse oximeter can be attached to a thin area of the caudal fin or other fin (Fig. 16.7). The pulse oximeter measures the oxygen saturation percentage of the blood flowing through the capillaries and indicates the pulse rate. This is helpful to determine if more aeration of the water is needed, including using pure oxygen from a canister to bubble through the water to increase the dissolved oxygen content. The pulse rate will decrease as the fish enters a deeper plane of anesthesia, so the pulse rate can be used to judge the depth of anesthesia. It is important to record the heart rate or pulse rate at the beginning of an anesthesia procedure to determine if the heartbeat is slowing down. Increase freshwater flow across the gills to lessen the anesthesia and increase the heart rate and pulse if it slows too much.

16.4 Surgery Techniques

Intracoelomic (abdominal) surgery is performed in fish through a ventral midline incision (Fig. 16.8).

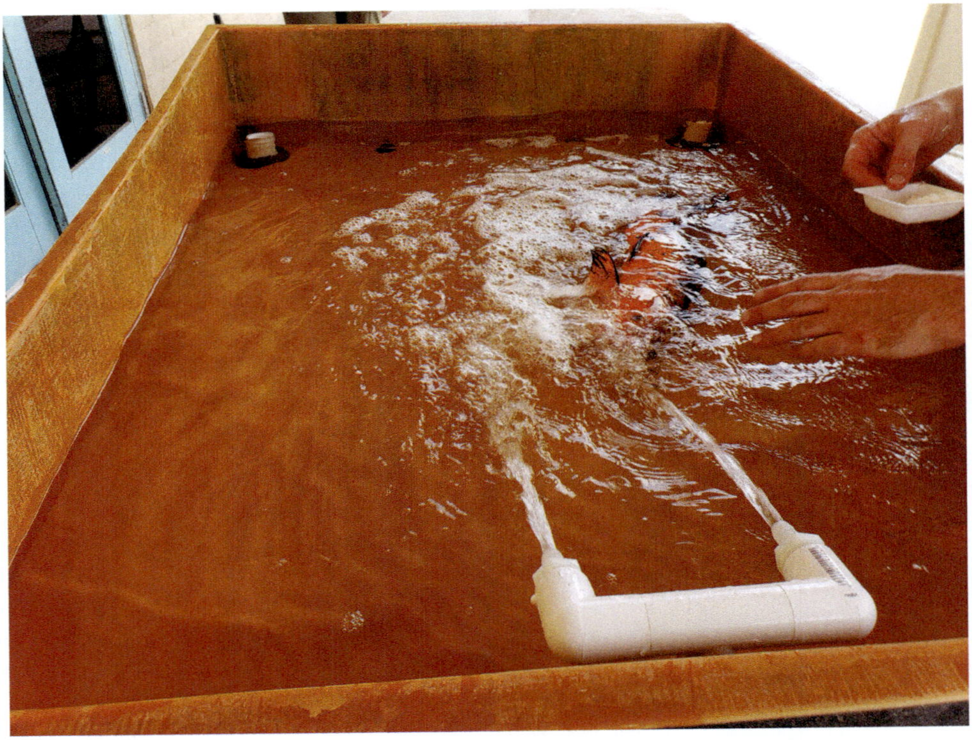

Fig. 16.5c. Anesthetic chamber made from a fiberglass tray. The water is pumped from a plastic bin under the surgery table and back out of the PVC tubes at the end of the tray. The height of the outlet tubes can be adjusted to control how deep the water is in the tray. This anesthetic induction chamber is also the surgery table, with a koi in the photograph being anesthetized for coelomic surgery. (Photograph by Sharmie Johnson.)

Table 16.1. Surgical supplies and equipment. (Lewbart, 2006.)

Ophthalmic or microsurgical pack
Suture material (4-0 to 2-0 absorbable monofilament most often used)
Sterile plastic surgical drape
Scalpel blades (#11 and #15)
Electrocardiogram machine
Pulse oximeter or Doppler
Recirculating water pump with tubing for anesthesia chamber
Aquarium air pump with tubing and air stones
Anesthetics (See Chapter 15, this volume)
Antibiotics (injectable)
Butorphanol (0.1–0.4 mg/kg IM)
Ketoprofen (2 mg/kg IM)
Triple antibiotic ointment
Povidone-iodine solution
Sterile ophthalmic lubricant
Silver sulfadiazine cream
Salt (1–3 g/l in recovery tank) for freshwater fishes

In large fish, such as koi, the scales along the incision line can be removed with forceps to facilitate a smooth incision. Alternatively, cutting through the scales can be done, then only removing those that are fragmented, leaving larger, mostly intact scales attached. Start the incision cranial to the vent and continue forward to the pectoral fin bones, as needed. The pelvic girdle may be separated with Mayo scissors or bone cutters if necessary. Gelpi retractors are helpful in keeping the coelomic incision open (Lewbart, 1998). Use gentle blunt dissection with the hemostats, Metzenbaum scissors, or gloved fingers to isolate the desired tissues. Ligate blood vessels as needed with 3-0 or smaller absorbable suture material. Stainless steel hemoclips may also be used for ligation. Bipolar cautery units are useful for small vessel hemostasis.

Successful coelomic surgeries have been performed on koi to remove both testicular and ovarian gonadal tumors, and enlarged egg masses (Saint-Erne, 2010b). Koi that have had difficulty spawning can have the

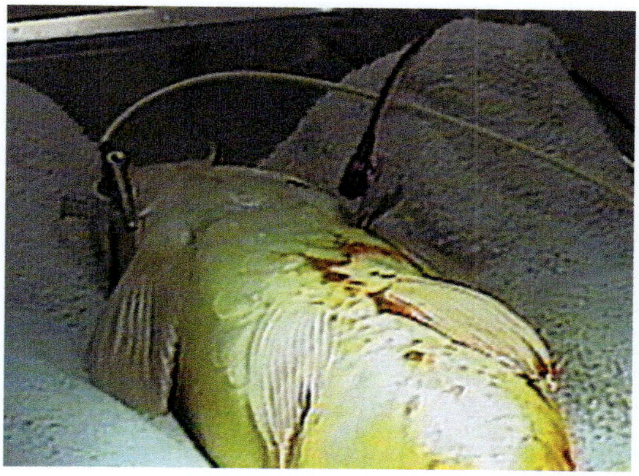

Fig. 16.6. Syringe needles inserted into muscles at the base of the pectoral fins of a koi (*C. rubrofuscus*) with ECG leads clamped to the metal of the needles. (Photograph by N. Saint-Erne.)

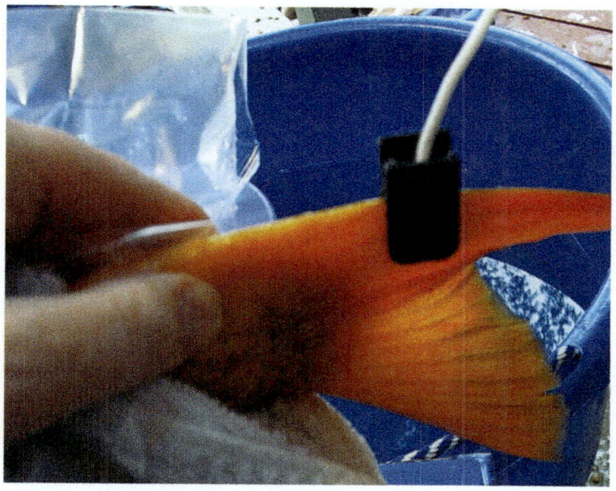

Fig. 16.7. Pulse oximeter on the caudal fin of a koi (*C. rubrofuscus*). (Photograph by N. Saint-Erne.)

ovaries removed surgically (Fig. 16.9). Gonadal tumors appear as large (as much as 10% of the total body weight in size), irregular, fibrous masses, and can often be diagnosed on radiographs. They can cause the abdomen to appear quite distended. These can be bluntly dissected free from fibrous attachments, using appropriate hemostasis. After removal, survey the internal organs to assess any damage from pressure necrosis or obstruction. The contralateral gonad should also be assessed.

Occasionally the gas bladder will become traumatized and distended, creating an appearance like an abdominal tumor. Radiographs or ultrasound examination will distinguish between an enlarged

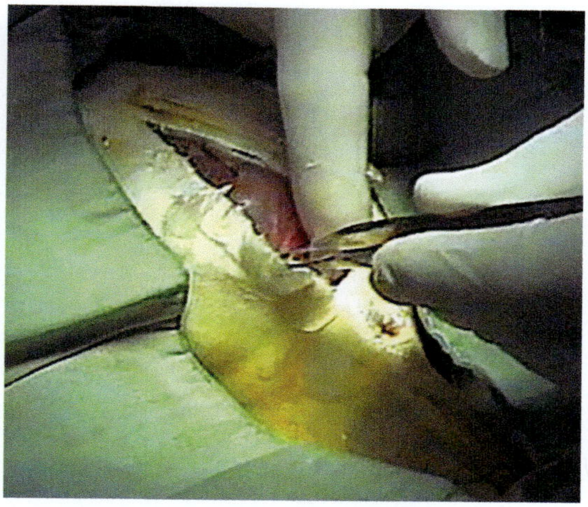

Fig. 16.8. Ventral midline incision on a koi (*C. rubrofuscus*) to remove a gonadal sarcoma. (Photograph by N. Saint-Erne.)

gas bladder and a tumor. The gas bladder in Cyprinids, such as goldfish and koi, consists of two compartments joined by an isthmus. The caudal compartment is connected to the esophagus by the pneumatic duct. The damaged compartment of the gas bladder can be isolated and ligated for removal. The cranial compartment when removed is ligated at the isthmus. The caudal compartment is ligated distal to the pneumatic duct attachment to the caudal compartment near the isthmus. The fish will gradually stabilize its buoyancy with the remaining portion of the gas bladder.

Sterile saline solution can be used to flush the coelomic cavity prior to closure. Filling the coelom with sterile saline solution will also minimize trapping gas into the coelom. Trapped air in the abdomen should be removed by aspiration after closing the muscles and before closing the skin. In smaller fish, the muscle layer and skin may be closed in one layer. For skin closure, use monofilament nylon or absorbable monofilament suture material with a swaged-on, reverse-cutting needle. Closure of the surgical incision is accomplished by a simple continuous or simple interrupted suture pattern (Fig. 16.10). Other suture patterns used for closure include cruciate sutures and Ford interlocking pattern. Remove the skin sutures in 2 to 4 weeks, or when the skin appears adequately healed (Fig. 16.11). Post-surgical pain management can be provided using butorphanol intramuscular injections.

Skin and fin wounds can be sutured using fine (3-0) monofilament nylon sutures. To repair split fin membranes, gently scrape the opposing edges

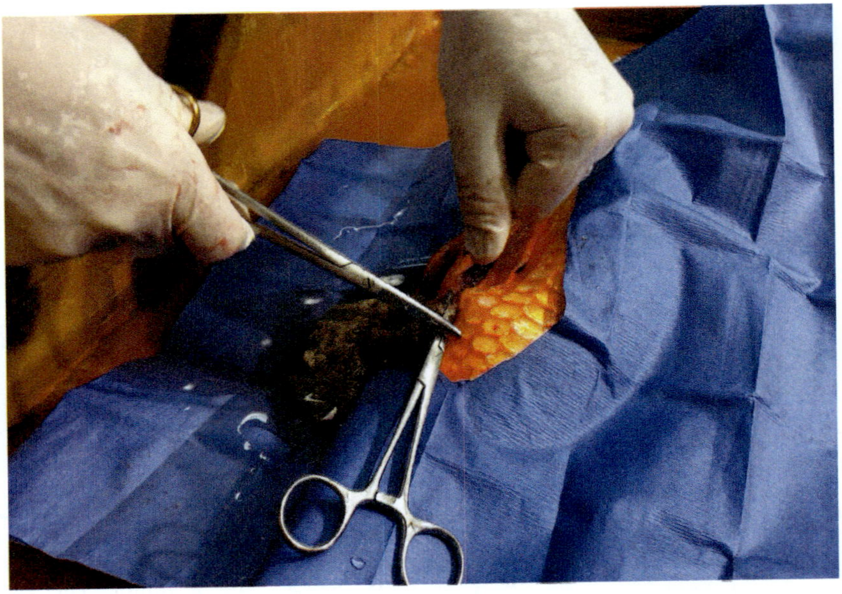

Fig. 16.9. Nick Saint-Erne performing a salpingohysterectomy on a koi (*C. rubrofuscus*). (Photograph by Sharmie Johnson.)

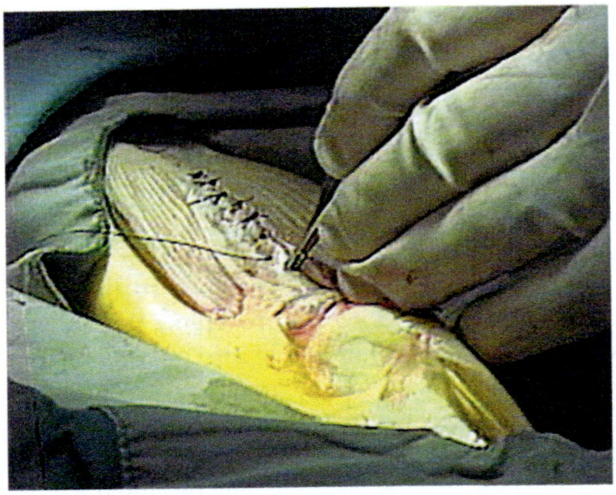

Fig. 16.10. Closure of the skin incision in a koi (*C. rubrofuscus*) using simple interrupted suture pattern. (Photograph by Donna Messina.)

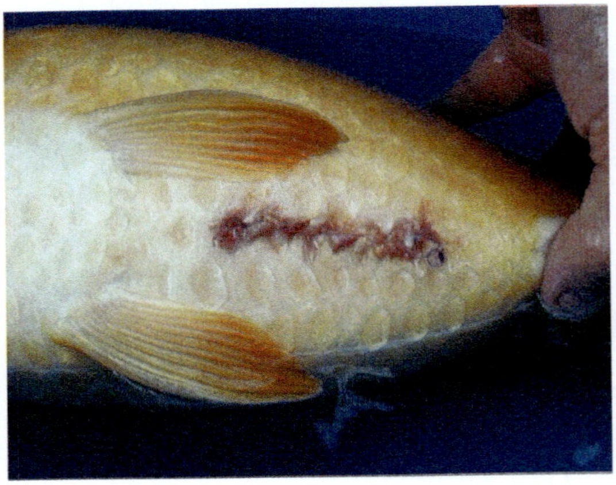

Fig. 16.11. A koi 2 weeks post-surgery presented to have the sutures removed. The incision is reddened but closed, and the inflammation will gradually diminish over a few weeks once the sutures are removed. (Photograph by N. Saint-Erne.)

with a scalpel blade to remove scar tissue and then tightly suture together the fin edges with a series of simple interrupted sutures (Figs 16.12a and b). Start at the base of the fin and work outward toward the edge of the fin. Incorporate one or more fin rays on each side to keep the sutures from tearing through the fin membrane. Apply Betadine solution topically to the fin before and after suturing. Remove the sutures in two weeks. Hyperplasia of the epithelium will grow over the suture sites but will regress after the sutures are removed, and it can be trimmed back at the time of suture removal.

Dermal tumors occur in fish on the skin and fins. They can be surgically excised while the fish is under anesthesia (Figs 16.13a, b and c). Dermal masses are sometimes difficult to completely excise and may recur if not fully removed (Harms and Lewbart, 2000). Due to the inelasticity of the skin of fishes,

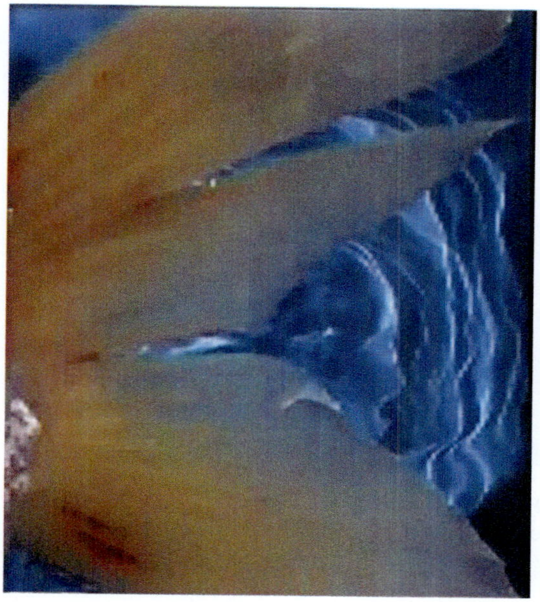

Fig. 16.12a. Split caudal fin on a koi (*C. rubrofuscus*). (Photograph by N. Saint-Erne.)

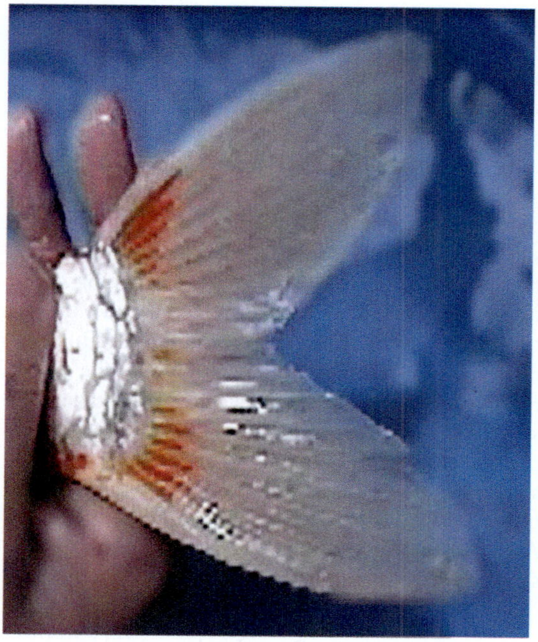

Fig. 16.12b. Caudal fin 8 weeks after repair surgery. The sutures were left in for 2 weeks, then removed. Initially, there was redness around the suture sites, but this regressed by 8 weeks post-surgery. (Photograph by N. Saint-Erne.)

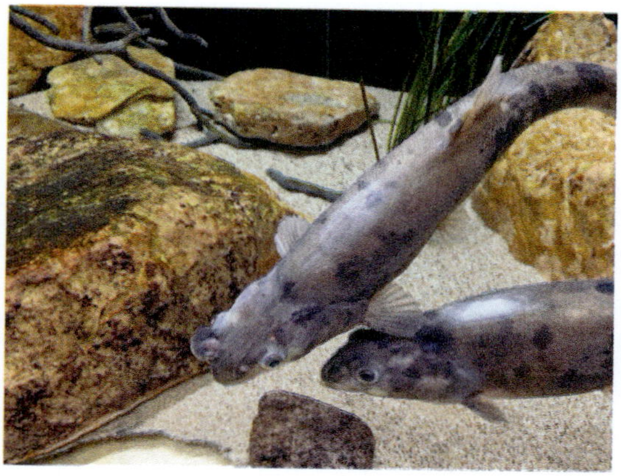

Fig. 16.13a. Roundtail chub (*Gila robusta*) with a dermal mass on its right nostril area. (Photograph by N. Saint-Erne.)

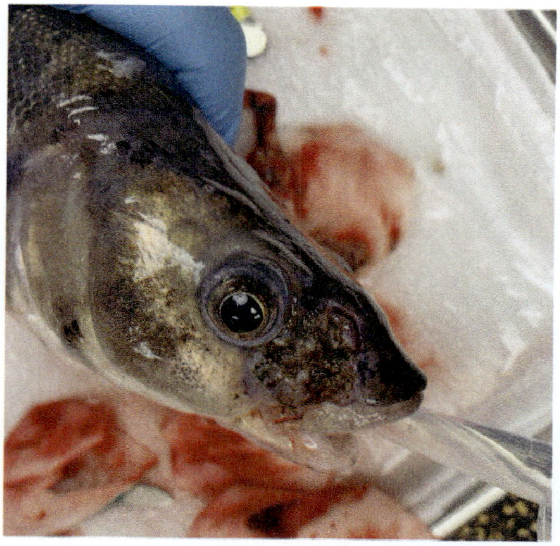

Fig. 16.13b. The growth was surgically removed, and the fish did well post-surgery, but the tumor started to regrow after 2 months. (Photograph by N. Saint-Erne.)

suturing skin wounds closed is not always possible, and healing by second intention is often necessary. Apply topical antibacterial ointments, such as silver sulfadiazine, on the wound daily during healing. When freshwater fish have open skin wounds, adding salt to the water at 0.1–0.3% (1–3 g/l) helps to minimize osmotic balances.

Oranda goldfish have a fibrous growth on top of the head called a "wen." Sometimes, the wen grows around the eyes (Figs 16.14a and b) or even overgrows large enough to occlude the opercular opening.

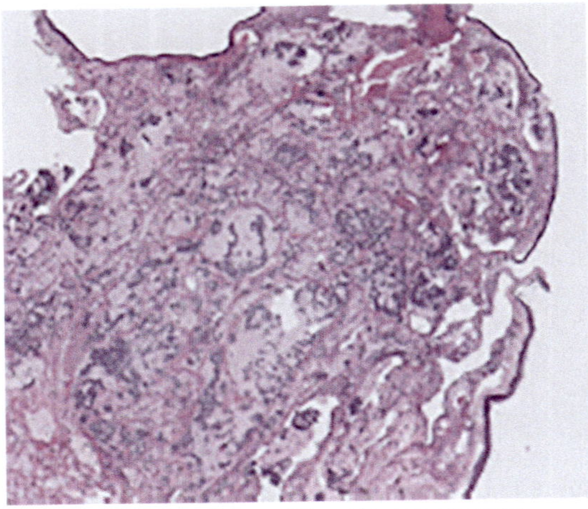

Low magnification of one of the adenocarcinomas

Fig. 16.13c. Histopathology image of the adenocarcinoma arising from the right nasal cavity that was removed from the roundtail chub. (Microphotograph by Ethan Biswell DVM MS Dipl ACVP.)

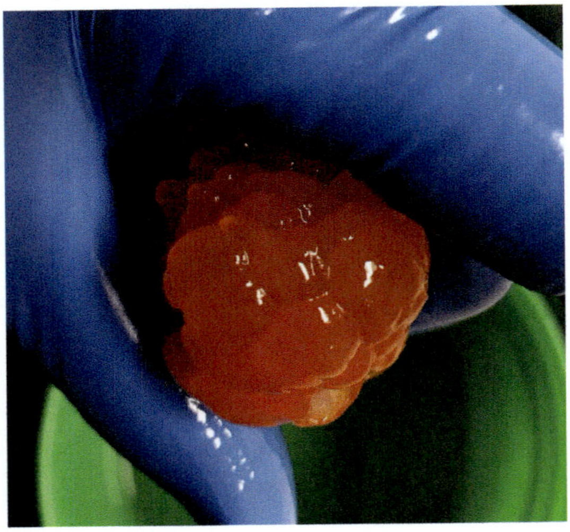

Fig. 16.14a. Oranda goldfish (*C. auratus*) with wen growing over face and covering the eyes. (Photograph by N. Saint-Erne.)

In these cases, the goldfish can be anesthetized, and the wen can be trimmed using iris scissors or a scalpel blade to remove the excess tissue from over the eyes or operculum. Topical disinfection with povidone-iodine before and after the surgery will reduce the risk of secondary bacterial or fungal infections. Fish that have the wen trimmed may

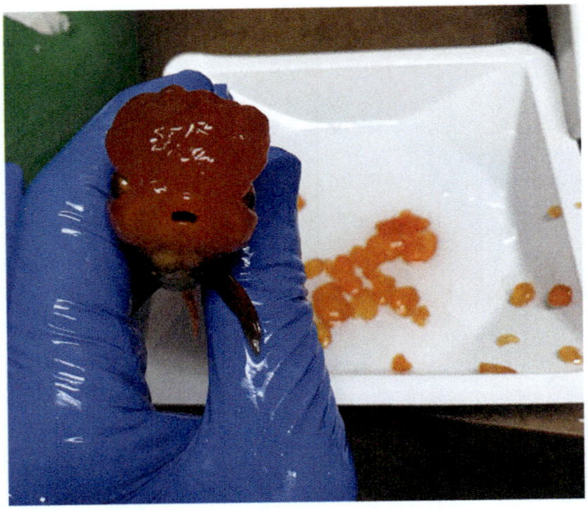

Fig. 16.14b. After carefully trimming the wen, the goldfish's eyes are uncovered. (Photograph by N. Saint-Erne.)

continue to have excessive growth of the wen and may need future treatment as well.

Eyes may require surgery after being injured by trauma, parasite infestation, cataracts, uveitis, or other diseases causing open wounds or exophthalmia (Sladakovic and Divers, 2021). Eye enucleation can be performed on an anesthetized fish positioned in lateral recumbency. Clean around the eye with a povidone-iodine solution. A shallow skin incision is made into the periocular skin around the orbit with a #11 scalpel blade, and then curved tenotomy or iris scissors (Fig. 16.15) are used to bluntly dissect the globe from the circumorbital sulcus (Harms and Lewbart, 2000). Transect the muscle attachments close to the globe, being careful not to damage the cranial nerves V and VII that transverse the ventrolateral orbital margin. The optic nerve is cut close to the globe, and the eye is removed. Electrocautery, direct pressure, or gelatin sponge can be used to stop any bleeding. Closing the limbic tissue over the optic nerve stump and eye socket bone will increase the rate of healing, leaving the socket to heal by secondary intention. Apply antibiotic ointment to the socket, until the skin grows over the surface.

16.5 Conclusion

Surgical techniques and procedures used in fish are not too different from those used in other animal species, and the surgical equipment is the same. The exception is the anesthetic delivery method, which

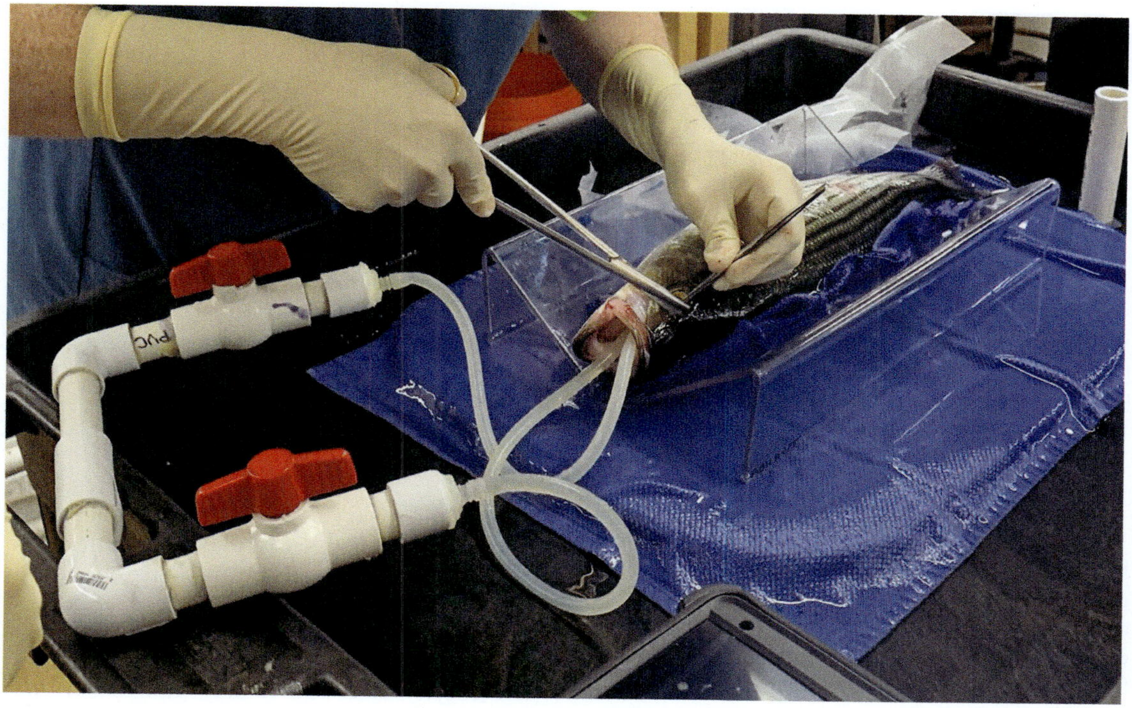

Fig. 16.15. Eye enucleation in a striped bass (*Morone saxatilis*), using scissors to separate the periocular skin around the orbit. (Photograph by N. Saint-Erne.)

can be easily and inexpensively constructed using an aquarium or plastic tub, a small water pump, and plastic tubing. Refer to the anesthesia instructions in Chapter 15 of this volume regarding fish anesthetics useful for surgery. After surgery, the fish should be kept in a clean environment, such as a hospital or quarantine tank, and provided antibiotics as needed to prevent wound infection. Once the surgical site has healed, the fish can be returned to the original aquarium or pond.

References

Harms, C. and Lewbart, G. (2000) Surgery in fish. In: Bennet, R.A. (ed.) *The Veterinary Clinics of North America–Exotic Animal Practice*. Vol. 3, No. 3. W.B. Saunders, Philadelphia, Pennsylvania, pp. 759–774.

Lewbart, G. (1998) Surgical removal of an undifferentiated abdominal sarcoma from a koi carp (*Cyprinus carpio*). *The Veterinary Record* 143, 556–558.

Lewbart, G.A. (2006) *A Brief Review of Advances in Fish Anesthesia, Analgesia, and Surgery*. Western Veterinary Conference Lecture Notes, Las Vegas, Nevada.

Saint-Erne, N. (2010a) Surgery. In: Saint-Erne, N. (ed.) *Advanced Koi Care*. 2nd edn. Erne Enterprises, Glendale, Arizona, pp. 53–57.

Saint-Erne, N. (2010b) Diagnostic techniques and treatments for internal disorders of Koi. In: Marshal, K. (ed.) *Veterinary Clinics of North America Exotic Animal Practice*. Vol. 13, No. 3. W.B. Saunders, Philadelphia, Pennsylvania, pp. 333–347.

Sladakovic, I. and Divers, S. (2021) Surgery and Endoscopy. In: Hadfield, C. and Clayton, L. (eds) *Clinical Guide to Fish Medicine*. Wiley, Hoboken, New Jersey, pp. 213–223.

17 Infectious Diseases

NICHOLAS SAINT-ERNE

Dr. Saint-Erne Consulting, PLLC, Phoenix, Arizona

Abstract

Infectious diseases are caused by bacteria, fungi, and viruses. These microorganisms can spread from one animal to another. In aquatic environments, many of the organisms are commonly present or ubiquitous and often are opportunist pathogens. The primary stressor is usually an injury, poor water quality, or parasitic infestations that lower the fish's immunity.

17.1 Signs of Infectious Disease in Fish

Infectious diseases are caused by microorganisms that can spread from one animal to another. There are many species of bacteria, fungi, and viruses that cause infectious diseases in freshwater and marine fish. In aquatic environments, many of the organisms are commonly present or ubiquitous and often are opportunist pathogens. Disease occurs secondary to tissue trauma caused by injury, parasites, or other stressful situations. Stress causes an initial release of the hormones epinephrine and glucocorticoids. Visible signs of stress include hyperventilation and there are other general behaviors that fish display which clearly indicate distress. These signs (Table 17.1) in fish can sometimes be due to poor water quality, or toxins in the water, but are often seen as a result of infections. This chapter will only cover the microorganisms that are commonly seen in ornamental fish species.

17.2 Viral Diseases

Viruses are submicroscopic infectious agents that replicate only inside the cells of a host organism, so are obligate intracellular pathogens. They carry either Ribonucleic Acid (RNA) or Deoxyribonucleic Acid (DNA) genetic material surrounded by a protein coat (Hoole *et al.*, 2001). They vary in size by species, typically 10–500 nm in length.

There are several significant viral infections of freshwater and marine fish that do not commonly occur in aquarium fish species. These include Viral Hemorrhagic Septicemia (VHS) and Infectious Hematopoietic Necrosis (IHN), both caused by *Novirhabdovirus*, Infectious Pancreatic Necrosis (IPN), caused by a *Birnavirus*, Infectious Salmon Anemia (ISA), caused by an *Isavirus*, Viral Erythrocyte Necrosis (VEN) caused by an *Iridovirus*, and Channel Catfish Virus (CCV) caused by a *Herpesvirus*. While currently not diagnosed in aquarium fish, it is important to know that other viruses are present and could potentially be seen in aquarium fish species. Below are the viral infections reported from aquarium fish species.

17.2.1 Herpes viruses

Cyprinid Herpes Virus 1 (Carp Pox) is not caused by a poxvirus but by *Herpesvirus cyprini*. It produces epidermal hyperplasia, causing superficial white- to pink-colored plaques on the skin and fins (Fig. 17.1). The lesions extend 1–2 mm above the surface of the skin and are usually smooth and firmly attached to the epithelium. Adjacent plaques may merge into larger raised areas. The skin lesions are benign and eventually slough. The disease is not fatal but can produce scarring. In severe cases, large areas of the body and fins can be covered with plaques. The fish swim and eat normally in most instances. It is considered contagious between fish, but in many cases, one or a few koi in a pond will be infected and the others show no signs of disease.

Corresponding author: DrSaintErne@gmail.com

© CAB International 2025. *The Handbook of Ornamental Fish Health and Welfare* (ed. N. Saint-Erne)
DOI: 10.1079/9781789246032.0017

Table 17.1. Signs of distress in fish. Author's own table.

- Fins clamping to the sides of the body
- Color changes (e.g. darkened color if stressed, paler skin caused by excess mucus production if parasitized)
- Flashing (scratching body on substrate or objects)
- Gasping (open mouth breathing, particularly at the water surface)
- Increased opercular movement rate (increased respiratory rate)
- Changes in normal behavior, such as reduced feeding or abnormal activity
- Redness to the fins or skin
- Cloudy or swollen eyes (pop-eye)
- Sores or ulcers on the skin
- Coelomic swelling (gonadal development, fluid accumulation, tumors, parasites)
- Scale loss or protruding from the body (lepidorthosis, or "pinecone" disease)
- Skeletal deformities
- Emaciation (nutritional deficiency, parasites, septicemia)
- Abnormal swimming
- Gill hyperplasia (toxins in the water, parasites, low pH)

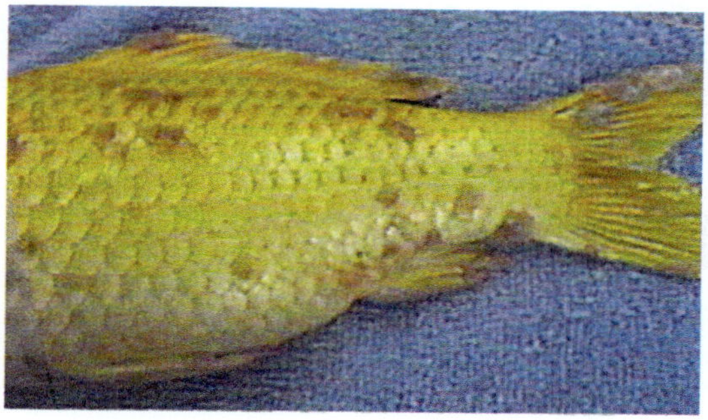

Fig. 17.1. Pink, raised, firm nodules of epidermal hyperplasia on the body and pectoral fin of a koi (*Cyprinus rubrofuscus*) caused by Carp Pox (CHV 1). (Photograph by N. Saint-Erne.)

The virus is transmitted by direct contact between an affected fish and a healthy fish. Overcrowding in the pond will increase the prevalence of the disease. It may be seasonal in occurrence and is more prevalent in cool water temperatures of 57–64°F/14–18°C, with regression often occurring as water warms in the spring to 68°F/20°C and above. Isolation of affected koi is suggested. It does not appear to affect goldfish. No treatments are completely effective against viruses, but the application of a topical disinfectant solution on the lesions may be helpful.

Cyprinid Herpes Virus 2 (Goldfish Hematopoietic Necrosis Virus) affects goldfish and gibel carp. The fish become lethargic, anorexic, and have pale gills and splenomegaly. Infection is most pathogenic at 68°F/20°C, with infections occurring below 59°F/15°C producing resistance to infection, and regression occurs at temperatures above 82°F/28°C (Baumgartner *et al.*, 2022). Diagnosis can be made by histopathology or polymerase chain reaction (PCR) testing of kidney or splenic tissues.

Cyprinid Herpesvirus 3 (Koi Herpesvirus) causes intranuclear inclusions in the cells of the hematopoietic (anterior) kidney and the gill epithelium of koi and common carp. The virus's envelope is 140–172 nm in diameter, with a hexagonal nucleocapsid. It was first diagnosed in koi in Israel and the United States in 1998. Affected koi are anorectic, lethargic, swim erratically, and have erythema of the skin and increased mucus production. On examination, the gills are pale and have severe necrosis (Fig. 17.2). Rapid mortality can occur after exposure, with incubation time dependent on temperature, approximately 30 days at 50°F/10°C and 3 days at 75°F/23.8°C.

The virus is highly contagious, transmitted even with brief contact, and can be spread via equipment such as nets and hoses. It causes a decreased immune response (immunosuppression), thereby allowing secondary bacterial infections to also occur, confusing the diagnostic process. Disease occurrence is temperature dependent, with signs present at 60–80°F/16–27°C. Warming affected fish above 82°F/28°C will stop the progression of disease, with the survivors becoming carriers and are resistant to further episodes. There is no specific treatment for the virus, but optimum water quality, high oxygen saturation, and treatment of secondary infections are all important in reducing mortalities. Quarantining and testing all new fish would reduce the spread of the disease to other fish.

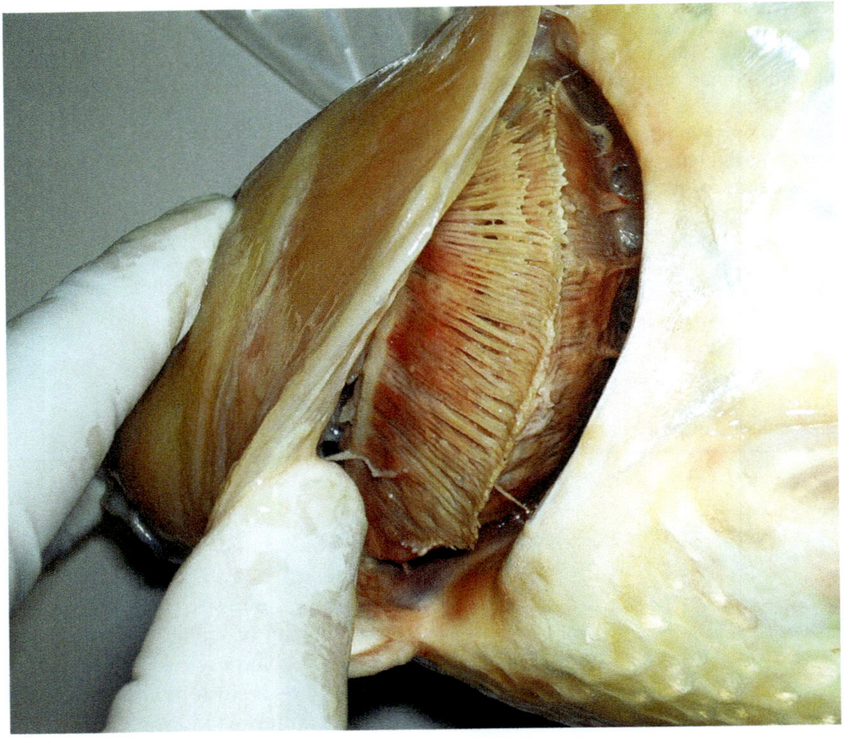

Fig. 17.2. Gills of a KHV-infected koi (*C. rubrofuscus*) showing necrosis of gill epithelium, exposing the cartilage of the gill filaments. (Photograph by N. Saint-Erne.)

17.2.2 Iridoviruses

The Iridovirus family of DNA viruses has many species that infect a variety of freshwater and marine fishes, causing many different types of diseases. Carp Gill Necrosis Iridovirus causes disease of common carp, caused by nonenveloped Iridovirus particles that measure 190–210 nm in diameter. The virus is found in cytoplasmic and intranuclear inclusions. The virus causes gill edema and necrosis, with discoloration and increased mucus production. Spinning Tilapia Syndrome is caused by an Iridovirus and is seen in tilapia cichlids. The fish, especially fry, swim erratically and are anorexic. The virus causes muscle and renal tubular necrosis. There is no known treatment, and affected fish should be isolated as soon as diagnosed.

Lymphocystis is a chronic dermal infection caused by an Iridovirus. The virus produces hypertrophy of the fibroblasts in the dermis of the fins and skin (Figs 17.3a and b). The fibroblasts enlarge and form white to gray-colored, papilloma-like growths. The virus is spread by direct contact and through fomites, such as nets. Affected fish should be isolated to prevent the spread of the virus. Increasing the water temperature may shorten the time of infection, as this viral disease is often self-limiting. Topical application of antibacterial ointment or diluted hydrogen peroxide has seemed to hasten the resolution of the fibrous growths. They can also be surgically excised.

Megalocytiviruses are another group of viruses from the Iridovirus family. They may cause lethargy, abnormal swimming, anorexia, and changes in the color of the skin. Some fish may get exophthalmia, dyspnea, and ascites. Clinical hematology may find hemolytic anemia with eosinophilic intracytoplasmic inclusion bodies in the erythrocytes. On necropsy, splenomegaly, renomegaly, hepatomegaly, and serosanguinous coelomic effusion may be seen. Diagnosis can also be confirmed with PCR testing.

17.2.3 Spring viremia of carp (infectious dropsy)

This fish disease of carp, koi, goldfish, and other cyprinids is caused by *Rhabdovirus carpio* (120 × 60–90 nm). It produces a wide variety of signs, including

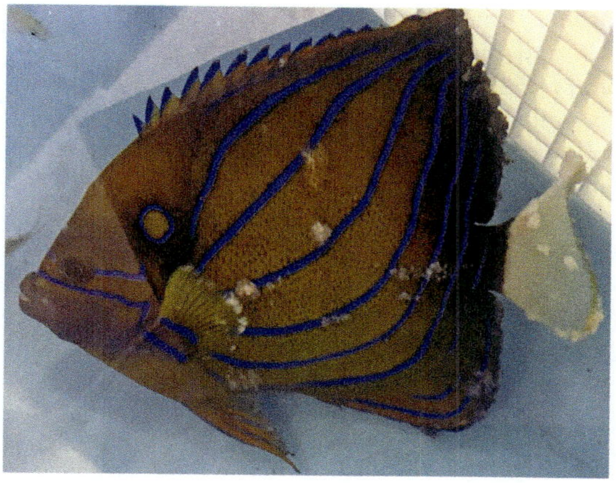

Fig. 17.3a. White, raised hypertrophic nodules on a Bluering angelfish (*Pomacanthus annularis*) caused by Lymphocystis virus. (Photograph by N. Saint-Erne.)

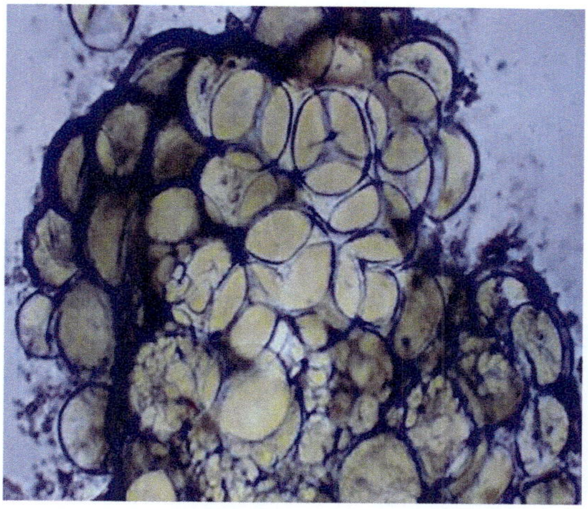

Fig. 17.3b. Microscopic examination of a fin biopsy sample from a fish with lymphocystis lesions showing the hypertrophy of dermal cells. (Microphotograph by N. Saint-Erne.)

a distended ascitic abdomen (dropsy), exophthalmia (pop-eye), inflamed and protruding vent, uncoordinated swimming, weak respiration, and hemorrhages on the gills and skin. The virus is shed in the feces, and the gills are the site of virus entry and primary replication. The virus will spread via the blood from the gills to the internal organs. Visceral hemorrhages and serosanguinous ascitic fluid are seen on necropsy. Eggs can be infected at breeding. Fish lice and leeches can also carry the virus between fish.

The disease is more severe in cold water temperatures, hence the prevalence of signs in spring, as the water temperature warms above 41°F/5°C. Warming the pond water up to 68°F/20°C will protect the fish from the virus. Ultraviolet (UV) irradiation of the pond water will inactivate the virus and help prevent its spread. Formalin added to the pond (25 mg/l) will also inactivate the virus. This is a World Organization for Animal Health reportable disease. Diagnosis can be made by virus isolation or PCR testing of tissue from organs or the brain. Depopulation may be required for affected fish.

17.2.4 Carp edema virus/Sleepy koi disease

Carp edema virus is a large, double-stranded DNA virus thought to belong to the Poxviridae family of viruses. Carp edema virus (CEV) can cause high mortality rates in wild and cultured common carp (*Cyprinus carpio*) and koi (*Cyprinus rubrofuscus*). Infected fish may exhibit hemorrhagic skin lesions with swelling (edema) of the underlying tissues, and thus the disease was originally named "viral edema of carp." The disease has also been referred to as "koi sleepy disease" (KSD) because infected fish become lethargic and unresponsive (Hesami, *et al.*, 2015). CEV disease was first described in Japanese koi in 1974 and since then has occurred in many parts of the world where Japanese koi were exported.

In CEV-infected fish, gill proliferation and thickening, or clubbing, may extend to the base of the gill filament and impair gill function. Enophthalmos and skin lesions can also occur. A definitive diagnosis requires specialized laboratory testing such as PCR that detects the DNA of CEV. In Japan, koi producers use 0.5% (5 g/l) salt in the water to prevent the disease after the young fish are moved from the earthen nursery ponds into cement-lined ponds for grading. Some producers also avoid harvest during periods when water temperatures are permissive for the disease (59–77°F/15–25°C). Always isolate and test sick fish showing suspect clinical signs of lethargy or gill hyperplasia.

17.3 Bacterial Diseases

Bacterial infections are often associated with poor water quality, high organic waste in the aquarium, handling and transportation of the fish, water temperature changes, hypoxia, parasite infestation, or other conditions that can lower the immunity of the fish. Most bacterial pathogens of fish are

Gram-negative aerobic rods. *Mycobacterium*, however, is a Gram-positive bacterial infection that causes chronic diseases in fish. Diagnosis is by isolation of the organism in pure culture from infected tissues and identification of the bacterial agent. Antibiotic sensitivity testing is recommended to determine the best medications for use with bacterial diseases (Petty *et al.*, 2022).

17.3.1 Bacterial hemorrhagic septicemia

This serious disease can be caused by several bacteria species, including *Aeromonas* and *Pseudomonas*, which are primarily in freshwater, and *Vibrio*, more common in marine fishes. Ulcerative lesions occur as the infection progresses, and mortality can increase if water quality is poor and parasites are not controlled. Antibiotic therapy is recommended if the fish are dying, but underlying stressors must be addressed for the antibiotics to help.

Aeromonas bacteria are almost always present in aquarium and pond water, and even on the fish itself. The organisms are Gram-negative, rod-shaped bacteria about 1 × 2.0–4.5 μm in size. They are motile, with a single polar flagellum. It is an opportunistic pathogen that proliferates when the fish are weakened or injured. Signs of infection include hemorrhages of the gills, erythema of the skin and fins (Fig. 17.4), loss of scales, and skin ulcers (Fig. 17.5). Eye swelling (exophthalmia) and abdominal swelling (dropsy) may also occur, secondary to circulatory disturbances and fluid accumulation. Infectious Dropsy of Carp (IDC) is caused by *Aeromonas hydrophila* and has signs of infection similar to Spring Viremia of Carp (Hoole *et al.*, 2001). Parasites such as fish lice and skin flukes cause skin wounds that can become infected with *Aeromonas* bacteria (Saint-Erne, 2010).

Vibrio bacteria are Gram-negative, motile, facultative anaerobic, curved rod (0.5 × 1.5–2.5 μm) bacteria. They most often occur in marine environments. Vibriosis causes hemorrhages and ulcerations of the skin, fin, and tail, and hemorrhagic degeneration of the internal organs. The signs in marine fish species are similar to those caused by *Aeromonas* in freshwater fish.

Treatment consists of antibiotic injections, antibiotics in the food or water, plus topical antimicrobial applications, such as povidone-iodine, silver sulfadiazine, or antibiotic ointments, directly on the skin ulcers (Fig. 17.6). Aquatic bacteria have become resistant to many antibiotics (especially amoxicillin, ampicillin, and tetracycline), so culture and sensitivity testing is necessary prior to choosing

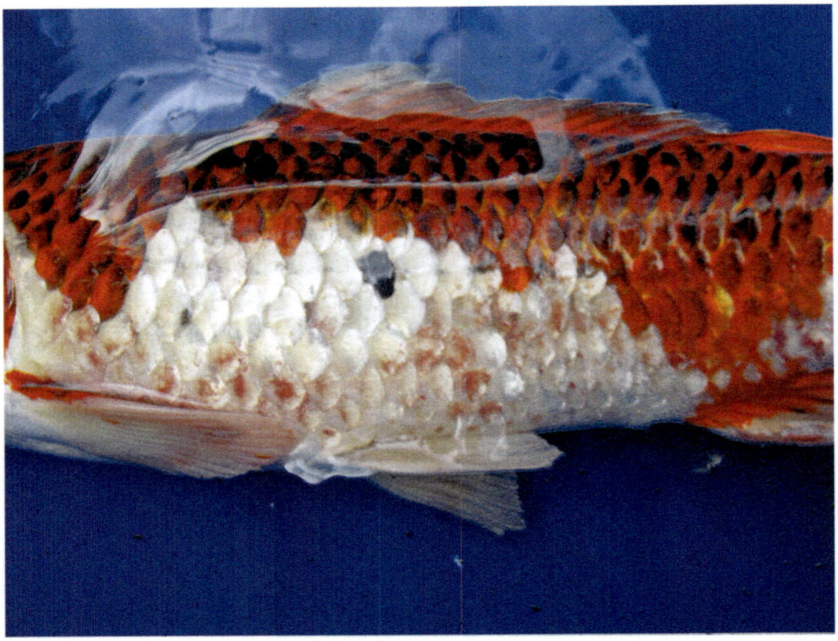

Fig. 17.4. Erythema of the pectoral fins and skin of a Sumigoromo koi (*C. rubrofuscus*). (Photograph by N. Saint-Erne.)

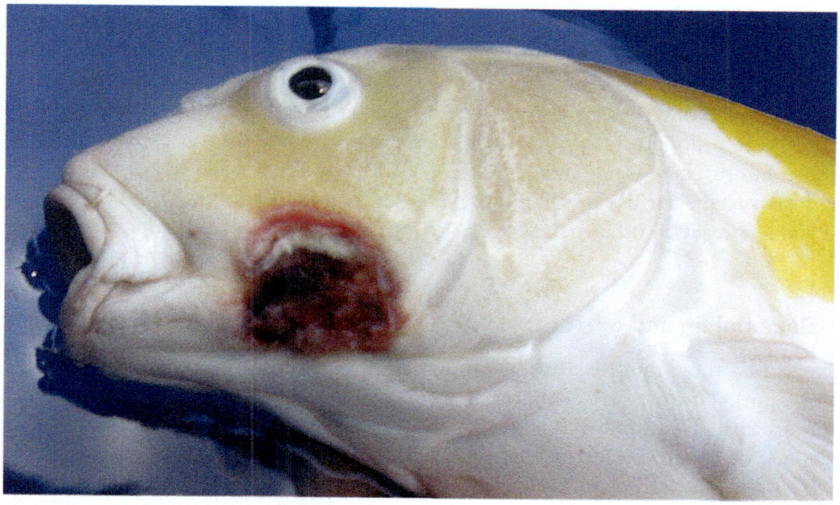

Fig. 17.5. Bacterial ulcer on the jaw of a Hariwake koi (*C. rubrofuscus*). (Photograph by N. Saint-Erne.)

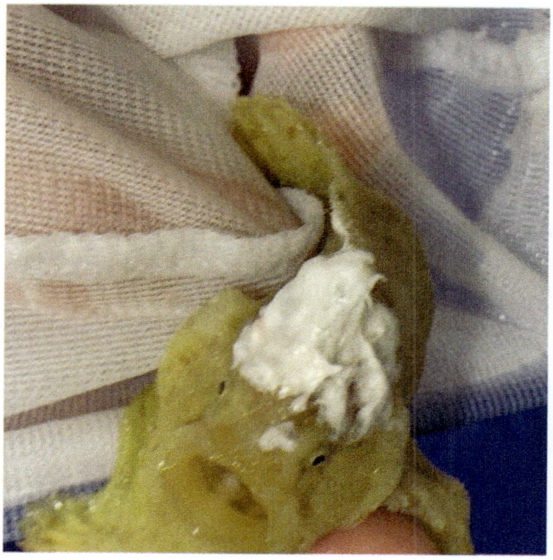

Fig. 17.6. Topical silver sulfadiazine ointment applied to a skin lesion of a frogfish (*Antennarius sp.*) that had *Vibrio alginolyticus* grown on a bacterial culture. (Photograph by N. Saint-Erne.)

an antibiotic. Water quality improvement is indicated for all disease conditions.

17.3.2 Erythrodermatitis (furunculosis, ulcer disease)

Aeromonas salmonicida achromogenes causes epithelial ulcers in salmonids (called furunculosis) and carp (called Carp Erythrodermatitis). It is a Gram-negative, non-motile, short rod (0.5 × 1.5 µm) bacterium. It occurs singly, in pairs, chains, or clumps. It is inactive in water temperatures below 40°F/4.4°C or above 68°F/20°C. Severe epizootics of this disease occur most frequently in outdoor koi and goldfish ponds in the spring when the water temperature is rising (increased bacterial growth), and the fish are stressed from over-wintering (decreased fish immunity). It is contagious and infected koi and goldfish should be isolated if possible.

It is marked by septicemia, causing skin erythema (redness), hemorrhages, ulcerations, scale protrusion (lepidorthosis), and pinkish, serosanguinous ascites. The redness also can occur on the base of the fins. Raised skin lesions (furuncles) may form first, which then ulcerate, exposing the underlying muscles (Figs 17.7a and b). Congestion and hemorrhage of the internal organs also occur, leading to necrosis of the liver and spleen. Blood culture is the best method for effective identification and sensitivity testing of *A. salmonicida achromogenes* in live fish. The kidney can be used to take a sample for bacterial culture during a necropsy of freshly dead fish.

Treatments with antibiotic (Azactam, Baytril, Fortaz, or NuFlor) injections have been effective, and it is recommended to apply a topical disinfectant (povidone-iodine, silver sulfadiazine, or antibiotic ointment) to the skin lesions. Tube-feeding a mixture of antibiotics and soaked, mashed fish food pellets can be used on larger fish in treatment tanks. Keep the water temperature in the treatment tank above 73°F/23°C to activate the fish's immune system. Prevent osmotic stress due to skin lesions by adding salt to freshwater aquariums to make a 0.1–0.3% salinity solution. There is a commercially available furunculosis vaccine for use in salmonids, which may have some efficacy in other fish species.

17.3.3 Bacterial fin and gill rot

This is usually caused by the Gram-negative, short (0.5–1 × 1.5–4 μm), motile, rod bacteria *Pseudomonas fluorescens*, *P. putida*, or *P. putrefaciens*, but *Aeromonas* or other species of bacteria can also be involved. Fin and tail erosions are the usual signs, but hemorrhages and skin ulcers sometimes occur, as seen with furunculosis. Some suspected cases of furunculosis have been found to be caused by *Pseudomonas* when cultured. A wet mount of infected organs or skin mucus may reveal motile bacilli that would quickly differentiate these bacteria from the non-motile *Aeromonas salmonicida*. Traumatic injuries to the fins often result in this secondary bacterial infection.

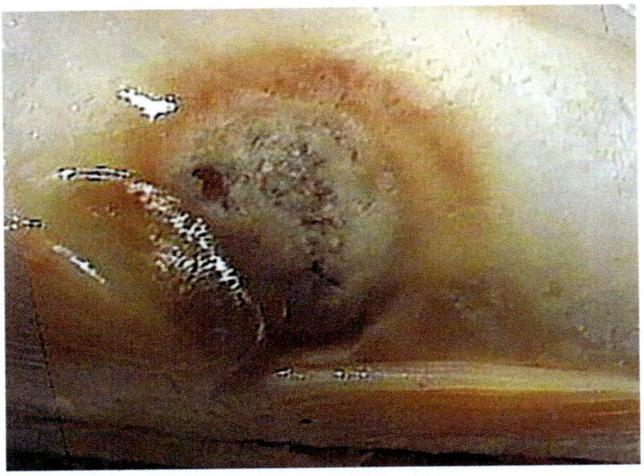

Fig. 17.7a. Furuncle surrounded by erythema on the side of a koi (*C. rubrofuscus*) above the pelvic fin. (Photograph by N. Saint-Erne.)

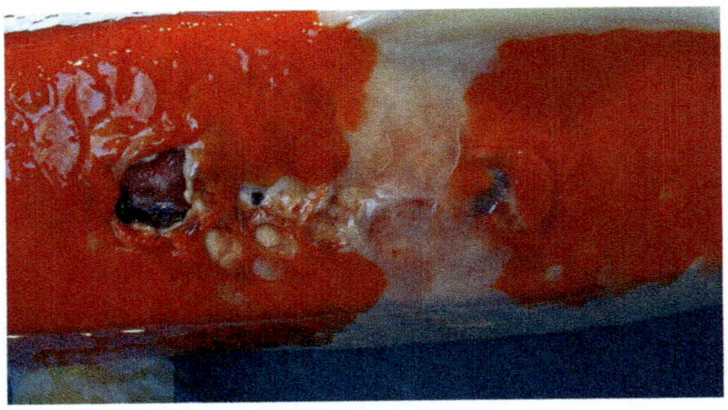

Fig. 17.7b. Skin ulceration and scale loss on a Kohaku koi (*C. rubrofuscus*). (Photograph by N. Saint-Erne.)

Treat with antibiotics in the food or water, antibiotic injections, and topical wound disinfection. Chloramine-T is often helpful in treating bacterial gill disease. Severely damaged fin margins can be trimmed off with a scalpel or sharp scissors, and the fin topically disinfected. This may hasten healing and fin regeneration. Fin rot is commonly associated with high bacterial populations in the environment due to accumulated wastes and poor water quality.

17.3.4 Columnaris (cotton disease)

Flavobacterium columnare (previously named *Flexibacter*) is a long (10–12 μm), thin, flexingly motile rod. It will grow in water from 39–95°F/4–35°C but is more pathogenic in water above 64°F/18°C. This opportunistic pathogen causes reddened areas on the skin with cottony white growths, often mistaken for a fungal infection. The lesions occur mostly on the lips and fins, and across the top of the caudal peduncle, forming a white area called "saddleback." On the surface of the fish, large masses of these bacteria will align themselves into "haystack" formations (Fig. 17.8). This allows

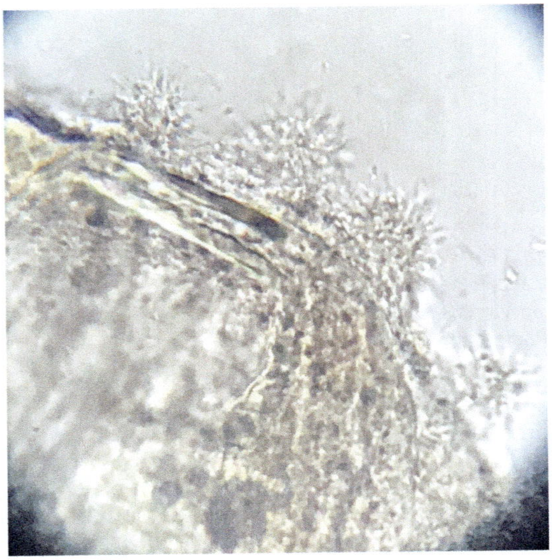

Fig. 17.8. Haystack appearance of *Columnaris* bacteria on a skin scrape biopsy. (Microphotograph by N. Saint-Erne.)

the diagnosis of *Flavobacterium* by microscopic observation of skin or fin biopsy samples. It often occurs on injured tissues. Most healthy fish are resistant to this infection, but it is particularly common in tilapia, goldfish, koi, and live-bearing fish (guppies, mollies, platys, and swordtails). Treat with antibiotics in the food and with copper sulfate baths. The disease is worse at higher water temperatures, so lowering the temperature may slow bacterial growth. Other stresses (poor water quality, parasites, trauma) predispose susceptible fishes to infection. Adding salt to freshwater (2–3 g/l) may be helpful as that reduces osmotic stress.

17.3.5 Edwardsiellosis

Edwardsiella ictaluri and *E. tarda* are Gram-negative, facultative anaerobic rods that can live in freshwater and marine environments and are commonly associated with disease in channel catfish. However, *E. ictaluri* (0.5 × 1.3 μm) has caused high mortality in zebrafish in research laboratories, and *E. tarda* (1.0 × 2.0–3.0 μm) infects marine as well as freshwater fish (Roberts, 2012). *Edwardsiella* is an obligate pathogen and can be transmitted orally by contact with infected fish, water, or feces. Clinical signs of disease include skin hemorrhages, pale gills, lethargy, and splenomegaly. On histopathology, bacteria frequently can be found in high numbers in the spleen, kidneys, nares, and forebrain. It can be isolated using standard bacterial culture media, but it is slow-growing (Petty *et al.*, 2022). Approved treatments in the United States for *Edwardsiella* include Sulfadimethoxine and Ormetoprim at 50 mg/kg BW given orally every 24 h for 5 days, and florfenicol at 10–15 mg/kg BW given orally every 24 h for 10 days (Hadfield, 2021a).

17.3.6 Francisellosis

Francisella bacteria can cause septicemia and granulomatous inflammation in fishes. These are Gram-negative, non-motile, aerobic coccobacilli (1.5 μm) that are facultatively intracellular, piscirickettsial-like organisms (Hadfield, 2021a). Transmission occurs by oral ingestion, and invertebrates may act as vectors. Clinical signs include lethargy, anorexia, spiral swimming, hemorrhages of the skin, exophthalmos, and gill hyperplasia with white nodules. Necropsy may show splenomegaly and renomegaly with white nodular granulomas and intracellular bacteria. Treatment with oral florfenicol 15–20 mg/kg BW in food every 24 h for 10 days may reduce mortalities. The existence of asymptomatic carrier fish can occur, with bacteria still in the spleen, once the clinical outbreak has subsided (Tamaru *et al.*, 2011).

17.3.7 Bacterial epitheliocystis

Epitheliocystis is caused by a Gram-negative, obligate intracellular bacterium in the order Chlamydiales, or possibly the phylum Proteobacteria. Epitheliocystis is seen in freshwater and marine aquarium fish, most frequently in discus (*Symphysodon* spp.), and oscars (*Astronotus ocellatus*). Infection involves the gills and occasionally the skin. Epitheliocystis should be suspected if colorless spherical structures (infected, hypertrophied cells) that have granular contents are seen on gill biopsy or skin mucus scraping. Histopathologic examination typically reveals basophilic hypertrophied cells. Clinical signs are variable, but heavily infected fish may be lethargic, anorexic, and dyspneic. Oral azithromycin or oxytetracycline has been used to successfully control infections.

17.3.8 Gram-positive bacterial infections

Streptococcus and related genera *Lactococcus*, *Enterococcus*, and *Vagococcus* are Gram-positive cocci bacteria, less than 2 μm wide, that form chains, which allows for a presumptive diagnosis. Infections are uncommon but can cause chronic disease that may continue for weeks, with only a few fish dying each day. A characteristic sign of *Streptococcus* infection is neurologic disease, often manifested by spinning or spiral swimming in the water. Brain and kidney cultures from suspect fish should be incubated on blood agar at 25°C for 24–48 h. Antibiotic therapy should be based on sensitivity testing. Erythromycin and florfenicol are often effective treatments. *Streptococcus iniae* has been isolated from tilapia and aquarium fish and has zoonotic potential. It frequently causes neurological signs in infected fish, including swimming in a spiral fashion.

17.3.9 Mycobacteriosis

Three species of mycobacteria are found in fish, *Mycobacterium marinum, M. fortuitum*, and *M. chelonae*. These are Gram-positive, acid-fast, non-motile coccobacilli measuring 1–10 μm in length by 0.2–0.6 μm wide. *Mycobacterium* may be a common constituent of the microflora in aquatic environments. Predisposing environmental factors that may increase infections include low dissolved oxygen, low pH, and high organic loads. The infection in fish may cause acute, necrotizing peritonitis, but more often causes a chronic granulomatous response. Fish with chronic wasting disease should be suspected of having mycobacteriosis (Baumgartner *et al.*, 2022). Transmission can occur through ingestion, so keeping the aquarium substrate clean of debris, and especially removing dead fish that may otherwise be eaten, is important in reducing the spread of mycobacteria.

Signs of disease in the fish include lethargy, anorexia, emaciation, skin lesions, exophthalmia, and ascites. Diagnosis is made by culturing the bacteria at 25–30°C for 3–4 weeks, and by acid-fast staining of affected tissues and examining them microscopically for the bacteria. PCR testing is often a more reliable diagnostic method. The granulomas can be seen microscopically in squash preparations of organs sampled at necropsy (Fig. 17.9) or through histopathology. Syngnathids (sea horses and pipefish) are highly susceptible, but the disease can be seen in any fish. Treatment is usually unrewarding, but a combination of enrofloxacin (10–14 mg/kg) and rifampin (10–20 mg/kg) can be tried. An infected aquarium should be disinfected before other fish are added.

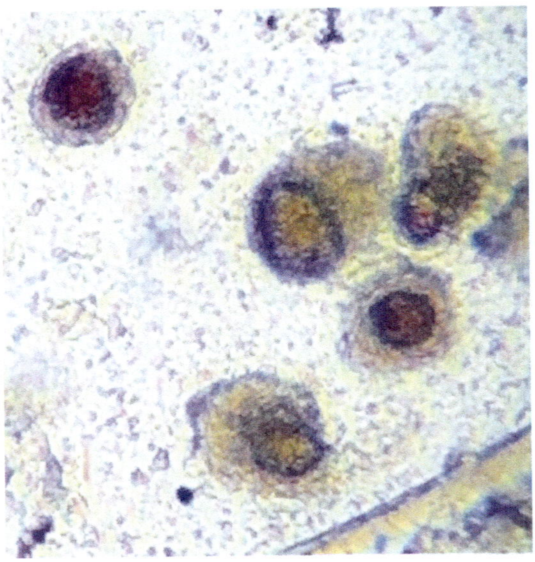

Fig. 17.9. *Mycobacterium* granulomas from the liver of a blue-green chromis (*Chromis viridis*). (Microphotograph by N. Saint-Erne.)

A zoonotic potential exists with mycobacteria, and people handling infected fish can get lesions on their hands from contamination of cuts or scrapes. This is known as "fish handler's disease." It is especially of concern in persons with immune deficiencies, who may develop respiratory disease in addition to localized skin infection. Wear examination gloves when handling fish or performing necropsies on fish suspected of having this or any other disease.

17.3.10 Bacterial swim bladder infections

Abnormalities of the swim bladder can occasionally be caused by bacterial infections, especially by *Aeromonas* in physostomous fish species. An infection that alters the pneumatic duct can allow water to enter the swim bladder, affecting the buoyancy of the fish. These fish lose their positive buoyancy as the air is replaced by water. They have difficulty swimming and often sit on the bottom of the aquarium or pond. They will even "hop" on the bottom rather than swim. There may be lesions on the abdomen and ventral fins from rubbing on the substrate (Figs 17.10a and b). The abdomen may appear enlarged due to abnormal distension of the swim bladder. A radiograph will help determine if water is in the swim bladder and differentiate it from a coelomic mass.

Treat affected fish by percutaneous aspiration of the fluid in the swim bladder while under anesthesia. For larger fish such as goldfish and koi, use a 22-gauge, 1½ inch (cm) long needle and place it through the body wall 1–2 cm below the lateral line at the caudal end of the coelomic cavity, which is before the vent. Angle the needle acutely forward, so it passes obliquely under the scales and through the

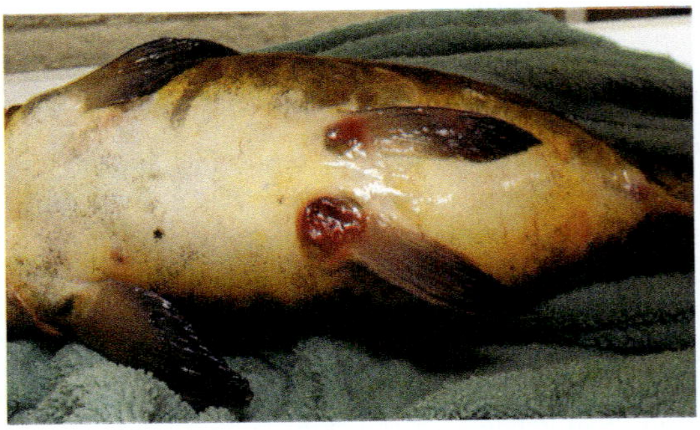

Fig. 17.10a. Chagoi koi (*C. rubrofuscus*) with lesions at base of pelvic fins from rubbing on bottom of pond due to negative buoyancy from a swim bladder infection. (Photograph by N. Saint-Erne.)

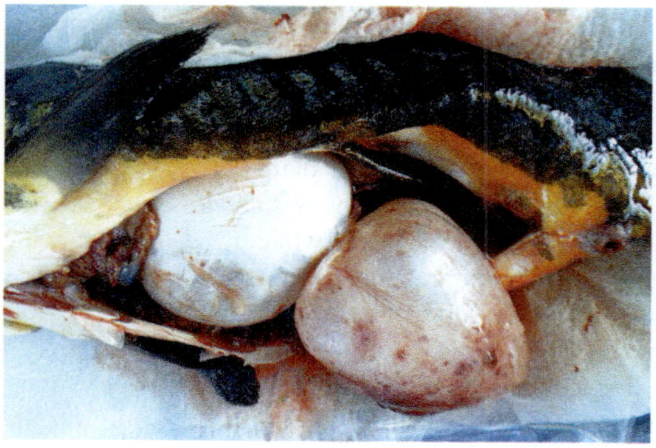

Fig. 17.10b. Necropsy of a Karasugoi koi (*C. rubrofuscus*) with internal hemorrhaging and overinflation of the gas bladder chambers. (Photograph by N. Saint-Erne.)

body muscle, and then into the caudal chamber of the gas bladder. Hold the fish out of the water with its head higher than the tail and aspirate all the fluid out of the swim bladder. Then inject an antibiotic, such as enrofloxacin (10–14 mg/kg), into the gas bladder by switching syringes on the inserted needle. Follow this with enough air injected into the bladder to produce slightly positive buoyancy. Press a finger over the skin as the needle is withdrawn to prevent pulling out any scales. Treat any abdominal skin lesions with topical antibacterial ointment. This process may need to be repeated weekly until no more fluid can be aspirated from the swim bladder.

17.4 Fungal Diseases

17.4.1 Oomycetes

Saprolegnia, Achlya, and *Aphanomyces* are aquatic oomycetes fungus-like eukaryotic microorganisms within the Stramenopiles Clade. They are filamentous and heterotrophic and can reproduce both sexually and asexually. They can produce infections in fish and their eggs. They are ubiquitous in aquatic environments, and often, fish are only secondarily infected when they are already suffering from an injury, bacterial infection, or parasites. These oomycetes occur as external pseudofungal infections in fish. They appear as white cottony tufts on the skin or gills and on fish eggs. These fungi can grow in water with up to 0.7% salinity, and in temperatures ranging from 32 to 96.8°F/0 to 36°C and in the pH range of 4.0–8.3. Microscopic examination shows transparent, aseptate, branching hyphae, about 20 μm in diameter (Figs 17.11a and b). The hyphae develop sporangia at their tips, which asexually produce spherical zoospores. Motile biflagellate primary zoospores (5 μm diameter) are released from the sporangium (100 μm long) on the tip of a mycelium. Each primary zoospore may encyst and divide internally to produce many secondary zoospores. Encysted nonmotile primary zoospores of *Achlya* cluster around the exit papilla of the sporangium while dividing. The zoospores attach to damaged tissue or other decaying organic matter and germinate to produce hyphae. On fish, the hyphae penetrate the skin and enter the skeletal muscle (Smith *et al.*, 2019).

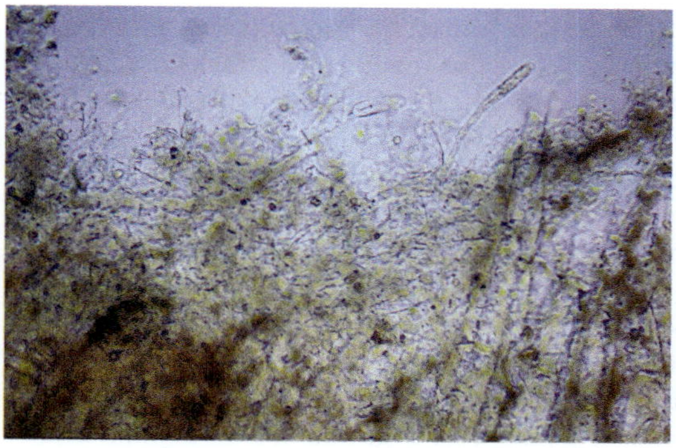

Fig. 17.11a. Mycelia seen on a fin biopsy examination of a Mexican longfin dace (*Agosia chrysogaster*). (Microphotograph by N. Saint-Erne.)

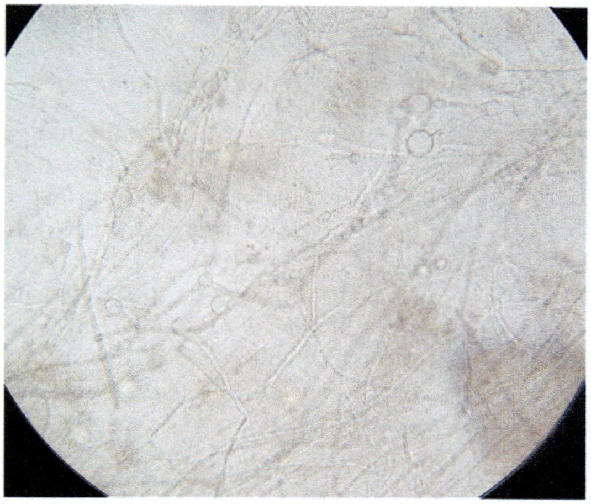

Fig. 17.11b. Hyphae seen on a skin scrape biopsy examination of a koi (*C. rubrofuscus*). (Microphotograph by N. Saint-Erne.)

Their growth usually occurs on tissue that has been previously damaged by trauma or other disease conditions. The hyphae produce proteolytic enzymes that cause the destruction of adjacent healthy tissue. The fungus also attacks unfertilized fish eggs but, once established, will spread to the viable eggs, causing their death by obstructing oxygen absorption with hyphae. Remove any white opaque eggs from the spawning mats, if possible, to prevent their decay and fungus proliferation.

Treatment consists of adding formalin/malachite solution or hydrogen peroxide to the water and using topical antifungal disinfectants (e.g. Betadine) on the affected skin. Oomycetes will proliferate in aquariums or ponds with large amounts of organic debris (dead plants and leaves, dead fish, uneaten food), so detritus removal and water changes are helpful. Prevent oomycetes growth on egg masses with methylene blue (0.25 mg/l of water daily for 3 days), or 3% hydrogen peroxide (0.25 ml/l of water).

17.4.2 Branchiomycosis (fungal gill rot)

Branchiomyces sanguinis and *B. demigrans* fungi invade the blood vessels of the gills, obstructing the flow of blood. Infected gill filaments become brownish with white or gray streaks and raised patches (Fig. 17.12). The gill filaments fuse together and have areas of avascular necrosis due to the fungal hyphae blocking the blood vessels of the gill. Gill biopsy of affected tissues will reveal telangiectasis and hyperplasia of gill lamellae. Affected fish become lethargic and anorexic and appear to be gasping.

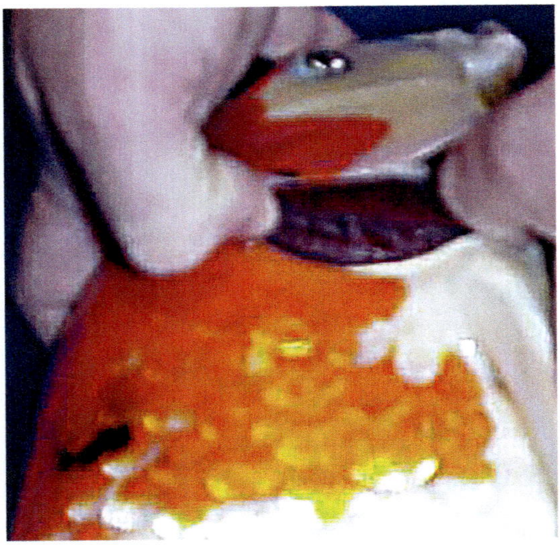

Fig. 17.12. White patches on a koi's gill filaments from *Branchiomyces* infection. (Photograph by N. Saint-Erne.)

Microscopically, sporangia on the fungal hyphae asexually produce non-motile spores (5–9 µm diameter), which are released into the water and will attach to the gill surface. The spores then germinate branched, aseptate hyphae (8–30 µm diameter) that penetrate the gill tissue. *Branchiomyces sanguinis* only grows within the gill capillaries, while *B. demigrans* will grow throughout the gill tissue and form masses of hyphae on the surface of the gills. This fungus grows in water temperatures of 57–95°F/14–35°C.

High levels of unionized ammonia in the water increase the incidence of fungal gill rot due to gill epithelial hyperplasia. Accumulation of organic debris in the pond, and suspended particulate matter, may also predispose fish to this infection. Death due to hypoxia can occur rapidly in affected fish, in as little as 2 days after infection. Mortality rates in affected fish can be high. Treat the water daily with methylene blue (0.25 mg/l water) or malachite green (0.10 mg/l water) and add salt to the water (0.3–0.5% salinity) until gill tissue is healthy. Prevent infections by keeping the water clean, reducing overcrowded conditions, and avoiding accumulations of decomposing organic matter.

17.4.3 Mesomycetozoea

This group of fungal-like organisms includes *Dermocystidium* and *Ichthyophonus*. They can occur in freshwater and saltwater. *Dermocystidium*, as the name implies, causes cysts in the dermis of the skin. The spore-filled hyphae infiltrate the skin and gills and form 1 mm raised nodules. These may be surgically removed to reduce the risk of spreading. Microscopic examination of a removed cyst will show many spores (3–15 µm diameter). Each spore has an eccentric nucleus, a large vacuole, and an inclusion body. *Ichthyophonus hoferi* spores are ingested by fish, mostly marine, but some freshwater fish have been infected (Hadfield, 2021b). Affected fish may become anorectic and emaciated. Muscle lesions appear, as may petechial hemorrhages of the skin. Diagnosis can be made by histopathology or PCR testing. Treat the skin with topical antifungal solutions such as Betadine or chlorhexidine and treat the water with antifungal dyes such as malachite green or methylene blue.

17.5 Conclusion

When a fish is exposed to an infectious disease, it is important to make a diagnosis and start treatment as quickly as possible. There are limited treatment options for viral infections, but medications can be used for bacterial and fungal infections. For all sick fish, morbidity, and mortality can be reduced by eliminating stressors. This includes moving affected fish into a quarantine or treatment tank, providing proper water quality at the preferred temperature, increasing aeration, and feeding high-quality foods. Nutritional support, if the fish are still eating, can be provided with additional vitamin C (500–1000 mg/kg BW) in the diet. Immune stimulants may also be helpful, such as beta-glucans at 1 g/kg food (0.1%) or allicin (garlic extract) at 5–10 g/kg food (0.5–1.0%) added to the diet for several weeks (Hadfield, 2021a).

Most bacterial infections in fish are secondary infections by bacteria that are ubiquitous in the aquatic environment. The primary stressor is usually an injury, poor water quality, or parasitic infestations that lower the fish's immunity. Treatment of microbial infections should be based on diagnostic tests, including bacterial culture and sensitivity testing, to ensure appropriate antibiotic medications are used. Pathogenic viruses, bacteria, and fungi can also be spread by handling fish or by fomites, such as nets. Proper quarantine programs and biosecurity measures will help reduce the risk of introducing pathogens into a fish population.

References

Baumgartner, W., Alcivar-Warren, A., Aydin, F.G., Bateman, K., Clinton, M. *et al.* (2022) Pathology of aquatic animal diseases. In: Urdes, L., Walster. C, and Tepper, J. (eds) *Fundamentals of Aquatic Veterinary Medicine*. Wiley, Oxford, pp. 73–98.

Hadfield, C.A. (2021a) Bacterial diseases. In: Hadfield, C. and Clayton, L. (eds) *Clinical Guide to Fish Medicine*. Wiley, Oxford, pp. 431–467.

Hadfield, C.A. (2021b) Fungal and fungal-like diseases. In: Hadfield, C. and Clayton, L. (eds) *Clinical Guide to Fish Medicine*. Wiley, Oxford, pp. 468–482.

Hesami, S., Viadanna, P., Steckler, N., Spears, S., Thompson, P. *et al.* (2015) *Carp Edema Virus Disease (CEVD)/Koi Sleepy Disease (KSD)*. FA189, School of Forest Resources and Conservation Program in Fisheries and Aquatic Sciences, UF/IFAS Extension, Gainesville, Florida.

Hoole, D., Bucke, D., Burgess, P. and Wellby, I. (2001) Cyprinid biology. In: Hoole, D., Bucke, D., Burgess, P. and Wellby, I. (eds) *Diseases of Carp and Other Cyprinid Fishes*. Blackwell Science, Oxford, pp. 8–20.

Petty, B.D., Francis-Floyd, R., and Yanong, R.P.E. (2022) Bacterial diseases of fish. In: *Merck Veterinary Manual*. Merck Sharp & Dohme, Rahway, New Jersey. Available at: https://www.merckvetmanual.com/exotic-and-laboratory-animals/aquarium-fish/bacterial-diseases-of-fish?query=bacterial%20diseases%20of%20fish (accessed 1 August 2024).

Roberts, H.E. (2010) Commonly observed clinical signs of stress in fish. In: Roberts, H.E. (ed.) *Fundamentals of Ornamental Fish Health*. Wiley-Blackwell, Ames. Iowa; 35.

Roberts, R.J. (2012) The bacteriology of teleosts. In: *Fish Pathology*. 4th edn. Wiley, Ames, Iowa, pp. 339–382.

Saint-Erne, N. (2010) Infectious diseases. In: Saint-Erne, N. (ed.) *Advanced Koi Care*. 2nd edn. Erne Enterprises, Glendale, Arizona, pp. 62–70.

Smith, P.A., Elliot, D.G., Bruno, D.W. and Smith, S.A. (2019) Skin and fin diseases. In: Smith, S.A. (ed.) *Fish Diseases and Medicine*. CRC Press, Boca Raton, Florida, pp. 97–117.

Tamaru, C., McGovern-Hopkins, K., Klinger-Bowen, R., Fox, B., Riggs, A. *et al.* (2011) *Detection of Asymptomatic Francisella spp. Carriers in Tilapia Cultured in Hawaii*. Center for Tropical & Subtropical Aquaculture Regional e-News, Honolulu, Hawaii.

18 Protozoan Parasites

AZUREEN ERDMAN

New River, Arizona

Abstract

Parasites are perhaps the most important and common cause of morbidity and mortality in captive aquatic species. Ciliates and flagellates are the most common causes of disease in ornamental fish and are the largest classification of protozoal parasites. Other protozoa include Myxozoa, microsporidia, and apicomplexans. Correctly diagnosing and treating protozoal parasites is important for maintaining healthy fish.

18.1 Diagnosing Protozoal Parasites

Parasites are perhaps the most important and common cause of morbidity and mortality in captive aquatic species (Austin, 2012). Diagnosis of protozoal infestations is best done by examination of a live fish, or a freshly dead refrigerated fish. Frozen specimens or fish dead for a prolonged period will not yield accurate samples. The soft-bodied protozoa will disappear rapidly from dead specimens. Consider taking samples and examining them tank side, or have clients bring the live fish into the clinic for examination. Either will yield more accurate results than taking and transporting samples to the laboratory (Saint-Erne, 2010).

Affected fish should have a small area of skin scraped and the mucus examined under a microscope. A small section of a fin and a few gill filament tips should also be clipped off for examination. Fresh, wet-mounted samples must be microscopically examined quickly to visualize the motility of many protozoa species. A blood sample can be drawn and checked for blood parasites. Feces should be examined for intestinal protozoa.

Even seemingly healthy fish may sustain a small number of protozoan parasites (Hoole *et al.*, 2001). Many of the protozoal parasites tend not to cause disease until the fish are immunocompromised, placed in poor environmental conditions, or the fishes' mucoid epithelial barrier is damaged, allowing these parasites to reproduce rapidly and become pathogenic (Plumb, 1999). However, when diagnosed, it is best to treat the aquarium to eliminate the protozoa and to not rely on only the fishes' immune system for their protection.

18.2 Ciliated Protozoa

18.2.1 *Ichthyophthirius multifiliis*

Ichthyophthirius multifiliis causes a disease of freshwater fish commonly called "Ich" or "white spot disease" (Scholz, 1999). The direct life cycle of Ich comprises three stages (Dickerson, 2012). The feeding stage (trophont) of this ciliate is 0.5–1.0 mm in diameter when on a fish. It is round to oval in shape, with many cilia covering its cell membrane (holotrichous). It contains a characteristic horseshoe-shaped macronucleus and a smaller round micronucleus. This horseshoe-shaped macronucleus is helpful in identifying the parasite under a microscope (Fig. 18.1). After feeding, the trophont drops off the host fish and forms a pseudocyst (tomont). This stage of the ciliate can exponentially multiply in number. One cell can divide into over 1000 new parasites, called tomites, inside of the tomont. The tomont will rupture and the tomites leave the cyst structure and become free-swimming theronts, 40–50 µm in length. The life cycle can take as little as 3 days or up to 6 weeks to complete, depending on environmental conditions and water temperatures.

Corresponding author: az.erdman@gmail.com

 © CAB International 2025.
DOI: 10.1079/9781789246032.0018

The mature trophonts are embedded in the gill epithelium or under the skin of the fish, forming visible white spots (Fig. 18.2). These trophonts will

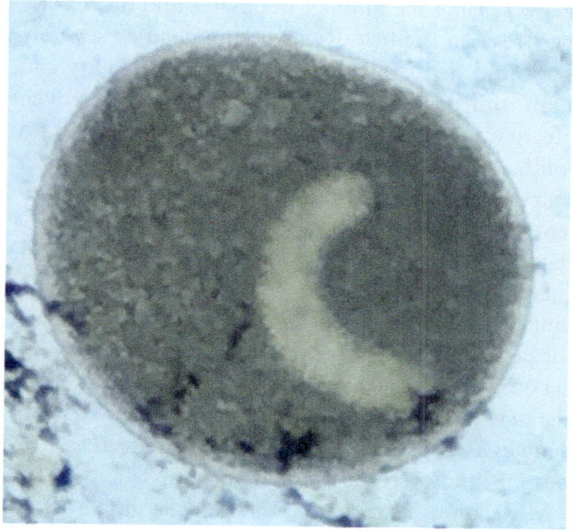

Fig. 18.1. Microscopic image of *Ichthyophthirius multifiliis* protozoan. (Microphotograph by N. Saint-Erne.)

feed on cellular debris and fluids, and grow to mature size, eventually leaving the fish and becoming tomonts. The tomont will attach to a surface in the aquarium, gravel, plants, or other décor items, where it then undergoes binary cell division. The tomites formed within the tomont will bore through the cyst wall and become motile theronts. These can only survive 2–3 days without a host. The pyriform, ciliated theronts will burrow into the skin, fins, and gills of fish in order to mature into trophonts, which starts the cycle over (Ewing and Kocan, 1992).

Populations housed under higher stress situations like hypoxic conditions, poor water quality, or high stocking densities are at higher risk for *I. multifiliis* outbreaks. Temperature affects the rate of parasite reproduction. The optimum temperature ranges for the reproduction of Ich parasites are between 16 and 23°C. At these temperatures, the entire life cycle can be completed within 6 days to 2 weeks, the faster time at the higher temperature. It has been shown that at 7°C the life cycle can take up to 40 days to complete. Higher temperatures

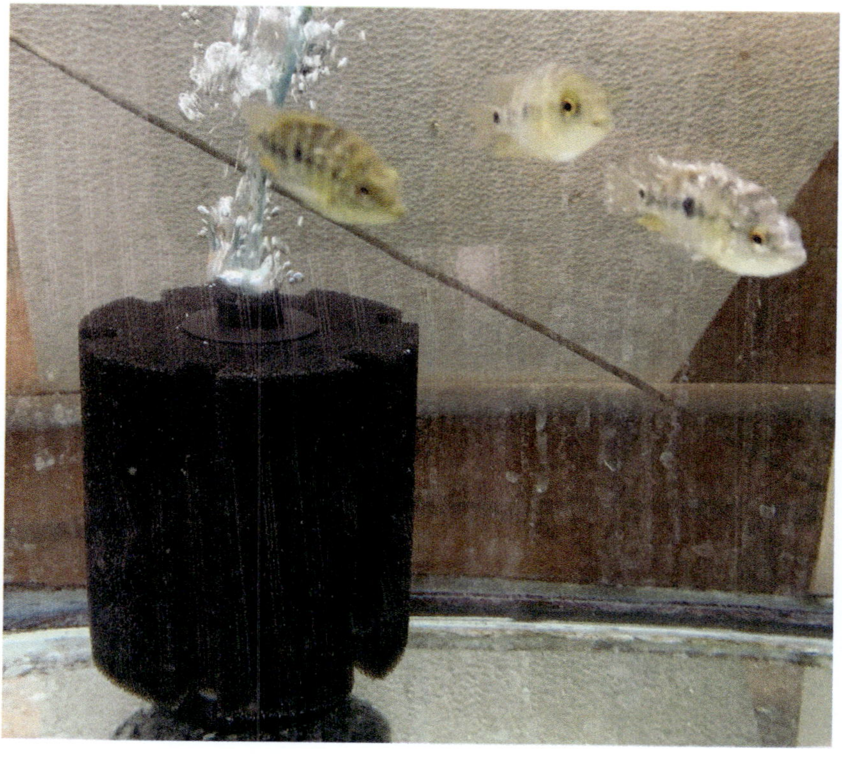

Fig. 18.2. Cichlid fish infested with white spot disease, or Ich, caused by the parasite embedded in the fish's epithelium, being treated in a quarantine tank. (Photo by N. Saint-Erne.)

allow for quick reproduction of the ciliate. However, *I. multifiliis* has been shown to stop multiplying at temperatures above 30°C. This can be useful and integrated as part of the treatment for fish that can tolerate higher water temperatures.

Clinical signs of this parasite include behavioral changes like flashing or rubbing on the bottom of the tank due to itching or irritation of the skin (Andrews *et al.*, 2002). Fish can swim erratically or violently. They may hold the fins against the body. If the gills are severely affected, the fish may stay near a water inlet or aeration source due to decreased ability to absorb oxygen across the inflamed gills. On physical examination, white spots can be seen on the skin, gills, fins, or cornea. Gills can appear swollen, pale, and covered in excessive mucous layers. Fish may show signs of sepsis, as the *I. multifiliis* will damage the epithelium and allow secondary bacterial infections to occur. In water temperatures ranging from 16–23°C, large numbers of acute mortalities can sometimes occur.

Diagnosis is based on the presence of *I. multifiliis* on gill biopsies (Fig. 18.3), mucus or skin scrapes, and fin clips (Noga, 2010). Small numbers, less than five parasites per low power field, may not be pathogenic, but when in high numbers disease is often present. Diagnosis can also be made on post-mortem examination by histopathology.

Management of outbreaks of *I. multifiliis* focuses on decreasing the number of ciliates and decreasing the stress on the fish. Remove any dead or severely moribund fish from the aquarium. If a facility can drain and dry the tank or pond, this has proven effective in killing the parasites. The bottom of a pond can be treated with quicklime. The water temperature can be increased to 30–32°C to prevent further parasite reproduction and then slowly decrease to the normal temperature range over 7 days. It is important to note that a drastic change in temperature is stressful to fish and this protocol may not be tolerated by some species. One of the options to combat outbreaks in a tank is to transfer the fish to a new tank every 12 h for 1 week. Repeated water changes and sediment cleaning can help decrease the tomonts and theronts in an aquarium.

Medications used to treat this parasite (Table 18.1) do not treat the embedded trophont or the encysted tomont. Therefore, chemical treatments need to be repeated for prolonged periods until the tomites emerge from the encysted tomont stage. There are many brands of commercial Ich medications available (Fig. 18.4).

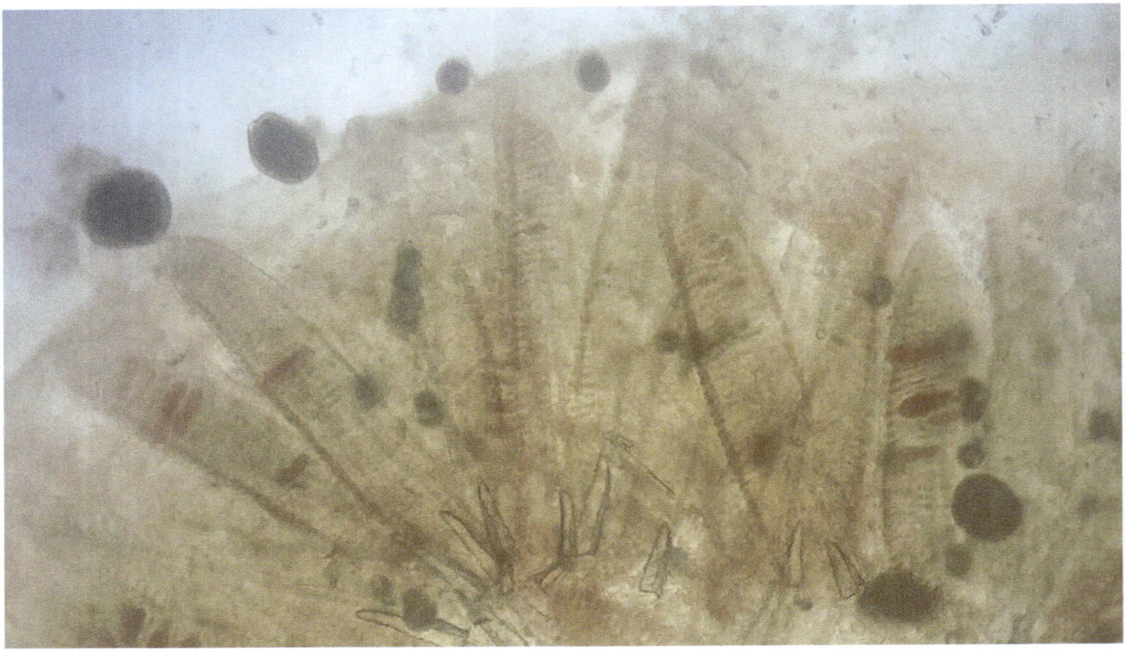

Fig. 18.3. Ich parasites of varying sizes on gill sample taken during a necropsy examination. (Microphotograph by N. Saint-Erne.)

Table 18.1. Treatments for Ichthyophthirius. Author's own table.

NaCl 1.5–2.5% for 10–30 min each 24 h (q24h) for 7 days
Potassium permanganate 2–4 mg/l as continuous treatment
Formalin 15–25 mg/l q48h for 1–4 weeks
Malachite green 0.1 mg/l for 1–4 weeks
Malachite green and formalin can act synergistically and are often used together
Toltrazuril 20–30 mg/l for 60-min dip q24h for three treatments (Loh, 2012)
Proto Pro containing Biokos at one tablet/50 l every other day for 3–6 treatments (Fig. 18.5)

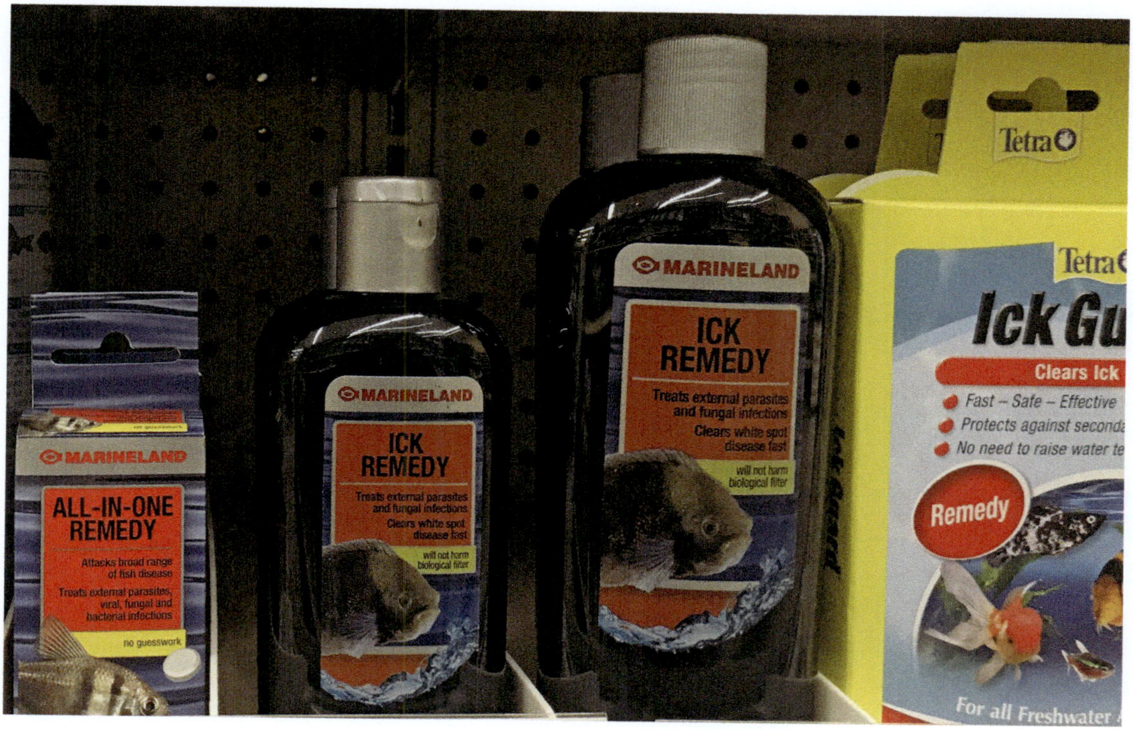

Fig. 18.4. Commercial products for treating Ich. (Photograph by N. Saint-Erne.)

Prevention for this ciliate is focused on quarantine protocols to prevent introduction into a fish system. A quarantine period of at least 7 days at a temperature of 24–28°C should be used for all new fish, plants, stones, and snails entering a system. It is important to maintain separate equipment or sterilize equipment between ponds and tanks to prevent further spread through fomites exposed to contaminated water.

18.2.2 *Cryptocaryon irritans*

Cryptocaryon irritans is known as "marine Ich" or "marine white spot" (Colorni, 1997). This ciliate has a lobed macronucleus. It appears pear shaped (pyriform) or club shaped, with cilia covering its body (holotrichous). It has a lifecycle like the freshwater *Ichthyophthirius* parasite. Though very similar to its freshwater counterpart, *I. multifiliis*, *C. irritans* has evolved in a convergent path and the two are not phylogenetically related. It swims by rotating slowly and "rolling" along. *C. irritans* can affect a large range of fish species. Elasmobranch are thought to be resistant to infestations.

Cryptocaryon irritans has a direct life cycle of four phases. The theront attaches to the host fish and within 5 min it invades the skin. The theront (25–60 μm in length) becomes a trophont that feeds on the host's body fluids and cells (Fig. 18.6). The trophont feeds for 3–7 days, reaching up to

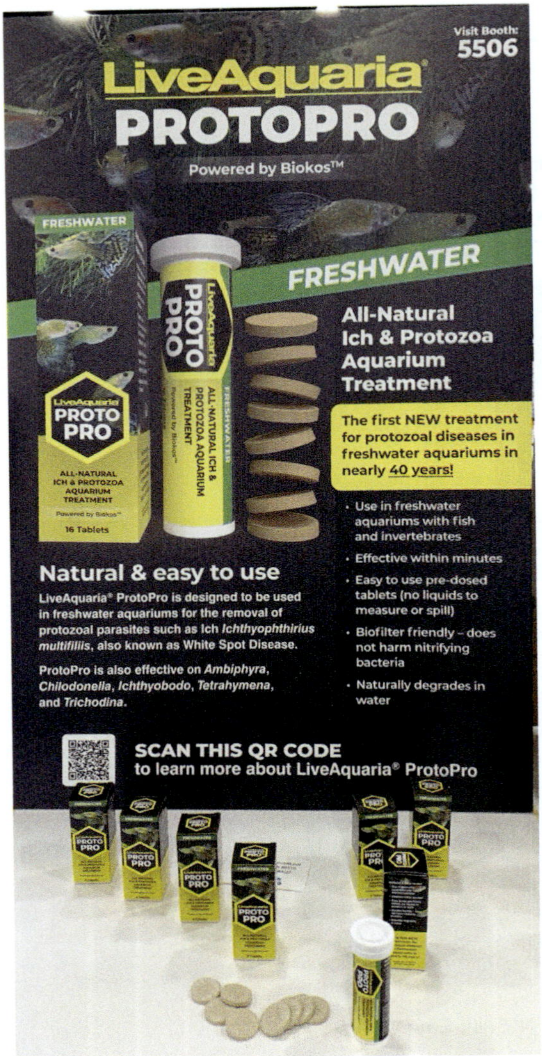

Fig. 18.5. ProtoPro is a new medication that breaks down the cell membrane of protozoa. (Photograph by N. Saint-Erne.)

450 μm in diameter, before leaving the fish, losing its cilia, and maturing into a protomont. The protomont adheres to the substrate for 2–18 h, when it will encyst and turn into a tomont. Two hundred or more tomites will form within the encysted tomont. The tomites will mature and excyst as free-swimming theronts. These will infest fish and start the cycle over. A theront that hasn't attached to a host within 6–8 h loses its infectivity quickly (Yanong, 2017). The life cycle generally takes 1–2 weeks when the temperatures range from 24–27°C. The length of the life cycle is temperature, salinity, and fish species dependent and has been shown to range from 6 days to 11 weeks. *C. irritans* can remain encysted and dormant for 4–5 months within an environment at 12°C. In these cases, when the temperature warms, it can then cause an outbreak. It has also been shown that the encysted state can survive for 2–4 weeks in hypoxic conditions.

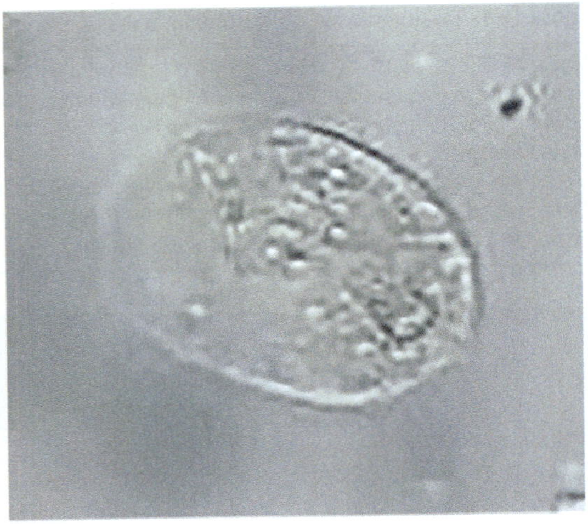

Fig. 18.6. *Cryptocaryon* trophont found on skin mucus biopsy of a powder blue tang (*Acanthurus leucosternon*). (Microphotograph by N. Saint-Erne.)

Infestations of *C. irritans* will appear as pinhead-sized white nodules on the fins, skin, and gills of the fish (Fig. 18.7). The white spots occur as the ciliates embed themselves in the epithelium. The ciliate will settle near the germinal layer within 5 min of attachment. The trophont will continue to grow and displace the overlying epithelial layers causing the white nodules. If embedded within the gills, it will settle along the basement membrane of the gill filament. If affecting the eyes, it will settle on the basement membrane of the cornea. Each nodule generally is caused by only one trophont. In severe infestations, multiple trophonts can be found within each white spot. Infested fish will have increased mucus production and skin discoloration. The fish may be anorexic. If the parasite settles on the gills, it can cause decreased oxygen exchange. The gills can appear pale, with mucus causing clumping of the lamellae (Cardoso *et al.*, 2019). Changes to the gills will cause fish to flare their operculum and swim near an aerator or the surface of the water. Fish may gasp at the surface of the water in respiratory distress. Fish will act irritated or itchy, showing fin tremors, flashing, hyperactivity, sudden darting, and irregular swimming. The fins can appear ragged, and the eyes can appear cloudy. Fish can develop immunity and can heal with no clinical signs in mild infestations. Immunity can take 6 months to occur. Fish that are immune can still act as carriers, allowing small numbers of protozoa to reproduce, and causing further outbreaks. Infestations will occur when fish are immunosuppressed due to poor water quality, drastic changes in temperature or salinity, overstocking, hypoxia, as well as many other factors.

Management of outbreaks focuses on decreasing the number of ciliates in the environment (Table 18.2) and decreasing stress. There are many commercial products available to use to treat Saltwater Ich (Fig. 18.8). Any water quality issues, overstocking, severe temperature changes, and other stressors need to be corrected. The use of UV sterilization may help decrease the number of free-swimming theronts. Ozone can be used to decrease ciliate populations, but limited information on effective doses is available. Encysted forms of the parasite can be removed by placing 1–2 cm of fine sand on the floor of the tank that can be suctioned out and replaced every 3–4 days for four changes.

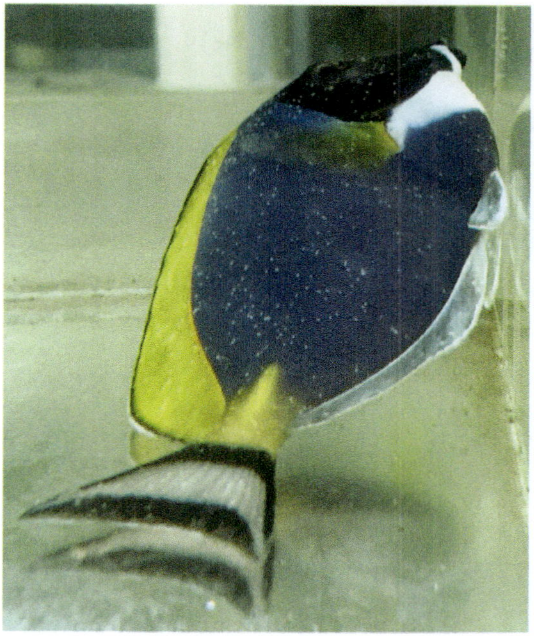

Fig. 18.7. Powder blue tang (*Acanthurus leucosternon*) infested with *Cryptocaryon* trophonts. (Photograph by N. Saint-Erne.)

Prevention is focused on not allowing *C. irritans* to enter the fish system. New fish, plants, and invertebrates should remain in quarantine for 3–6 weeks at 24–27°C. While in quarantine, species can be moved four times in 3-day intervals to a new tank. The tanks should be cleaned and dried in between uses. Equipment, décor, plants, and coral should not be moved between tanks, as they can act as fomites. If equipment must be reused for quarantine tanks, it should be disinfected prior to transferring. Disinfection of nets or other equipment can include submersion in fresh water for 3 h, soaking in 60 mg/ml chlorine for 24 h or soaking in 100 mg/l benzalkonium chloride. If seawater is being used as the water source, it should be stored for at least 24 h prior to entering the system as the free-living theronts become much less infective after that time.

18.2.3 *Chilodonella*

Multiple *Chilodonella* ciliate species have been reported, however not all have been found to be pathogenic. *Chilodonella uncinate* and *C. cucullulus* have been found on wild-caught fish with no clinical signs of disease. Both *C. hexasticha* and *C. piscicola* have been reported in disease outbreaks (Bastos Gomes *et al.*, 2017). Differentiation between the species is made based on the measurements of the macronucleus and micronucleus. In general, all species have an oval and flattened body shape (Fig. 18.9), considered somewhat heart- or

Table 18.2. Treatments for *Cryptocaryon*. Author's own table.

Formalin 25 mg/l q48h for 1–4 weeks
Malachite green 0.1 mg/l for 1–4 weeks
Malachite green and formalin can act synergistically and are often used together
Copper sulfate 0.15–0.20 mg/l (caution with invertebrates and elasmobranchs, also requires daily testing and retreatment due to loss through binding and precipitation in high salinity water)
Hypo-salinity bath (8–10 mg/l) for 3 h, 3 days in a row; not tolerated by all species of fish, and depending on strain of *Cryptocaryon* may not respond
Chloroquine 10–20 mg/l for 1–2 weeks (Loh, 2012).

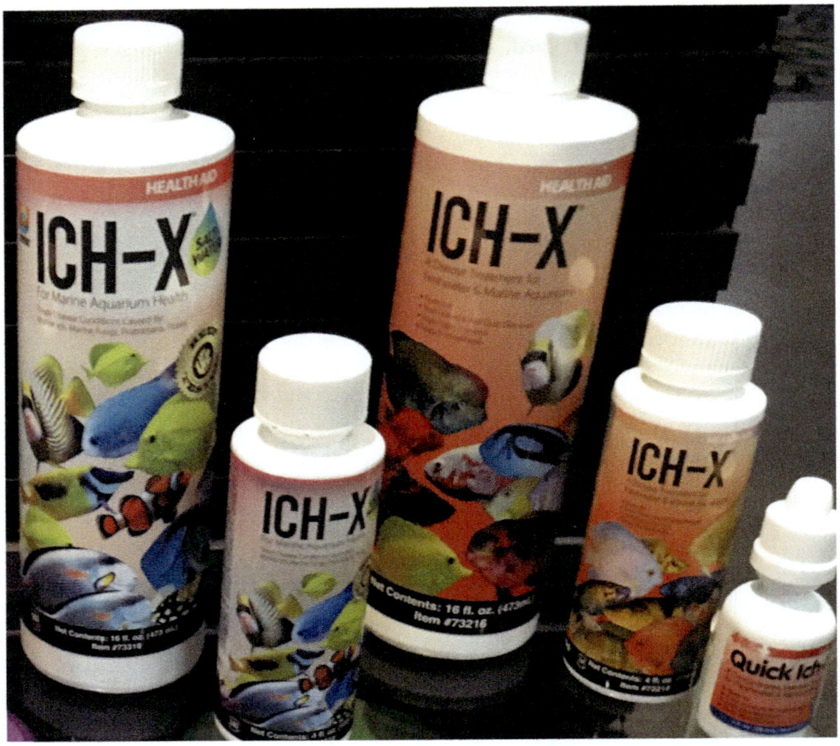

Fig. 18.8. Commercial medications that are used to treat Saltwater Ich. (Photograph by N. Saint-Erne.)

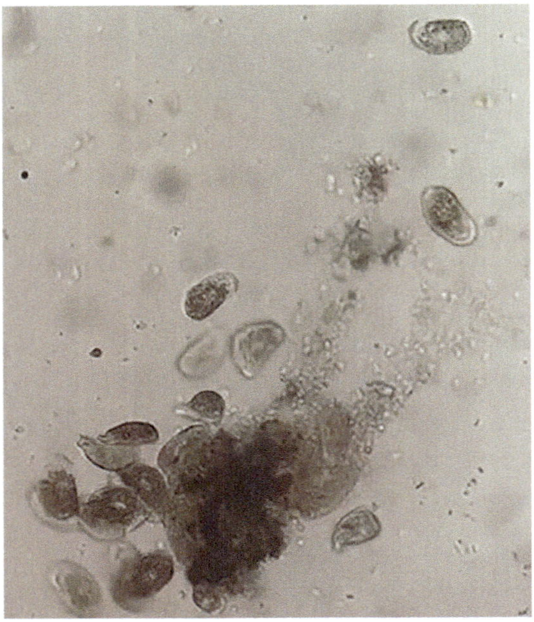

Fig. 18.9. Group of *Chilodonella* found on skin mucus biopsy examination. (Microphotograph by N. Saint-Erne.)

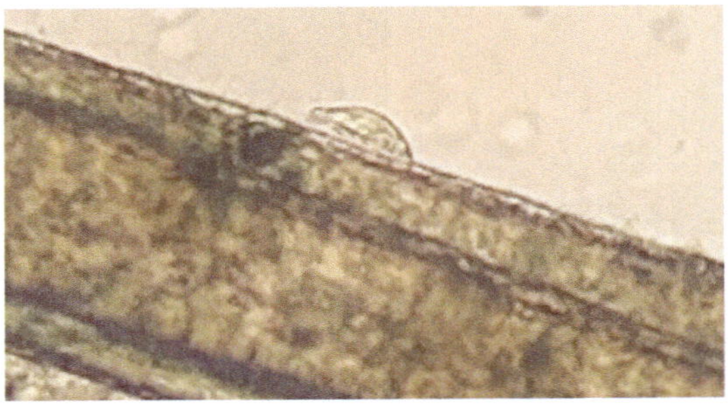

Fig. 18.10. Side view of a *Chilodonella* found on fin biopsy examination. (Microphotograph by N. Saint-Erne.)

bean-shaped, with parallel rows of cilia and a notched side (Bastos Gomes *et al.*, 2016). When viewed from the side, they are flattened ventrally and appear to have a lip on the anterior end (Fig. 18.10). *Chilodonella* are very large in size (30–80 μm × 20–62 μm) and tend to swim rapidly with an erratic swimming pattern. They are found in freshwater environments.

Chilodonella reproduces through binary fission, a form of asexual reproduction, and through conjugation, a form of sexual reproduction. *Chilodonella* will continue to rapidly reproduce asexually in the presence of large food sources and even in low-oxygen environments. Their population can double within hours.

This ciliate species attaches to the skin, fins, and gills and feeds on the epithelial cells around its attachment point. This can cause severe tissue lesions and excessive mucus production. Lesions can include epithelial hyperplasia, gill hypertrophy, and lamellar fusion of the gills (Klinger and Floyd, 2013). Clinical signs are associated with irritation and damage of the epithelium and changes in the gills (Valladão *et al.*, 2019). Fish can show flashing and rubbing on the surfaces of the tank. A fish can exhibit gasping behavior associated with increased mucus production on the gills and decreased oxygen transfer. Severe cases result in mortality. Mild clinical signs can involve anorexia, hypoxia, skin depigmentation, ulceration of the epithelium, scale loss, and swimming slowly near the surface.

Infestations with this flagellate are most commonly associated with high ammonia levels, accumulation of organic material, and large variations in water temperature. *Chilodonella hexasticha* is more commonly seen in temperatures ranging from 26°C to 31°C. *Chilodonella piscicola* prefers a colder environment and has an optimum temperature range between 4°C and 20°C.

Treatment involves adding medications to the water or placing the fish in a small container of aerated, medicated water for a short time (Table 18.3). Prevention of *Chilodonella* is centered around good quarantine protocols, providing good water quality, and decreasing stress.

18.2.4 *Brooklynella*

Brooklynella hostilis is the marine equivalent of *Chilodonella*. *Brooklynella* has a bean- or kidney-shaped body (36–86 μm × 32–50 μm) and can be seen slowly moving in a gliding fashion using the cilia located on its ventral surface (Fig. 18.11). The parasite is dorsal-ventrally flattened in appearance and has a notch at one end (Lom and Corliss, 1971). It contains a visible opening for its cytopharyngeal tube and contains one oval macronucleus. *Brooklynella* reproduces through binary fission and can be found as part of the normal water microorganisms. In small numbers, less than five per lower power field, it can sometimes be considered normal. Outbreaks of *Brooklynella* are reported with environmental stress, trauma, high concentrations of ammonia, elevated temperatures, overcrowding, poor water quality, and hypoxia.

Table 18.3. Treatment options for *Chilodonella*. Author's own table.

Treatment
Copper sulfate 0.15–0.20 mg/l for 3 days
Formalin 25 mg/l q48h for 2–3 treatments
Formalin 150 mg/l dip for 60 min
Hydrogen peroxide 200 mg/l dip for 30 min
NaCl 10 mg/l dip for 60 min
Potassium permanganate 2–10 mg/l dip for 60 min (Loh, 2012)

Brooklynella favors attachment to the gills primarily, but in heavy infestations, it can be found on the skin as well. Clinical signs are often due to changes in the gills. The parasite will cause increased mucus production, gill hypertrophy and hyperplasia, and visible petechia or hemorrhage on the gills (Lom and Nigrellia, 1970). Due to these changes, the fish may have decreased oxygen exchange and show signs of respiratory distress by gasping at the surface of the water (piping) or staying near the water inlet or aeration sources. Once the parasite moves to the skin it can cause ulcerative lesions, creating petechiae and erythema around the ulcers.

Diagnosis is made with a skin scrape or gill biopsy. The parasite can be eradicated through freshwater dips, formalin baths, or prolonged immersion in a mixture of formalin (25 mg/l) and malachite green (0.10 mg/l), as used to treat

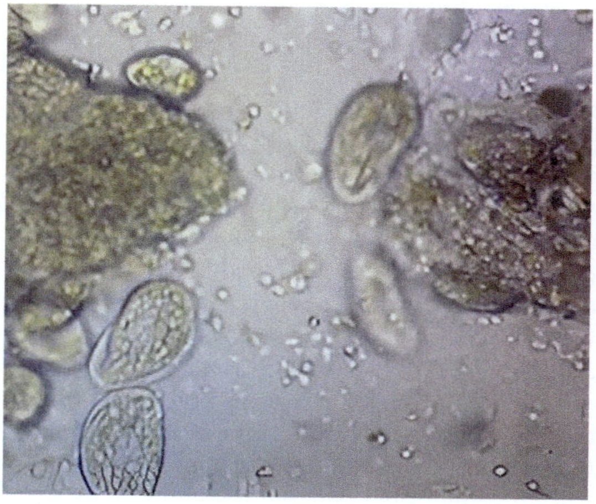

Fig. 18.11. *Brooklynella* from a skin mucus biopsy examination of a marine fish. (Microphotograph by N. Saint-Erne.)

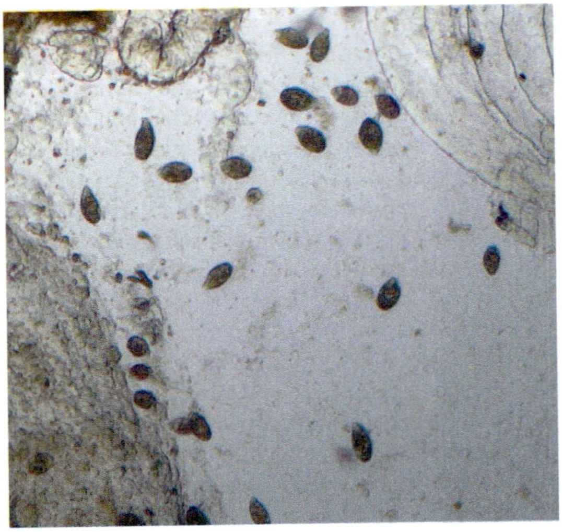

Fig. 18.12. *Tetrahymena* seen on a skin scrape biopsy from a guppy (*Poecilia reticulata*). (Microphotograph by N. Saint-Erne.)

Cryptocaryon. Prevention is centered around decreasing stress, maintaining a sustainable stocking density, and maintaining good water quality within a system.

18.2.5 *Tetrahymena*

Tetrahymena is a free-living ciliate found within the environment as part of the normal freshwater microorganisms. Its body is teardrop- or pear- (pyriform) shaped, and 55 µm × 30 µm in size (Fig. 18.12). It swims by rotating along its long axis, which can appear like a spiraling football. The body of this parasite is covered with cilia. The number of cilia meridians can help with identification. *Tetrahymena pyriformis* lacks a caudal cilium and has 20–30 ciliated meridional kineties (Woo, 2006). *Tetrahymena corlissi* has 25–31 ciliated meridional kineties and a long caudal cilium. It reproduces by binary fission, with the cell splitting into a front and back half, creating two separate protozoa (Fig. 18.13).

Tetrahymena lives in the organic debris found within the aquarium (Ponpornpisit *et al.*, 2000). Outbreaks most commonly occur in temperatures between 25°C and 30°C and a pH between 6.0 and 8.0. As with many other protozoan parasites, poor water quality conditions, stressful situations, drastic changes in temperature, and heavy organic material concentrations will predispose a population to an outbreak (Pimenta Leibowitz *et al.*, 2005).

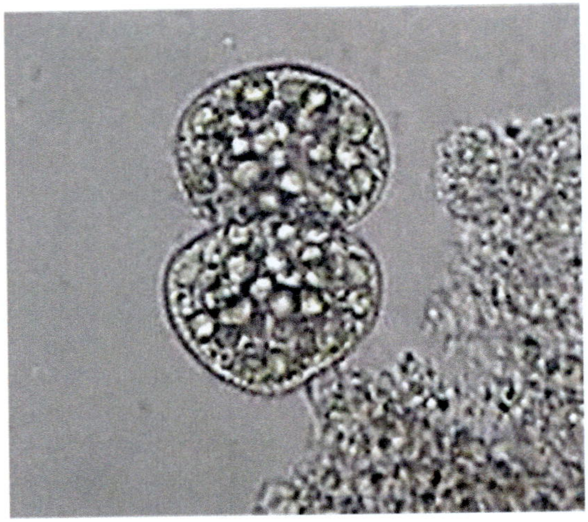

Fig. 18.13. *Tetrahymena* in the process of splitting into two by binary fission. (Microphotograph by N. Saint-Erne.)

Tetrahymena species often affect guppies and cause up to 100% mortalities during outbreaks (Sharon *et al.*, 2014). It has been reported to cause disease in other species with lower morbidity and mortality rates. *Tetrahymena* has been noted to colonize the periorbital region and cause white patches on the epithelium in those areas. Periorbital disease causes exophthalmia and lesions that are referred to as the "spectacle eye" (Leibowitz and Zilberg, 2009). This ciliate can be found in the bloodstream and once found systemically can be seen in most organs within the body. It is important to note that *Tetrahymena* is part of the normal tank microorganisms and can be found on dead fish at the bottom of the tank incidentally. Diagnosis is made by sampling live and moribund fish with gill biopsy and mucus scrapings.

Treatment protocols include a formalin bath. Once the parasite has gone systemic, albendazole, niclosamide, and chloroquine dips have been shown to improve survivability but not eliminate the disease. Prevention is centered around good quarantine protocols, providing good water quality, removing wastes and debris from the aquarium substrate, and decreasing stress.

18.2.6 *Uronema*

Uronema marinum is the marine equivalent of *Tetrahymena*. *Uronema* is elongated (30–50 µm long) with a rounded posterior and bluntly pointed anterior end (Fig. 18.14). The buccal cavity runs from the anterior end of the ciliate to the posterior and incorporates more than half the length of the organism. The attachment organ, also known as the cystome, is irregular in shape. The ciliate contains a central oval macronucleus and a single micronucleus. The cilia are arranged in 13–16 bipolar meridians. *Uronema* can survive and reproduce in temperatures between 10°C and 30°C with a preferred temperature range between 25°C and 30°C. Reproduction is affected by the bacterial populations within the tank that are a food source for the ciliates. Reproduction can occur within a large range of salinity, from 5 PPT to 31 PPT (Crosbie and Munday, 1999).

Clinical signs include hemorrhage of the epithelium with an area of depigmentation and erosion or ulceration (Fig. 18.15). Fish can become lethargic (Cheung *et al.*, 1980). When invading the gills, it can move into the capillaries and block blood flow causing aneurysms and detachment of the lamellae. When invading muscle tissue, it will preferentially invade highly vascularized red muscle tissue. In sea horses, it has been noted to become systemic without causing any cutaneous lesions. Diagnosis is made through microscopic examination of skin mucus or biopsy of the gills and through histopathology on post-mortem necropsy.

Treat *Uronema* with medications used for *Cryptocaryon*. Prevention is centered around good quarantine protocols, providing good water quality, removing debris from the aquarium, and decreasing stress.

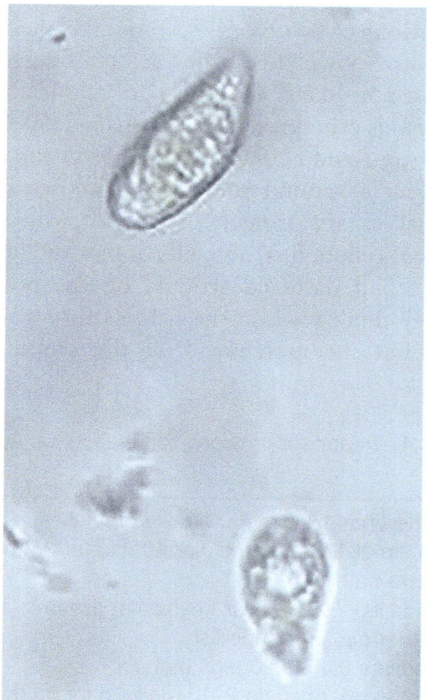

Fig. 18.14. *Uronema* found on skin mucus biopsy of a saltwater fish. (Microphotograph by N. Saint-Erne.)

18.2.7 *Trichodina*

Trichodina is a peritrichous protozoa that can be found in both freshwater and saltwater environments. All trichodinids are essentially commensals and are a normal part of aquatic microorganisms (Woo, 2006). In low numbers, less than five per low power field, they may be nonpathogenic on fish. High numbers and clinical signs signify it may be the cause of the patient's disease. Ciliates within this species are ventrally flattened and round. The body is saucer-shaped with a spiral ring of cilia along the margin and one ring of cilia near the mouth (Figs 18.16a and b). There are hook-like projections from a ring of denticles that converge near the center. The denticles support the body.

Trichodina reproduce through binary fission. There is some host-specificity with different species of trichodinids. *Trichodina acuta* (35–60 µm diameter) is found mainly on the skin of most freshwater fish. *T. heterodentata* (38–82 µm diameter) is mostly reported in cichlids, cyprinids, gobiids, and poecilids. *T. centrostrigeata* (29–49 µm diameter) is found mainly on the gills of several freshwater species,

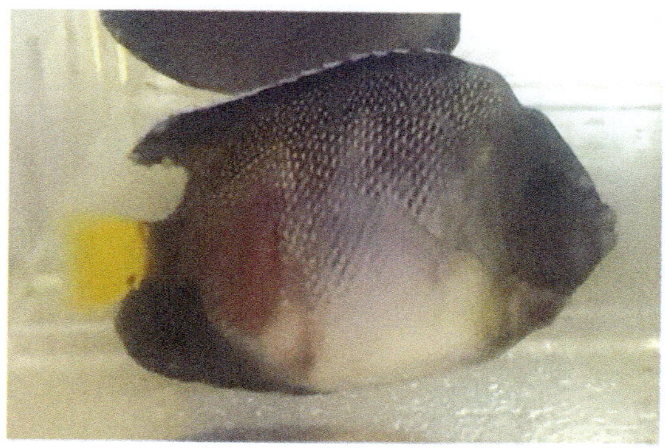

Fig. 18.15. Yellowtail Angelfish (*Apolemichthys xanthurus*) with skin lesions associated with *Uronema*. (Photograph by N. Saint-Erne.)

mostly cichlids. *T. jadranica* (18–35 µm diameter) has been found on the gills of marine and freshwater fishes. *T. reticulata* (31–57 µm diameter) shows specificity for goldfish and carp. Related trichodinids include the genera *Hemitrichodina*, *Vauchomia*, *Paratrichodina*, *Tripartiella*, *Trichodonella*, and *Dipartiella*. These are similar protozoa that are found in fresh and saltwater fishes (Woo, 2006).

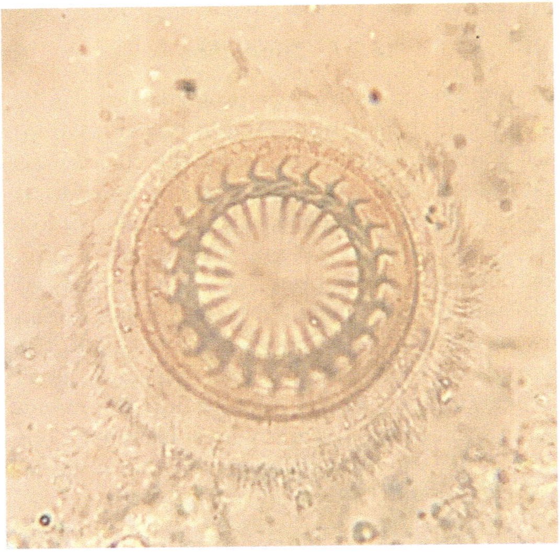

Fig. 18.16a. Cilia around the margin of the body and inner ring of denticules of a *Trichodina* protozoan. (Microphotograph by N. Saint-Erne.)

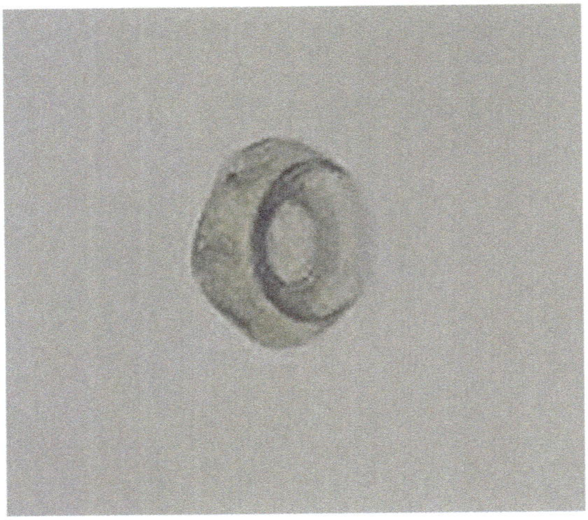

Fig. 18.16b. Side view of *Trichodina* showing its saucer-shaped body. (Microphotograph by N. Saint-Erne.)

Trichodina species target the gills and skin. In some cases, it has been found in the urinary bladder and oviducts without significant corresponding disease or signs. Clinical signs are caused by the parasites feeding on the mucus and detritus covering the gills and skin, creating ulcerations and damage to the epithelial layers and mucoid barrier. Clinical signs include ulcerative skin lesions, increased mucous production, anorexia, emaciation, and lethargy. Mortalities are often caused not by the ulcerative lesions but by the secondary infections that gain a foothold through the damaged epithelium.

Trichodina can occur in higher numbers with poor water quality, water pollution, or in farm systems that bring in water from rivers or oceans. Heavy infestations are often associated with large amounts of organic debris within the tank, allowing for a larger food source for the ciliates or heavy levels of pollutants (Aksit *et al.*, 2008). Treatment includes medications listed in Table 18.4. Prevention is centered around good quarantine protocols, providing good water quality, and decreasing stress.

18.2.8 *Ambiphrya*

Ambiphrya is a sedentary ciliate that is a normal part of the water microorganisms. On microscopic examinations of fish biopsies, in numbers less than five per low power field, they are considered normal and not likely the cause of clinical signs. *Ambiphrya* is cylindrical or barrel-shaped (50–95 µm × 40–61 µm) and contains oral cilia on top and a band of cilia around the middle, known as the equatorial ciliary fringe, or ciliary girdle. They attach to the skin, fins, and gills of fish and hold on with a broad flattened scopula on the posterior end. They don't feed on the fish, as they are filter feeders, but the attachment of the scopula can

Table 18.4. Treatment protocols for *Trichodina*. Author's own table.

Correct the underlying water quality problem
Formalin dip at 170–250 mg/l for 60 min, or 25 mg/l long-term bath
Salt bath at 1.5–3.0 PPT for freshwater fish, freshwater dip for marine fish
Copper sulfate 0.15–0.20 mg/l baths
Potassium permanganate 2–10 mg/l dip for 60 min (Loh, 2012)
UV irradiation at 2.2×10^6 µWs/cm^2 within the filter system to kill protozoa

cause epithelial damage. The macronucleus is long, thin, and ribbon shaped (Woo, 2006).

This ciliate tends to be nonpathogenic until there are heavy organic loads, poor water quality, high stocking densities, or stress causing the fish to be immunocompromised. Because of their affinity to attach to the gills, in high numbers this ciliate can inhibit oxygen exchange, causing the fish to gasp or gape at the surface (piping) due to respiratory distress. Fish may congregate around the water inlet and aeration sources. Fish can appear hyporexic, anorexic, lethargic, and have abnormal swimming patterns. As this ciliate is a normal part of the water flora, prevention of outbreaks is centered around decreasing stress, providing good water quality, reducing organic debris in the aquarium, and proper quarantine protocols to reduce introduction. Treatment during an outbreak includes copper sulfate or potassium permanganate baths.

18.2.9 *Coleps*

Coleps species are considered a nonpathogenic normal part of the water system. This ciliate becomes pathogenic in poorly managed and heavily stocked populations (Székely and Bereczky, 1992) that are undergoing stress from low oxygen, poor water quality, or changes in temperature. *Coleps* prefer to target dead fish or organic detritus material, but in heavy numbers can be found on living individuals. Reports of outbreaks for this ciliate have shown mortalities in young fry, and it is suspected it will cause disease only in the weak, small, or young. *Coleps* have a barrel-shaped body (100–250 μm in length) that is covered by lamellae that are concentrically arranged and hardened with calcium deposition. The cilia surround the cytostome, the attachment stalk, and are located on the anterior end. Depending on the species, cilia can arise from the posterior end as well. *Coleps* attach to the epithelium via a cytostome. It can cover the fish's body surface, gills, and fins in heavy infestations, creating ulcerative skin lesions, proliferation of gills, and a ragged appearance to the fins (Wooster and Bowser, 1994).

18.2.10 *Apiosoma*

Apiosoma is a sedentary ciliate that is a common water microorganism. In low numbers, less than five per low power field, it is considered nonpathogenic when found on biopsy samples. It has a vase-shaped body, 60–110 μm long. It contains a conical or triangular macronucleus and a small round micronucleus. Cilia are located around the mouth. It has a narrow base (scopula) used for attachment to a substrate, which could be a fish. *Apiosoma* attaches to the skin, fins, and gills and can block oxygen exchange when present in high numbers. This ciliate can become an opportunistic pathogen with situations of overcrowding, overfeeding, stress, and heavy levels of organic matter. Clinical signs include respiratory distress and signs of low-oxygen levels due to the hyperplasia of the gill tissue with excessive mucus production. The site of attachment can also become infected with bacteria or fungi.

18.2.11 *Epistylis*

Epistylis, previously referred to as *Heteropolaria*, is considered commensal, as it feeds on organic material in the water, and becomes opportunistic on fish in situations with high stocking densities, poor water quality, or other stressful events. *Epistylis* has a direct life cycle and undergoes budding to reproduce. The body, called a zooid, can contract, and has a retractile peristomal lip. The zooid (40–80 μm × 20–30 μm) is cylindrical and elongated if stretched. If the zooid is contracted, it can appear conical or round in shape. The cytoplasm is clear, containing many vacuoles and a macronucleus that is band-shaped (Foissner *et al.*, 1985). There are cilia around the mouth. The free-swimming life stage is called a teletroch. During this life stage, the ciliate is ellipsoidal and flattened. It attaches to the substrate with a scopula that produces a long, noncontractile stalk bearing the zooid. The stalks can dichotomously branch allowing the zooids to grow in colonies (Fig. 18.17). The stalks prefer to attach to hard, calcified surfaces like the scales and spines of fins.

Infested fish will appear with white, tuft-like growths similar in appearance to a fungal infection. Ulcerations can occur at the attachment point and allow for opportunistic bacteria to create secondary infections. "Red sore disease" is an *Aeromonas* infection secondary to an *Epistylis* infestation. Salt is very effective for treating *Epistylis* and can be administered as a 0.02% long-term salt bath or a 3% short salt dip.

18.2.12 *Trichophrya*

Trichophrya, also described as *Capriniana piscium*, is a suctorial ciliate that appears oval or elongated, up to 100 μm long. *Trichophrya* can have feeding

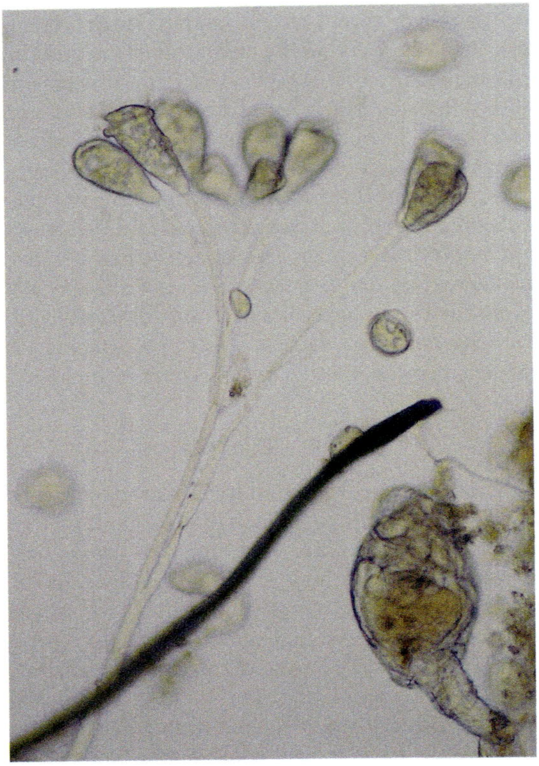

Fig. 18.17. Colony of *Epistylis* on a common stalk. There is a rotifer in the lower right corner of the photograph. (Microphotograph by N. Saint-Erne.)

tubes (suctorial tentacles) that protrude from the body at times, creating a pincushion appearance. Orange to brown granules can be found within the body of *Trichophrya*. This ciliate has a direct lifecycle and reproduces by endogenous budding (Woo, 2006). It feeds on ciliophorans and not on the fish itself. It is considered commensal and a normal part of the environment but in heavy numbers can colonize the gills causing increased mucus production and hypertrophy of the gill tissues. Fish will clinically appear in respiratory distress, or with clinical signs of hypoxia due to decreased oxygen exchange across the gill surface. Outbreaks of this ciliate are seen with heavy levels of organic matter in the environment. Copper sulfate baths are effective in treating this ciliate.

18.3 Flagellated Protozoa

18.3.1 *Hexamita*

Flagellated protozoa (Mastigophora) have one or more whip-like flagellae used for locomotion. *Hexamita* is a diplomonad flagellate closely related to the genus *Spironucleus* protozoa. *Hexamita* and *Spironucleus* have been reported in angelfish (Poynton *et al.*, 1995). Three species of *Hexamita* are reported to affect fish: *H. salmonis*, *H. truttae*, and *H. intestinalis*. *H. salmonis* affects salmonid fishes. *H. truttae* and *H. intestinalis* have been reported in a wide range of species. *Hexamita* is egg shaped or teardrop shaped (up to 20 μm long) and has eight total flagella: three pairs of anterior flagella used for locomotion and one pair of posterior recurrent flagella. Within the cell are two oval nuclei in the middle portion of the body. It reproduces through binary fission and can therefore reproduce rapidly. It will form an oval cyst as it divides, which will release two trophozoites after division. Transmission occurs through ingestion of contaminated material and water containing cysts or trophozoites. The trophozoites live in the lumen of the intestines, and trophozoites and cysts are normally voided with feces. Outbreaks occur during times of stress, overcrowding, poor water quality, and drastic temperature changes.

Hexamita can live in rich organic water or as an intestinal parasite (Woo, 2006). *Hexamita* will target the intestines and gallbladder but can also be found on the epithelium. Gastrointestinal clinical signs include anorexia, emaciation, yellow mucoid stools, diarrhea, and lethargy (Williams *et al.*, 2011, 2013). If invading the gills, it can cause pallor, hyperplasia of the gills, and increased mucus production. Ulcerative lesions can be seen on the fins and head. Some fish will exhibit abnormal swimming patterns. If the liver and gall bladder are involved, the fish may exhibit coelomic distension, petechiae, and ascites. Diagnosis is made microscopically from a fecal sample direct smear or skin scrape examination.

Proper quarantine protocols to prevent the introduction of this flagellate into the fish system are very important. Preventing stress and providing a good living environment for fish is the key to preventing outbreaks. Treatment options are listed in Table 18.5.

18.3.2 *Spironucleus*

Spironucleus is a diplomonad binucleate flagellated protozoa. They are considered commensal organisms that are usually found within the GI tract of fish. *Spironucleus barkhanus*, *S. salmonicida*, *S. salmonis*, *S. torosa*, and *S. vortens* have all been reported to cause disease within fish. *S. vortens*, common in angelfish and discus, is presumed to be the cause of "hole-in-the-head" disease in cichlids (Woo, 2006). *Spironucleus* are pyriform or spherical in shape (Fig. 18.18). There are two flagella located on the posterior body, and six anterior flagella arranged in two groups of three flagella. Each parasite will contain a paired set of nuclei located very close to each other in the narrow anterior end of the body. The nuclei are elongated and taper on the anterior end. Transmission of *Spironucleus* occurs through the fecal-oral route and is considered to only cause disease in immunocompromised fish.

These parasites have a direct life cycle, and they reproduce through binary fission. The motile parasitic trophozoite is considered the infective or feeding stage. This form can encyst, allowing the parasite to become resistant to environmental changes such as swings in temperature, hypoxic situations, and pH changes. Both the trophozoite and cysts are shed within the feces (Williams *et al.*, 2011, 2013). The trophozoites can survive for up to 36 days if encased and protected by fecal matter. Once trophozoites enter the water column without access to the host and protection of feces, they will die within hours. The encysted life stage is thought to be the cause of water-borne transmission outbreaks due to its ability to survive long periods in the environment.

Large numbers of *Spironucleus* flagellates colonizing the intestinal tract can lead to two forms of disease: coelozoic and histozoic. The coelozoic form is the intestinal infestation. Clinical signs of the coelozoic form include mostly gastrointestinal signs. Fish will be hyporexic or anorexic and have visible signs of weight loss and lethargy. They might exhibit signs of enteritis like the presence of dark colored or stringy feces. Fish can have pale gills, or be swimming in unusual patterns, often seen swimming on their sides or staying around the aeration sources. They may exhibit ascites. The histozoic form of this disease is considered the systemic infestation. In discus, angelfish, and other cichlids, this can present as "hole-in-head disease." Fish will exhibit necrotic lesions in the head region and along the lateral line organ. The necrotic lesions are usually bilateral and symmetric. Systemically, the flagellate can be found within granulomatous lesions within the heart, liver, or kidneys. Internal hemorrhage has been noted with the histozoic form of this disease.

Treatments for *Spironucleus* can include those medications used for *Hexamita* (Table 18.5) or treatments added to the water (Table 18.6; from Sangmaneedet and Smith, 1999). Prevention is key to this disease. Proper quarantine protocols with screening fecal examinations can help prevent introduction. Some fish are asymptomatic and can

Table 18.5. Treatment protocols for *Hexamita*. Author's own table.

Treatment
Metronidazole 5 mg/l in water for 3 h every 48 h for three treatments, or 25–50 mg/kg PO q24h for 5–10 days (Tojo and Santamarina, 1998)
Benzimidazole, ronidazole, secnidazole, at 2–5 g/kg feed for 2 days
Abendazole, aminosidine, diethylcarbamacine, nitroscanate 40 g/kg feed for 2 days
Magnesium sulfate 0.2–0.3% in diet for 3 days (Sangmaneedet and Smith, 1999)
Carbarsone in diet for 3 days at 0.2% concentration

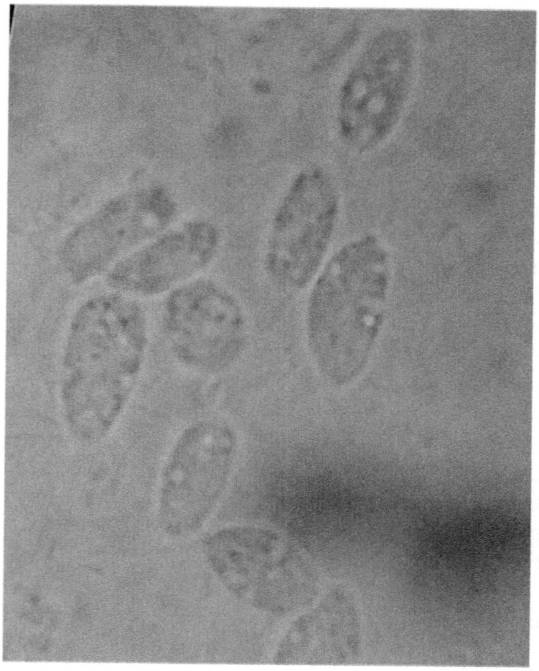

Fig. 18.18. *Spironucleus* flagellated protozoa from the intestines of an angelfish (*Pterophyllum scalare*). (Microphotograph by N. Saint-Erne.)

Table 18.6. Treatment options for *Spironucleus*. Author's own table.

Treatment
Metronidazole 6 mg/l in aquarium water
Dimetridazole 4 mg/l in aquarium water
Mebendazole 0.5 mg/l in aquarium water

act as carriers. Outbreaks are associated with overcrowding, temperature fluctuations, poor water quality, and other stressful conditions. Because of this, the focus should be on providing good living conditions and decreasing stress within a population of fish.

18.3.3 *Ichthyobodo*

Ichthyobodo necator and *I. pyrformia* have been identified as pathogens in fish. *Ichthyobodo necator* was previously known as *Costia necatrix* (Woo, 2006) and infestations from it are often still referred to as "Costia" to avoid confusion with *Ichthyophthirius*. *Ichthyobodo* has a direct life cycle that requires a host to complete. The free-swimming saprophagous life stage is pyriform in shape (5–18 μm long) and has two flagella (though it can be seen as having four during longitudinal binary division). The flagella extend from within the anterior groove that runs on two thirds of the ventral surface. This free-living version has a round to oval nucleus. During the saprophagous stage, it feeds on detached and decaying material on the bottom of the tank or pond. Once attached to the host by a pointed cytostome at its anterior end, it becomes elongated in shape with less prominent flagella. This form will look like a "comma" (Bruno *et al.*, 2006). During stressful environment changes, the free-living stage can encyst within the environment and increase its ability to survive. It can survive in a pH of 4.5–7.5, temperatures ranging from 2–38°C, and high salinity environments. It can be found infesting both fresh and saltwater fish species. *Ichthyobodo* is transmitted through water and on fomites (Robertson, 1985). Outbreaks occur during times of stress, poor nutrition, overcrowding, and poor water quality and when there is damage to the epidermis.

Ichthyobodo prefers to attach to the skin and gills of the host (Fig. 18.19). Its preferred sites are the skin around the dorsal fin and tips of lamellae on the gills. Clinical signs include pale areas with large amounts of mucus on the surface of the epidermis, causing a blue discoloration seen on physical exam. Gills could appear pale and swollen or hyperplastic, with excessive mucus production. An affected fish may flash or rub on the surfaces of rocks or aquarium ornaments. Fish can become anorexic or lethargic. Diagnosis is made on skin scrape and gill biopsy. It is important to note studies have shown that if left for 10 min on a slide, *Ichthyobodo* will detach from tissue and be seen free swimming. The parasite will die within 30 min of detachment, making it important to microscopically examine the biopsies quickly after attaining the samples. Treatment methods are listed in Table 18.7, which also can be used for other species of external flagellated protozoa.

18.3.4 *Cryptobia*

Seven species of *Cryptobia* have been associated with the gastrointestinal tract of fish; only *C. iubilans* is reported to be pathogenic and parasitic. *Cryptobia* are common infestations in cichlid species but can be found in many species of freshwater and marine fish. This flagellate is elongated (14–23 μm long) with narrower ends and two flagella. The shorter anterior flagellum is free, while the recurrent flagellum is attached along the body and ends as a free flagellum at the posterior end (Woo, 2006). This flagellate can be found in the gills, on the body surface, within the intestines and in the blood vessels. It attaches to

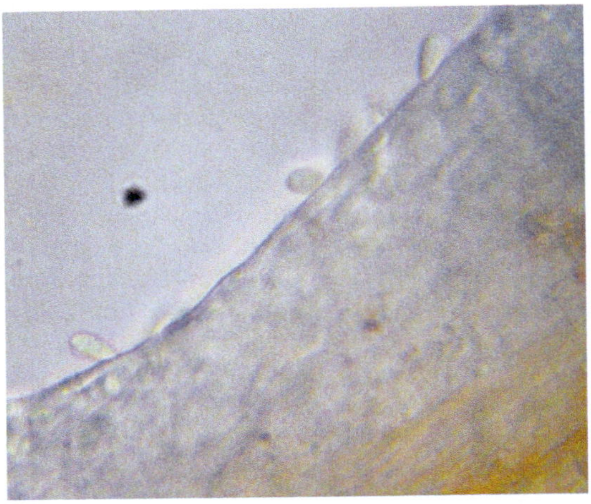

Fig. 18.19. *Ichthyobodo* attached to epithelium of a koi (*C. rubrofuscus*). (Photo by N. Saint-Erne.)

Table 18.7. Treatment protocols for *Ichthyobodo*. Author's own table.

Formalin 250 mg/l for a 1-h dip, remove fish sooner if appearing stressed
Formalin 25 mg/l for 24-h bath
NaCl 10–15 g/l for 30 min, or 2 g/l for 10 h
Copper sulfate 2 mg/l for 4 h q48h two times (Mitchell *et al.*, 2008)
Potassium permanganate 2–10 mg/l dip for 60 min (Loh, 2012)

epithelial surfaces by its posterior flagellum. Ingesting dead affected fish is one way for fish to become infested, but transmission through the water can occur (Woo, 2006). Leeches can transmit the hematozoic form of *Cryptobia* between fish.

Cryptobia has been implicated as a potential cause of "Malawi bloat," but its importance in this syndrome is unclear (Mayer and Donnelly, 2013). Heavy infestations can cause significant mortality. Clinical signs include emaciation, lethargy, or fish that have areas of dark skin pigmentation. Providing good nutrition and minimizing stress within the fish population is key to preventing and treating clinical signs associated with *Cryptobia*. Infestations have been noted to spontaneously resolve once the environmental factors causing stress are addressed. Chemical treatment involves treating with a formalin bath or treatments used with other protozoa.

18.3.5 *Trypanosoma* and *Trypanoplasma*

Trypanosomes can occur in fresh and salt water. They have a free flagellum at the anterior end. These flagellated blood parasites live within the circulatory system of fish and can be found in the gills. They can cause obstructions in the blood vessels of the gills. They can multiply rapidly by binary fission in the blood (Woo, 2006). Their preferred optimum temperature is 20°C, but they will multiply at temperatures from 10°C to 30°C. Signs of infestation in fish include anorexia, lethargy, weight loss, anemia, and ascites (Saint-Erne, 2010). They are spread between fish by leeches. Diagnosis is made by examining blood smears and gill biopsies under a microscope. The organisms appear as undulating flagellated protozoa moving rapidly among the red blood cells. Collect the blood from the gill biopsy or from the caudal vein ventral to the spine in the caudal peduncle. Prevent the disease by controlling leeches in the pond or aquarium.

18.4 Dinoflagellate Protozoa

18.4.1 *Piscinoodinium*

The genus for these protozoa was originally named *Oodinium* but differences in morphology among the species prompted the original genus to be divided into several genera. *Piscinoodinium* is very similar to the saltwater parasite *Amyloodinium* but causes disease in freshwater fish. It is highly pathogenic and can cause 100% mortality in some cases. It is commonly known as "freshwater velvet disease," due to the velvety-looking texture of the affected fish's skin. Both *Piscinoodinium limneticum* and *P. pillulare* have been identified as pathogens (Florindo *et al.*, 2017). The lifecycle of this species starts as free-swimming dinospores within the water that attach to the host fish. Once attached, they become sessile, saclike trophonts that feed on the epithelium of the host. It will preferentially attach to the skin, gills, fins, esophagus, and intestinal lining. The trophont is a non-motile, pyriform- to oval-shaped organism that is yellow to green in color. After feeding, the trophont drops off the fish to form a cyst (tomont) and divides asexually within the cyst. The cyst opens to release dinospores that will infest other fish. Dinospores have two flagella to allow them to swim in the water. It can reproduce quickly in environments with low dissolved oxygen, high stocking densities, and high organic matter concentrations within the aquarium or pond.

Generally, this dinoflagellate causes cutaneous clinical signs. Infestations within the epidermis will cause excessive mucus production, patches of dark coloration of the integument, visible ulcerations, a golden "velvet"-like color, and tattered fins. Infestations in the gills cause hyperplasia and damage to respiratory epithelium (Paul *et al.*, 2018). In some cases, fin erosion and generalized petechiae have been reported (Gomes *et al.*, 2018). Fish may swim slowly, acting weak and lethargic. Diagnosis can be made through physical examination for the presence of rust-colored lesions (Ferraz and Sommerville, 1998). Skin cytology and gill biopsy cytology can be helpful with identification. In one study, diagnosis was made by taking a gill arch from a dead fish and placing it in a transparent vial with pond water. The vial was then shaken gently for 3 min and then rested for 30 min to allow sediment to form. The parasite can be identified within the sediment layer.

Treatments are listed in Table 18.8. Clearing an infestation completely can be difficult because the parasite can reside in the GI tract and escape exposure to treatments.

Table 18.8. Treatments for *Piscinoodinium*. Author's own table.

Formalin 25 mg/l bath treatment
Darkening the tank to prevent photosynthesis by the dinoflagellates
Prolonged salt treatment at 0.1–0.3% (1–3 PPT) salinity for freshwater fish

18.4.2 *Amyloodinium*

Amyloodinium ocellatum is commonly known as marine velvet disease. It causes serious morbidity and mortality in brackish and marine fish. It can infest both elasmobranchs and teleost fishes (Woo, 2006). It is a dinoflagellate that is a free-living member of planktonic communities, but part of its lifecycle is parasitic (Smith and Schwarz, 2019). The free-swimming and photosynthetic dinospore (8–13 µm long) can attach to a host fish. The dinospore differentiates into a trophont (350 µm long), which feeds on epithelium. *Amyloodinium* trophonts are oval- to pear-shaped and are brown to gold in color. They attach to the host with rhizoids, a hook-like anchoring organ. The trophont matures and detaches as a tomont, or dividing stage, and creates a cyst. As many as 256 dinospores develop within the cyst and then excyst, or hatch, and enter the environment. The life cycle can be completed in 7–20 days and is temperature dependent, with the ideal temperature being between 18°C and 30°C. They stop dividing at temperatures lower than 16°C. The lifecycle slows and the survival rate decreases with an increase in salinity. Ideal salinity for the dinospores ranges between 12 and 50 PPT (Paperna, 1984).

Amyloodinium targets the gills and in heavy infestations can affect skin and eyes. Clinically the fish will appear with a gold velvety appearance on their epithelium. Severe infestations can cause gill hyperplasia, inflammation, hemorrhage, and necrosis in areas of attachment. Diagnosis is made by physical exam, gill biopsy, or skin scrape.

Treatment focuses on both chemical treatment (Table 18.9) and cleaning the tank of encysted tomonts. UV and ozone can be used in the filtration system to reduce the dinospores. Cleaning the bottom of the tank to remove encysted parasites is effective in decreasing the tomonts. Physical filtration can help decrease parasite load with diatomaceous earth filters, micro screen, drum, or bead filters of 50 µm filtering capacity. It is important to note that no chemicals affect the encysted tomonts. Therefore, any treatments will require repeat dosing every 3–10 days, depending on the water temperature.

Table 18.9. Treatment options for *Amyloodinium*. Author's own table.

Treatment
Formalin 25 mg/l long-term bath
Hydrogen Peroxide 25 mg/l
Freshwater dips 3–5 min long
Copper sulfate 0.15 mg/l for 10–14 days
Chloroquine 10 mg/l for 10 days (Loh, 2012)

18.5 Apicomplexa

Apicomplexa protozoa occur in many animal species and are among the most harmful pathogens in warm-blooded species. Apicomplexa parasites infest both marine and freshwater fish species. These parasites have a special cell organelle, called the apical complex, which facilitates invasion into the host cell. They can form spores and oocysts. There are two major groups: Coccidia, which are primarily intestinal parasites and produce resistant oocysts in the host, and Adeleid, which are blood parasites.

18.5.1 Adeleid

Adeleid blood parasites have merogonic and gamogonic stages in fish hosts, while spore formation occurs in parasitic annelids (leeches) or insects. *Haemogregarina*, *Cyrilia*, *Desseria*, *Dactylosoma*, *and Babesiosoma* are genera of Apicomplexa protozoa that can be found within the bloodstream as hemoparasites. In general, fish are asymptomatic. These parasites are often incidentally found on blood smear examinations.

18.5.2 Coccidia

Coccidia protozoa are obligate intracellular parasites that undergo reproduction through sporulation within the epithelium of target cells. Many individuals can be asymptomatic with active infestations. Severely affected fish are thin and depressed. Their feces are often yellowish. Microscopic examination of the feces will reveal the coccidia oocysts (20–40 µm). Each oocyst contains four sporocysts, each of which contains two sporozoites. The sporozoite development is divided into merogony, gamogony, and sporogony. Merogony begins with the invasion of the host cell by the sporozoite, which then begins to grow and changes into a meront. In the meront, merozoites are formed and then released to invade other cells. The merozoites form macrogamonts and microgamonts, in which numerous microgametes develop. The macrogamonts develop into an oocyst. The zygote in the oocyst divides and forms sporocysts, in which sporozoites develop (Woo, 2006).

Cryptosporidium is a genus of coccidia that has 29 species that target fish (Bolland *et al.*, 2020). *Cryptosporidium scophthalmi*, *C. molnari*, *C. bollandi*, *C. nasorum*, and *C. huwi* have all been demonstrated in fish (Golomazou and Karanis, 2020). In addition to the fish-specific versions, the mammalian genotypes that target rats have been reported in fish. This occurs where contamination of an aquatic environment with agricultural runoff and sewage has occurred.

Clinical signs are based on the target organ involved. In most coccidia species, the intestinal tract is the target organ, but *Cryptosporidium* can be found in other organs. The reproductive tract, liver, spleen, and swim bladder have all been reported with various severity of clinical signs. In cases of gastritis, inflammation is severe, and necrosis of gastric mucosal epithelium is noted. When targeting the liver and bile ducts, it can cause fibrosis of the bile ducts and necrosis of adjacent hepatic cells. In cases where the target tissue was the liver, it appeared brown with severe granulomatous inflammatory lesions. Secondary signs of liver failure were seen as superficial hemorrhages in the skin and hyperemia of the gills. The spleen can appear swollen and irregular. Angelfish larvae have shown infestations can cause emaciation, stunted growth, and coelomic distension from organomegaly and ascites. Fish can appear anorexic and listless. In some cases, *Cryptosporidium* has been noted to travel systemically, causing granulomatous lesions throughout the gills, liver, kidneys, spleen, intestines, and subcutaneous layers.

Goussia guamaensis is a specific coccidia that has been found in the swim bladder, liver, spleen, and kidneys of fish from Africa and Asia. In species from the Amazon River basin, it targets the stomach, intestines, liver, and swim bladder. *Calyptospora* is a genus containing six species, including *Calyptospora spinosa*, *C. serrasalmi*, *C. funduli*, and *C. paranaidji*. This genus of coccidia target fish from the Amazon River basin and affects the liver (Negrão *et al.*, 2019). It has also been found in the gallbladder and pancreas. It seems to have a higher prevalence in the carnivorous fish species. The liver of infected individuals will appear swollen and pale in appearance.

Eimeria species have been reported in teleost fish and elasmobranchs. *Eimeria* species have a direct life cycle that is completed within a single host. The *Eimeria* life cycle has an exogenous phase, where the oocysts are excreted into the environment, and an endogenous phase, where parasite development occurs in the host's intestines. Parasite transmission occurs orally by contact with contaminated feces. General clinical signs include emaciation, hyperoxia, lethargy, and death. Mucoid, yellow feces may also be seen in affected fish (Smith and Roberts, 2010). The target organs vary between species of *Eimeria*, with the serosal surface and gastrointestinal tract (Silva *et al.*, 2019) being the most commonly reported sites.

Diagnosis of coccidia infestations can be made through fecal examination, intestinal sampling on necropsy, and histopathology. On post-mortem examination, the gastrointestinal tract can appear gas-distended with white-colored feces. The liver can appear swollen, irregularly shaped, or pale (Silva *et al.*, 2020). The spleen may appear irregular and swollen. The parasite may be found within the coelomic cavity or seen within other non-target organs on histopathology of coelomic tissues.

Amprolium chloride fed at a dose of 5 mg/kg BW every other day for three doses has been reported to be an effective treatment for coccidia infestations (Woo, 2006). It is important to follow a proper quarantine period and screening protocol to prevent introduction within a system. Minimizing stress within a population can help prevent outbreaks. Populations at high risk for infestation include those living in poor water quality environments, high stocking densities, and other stressful conditions that are often seen with intensive aquaculture practice.

18.6 Microsporidia

Microsporidia are unicellular organisms living as intracellular, spore-forming parasites. Transmission occurs through ingestion of spores (2–10 μm long). There is suspected to be a vertical transmission component. The fish will ingest a thick-walled spore that contains a sporoplasm. The sporoplasm is released and migrates to its target organ depending on the species of microsporidian. The sporoplasm then undergoes proliferation as a merogony creating many meronts through binary fission. Meronts will mature into sporonts that will then produce sporoblasts, which mature into spores, through the process of sporogony. Spores are released through rupturing of the cyst, host death, or predation.

Microsporidia that infest the intestines of marine and freshwater fishes belong to the genera *Glugea* and *Loma*. The microsporidia that infest muscle tissues are from the genera *Pleistophora*, *Heterosporis*,

Kabatana, and *Microsporidium*. *Pleistophora hyphessobryconis* occurs commonly in freshwater aquarium fish (Woo, 2006). It has been called "Neon Tetra Disease" because of its prevalence in this species, but it occurs in other fish as well, including zebrafish used in research laboratories (Sanders *et al.*, 2010). The spores are ovoid, 4 µm × 6 µm in size. Infected skeletal muscle tissues appear as whitish patches under the skin. The parasite may spread from the muscles to other organs in the body.

Clinical signs of an infestation are based on the target organ location. Fish can exhibit emaciation, spinal deformities, organ dysfunction, ascites, and white to yellowish growths or nodules. The cells of the target organ will hypertrophy around the parasite and create a xenoma, the whitish cyst-like structure encapsulating the parasite. Diagnosis is made by observing the spores under a wet mount preparation of the nodules, or by using histology post-mortem. Prevention is key for this disease and a proper quarantine protocol can help prevent the introduction of the parasite into a fish system. Treatment with Toltrazuril (Bayer) 5–20 mg/l of water as a 1–4-h dip in well-aerated water has been suggested. The best recommendations are to depopulate and disinfect the pond or tank to prevent further infestation.

18.7 Myxozoa

The phylum Myxozoa was originally classified as protozoa, but studies suggest they may be Metazoa since they have multicellular spores. Myxozoa are obligate parasites that require the host's tissues to continue their lifecycle. They can be histozoic (infesting body tissues) or coelozoic (infesting inside the body cavity), and most organs of a fish can be infested (Woo, 2006). They are spore-forming organisms and have an indirect lifecycle that involves the fish and an invertebrate definitive host, in most cases an oligochaete worm.

The spore size in fish hosts is usually 10–20 µm in length. Spores are released from the fish and are ingested by the invertebrate host, where the valves of the spore split to release the infective sporoplasm. The sporoplasm penetrates between the epithelial cells of the intestines of the invertebrate host. Two sporoplasms fuse together in a form of sexual reproduction that undergoes three phases: schizogony, gametogamy, and sporogony. In the infective stage, the actinospore (from oligochaetes) or malacospore (from bryozoan hosts), is released into the environment from the invertebrate host through defecation or on the death of the host. The actinospore then attaches to a fish using polar filaments. The actinospore releases a sporoplasm that penetrates the fish's epidermis and travels to its target organ. Once the target organ is reached by the sporoplasm, the parasite will become a trophozoite, which then matures into the asexually reproducing plasmodium stage. Within the plasmodium, the myxospores will begin to form. The myxospores are released into the environment through rupture of the cyst, death, and decay of the host or through predation and passing the myxospores through the feces into the water. Myxospores can last in the environment for up to 1 year. Ingestion of myxospores by oligochaetes continues the life cycle.

Myxozoa are not pathogenic in low numbers, but in heavy infestations can cause high mortalities. *Myxobolus cerebralis* has been seen in salmonids, with a predilection for rainbow trout (Noble and Summerfelt, 1996). Spores for this organism are oval with two bipolar capsules. Infestations cause a whirling swimming pattern due to damage to the cartilaginous aspect of the ear. Clinically a dark patch along the caudal one-third dorsum of the body can be observed due to damage of the sympathetic nerves. In some cases, fish can be seen with vertebral malformations and malformed jawbones causing malocclusion due to invasion of the cartilage in those regions. Transmission occurs through the ingestion of spores, which then migrate to the cartilage. Spores will develop in 90 days at 17–16°C and 120 days at 12–13°C. Prevention involves minimizing exposure to the intermediate host, the tubifex worm. Raise salmonids in concrete raceways. When this is not possible, disinfect the organic bed with lime prior to restocking.

Myxobolus koi forms cysts in the gills of koi and other carp species. This can cause hypertrophy of the branchial epithelium and clubbing of the gill filaments. Spores measure 12–15 µm × 5–9 µm and contain two equal-sized polar capsules (Fig. 18.20). Each polar capsule contains a coiled polar filament that is extended from the spore and used for locomotion when the mature spore is released from the fish (Woo, 2006). The spores are released when the fish dies and remain stable in the pond environment

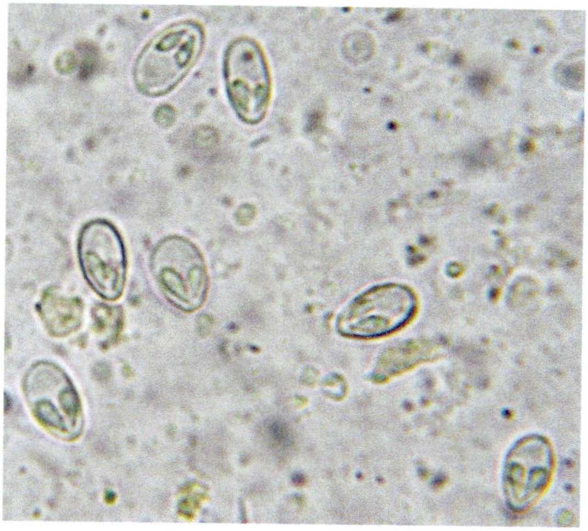

Fig. 18.20. *Myxobolus koi* from the gills of a koi (*C. rubrofuscus*). (Microphotograph by N. Saint-Erne.)

for a year. Eventually, the spores are ingested by an intermediate host (an oligochaete worm). Once ingested by the intermediate host, the valves of the spore open, releasing the sporoplasm. The sporoplasm then transforms into the infective actinospore stage in the worm. These wait to enter the fish host by ingestion of the worm. Once inside the fish host, the actinospore develops into a plasmodium that migrates to its specific tissue site in the fish (the cartilage of the gill filament). In the gill cartilage, the plasmodium grows and produces many spores that are released into the fish's tissue. In some cases, the plasmodium and the spores do not cause much tissue damage, and the fish acts normally. In severe infestations, there can be damage to the gill filaments causing noticeable lesions and gill necrosis. Eliminating live worms in the pond would prevent the completion of the parasite's life cycle and its spread to the other fish (Saint-Erne, 2010).

Hoferellus carassii (*Mitraspora cyprini*) causes "kidney bloater disease" in goldfish and can infect common carp. The fish are infested by ingesting spores in the water, and the sporoplasm leaves the spore, penetrates through the intestinal mucosa, and circulates through the blood system. When passing through the kidney blood vessels, it penetrates the epithelial cells of the renal tubules. There, it reproduces asexually before releasing spores that pass into the water with fish urine. The spores are shed in the urine on a seasonal basis, with their release usually occurring in late winter. The protozoa's multiplication causes kidney enlargement and ultimate kidney failure. Grossly, the fish will look bloated, and on necropsy one or both kidneys will be greatly enlarged. Histopathology of affected kidney tissue reveals papillary cystic hyperplasia and protozoal trophozoites visible in the kidney tubules.

Tetracapsula has been noted to cause proliferative kidney disease and has occurred in multiple species, including zebrafish. *Tetracapsula bryosalmonae* is presporogonic in the blood and interstitial kidney and is sporogonic in the kidney tubules. It causes swelling of the kidney and spleen, pale gills, darkened areas of the body, ascites, and exophthalmia. Clinically, enlargement of the kidney can be noted on a necropsy exam. The highest level of mortalities is noted in warmer temperatures.

Other forms of Myxozoa that have been recorded include *Chloromyxum*, which have been noted to cause granulomatous disease in the GI tract and kidneys, creating a fish that is chronically emaciated. The spores appear more rounded to walnut shape, with four polar capsules present. *Kudoa*, or *Unicapsula seriolae*, has been noted to cause myoliquefication in marine fish after death. Spores for this myxozoan appear as a four-pointed star. *Henneguya* has been noted to target the epidermis and causes increased mucus production. The spores appear elliptical in shape with two long tails. *Henneguya ictalurid* is a major disease of channel catfish and can result in high mortalities due to granulomatous inflammation of the gills. Many other Myxozoa species have been noted to target the swim bladder, liver, brain, skin, and muscle in a variety of species.

Diagnosis is made on the cytology of the tissues and finding the spores. Often, diagnosis is made through squash-prep slides, or on histopathology post-mortem. Polymerase Chain Reaction (PCR) tests have been developed to detect Myxozoa parasites. There isn't an effective treatment. Fumagillin given orally at 3 mg/kg BW for 6 days can slow the progression of disease but doesn't eliminate the infestation. Prevention is key for this disease. Removal of dead fish from the water is critical to limit the release of spores from the dead fish. Draining, drying, and then liming of fishponds reduce the numbers of both myxospores and oligochaete worms. Avoid feeding live tubifex worms to fish, as they can be the source of infestation. Once an infestation is noted, it is better to depopulate the affected fish.

18.8 Conclusion

Protozoa are a major health concern in aquaculture and eliminating them from fish is an important goal for aquatic veterinarians. There is still a considerable amount of information that we don't know about protozoa. Molecular genetics will play an important role in the future for a better understanding of the taxonomy, reproduction, and life cycles of protozoan parasites. More research must be done on treatment methods to reduce these parasites that cause high economic loss in both food and ornamental fish.

References

Aksit, D., Falakali-Mutafi, B., Gocmen, B. and Gurelli, G. (2008) A preliminary observation on *Trichodina* sp. (Ciliophora: Peritricha) on the gills of limpets (*Patella* spp.) in Antalya (Turkey). *North-Western Journal of Zoology* 4(2), 295–299.

Andrews, C., Exell, A. and Carrington, N. (2002) *The Interpet Manual of Fish Health*. Interpet, Surrey, UK.

Austin, B. (2012) *Infectious Disease in Aquaculture: Prevention and Control*. Woodhead, Philadelphia, Pennsylvania.

Bastos Gomes, G., Jerry, D.R., Miller, T.L. and Hutson, K.S. (2016) Current status of parasitic ciliates *Chilodonella* spp. (Phyllopharyngea: Chilodonellidae) in freshwater fish aquaculture. *Journal of Fish Diseases* 40(5), 703–715.

Bastos Gomes, G., Miller, T.L., Vaughan, D.B., Jerry, D.R., McCowan, C. *et al.* (2017) Evidence of multiple species of *Chilodonella* (Protozoa, Ciliophora) infecting Australian farmed freshwater fishes. *Veterinary Parasitology* 237, 8–16.

Bolland, S.J., Zahedi, A., Oskam, C., Murphy, B. and Ryan, U. (2020) *Cryptosporidium bollandi* n. sp. (Apicomplexa: Cryptosporidiiae) from angelfish (*Pterophyllum scalare*) and Oscar fish (*Astronotus ocellatus*). *Experimental Parasitology* 217, 107956.

Bruno, D., Nowak, B. and Elliott, D. (2006) Guide to the identification of fish protozoan and metazoan parasites in stained tissue sections. *Diseases of Aquatic Organisms* 70, 1–36.

Cardoso, P.H.M., Soares, H.S., Martins, M.L. and Balian, S.C. (2019) *Cryptocaryon irritans*, a ciliate parasite of an ornamental reef fish yellowtail tang *Zebrasoma xanthurum*. *Revista Brasileira de Parasitologia Veterinária* 28(4), 750–753.

Cheung, P.J., Nigrelli, R.F. and Ruggieri, G.D. (1980) Studies on the morphology of *Uronema marinum* Dujardin (Ciliatea: Uronematidae) with a description of the histopathology of the infection in marine fishes. *Journal of Fish Diseases* 3(4), 295–303.

Colorni, A. (1997) *Cryptocaryon irritans* Brown 1951, the cause of "white spot disease" in marine fish: an update. *Aquarium Science and Conservation* 1, 217–238.

Crosbie, P. and Munday, B. (1999) Environmental factors and chemical agents affecting the growth of the pathogenic marine ciliate *Uronema nigricans*. *Diseases of Aquatic Organisms* 36, 213–219.

Dickerson, H.W. (2012) *Ichthyophthirius multifiliis*. In: Woo, P. and Buchmann, K. (eds) *Fish Parasites*. CAB International, Wallingford, UK, pp. 55–72.

Ewing, M.S. and Kocan, K.M. (1992) Invasion and development strategies of *Ichthyophthirius multifiliis*, a parasitic ciliate of fish. *Parasitology Today* 8(6), 204–208.

Ferraz, E. and Sommerville, C. (1998) Pathology of *Piscinoodinium* sp. (Protozoa: Dinoflagellida), parasites of the ornamental freshwater catfishes *Corydoras* spp. and *Brochis splendens* (Pisces: Callichthyidae). *Diseases of Aquatic Organisms* 33, 43–49.

Florindo, M., Jeronimo, G., Steckert, L., Acchile, M., Tavares Goncalves, E. *et al.* (2017) Protozoan parasites of freshwater ornamental fish. *Latin American Journal of Aquatic Research* 45(5), 948–956.

Foissner, W., Hoffman, G.L. and Mitchell, A.J. (1985) *Heteropolaria colisarum* Foissner & Schubert, 1977 (Protozoa: Epistylididae) of North American freshwater fishes. *Journal of Fish Diseases* 8(2), 145–160.

Golomazou, E. and Karanis, P. (2020) Cryptosporidium species in fish: an update. *Environmental Sciences Proceedings* 2(1): 13.

Gomes, A.L.S., Costa, J.I. da, Benetton, M.L.F., Bernardino, G. and Belem-Costa, A. (2018) A fast and practical method for initial diagnosis of *Piscinoodinium pillulare* outbreaks: piscinootest. *Ciência Rural* 48(7). doi:10.1590/0103-8478cr20170680.

Hoole, D., Bucke, D., Burgess, P. and Wellby, I. (2001) *Diseases of Carp and Other Cyprinid Fishes*. Blackwell Science, Oxford.

Klinger, R.E. and Floyd, R.F. (2013) Introduction to freshwater fish parasites. Available at: https://extension.rwfm.tamu.edu/wp-content/uploads/sites/8/2013/09/Introduction-to-Freshwater-Fish-Parasites.pdf (accessed 12 November 2020).

Leibowitz, M.P. and Zilberg, D. (2009) *Tetrahymena* sp. infection in guppies, *Poecilia reticulata* Peters: parasite characterization and pathology of infected fish. *Journal of Fish Diseases* 32(10), 845–855.

Loh, R. (2012) *Fish Vetting Medicines*. Loh Publishing, Perth, Australia.

Lom, J. and Corliss, J.O. (1971) Morphogenesis and cortical ultrastructure of *Brooklynella hostilis*, a dysteriid ciliate ectoparasitic on marine fishes. *The Journal of Protozoology* 18(2), 261–281.

Lom, J. and Nigrellia, R.F. (1970) *Brooklynella hostilis* n. g., n. sp., a pathogenic cyrtophorine ciliate in marine fishes. *The Journal of Protozoology* 17(2), 224–232.

Mayer, J. and Donnelly T.M. (2013) Gastrointestinal protozoal parasites. In: Mayer, J. and Donnelly T.M. (eds) *Clinical Veterinary Advisor: Birds and Exotic Pets*. Elsevier, St. Louis, Missouri, pp. 28–29.

Mitchell, A.J., Darwish, A. and Fuller, A. (2008) Comparison of tank treatments with copper sulfate and potassium permanganate for sunshine bass with ichthyobodosis. *Journal of Aquatic Animal Health* 20(4), 202–206.

Negrão, M.C., da Silva, M.R.L., Videira, M.N. and Viana, L.A. (2019) Prevalence and molecular characterization of Calyptospora parasites, Overstreet, Hawkins and Fournié, 1984 (Apicomplexa: Calyptosporidae) in fishes from the eastern Amazon, Brazil. *Parasitology International* 73, 101975.

Noble, A.C. and Summerfelt, S.T. (1996) Diseases encountered in rainbow trout cultured in recirculating systems. *Annual Review of Fish Diseases* 6, 65–92.

Noga, E.J. (2010) *Fish Disease: Diagnosis and Treatment*. Wiley, Ames, Iowa.

Paperna, I. (1984) Reproduction cycle and tolerance to temperature and salinity of Amyloodinium ocellatum (Brown, 1931) (Dinoflagellida). *Annales de Parasitologie Humaine et Comparée* 59(1), 7–30.

Paul, T., Mandal, J., Dasgupta, M., Sarkar, G., Karmakar, D. *et al.* (2018) A preliminary study on prevalence of parasites in ornamental fish, *Carassius auratus* (gold fish). *International Journal of Engineering, Science and Mathematics* 7(1), 74–83.

Pimenta Leibowitz, M., Ariav, R. and Zilberg, D. (2005) Environmental and physiological conditions affecting *Tetrahymena* sp. infection in guppies, *Poecilia reticulata* Peters. *Journal of Fish Diseases* 28(9), 539–547.

Plumb, J.A. (1999) Overview of warmwater fish diseases. *Journal of Applied Aquaculture* 9(2), 1–10.

Ponpornpisit, A., Endo, M. and Murata, H. (2000) Experimental infections of a ciliate *Tetrahymena pyriformis* on ornamental fishes. *Fisheries Science* 66(6), 1026–1031.

Poynton, S.L., Fraser, W., Francis-Floyd, R., Rutledge, P., Reed, P. and Nerad, T.A. (1995) *Spironucleus vortens* N. Sp. from the freshwater angelfish *Pterophyllum scalare*: morphology and culture. *The Journal of Eukaryotic Microbiology* 42(6), 731–742.

Robertson, D.A. (1985) A review of *Ichthyobodo necator* (Henneguy, 1883) an important and damaging fish parasite. In: Muir, J.F. and Roberts, R.J. (eds) *Recent Advances in Aquaculture*. Vol. 2. Springer, Boston, Massachusetts, 1–30. doi:10.1007/978-1-4684-8736-7_1.

Saint-Erne, N. (2010) Protozoal parasites. In: Saint-Erne, N. (ed.) *Advanced Koi Care*. 2nd edn. Erne Enterprises, Glendale, Arizona, pp. 73–79.

Sanders, J., Lawrence, C., Nichols, D., Brubaker, J., Peterson, T. *et al.* (2010) *Pleistophora hyphessobryconis* (Microsporidia) infecting zebrafish (*Danio rerio*) in research facilities. *Diseases of Aquatic Organisms* 91(1), 47–56. doi:10.3354/dao02245.

Sangmaneedet, S. and Smith, S. (1999) Efficacy of various chemotherapeutic agents on the growth of *Spironucleus vortens*, an intestinal parasite of the freshwater angelfish. *Diseases of Aquatic Organisms* 38, 47–52.

Scholz, T. (1999) Parasites in cultured and feral fish. *Veterinary Parasitology* 84(3–4), 317–335.

Sharon, G., Pimenta Leibowitz, M., Chettri, J.K., Isakov, N. and Zilberg, D. (2014) Comparative study of infection with *Tetrahymena* of different ornamental fish species. *Journal of Comparative Pathology* 150(2–3), 316–324.

Silva, M.F., Araújo, R.S., Silva, D.T., Sanches, O., Hamoy, I. and Matos, E. (2019) Gastric coccidiosis in *Thoracocharax stellatus* caused by *Goussia guamaensis* n. sp. (Apicomplexa: Eimeriidae) from the Amazon region. *Journal of Fish Diseases* 42(6), 905–912.

Silva, M.F., Orlanda, J.F.F., Araújo-Costa, M.J., Hamoy, I. and Matos, E. (2020) Hepatic coccidiosis in *Triportheus angulatus* Spix & Agassiz, 1829 (Characiformes: Triportheidae), a tropical fish from the Eastern Brazilian Amazon, with the description of a new species of *Calyptospora* (Apicomplexa: Calyptosporidae). *Journal of Eukaryotic Microbiology* 67(3), 352–358.

Smith, S. and Roberts, H. (2010) Parasites of fish. In: Robers, H. (ed.) *Fundamentals of Ornamental Fish Health*. Wiley, Ames, Iowa, pp. 102–112.

Smith, S. and Schwarz, M. (2019) Getting acquainted with *Amyloodinium ocellatum*. Virginia Cooperative Extension. Available at: https://www.pubs.ext.vt.edu/600/600-200/600-200.html (accessed 15 December 2020).

Székely, C. and Bereczky, M. (1992) An unusual case of disease in pet fish stocks caused by *Coleps* sp. (Protozoa: Kinetoflagminophorea). *Diseases of Aquatic Organisms* 13, 143–145.

Tojo, J. and Santamarina, M. (1998) Oral pharmacological treatments for parasitic diseases of rainbow trout *Oncorhynchus mykiss*. I: *Hexamita salmonis*. *Diseases of Aquatic Organisms* 33, 51–56.

Valladão, G.M.R., Pereira, M.M., Gallani, S.U. and Pilarski, F. (2019) A massive *Chilodonella hexasticha* infestation associated with yellowtail tetra *Astyanax lacustris* mortality in aquaculture: identification and pathology. *Aquaculture Research* 50(7), 2019–2022.

Williams, C.F., Lloyd, D., Poynton, S.L., Jorgensen, A., Millet, C. and Cable, J. (2011) *Spironucleus* species: economically important fish pathogens and enigmatic single-celled eukaryotes. *Journal of Aquaculture Research and Development* S2:002. doi:10.4172/2155-9546.S2-002.

Williams, C.F., Vacca, A., Lloyd, D., Schelkle, B. and Cable, J. (2013) Non-invasive investigation of *Spironucleus vortens* transmission in freshwater angelfish *Pterophyllum scalare*. *Diseases of Aquatic Organisms* 105(3), 211–223.

Woo, P.T.K. (2006) *Fish Diseases and Disorders, Vol. 1 Protozoan and Metazoan Infections*. 2nd edn. CAB International, Wallingford, UK.

Wooster, G.A. and Bowser, P.R. (1994) Unusual infection of rainbow trout *Oncorhynchus mykiss* by the protozoan *Coleps* sp. (Ciliophora: Prostomatea) in a closed recirculation aquaculture system. *Journal of the World Aquaculture Society* 25(4), 566–570.

Yanong, R.P.E. (2017) Cryptocaryon irritans infections (marine white spot disease) in fish. Available at: https://edis.ifas.ufl.edu/fa164 (accessed 22 January 2021).

19 Metazoan Parasites

Azureen Erdman

New River, Arizona

Abstract

Parasites are potentially the most economically significant pathogens in aquaculture. The most commonly encountered parasites are protozoa; however, multicellular (metazoan) parasites can cause significant morbidity and mortality as well. This chapter covers monogenean, digenean, acanthocephalan, nematode, tubularian, cestode, and crustacea that have been identified as fish parasites, the clinical signs they can cause, and how to treat infestations.

19.1 Monogenean Flatworms

The phylum Platyhelminthes (flatworms) is divided into four classes: Monogeneans, Trematodes, Turbellaria, and Cestodes. Platyhelminthes is the second largest group of fish parasites, after the protozoal parasites. Monogenean flatworms are characterized and identified based on their posterior attachment organ (opisthaptor), the presence of eyespots in some species, and the mode of reproduction (Klinger and Floyd, 2013). These parasites all have a direct lifecycle. Some reproduce with eggs, and some are live-bearing. Some are hermaphrodites and can self-fertilize. Clinical signs of a monogenean infestation can vary; however, most will cause flashing—or rubbing the body on the substrate—in their teleost hosts. Fish can show signs of lethargy, clamped fins, and excess mucus production. Physical lesions can include cutaneous ulcers and scale loss. Treatment for monogenean infestations can include formalin, praziquantel, or potassium permanganate bath treatments. Fresh or saltwater baths have been reported to be effective. In large-scale farms, praziquantel in the feed, organophosphate baths, and hydrogen peroxide baths are used. Control using cleaner fish has been tried (Becker and Grutter, 2004).

Monogeneans are divided into two subclasses. Monopisthocotylea includes the families Gyrodactylidae, Dactylogyridae, Capsalidea, and Ancyrocephalidae. Polyopisthocotylea includes *Discocotyle*, *Allobivagina*, *Heteraxin*, and *Microcotyle*. Monopisthocotylea have a single attachment organ with several large hooks and peripheral hooklets. These parasites feed on host cuticle and epithelium. This creates focal areas of cutaneous irritation, hyperemia, hyperplasia, and increased mucus in the areas of attachment (Roberts *et al.*, 2009). Parasites from the subclass Polyopisthocotylea have adhesive suction organs that adhere to the integument, allowing them to attach and feed on blood (Rubio-Godoy, 2007). They cause less localized damage but can in high numbers cause severe anemia in a fish.

19.1.1 *Gyrodactylus*

Gyrodactylus is a genus within the Monopisthocotylea subclass. It is identified by its pair of large anchors and 16 marginal hooklets within the posterior attachment organ, known as the opisthaptor. They have no eyespots, and an embryo with hooks is often visible microscopically within the adult (Fig. 19.1). They are hermaphroditic and give birth to live young, one at a time (Fig. 19.2). The young are parasitic immediately after birth (Saint-Erne, 2010). Only 60% of *Gyrodactylus* species were reported to preferentially choose one species of host (Harris *et al.*, 2004). The remaining have been identified on a wide range of freshwater and marine hosts. *Gyrodactylus* is also known as the "skin fluke" and tends to adhere to the skin and fins, but sometimes

Corresponding author: az.erdman@gmail.com

© CAB International 2025.
DOI: 10.1079/9781789246032.0019

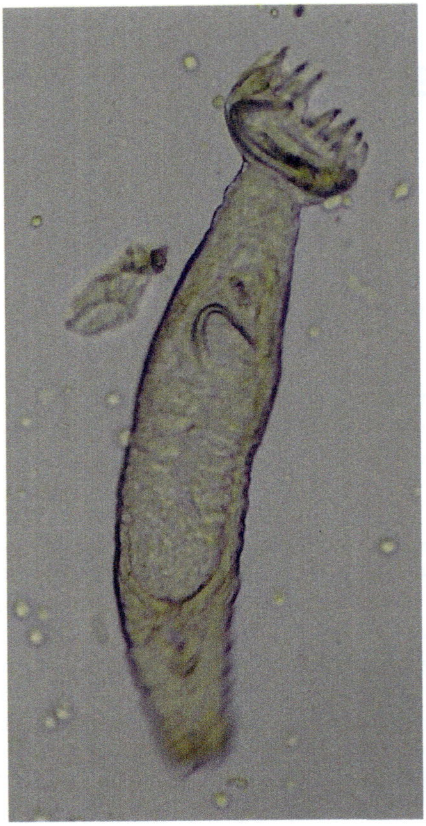

Fig. 19.1. *Gyrodactylus* with hooks of folded embryo visible within its body. (Microphotograph by N. Saint-Erne.)

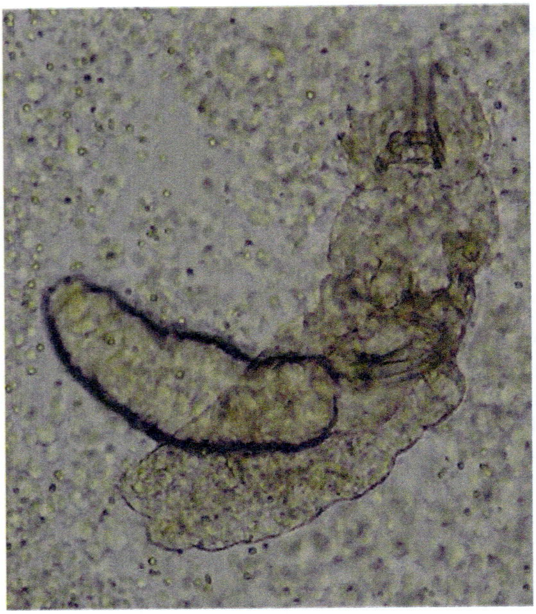

Fig. 19.2. *Gyrodactylus* giving birth. The hooks of the embryo are still within the parent's body. (Microphotograph by N. Saint-Erne.)

is found on the gills as well. It is transmitted through direct contact with infested fish. The infectious larvae (oncomiracidium) have been seen "hanging in the water column" in an ideal position to allow them to attach to a new host as the fish swim by (Cable *et al.*, 2002). It can also be spread by indirect contact with fomites, like substrate, nets or other equipment, and caretakers that are contaminated with larvae (Soleng *et al.*, 1998).

Most *Gyrodactylus* are live-bearing (viviparous). In these viviparous parasites, three generations of parasites can sometimes be actively growing. The unborn larva within the adult may already be gravid. The larva will be born and can give birth to the already-growing daughter within 24 h. This allows them to rapidly reproduce in a closed fish system. A few within this order are egg layers. The egg-laying *Gyrodactylus* attach the eggs to their skin with a strong adhesive until they hatch.

Clinical signs are caused by the parasite feeding on the epithelial layers of the fish (Fig. 19.3). Fish can appear with hyperemic ulcerative lesions or have dark necrotic skin lesions. There will be an increase in mucus production. Fish can be seen flashing and rubbing against objects within the tank. Parasite attachment on the gills will cause clubbing secondary to the hyperplasia and increased mucus production within the gills. Erosions can be seen on the fins. Fish can appear lethargic and have decreased appetite. Treatments for these include formalin baths and salt water dips (Francis-Floyd, 2019).

19.1.2 *Dactylogyrus, Pseudodactylogyrus, Cleidodiscus*

Dactylogyrus, and similar flukes *Pseudodactylogyrus*, *Cleidodiscus* are classified within subclass Monopisthocotylea. These parasites are considered "gill flukes," as they primarily attach to the gills. They are identified with 2–4 eyespots near the anterior of the body, an opisthaptor with a pair of large anchor hooks, and 12, 14, or 16 marginal hooklets, depending on the species. There are 971 species that have been identified within the *Dactylogyrus* genus (Dove and Ernst, 1998). Of these 971 species, 95%

have been found to preferentially choose a host within the Cyprinidae family. Parasites within this family are egg layers (oviparous). These eggs (40 μm) are very sticky, may have hooklets on the end, and can easily become trapped in gill mucus, filter media, and substrates within the tank (Fig. 19.4). The eggs hatch in 2–3 days, releasing an oncomiracidium that swims to find a fish host within 24 h. Eggs are impervious to treatment, making it hard to remove them from the water and equipment once an infestation occurs. These parasites have been shown to have the highest success hatching at 20°C. The whole life cycle can be completed in 8–11 days at 20°C, allowing for a population of fish to become quickly infested with heavy numbers (Fig. 19.5). Transmission involves direct contact with infested individuals or with equipment or humans not properly disinfected when moving among aquariums.

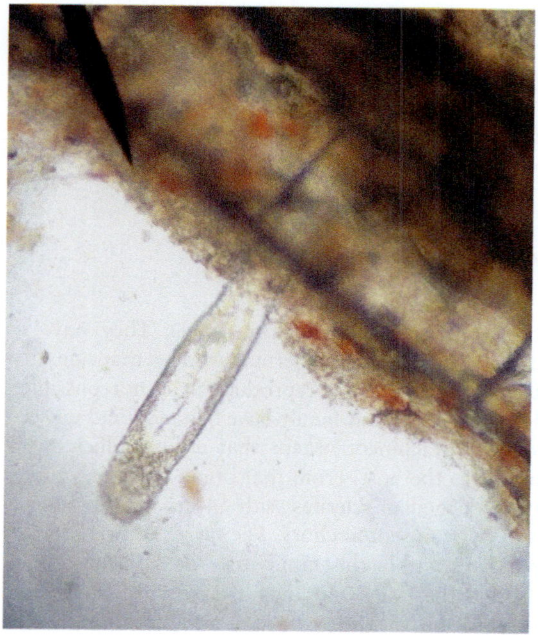

Fig. 19.3. Skin fluke attached to the margin of a caudal fin. (Microphotograph by N. Saint-Erne.)

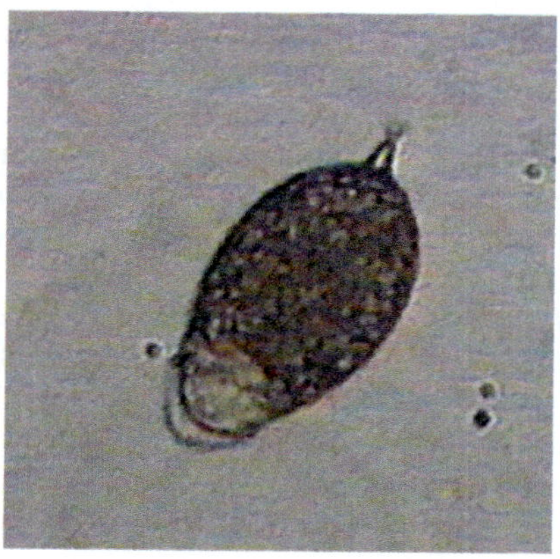

Fig. 19.4. Gill fluke egg with hooklet. (Microphotograph by N. Saint-Erne.)

Due to their preference to adhere to the gills, most of the clinical signs involve changes to the gills or the ability to respire. Fish can be seen crowding around the water inlet or at the surface. They may have an increase in respiration, or in severe cases, be seen gasping at the surface of the water. Fish can have a decrease in appetite. They may appear in poor body condition. The gills themselves can have a loss of architecture as clubbing occurs secondary to hyperplasia of the tissue and increased mucus production (Fig. 19.6). The parasites can affect the fish's immune response and allow for secondary bacterial infections to occur. Most commonly *Flavobacterium* infections are reported (Zhang *et al.*, 2015). Treatment can include salt baths, formalin baths, or mebendazole baths.

Pseudodactylogyrus affects the gills of eels. Two species have been reported, *P. bini* and *P. anguillae* (Katahira *et al.*, 2012). Both species are noted to feed on the mucous layer and epithelial cells causing irritation and damage to the gills as it feeds. *P. bini* is identified as being shorter and stouter. It is more often found in the distal or central aspects of gill filaments

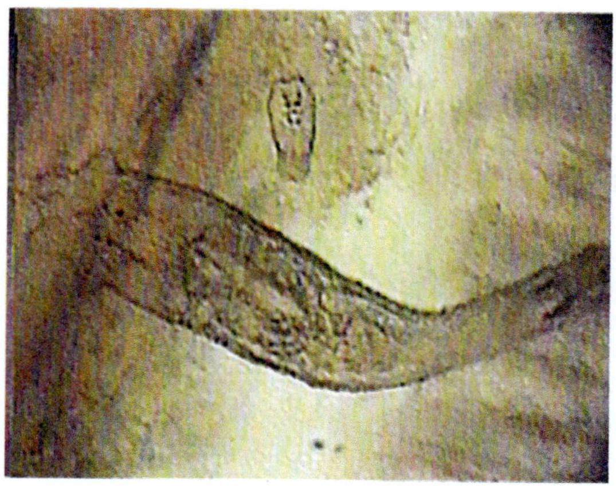

Fig. 19.5. Newly hatched gill fluke next to an adult, seen on a gill biopsy examination. (Microphotograph by N. Saint-Erne.)

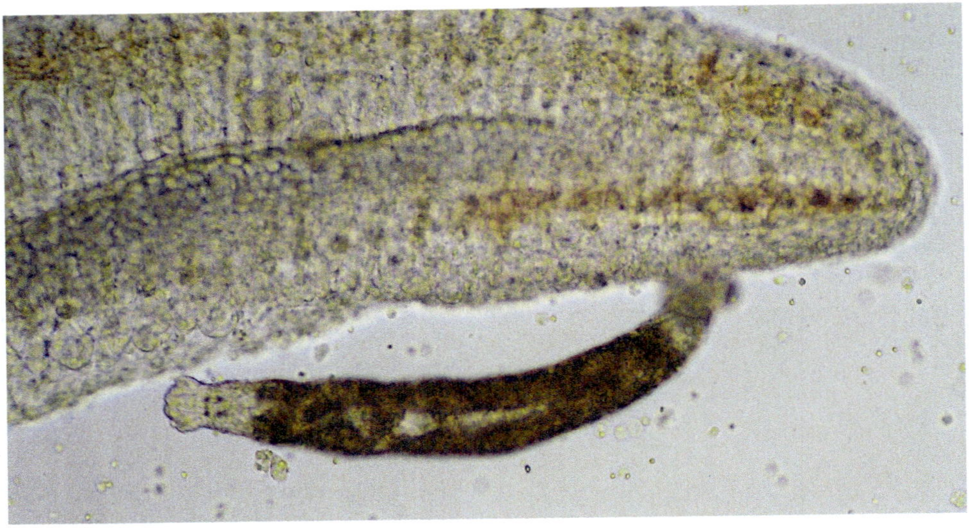

Fig. 19.6. Gill fluke seen on a gill biopsy examination. (Microphotograph by N. Saint-Erne.)

and prefers the anterior gill arches. *P. anguillae* favors the proximal aspect of the gill filaments and is more commonly found on the posterior gill arches. *P. bini* is more sedentary, whereas *P. anguillae* is often found moving actively on the gill surface, and on cytology when looking at a gill biopsy. This parasite has a direct life cycle and is oviparous (Buchmann *et al.*, 1987). Eggs are released within the water column. At temperatures up to 28°C eggs will be released. Larvae, known as oncomiracidia, hatch at an ideal temperature between 19°C and 26°C. It has been noted that in temperatures ranging from 20°C to 22°C the larvae will die within 2–5 h if they do not attach to a host fish. The oncomiracidia attaches to the host and develops into an adult in 7–9 days. Infested eels will swim slowly, act lethargic, and gather in areas with low water currents. In severe cases, hyperemia will occur around the face and gills. The parasite will cause clubbing of the gills due to hyperplasia of the tissue and increased mucus production. In cases with severe gill damage eels can be noted to be hemorrhaging from the gills. Formaldehyde and sodium chloride have been used to treat these parasites. Potassium permanganate baths have been reported as useful, but it only decreased the population of the parasites by 50%.

19.1.3 Capsalidea

Capsalidea is a family of Monogenea in the Monopisthocotylea subclass, and 200 species have been reported (Whittington, 2004). They have a direct life cycle and are hermaphrodites that can self-fertilize when sexual reproduction is not possible. Parasites within this family have flattened, and saucer-shaped attachment organs that use an adhesive to attach to the host. From that organ protrudes three pairs of median sclerites with 14 marginal hooklets and two pairs of anchors. The target organs for the parasites within this family are the skin and areas around the eyes. Capsalids are oviparous and can produce up to 80 eggs a day and start producing eggs between 4 and 21 days of age. Eggs will have a linear string-like appendage that has an adhesive droplet at the end, allowing them to adhere to structures within the environment. The eggs hatch in 5–8 days at 23°C. Once in a fish system, Capsalids are difficult to remove, and due to their ability to self-fertilize, they can multiply rapidly. Clinical signs can include extensive visible erosions and ulcerations. *Entobdella* has been reported in both elasmobranchs and teleosts. *Dermophthirius* has been reported in lemon sharks (Cheung and Ruggieri, 1983).

Neobenedenia species have been reported to cause cutaneous and ocular lesions in marine tropical fish, as they graze on the epidermis and mucus layer. They are characterized by a large circular opisthaptor with three pairs of curved anchors on the posterior aspect of the body and two small suckers on the anterior end. *Neobenedenia* flukes are also known as the "marine flukes." There have been over 100 species reported, most of which have been found to have a low host specificity. Species within this genus have a high reproduction rate and environmentally resilient eggs. It has been shown that they can reach sexual maturity within 10 days and can produce on average 190 eggs per day in optimum conditions. Since they can self-fertilize, a single isolated *Neobenedenia* within an environment can produce over 3000 infective larvae within 2 weeks. Eggs are laid within the first few hours of darkness. The larvae will hatch within the first 3 h of daylight. As the larvae only live without a host for 24–48 h this gives the larvae the best chance of finding and attaching to a host as the fish become more active in the daylight. Hatching is salinity and temperature dependent (Ellis and Watanabe, 1993; Brazenor *et al.*, 2018). About 80% of the eggs will hatch when the water temperatures range between 26°C and 32°C. However, the warmer the water, the shorter the lifespan of the larvae (Dinh Hoai and Hutson, 2014). Eggs themselves do not hatch in water with a salinity of less than 11% (Brazenor and Hutson, 2015). Once the eggs are laid, a ciliated larva (oncomiracidium) develops within. The oncomiracidium will emerge and swim to locate a host. Once adhering to the host, they migrate to the preferred sites, including the eyes, fins, and dorsal or ventral extremities. Treatment for these parasites includes praziquantel (Morales-Serna *et al.*, 2018), formalin, mebendazole, and cleaner fish (Cowell *et al.*, 1993), fresh water baths, or placing the fish in a low salinity environment for 5 days. Praziquantel is shown to be less effective in *Neobenedenia* than it is in *Benedenia* and may require higher doses or longer treatment lengths when treating *Neobenedenia* outbreaks (Fig. 19.7).

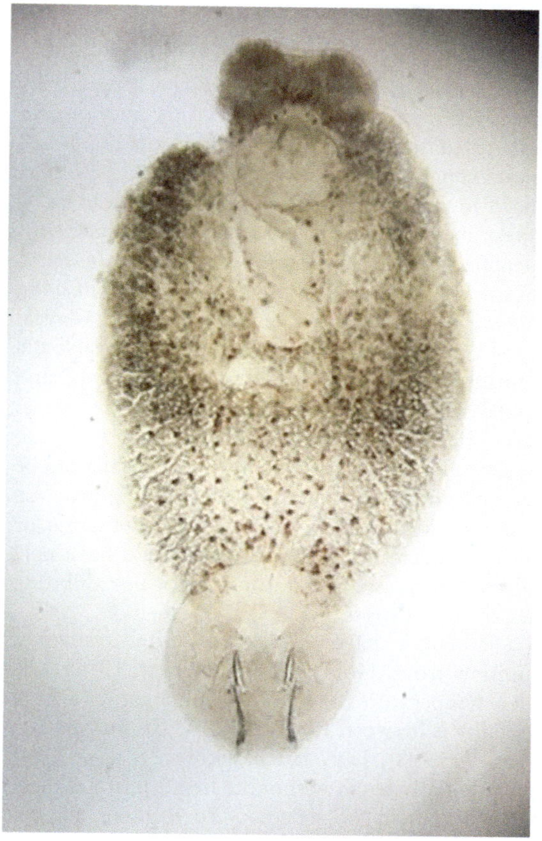

Fig. 19.7. Monogenean *Neobenedenia* found on a blue tang (*Paracanthurus hepatus*). (Photo by Robert Martinez.)

Benedenia has over 70 described species within the genus (Whittington, 1996). These parasites are identified with a large circular opisthaptor on the posterior body with two pairs of curved anchors and two small suckers on the anterior end. The body is flattened and leaf-shaped. Like *Neobenedenia*, they cause cutaneous ulcerations and very similar clinical signs. *Benedenia* species are located on the epithelium, with no ocular lesions. They have a direct life cycle like *Neobenedenia* and can affect a wide range of hosts. Treatments include praziquantel (Hirazawa *et al.*, 2013), formalin, mebendazole, and cleaner fish.

19.1.4 Ancyrocephalidae

Ancyrocephalidae is a family within the Monopisthocotylea subclass. They are closely related to the dactylogyrids and not selective for their host species. They can be found on the gills or in the esophagus and pharynx of freshwater, marine, and brackish fish. *Neodiplectanotrema*, *Diplectanotrema*, and *Pseudempleurosoma gibsoni* have been found in the esophagus and pharynx of fish (Santos *et al.*, 2001). *Paradiplectanotrema* has been reported in the esophagus of marine fish. *Enterogyrus* has been found within the stomach of African and Asian cichlid species. This family of parasites has a slender body with a single pair of glands on the head that extend to the parasite's pharynx. They are identified by two eyespots, two pairs of hamuli, and 12–14 marginal hooklets. They are oviparous and have a direct life cycle. Treatment is similar to treating *Dactylogyrus* and can include salt baths, formalin, or mebendazole treatments.

19.1.5 Polyopisthocotylea

Polyopisthocotylea is a subclass within the monogenean class. These parasites are characterized by their series of adhesive suckers that they use to adhere to the integument to feed on the host's blood supply. Because these parasites feed on blood, they can cause less visible skin lesions but can cause severe anemia in their host. Multiple genera have been identified in this subclass *Discocotyle*, *Allobivagina*, *Heteraxin*, *Heterobothrium*, *Neoheterobothrium*, *Allobivagina*, *Heteraxine,* and *Microcotyle*. Clinical signs are respiratory distress and anemia. Visible gill damage can include increased mucus production and epithelial hyperplasia with secondary clubbing. In heavy infestations, hemorrhage and aneurysms can be seen. Hosts with moderate to severe anemia can be seen gasping at the surface, congregating near the water intake or aeration source, acting lethargic, or showing decreased appetite. They could have pale gills and increased respiratory rate or be exhibiting respiratory distress.

Discocotyle have been reported in freshwater rainbow trout (Noble and Summerfelt, 1996). The ideal temperature range for egg hatching with 92% viability is between 13°C and 18°C (Gannicott and Tinsley, 1998). Eggs hatch within 28 days. Eggs preferentially hatch within the first 2 h of darkness when host fish are sedentary to facilitate attachment of the greatest number of oncomiracidia as possible. *Microcotyle* are reported in the gills of marine butterflyfish and angelfish. Reports have shown mortalities up to 90% (Sanz, 1992). These mortalities are due to anemia and asphyxiation, or sepsis from secondary bacterial infections. Praziquantel, mebendazole, and formalin baths are reported to be effective in treating Polyopisthocotylea parasites (Katharios *et al.*, 2006).

19.2 Digenean Trematodes

The digenean trematodes contain over 6000 described species. They are typically identified in wild fish and less commonly seen in captive species because they require multiple hosts to complete their life cycle. This class of Platyhelminthes parasites has a complex indirect lifecycle. Adult stages of many of the species infest the gastrointestinal tract of the definitive host. Control of these parasites focuses on preventing the continuation of the lifecycle. This is achieved through controlling access by birds (the definitive host) to ponds and getting rid of the first intermediate snail hosts with molluscicides. Fish can be treated with praziquantel to eliminate the trematodes. Intramuscular praziquantel injections (25 mg/kg body weight [BW], one time) may eliminate the encysted metacercaria (Saint-Erne, 2010).

Centrocestus formosanus is a digenean trematode that causes gill disease. Its first intermediate host is a snail, with the second intermediate host being the fish (Iaria *et al.*, 2019). The definitive host is a mammal or a piscivorous bird, commonly reported as being the green heron and great egret. Eggs are laid in the definitive host's intestinal tract and pass into water with feces. The eggs hatch, releasing miracidia, or the eggs are ingested by snails. The miracidia develop into cercariae within snails. The cercaria leaves the snail and penetrates a fish where it encysts and develops into a metacercaria. The fish is then ingested by the final host, and the parasite matures within the mammal or bird's gastrointestinal tract. Physical changes seen on examination of a fish with this parasite are associated with the parasite's affinity for the cartilage tissue. Within the intermediate fish host, the parasite migrates into the gill tissue, specifically the cartilage, and matures to a metacercaria causing proliferation of the cartilage in the gill arch (Fig. 19.8). This can cause dilated gill filaments with adhesions between gills, as well as hyperemic gills. In severe cases, fish will appear in respiratory distress.

Posthodisplostomum minimum is known as the "white grub" (Lane *et al.*, 2015). These parasites

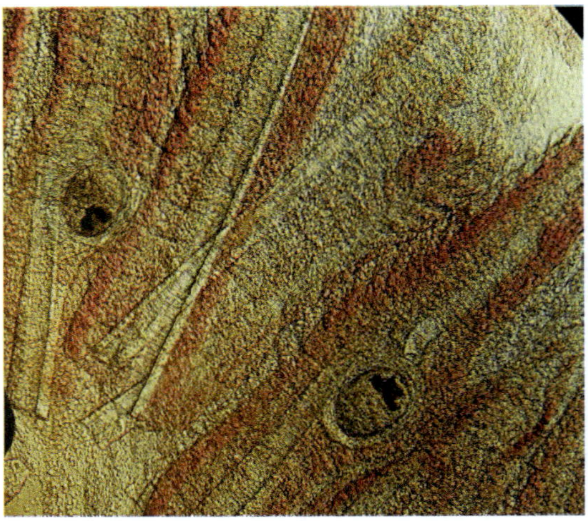

Fig. 19.8. Two Digenean flukes encysted in gill tissue of a dragon goby (*Gobioides broussonnetii*). (Microphotograph by N. Saint-Erne.)

are found within the visceral tissue of their intermediate fish host. Very similar to *Centrocestus*, the larvae (cercariae) live in snails. The cercariae will leave the snails and penetrate fish where they encyst as metacercaria within the visceral tissues (Fig. 19.9). The intermediate fish host is then ingested by birds where they will excyst and mature while living in the intestines of the definitive bird host. *P. minimum minimum* has been reported to specifically infest fish within the Cyprinidae family. *P. minimum centrarchi* has been reported to infest the Centrarchidae family specifically.

Clinostomum marginatum, also known as the "yellow grub," prefers to encyst in the muscle (Calhoun *et al.*, 2019). There are over 60 recognized species. This parasite is carried by birds that defecate eggs into the aquatic environment. The eggs hatch into miracidia, which penetrate snails and turn into sporocysts. Free-swimming cercariae are released from the snail and attach to fish or amphibian intermediate hosts, where they penetrate into the muscle. The fish or amphibian hosts are ingested by piscivorous birds, and the lifecycle continues (Plumb, 1999).

Diplostomulum spathaecum, also known as the eye fluke, has the same life cycle. The metacercaria of this genus prefer to settle in the eyes of catfishes and centrarchids. Clinical signs are associated with blindness and inability to hunt. Fish can be thin, lethargic, and anorexic. They may swim erratically or bump into surfaces, with an inability to catch prey.

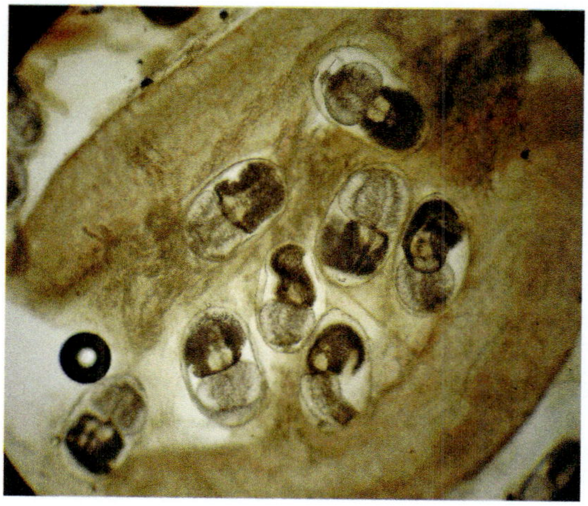

Fig. 19.9. Digenean flukes in visceral tissue of a rosy red minnow (*Pimephales promelas*). (Microphotograph by N. Saint-Erne.)

Cryptocotyle lingua is also commonly called "black-spot disease" due to the accumulation of the melanocytes at the site of infestation. The lifecycle is the same as other digeneans. Large operculated eggs are defecated out of the final bird host. The egg hatches into a miracidium and infests a snail. Cercariae develop within the snail and are released, where they penetrate the intermediate fish hosts. It matures into a metacercaria producing a cyst within the fish. The fish gets eaten by the final host and it differentiates into an adult that produces eggs and continues the cycle. Clinical signs are based on migration of the parasite and encysting of the parasite. The cercariae can cause hemorrhage and necrosis during migration through the fish host. The encysted metacercariae appear raised and dark, with melanocytes within the tissue. Encysted metacercariae can cause disfigurement and be esthetically unpleasing but are often otherwise not pathogenic. They can be found encysted in the eye, muscle, gills, or viscera of fish tissue.

Sanguinicola (blood flukes) are a genus of digenean trematodes that use fish as its final host. It lives in the blood vessels, heart, and gills. The blood flukes mature to adults in the fish, and are dioecious, with male and female genders. Mature adults copulate and eggs are released into the bloodstream (Hadfield and Clayton, 2021). Its triangular-shaped eggs can cause blockages in the circulatory system. The eggs hatch, releasing miracidia that penetrate through the gills and enter the water in search of their intermediate host, a mollusk. After developing to the cercarial stage in the mollusk, they return to the fish and reenter the gills. They reach sexual maturity in the gills and deposit eggs. Gill damage occurs from the larval penetrations and from blood vessel blockages. Secondary bacterial infections can occur in the necrotic tissues. Praziquantel given orally at 7.5–15 mg/kg BW q24h for 3 days has eradicated adult blood flukes in the fish.

19.3 Turbellaria

Turbellaria is a class of ciliated flatworms containing over 4500 species. The majority of Turbellaria are nonparasitic predators, but a few aquatic species are parasitic. There are two well-described Turbellaria that parasitize marine fish: *Paravortex* and *Ichthyophaga*. Both are reported to cause disease in marine fish known as "black-spot disease" or "tang disease" (Cannon and Lester, 1988). They have a direct life cycle with a free-living phase

(Justine *et al.*, 2009). Both species are known to be hermaphrodites. The larva will encyst on the host fish's skin and gills and become covered by a capsule from the fish's epithelia, which usually becomes pigmented with melanin, forming a black spot. Once mature, they rupture out of the fish and form a cocoon. The young are produced within the adult while cocooned. The adult ruptures open and the young are released to find a fish host on which to attach. Treatments for Turbellaria include praziquantel, organophosphate, formalin, and freshwater baths.

Ichthyophaga, also known as *Piscinquilinus*, is identified by eyes on their anterior end and the pharynx on the posterior end of the body. The body shape is ovoid with a thin body wall. They are fully ciliated around the body. The eyespots are shaped like brown clovers on microscopic exam. The capsule overlying the encysted *Ichthyophaga* larva is thick and fibrous and is pigmented with melanin. Each thick capsule contains a white-colored worm that is 2–4 mm in length.

Paravortex are viviparous and the life cycle can take only 10 days to complete (Hadfield and Clayton, 2021). They are identified by the eyes and pharynx on the anterior end of the body. The body is elongated and spherical or spindle-shaped with two eyespots. *Paravortex* are completely covered in cilia. They have been reported to affect mostly tangs but have been found in other tropical marine species. The larvae encyst on the fish, creating an acute hemorrhagic dermatitis with epithelial hyperplasia. Melanocytes will be found within the hyperplasia, creating a hyperpigmented nodule. Each nodule of this species contains one worm within a thin epidermal pocket, rather than the thick fibrous capsule seen with *Ichthyophaga*. The parasitic larva encysts and feeds on the fish for about 6 days, and then it falls off and forms a cocoon. The young are created within the cocooned adult. The adult body ruptures and up to 160 young are released.

19.4 Cestodes

Cestodes are tapeworms and can be found in many organs within many hosts. Most of these parasites have a complex lifecycle involving at least one but often two intermediate hosts. They are identified by their segmented bodies and their attachment organ. The body segments are called proglottids. The attachment organ is known as a scolex. In general, the larvae of cestodes cause damage, as they migrate through the muscle. Fish serve as definitive hosts for some species of tapeworms that live in their intestinal tracts (Fig. 19.10). The adults of the tapeworms *Bothriocephalus acheilognathi* and *Caryophyllaeus fimbriceps* can be found in fish intestines. Fish also are secondary intermediate hosts for larval stages (plerocercoids) of tapeworms such as *Ligula intestinalis*, which encyst in their muscles and abdomen. Treatment for most cestodes is praziquantel as a 10 mg/L bath for 1–3 h. Control and prevention involve identifying the intermediate hosts and controlling those.

Ligula cestodes have been noted to cause peritoneal adhesions and pressure atrophy of organs once they infest the peritoneal cavity. *Gilquinia squali* targets the eyes and causes blindness. This creates fish that are unable to find food and feed. *Acanthobothrium* has been noted as an incidental finding in the spiral valve of asymptomatic elasmobranchs (Rica *et al.*, 1995).

Bothriocephalus acheilognathi is known as the Asian tapeworm or Japanese tapeworm (Scholz, 1999). It has been researched extensively as it is zoonotic when undercooked fish meat is ingested. This tapeworm is found to live in the anterior intestine of fish within the *Cyprinidae* family, channel catfish, discus, livebearers, killifishes, and angelfish. It is large (up to 20 cm) and has a prominent head end (scolex) that has a groove (bothria) on each side. The segments (proglottids) are rectangular. The adult tapeworm can damage or even obstruct

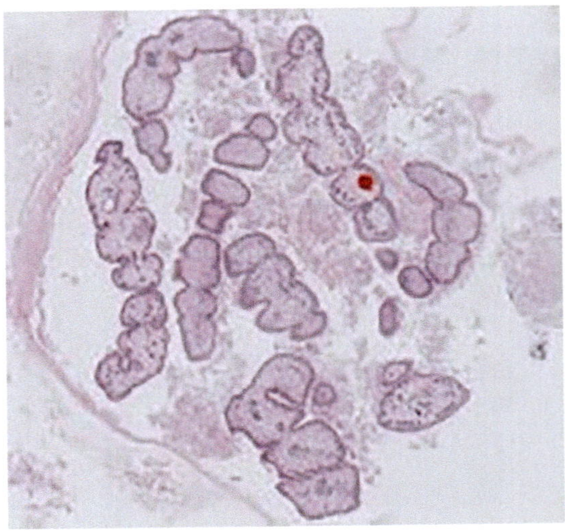

Fig. 19.10. Histopathology image of tapeworms in the intestines of a Gila chub (*Gila intermedia*). (Microphotograph by Ethan Biswell DVM MS Dipl ACVP.)

the anterior intestines. Clinical signs of cestode infestation in fish include anorexia, weight loss, swollen abdomen, lethargy, and muscle loss. Fish become infested with this tapeworm by ingesting copepod crustacea (the intermediate host) that contain plerocercoids. Treat with praziquantel injection (25 mg/kg BW) or with praziquantel 0.50% medicated food; prevent by not feeding live copepods to the fish. Treat the pond with antiparasitic medications used for crustacean parasites (e.g. trichlorfon) to eliminate copepods in the pond.

Caryophyllaeus fimbriceps is a non-segmented tapeworm that is parasitic in the intestines of fish. Its intermediate hosts are oligochaete worms of the genera *Tubifex* and *Limnodrilus*. Eating the worm host infests the fish. Large numbers of tapeworms can cause intestinal inflammation and weight loss. Treat with praziquantel 0.50% added to the food. Avoid feeding live oligochaete worms to fish (Saint-Erne, 2010).

19.5 Acanthocephala

Acanthocephala are also known as "spiny-headed worms" (Nicholas, 1973). There are approximately 1100 species, of which nearly half are found as adults in the intestines of fishes. They are identified by the hooks and proboscis of their attachment organs (Richardson, 2013). On the anterior portion of these parasites is a proboscis armed with recurved hooks aligned in a longitudinal or spiral pattern. These worms can affect a wide range of hosts. They are white to slightly yellow in color and sexually dimorphic. They require a vertebrate definitive host and arthropods as the intermediate hosts. Mating occurs in the definitive fish host's intestines. Eggs are passed in the feces and ingested by an intermediate host, often a crustacean. Acanthors hatch from the eggs. Then, the acanthor penetrates through the intermediate intestines as an acanthella, where it encysts as a cystacanth in the serosa. Once the intermediate host is ingested, the cystacanth activates in the final fish host and matures into the adult (Woo, 2006). These worms contain no digestive tract. They use the hooked proboscis to attach inside the intestines of the fish. They absorb predigested nutrients directly across the tegument. Very little pathology is associated with this parasite unless they are in heavy numbers, in which cases they have been reported to cause ill-thrift, lethargy, and anorexia. Treatment with loperamide at 50 mg/kg BW given orally for 3 consecutive days has been used.

19.6 Nematodes

The phylum Nematoda, also known as roundworms, encompasses a very large number of species of worms. Unlike flatworms, they have tubular digestive systems with openings at both ends. Nematodes have successfully adapted to nearly every ecosystem: from marine to freshwater, and in soil, and they are found from the polar regions to the tropics, as well as from the highest to the lowest of elevations. The many parasitic forms include pathogens in most plant and animal species. Clinical signs that occur in fish infested with roundworms include anemia, lethargy, poor weight gain, failure to thrive, and a decrease in reproductive rates.

19.6.1 Anguillicoloid nematodes

Anguillicoloides is a Dracunculoidea nematode that is specific to eels (Koie, 1991). *Anguillicoloides* genus contains five species, all of which are oviparous. These worms target the swim bladder and degrade hemoglobin, causing hypoxia signs. With an indirect lifecycle, planktonic crustacea (copepods and ostracods) are the intermediate hosts and eels are the final hosts. The life cycle of *Anguillicoloides crassus* begins when the adult nematode releases thousands of eggs in the eel's swimbladder. The eggs hatch within the eel, and the larvae leave the swim bladder through the pneumatic duct, then enter the gastrointestinal tract of the eel. Larvae are passed out into the water with the host's feces and then they penetrate into a copepod. The copepod is ingested by an eel, and the larvae migrate through the intestinal wall, body cavity, and into the swim bladder of the eel (De Charleroy *et al.*, 1990). With low numbers of worms, eels are often asymptomatic and are found to have a fibrotic swim bladder on necropsy. In heavy infestations, eels can be easily stressed during handling. They will be at higher risk for secondary bacterial infections. Both acute hemorrhage into the swim bladder and rupture of the swim bladder have been reported. In large populations, a decreased growth rate has been seen. Treatments include fenbendazole, levamisole, and piperazine. However, once a parasite is encysted in the swim bladder it is difficult to eliminate.

19.6.2 Anisakidae nematodes

Contracaecum is a genus of parasitic nematodes from the family Anisakidae. These nematodes are parasites of the stomach or small intestines of fish-eating mammals and birds (Lymbery *et al.*, 2002). The eggs and the successive stages of their larvae use invertebrates and fishes as intermediate hosts. It is the only genus in the family Anisakidae that can infect terrestrial, marine, and freshwater animals. The adult roundworms live in the paratenic host's GI tract. The eggs are shed in feces and hatch in the water. The larvae are ingested by invertebrates within the environment, and then those invertebrates are ingested by the fish as a secondary host in the lifecycle. Within the fish, *Contracaecum* targets the liver and tissue adjacent to the dorsal aorta. They can cause death in fish that are in poor condition, or when the worms migrate into cardiac tissue. *Contracaecum* larvae can infest humans. The human infestation of Anisakidae nematodes such as *Contracaecum* is called anisakiasis.

19.6.3 Ascarid nematodes

Ascaridida is an order of nematodes that have an indirect lifecycle where fish are the intermediate host, or a paratenic host, with encysted larvae in their muscles or viscera. Ascarids in the genus *Eustrongylides* encyst in the muscle and coelom of fish. Eustrongylides are typically very long, coiled, and red (due to presence of hemoglobin). They have an indirect lifecycle with a definitive host being a wading bird. The first intermediate host is oligochaetes and other worms. Affected fish typically have bloated abdomens (dropsy), as the nematodes frequently migrate into the body cavity from the gut. In small numbers, these roundworms often cause no mortalities but can decrease the ability to sell fish for food. Control of these parasites involves targeting the intermediate hosts and preventing birds from having access to the fish ponds.

19.6.4 Camallanid nematodes

Camallanus worms are small, red, thread-like worms (Fig. 19.11) that can be seen protruding from the anus of their host (Kim *et al.*, 2002). If disturbed, the worm will retreat into the fish's intestines. They have been commonly reported in guppies, angelfish, discus, and other cichlids (Fig. 19.12). They have an indirect lifecycle and are ovoviviparous, as females

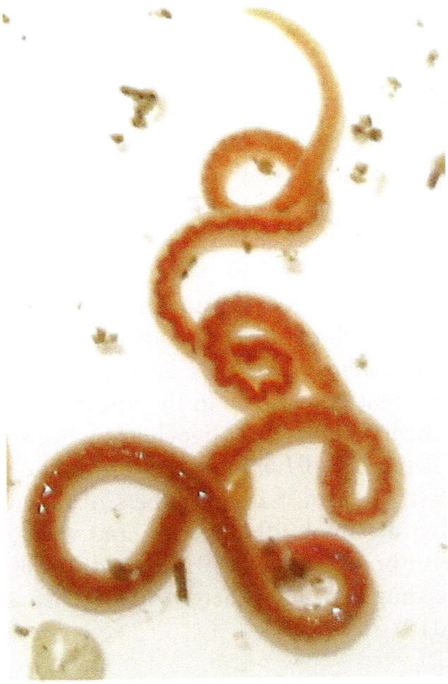

Fig. 19.11. *Camallanus* worm removed from the intestines of a fish during necropsy. (Photograph by N. Saint-Erne.)

incubate the eggs, which hatch into larvae within their bodies. The larvae are released into the water with the fish's feces and are ingested by a crustacean, usually a copepod. Within the copepod, the larvae further develop. After the copepod-containing larvae are eaten by the fish, the larvae migrate into the fish's intestines, there developing into reproductive adults (Yanong, 2017). These worms can cause emaciation due to gastrointestinal ulcerations. Treatment is with fenbendazole 25–50 mg/kg BW, added to the food or as a bath treatment.

19.6.5 Capillariidae nematodes

The Capillariidae family includes many genera of parasitic nematodes. *Capillaria pterophylli*, a parasite found in the GI tract of angelfish. *Capillostrongyloides ancistri* has been reported in bushy-mouth catfish. *Pseudocapillaria tomentosa* has also been reported in a variety of hosts. In general, these worms cause chronic wasting or poor weight gain in heavy numbers. They cause severe inflammation in the fish host's gastrointestinal tract and visceral cavity, as these worms can migrate through tissues to their target organ. In zebrafish, they have been reported to cause neoplasia and

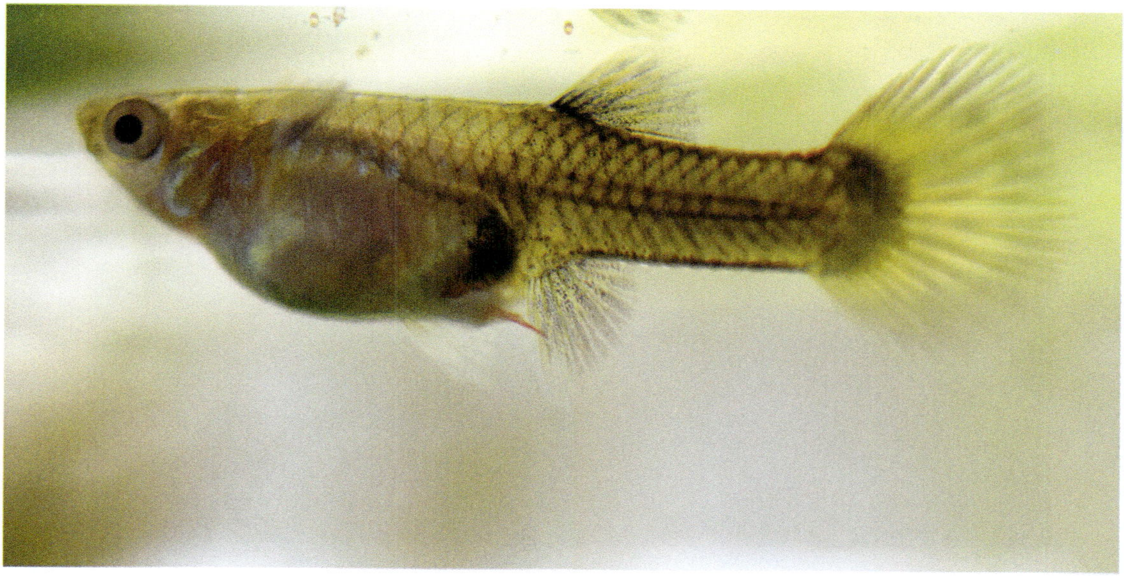

Fig. 19.12. Female Guppy (*Poecilia reticulata*) with a parasitic nematode, *Camallanus cotti*, protruding from her vent. https://commons.wikimedia.org/wiki/File:190729_Guppy_01.jpg BlueBreezeWiki, CC BY-SA 3.0.

tumor formation. They have become a problem in zebrafish research laboratories, as they can affect the outcome of a research study, depending on the purpose of the study. Up to 10% of research facilities were found to have *Capillostrongyloides* within their fish stock. Mortalities are not common but have been reported in heavy infestations.

Capillariidae species have direct life cycles and can spread from one fish to another by ingestion of infective larvae. *Capillaria* is a long, thin roundworm found within the fish's intestines (Fig. 19.13). Its attachment to the wall of the intestines can lead to areas of necrosis and secondary bacterial infections. It may reduce growth rate and reproductive ability of the fish. Feces of affected fish may contain excessive mucus. Diagnosis can be made by finding the operculated eggs during a microscopic examination of a fecal sample (Fig. 19.14). Ova with bipolar caps will be seen in infested fish fecal material. It may take *Capillaria pterophylli* eggs up to 3 weeks at 20–23°C before they contain embryos developed enough to be infective when ingested by a fish. The length of time required from infection until the mature adult parasites are producing eggs or larvae is approximately 3 months at these temperatures. Even though *Capillaria* species have direct life cycles, a tubifex worm may act as a paratenic host and carry infective stages of *Capillaria*. In the laboratory setting, it has been shown that *Capillostrongyloides* can spread by direct transmission (Kent *et al.*, 2002).

Treat with fenbendazole 0.25% in the food for 2 days, and then repeat treatment in 2 weeks. Recheck the fecal sample to evaluate treatment success. Repeat treatment as necessary (Saint-Erne, 2010). Other treatment options include mebendazole, trichlorfon, emamectin, ivermectin, and levamisole (Collymore *et al.*, 2014). It is important to note brood stock may become sterile when levamisole is used. Other reported effective protocols include fenbendazole at 0.125 mg/l fed to artemia, then feeding the artemia to the fish. However, treatment with fenbendazole caused malformed or dead embryos after treatment initially, but the breeders produced normal clutches the next breeding cycle. Control within a population can involve bleach treatment of fish eggs or depopulating and restocking from a pathogen-free stock. It has been shown that UV treatment of the water can decrease the parasite load (Kent *et al.*, 2019).

19.7 Leeches

Leeches are annelid worms that are closely related to the oligochaetes, which include the earthworm. They have muscular segmented bodies that can

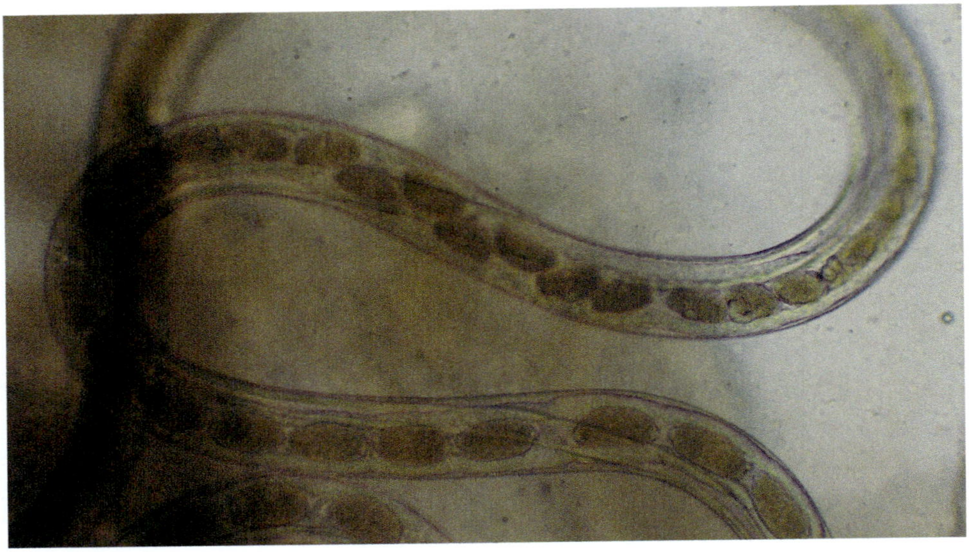

Fig. 19.13. *Capillaria* worm carrying eggs. (Microphotograph by N. Saint-Erne.)

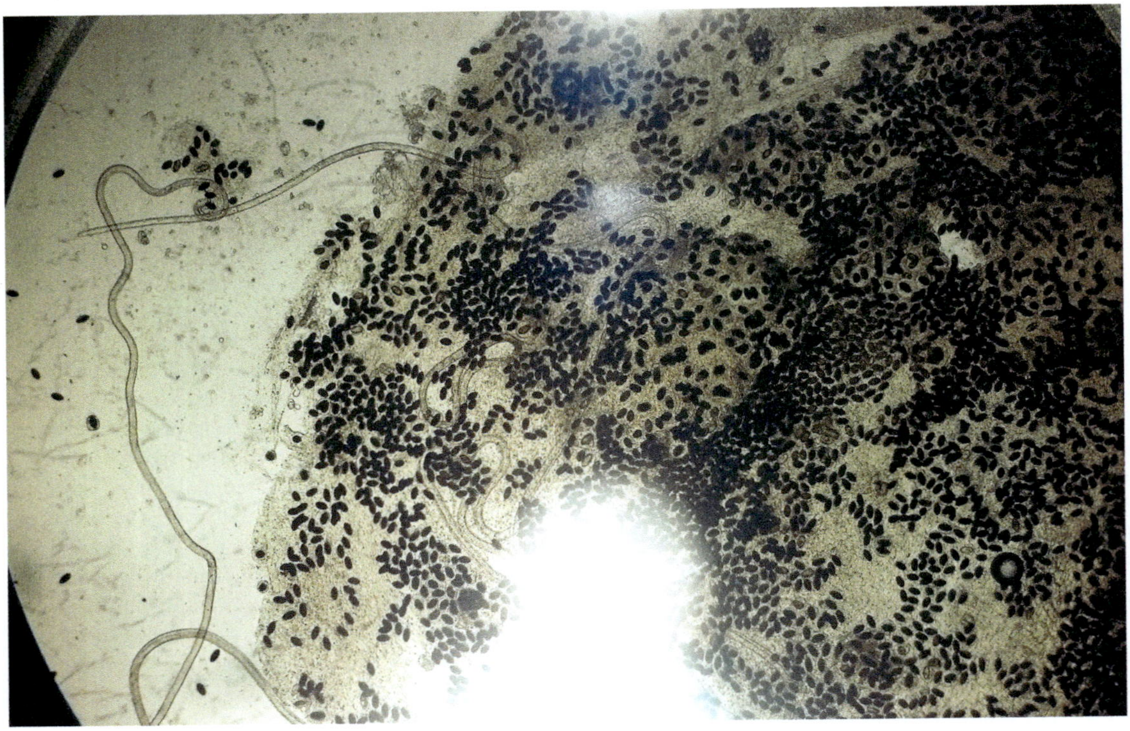

Fig. 19.14. *Capillaria* worms and massive number of eggs from the intestines of a fish, found on necropsy. (Microphotograph by N. Saint-Erne.)

lengthen and contract by use of suckers at both ends (Fig. 19.15). There are over 680 species of leeches, with about 100 marine species, 480 freshwater, and 100 terrestrial species (Sket and Trontelj, 2008). Not all species of leeches are parasitic, but parasitic species are hematophagous. Leeches are hermaphroditic, and mating may occur on or off the fish host. After feeding, the adult leech lays eggs within a cocoon that it attaches to the substrate or plants. When the eggs hatch, the juvenile leeches must find a fish for feeding but can live for a week or more before feeding. These parasitic annelid worms are not commonly seen in the ornamental fish market, but when they occur in heavy numbers, leeches can cause severe anemia and secondary bacterial infections. They are more often seen in wild-caught or pond-raised fish. Affected fish can appear listless, lethargic, and hyporexic. They may swim in an agitated fashion. Reddened areas on the skin can be a sign of previous attachment points of leeches, as they secrete anticoagulants to prevent blood from clotting at a feeding site.

Leeches can be vectors for viral infections, as well as *Cryptobia* and *Trypanosoma* parasites. Leeches should be picked off fish when seen, and the skin swabbed with a disinfectant. Soaking affected freshwater fish in a 2–3% salt solution for 10–20 min will cause the leeches to drop from the host. Trichlorfon at 0.25–0.50 mg/l added to the water will kill leeches in a fish pond (Saint-Erne, 2010). In heavily infested environments, the pond or tank can be drained, dried, and treated with lime and allowed to remain dry for a few weeks.

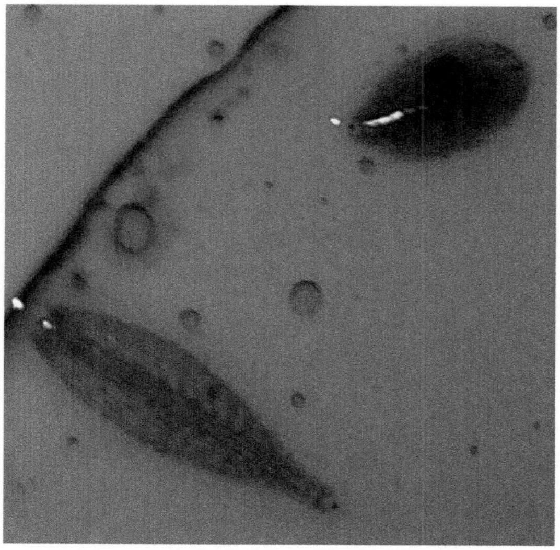

Fig. 19.15. Two leeches, one is extended using the suckers at each end of the body, and one is contracted. (Photograph by N. Saint-Erne.)

19.8 Crustacea

Crustacea are a subphylum of the Arthropods. The crustacean class Copepoda contains anchor worms (*Lernaea*) and gill maggots (*Ergasilus*). The Branchiura class encompasses crustacean parasites commonly known as fish lice (*Argulus*). Pentastomida is a subclass of the Crustacea (Kabata, 1970).

Pentastomids are vermiform, obligate parasites that have a mouth flanked by two paired hooks. All species attain sexual maturity in the respiratory tract of vertebrates; 70% of the definitive hosts are snakes, followed by crocodiles, lizards, amphibians, and turtles. Two species occur in marine birds, and one occurs in the nasopharynx of canines. Intermediate hosts include fish, amphibians, lizards, snakes, insects, and mammals, although a few species may have a direct life cycle (Riley, 1983). About 130 species of pentastomids are known; all are obligate parasites. Pentastomids are worm-like animals 1–14 cm in length. The female is larger than the male. The anterior end of the body bears five protuberances, four of which are clawed legs, while the fifth bears the mouth. The body is segmented and covered in a chitinous cuticle. Infestations have been found in several families of fish including the Cichlidae (tilapia), Cyprinidae (danios), Cyprinodontidae (flagfish), and Poecilidae (mosquito fish, swordtails, mollies, platys, guppies). Pentastomids in fish resemble small white, segmented worms. However, they are more closely related to *Argulus* fish lice.

Pentastomids have an indirect life cycle, where fish are the intermediate host. Adults of the pentastomid species that infest fish are found in reptiles, which are their final hosts. The adult stages of the parasite are found in the respiratory systems of reptiles, usually within the lungs and/or trachea. The adult pentastomids in the reptile deposit eggs that are coughed up, swallowed, and then passed through the reptile's gastrointestinal tract, where they are deposited into the water in the feces. The eggs develop into the infective stage and, after being eaten by the fish, the larvae hatch out and grow within the fish. After infected fish are eaten by the final reptile host, the parasite perforates the intestinal wall, migrating through the body to the lungs. When the pentastomid matures, the life cycle is completed.

Pentastomids can be found encapsulated in many different locations within fish, producing swellings of the skin, muscle damage, and organ damage. Primary prevention of pentastomid infestations in fish requires control of the final hosts: aquatic turtles, water snakes, and alligators. Fish in ponds with any of these predators may be susceptible to pentastomid infections (Yanong, 2019).

Lernaea are also commonly known as "anchor worms." It is frequently seen in freshwater species, most commonly in koi and goldfish (Fig. 19.16). These copepod crustacea have free-swimming larval stages. Once mature, the adult male (170 × 780 μm) will mate with a female and then die. The mature female may be up to 4 cm long. The fertilized female develops an anchor-shaped head, which it embeds into the skin of the host fish (Fig. 19.17). This causes a reddened sore, which may become secondarily infected with bacteria. The female develops two large egg sacs on its external end, containing several hundred eggs each. The egg sacs are shed when the eggs are ready to hatch. The nauplii hatch from the eggs and break out of the egg sac. The female will then develop new egg sacs. At the optimal temperature of 25°C, egg sacs are produced every 2 weeks. Temperatures below 14°C inhibit their reproduction. In winter, anchor worms can hibernate in the pond and cause an epidemic in early spring as the temperature warms (Saint-Erne, 2010). Treat by gently extracting the parasite with forceps, being careful not to leave any of the anterior anchor behind. Treat the wound with topical disinfectant. Trichlorfon organophosphate or Dimilin can be used to kill the free-living juvenile stage. Lernaea are also inhibited by 2% salt solutions for short duration (10–20 min) baths.

Ergasilus copepods (gill maggots) attach to fish's gill filaments with specialized claws formed from the second pair of antennae. Only the gravid female is parasitic. After mating with a free-swimming male, the female finds a host on which to feed while developing eggs. The two large white egg sacs that develop on the female's posterior resemble maggots. Each egg sac can contain more than 100 eggs. The eggs are retained in the female's egg sacs until they hatch. After hatching, the juveniles are free-living in the water until they mature and mate. Treat with trichlorfon (0.25 mg/l) or Dimilin (0.13 mg/l) once weekly for three doses. They are not a problem in small numbers, but heavy infestations can cause severe focal damage.

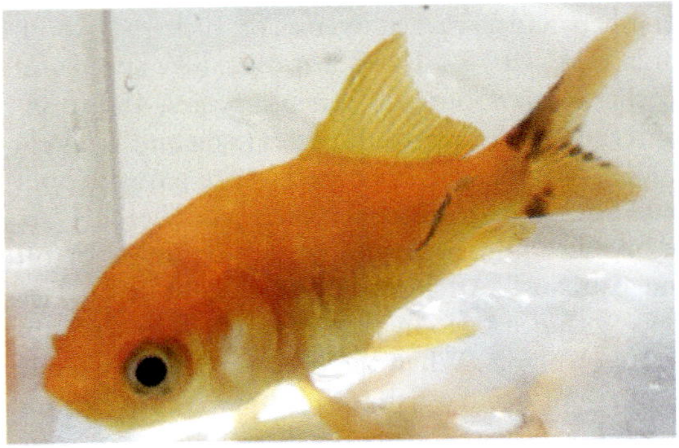

Fig. 19.16. Female anchor worm attached to the side of a goldfish (*Carassius auratus*). (Photograph by N. Saint-Erne.)

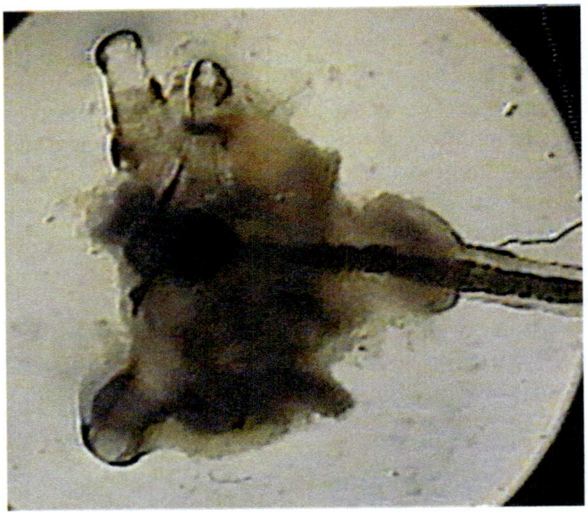

Fig. 19.17. Photograph of the anchor portion of the anchor worm that embeds under the skin of the fish. (Microphotograph by N. Saint-Erne.)

Argulus (fish lice) are found on the skin and in heavy numbers will cause ulcerations and resulting secondary bacterial infections. These are oval, flattened Branchiurans with two prominent compound eyes, two sucking discs, and a stylet anterior to the mouth (Fig. 19.18). This stylet repeatedly pierces the skin of the fish and releases

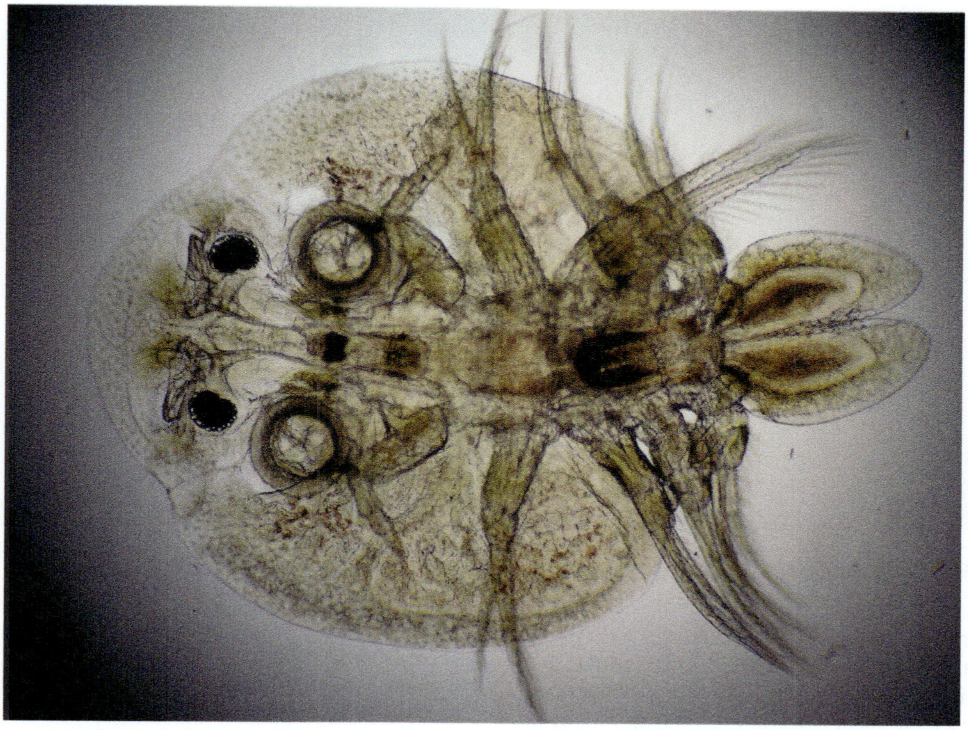

Fig. 19.18. *Argulus* under 40× magnification on a microscope. (Microphotograph by N. Saint-Erne.)

toxic secretions. They feed on the tissue fluids released by this trauma. The feeding habits of fish lice create local hyperemia, hyperpigmentation, epidermal hyperplasia, dermal hemorrhage, and loss of scales. These lice can act as vectors for viral disease in fish. Affected fish flash frequently. Skin ulcers from secondary bacterial or fungal infections are common in fish affected with *Argulus*.

The adult female fish louse lays a thin strip of eggs on submerged objects near the water surface. After laying eggs the female will swim away to find a fish host. The eggs hatch in 2–8 weeks depending on temperature. The larvae must attach to a fish to feed within the first 3 days but can swim between fish after feeding. They are freely moving on the host and swim well. They mature in 3–6 weeks. Adults can grow to 1 cm long. Reproduction ceases in temperatures below 14°C.

Argulus are seen mostly in koi and goldfish raised in ponds (Fig. 19.19). For best control, treat the pond with trichlorfon (0.25 mg/l) on a weekly basis for 4–8 weeks. Dimilin (0.13 mg/l) and lufenuron (409.8 mg tablet/1000 gallons) have also been used for control of fish lice.

19.9 Mollusk Parasites

The larvae (glochidia) of freshwater bivalve mollusks (clams) of the family Unionidae attach to the fins and gills of fish. There they feed by osmotic absorption from the surrounding tissue. After a feeding period of several months, they drop off and mature. Not placing freshwater clams into the aquarium or pond will prevent this temporary parasite.

19.10 Conclusion

Metazoan parasites are multicellular eukaryotic organisms that can cause significant lesions in ornamental fish. There are several phyla of Metazoa that contain species that parasitize fish, including Platyhelminthes (Classes: Monogenea, Digenea,

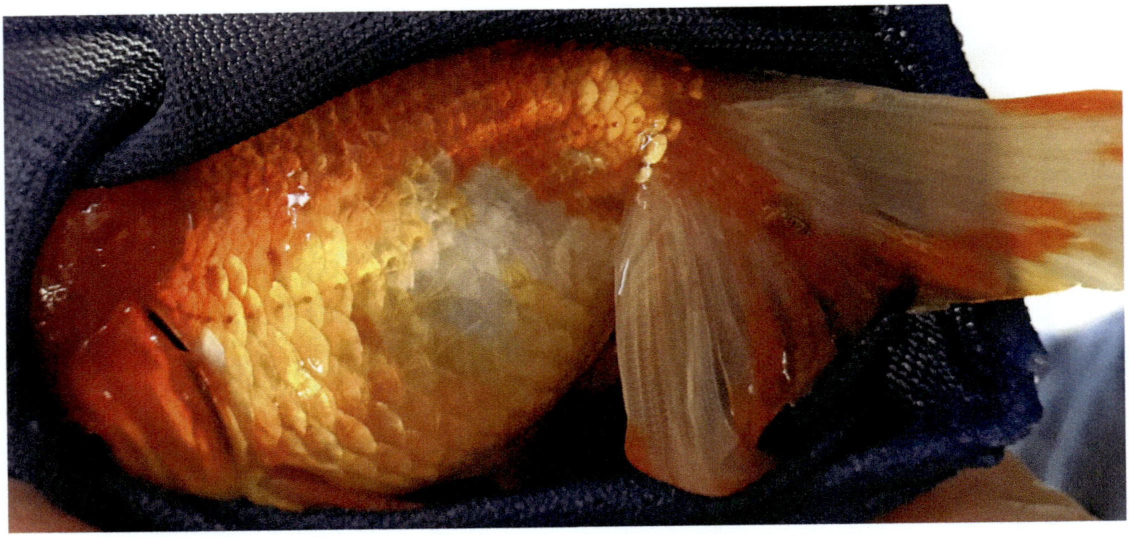

Fig. 19.19. *Argulus* on the caudal fin of an oranda goldfish (*C. auratus*). (Photograph by N. Saint-Erne.)

Turbellaria, Cestoda), Acanthocephala, Nematoda, Annelida, Arthropods (Crustacea), and Mollusk. It is important to properly diagnose fish diseases and identify the etiologic agent. Parasites can spread rapidly in some cases and require the appropriate treatments to eliminate them from the pond or aquarium.

References

Becker, J.H. and Grutter, A.S. (2004) Cleaner shrimp do clean. *Coral Reefs* 23, 515–520.

Brazenor, A.K. and Hutson, K.S. (2015) Effects of temperature and salinity on the life cycle of *Neobenedenia* sp. (Monogenea: Capsalidae) infecting farmed barramundi (*Lates calcarifer*). *Parasitology Research* 114(5), 1875–1886.

Brazenor, A.K., Saunders, R.J., Miller, T.L. and Hutson, K.S. (2018) Morphological variation in the cosmopolitan fish parasite *Neobenedenia girellae* (Capsalidae: Monogenea). *International Journal for Parasitology* 48(2), 125–134.

Buchmann, K., Mellergaard, S. and Køie, M. (1987) *Pseudodactylogyrus* infections in eel—a review. *Diseases of Aquatic Organisms* 3, 51–57.

Cable, J., Scott, E.C.G., Tinsley, R.C. and Harris, P.D. (2002) Behavior favoring transmission in the viviparous monogenean *Gyrodactylus turnbulli*. *The Journal of Parasitology* 88(1): 183.

Calhoun, D.M., Leslie, K.L., Riepe, T.B., Achatz, T.J., McDevitt-Galles, T. *et al.* (2019) Patterns of *Clinostomum marginatum* infection in fishes and amphibians: integration of field, genetic, and experimental approaches. *Journal of Helminthology* 94:e44. doi:10.1017/S0022149X18001244.

Cannon, L. and Lester, R. (1988) Two turbellarians parasitic in fish. *Diseases of Aquatic Organisms* 5, 15–22.

Cheung, P.J. and Ruggieri, G.D. (1983) *Dermophthirius nigrellii* n. sp. (Monogenea: Microbothriidae), an ectoparasite from the skin of the lemon shark, *Negaprion brevirostris*. *Transactions of the American Microscopical Society* 102(2): 129.

Collymore, C., Watral, V., White, J.R., Colvin, M.E., Rasmussen, S. *et al.* (2014) Tolerance and Efficacy of Emamectin Benzoate and Ivermectin for the Treatment of *Pseudocapillaria tomentosa* in Laboratory Zebrafish (*Danio rerio*). *Zebrafish* 11(5), 490–497.

Cowell, L., Watanabea, W., Head, W., Grovepd, J. and Shenkepjb, J. (1993) Use of tropical cleaner fish to control the ectoparasite *Neobenedenia melhi* (Monogenea: Capsalidae) on seawater-cultured Florida red tilapia. *Aquaculture* 113, 189–200.

De Charleroy, D., Grisez, L., Thomas, K., Belpaire, C. and Ollevier, F. (1990) The life cycle of *Anguillicola crassus*. *Diseases of Aquatic Organisms* 8, 77–84. Available at: https://www.int-res.com/articles/dao/8/d008p077.pdf (accessed 24 November 2019).

Dinh Hoai, T. and Hutson, K.S. (2014) Reproductive strategies of the insidious fish ectoparasite, *Neobenedenia* sp. (Capsalidae: Monogenea). *PLoS ONE* 9(9): e108801.

Dove, A.D.M. and Ernst, I. (1998) Concurrent invaders—four exotic species of Monogenea now established on exotic freshwater fishes in Australia. *International Journal for Parasitology* 28(11), 1755–1764.

Ellis, E. and Watanabe, W. (1993). The effects of hyposalinity on eggs, juveniles and adults of the marine monogenean, *Neobenedenia melleni*, Treatment of ectoparasitosis in seawater-cultured tilapia. *Aquaculture* 117, 15–27.

Francis-Floyd, R.K. (2019) *Monogenean Parasites of Fish*. Available at: https://edis.ifas.ufl.edu/fa033 (accessed 20 November 2020).

Gannicott, A.M. and Tinsley, R.C. (1998) Environmental effects on transmission of *Discocotyle sagittata* (Monogenea): egg production and development. *Parasitology* 117(5), 499–504.

Hadfield, C. and Clayton, L. (2021) *Clinical Guide to Fish Medicine*. Wiley, Hoboken, New Jersey.

Harris, P.D., Shinn, A.P., Cable, J. and Bakke, T.A. (2004) Nominal species of the genus *Gyrodactylus* von Nordmann 1832 (Monogenea: Gyrodactylidae), with a list of principal host species. *Systematic Parasitology* 59(1), 1–27.

Hirazawa, N., Akiyama, K. and Umeda, N. (2013) Differences in sensitivity to the anthelmintic praziquantel by the skin-parasitic monogeneans *Benedenia seriolae* and *Neobenedenia girellae*. *Aquaculture* 404–405, 59–64.

Iaria, C., Migliore, S., Macri, D., Bivona, M., Capparucci, F. *et al.* (2019) Evidence of *Centrocestus formosanus* (Nishigori, 1924) in Zebrafish (*Danio rerio*). *Zebrafish* 16(6), 522–526.

Justine, J., Leblanc, P., Keller, F. and Lester, R. (2009) Turbellarian black spot disease in bluespine unicornfish *Naso unicornis* in New Caledonia, caused by the parasitic turbellarian *Piscinquilinus* sp. *Diseases of Aquatic Organisms* 85, 245–249.

Kabata, Z. (1970) *Diseases of Fishes, Book 1: Crustacea as Enemies of Fishes*. T.F.H. Publications, Neptune, New Jersey.

Katahira, H., Mizuno, K., Umino, T. and Nagasawa, K. (2012) Influence of host habitat on the occurrence of gill monogeneans *Pseudodactylogyrus* spp. on wild Japanese eels *Anguilla japonica*. *Diseases of Aquatic Organisms* 100(1), 43–49.

Katharios, P., Papandroulakis, N. and Divanach, P. (2006) Treatment of *Microcotyle* sp. (Monogenea) on the gills of cage-cultured red porgy, *Pagrus pagrus* following baths with formalin and mebendazole. *Aquaculture* 251(2–4), 167–171.

Kent, M., Bishop-Stewart, J., Matthews, J. and Spitsbergen, J. (2002) *Pseudocapillaria tomentosa*, a nematode pathogen, and associated neoplasms of zebrafish (*Danio rerio*) kept in research colonies. *Comparative Medicine* 53(4), 354–358.

Kent, M.L., Watral, V., Villegas, E.N. and Gaulke, C.A. (2019) Viability of *Pseudocapillaria tomentosa* eggs exposed to heat, ultraviolet light, chlorine, iodine, and desiccation. *Zebrafish* 16(5), 460–468.

Kim, J.-H., Hayward, C.J. and Heo, G.-J. (2002) Nematode worm infections (*Camallanus cotti*, Camallanidae) in guppies (*Poecilia reticulata*) imported to Korea. *Aquaculture* 205(3–4), 231–235.

Klinger, R.E. and Floyd, R.F. (2013) *Introduction to Freshwater Fish Parasites*. Available at: http://edis.ifas.ufl.edu/FA041 (accessed 12 November 2020).

Koie, M. (1991) Swimbladder nematodes (*Anguillicola* spp.) and gill monogeneans (*Pseudodactylogyrus* spp.) parasitic on the European eel (*Anguilla anguilla*). *ICES Journal of Marine Science* 47(3), 391–398.

Lane, B., Spier, T., Wiederholt, J. and Meagher, S. (2015) Host specificity of a parasitic fluke: is *Posthodiplostomum minimuma* centrarchid-infecting generalist or specialist? *Journal of Parasitology* 101(1), 6–17.

Lymbery, A., Doupé, R., Munshi, M. and Wong, T. (2002) Larvae of *Contracaecum* sp. among inshore fish species of southwestern Australia. *Diseases of Aquatic Organisms* 51, 157–159.

Morales-Serna, F.N., Chapa-López, M., Martínez-Brown, J.M., Ibarra-Castro, L., Medina-Guerrero, R.M. and Fajer-Ávila, E.J. (2018) Efficacy of praziquantel and a combination anthelmintic (Adecto®) in bath treatments against *Tagia ecuadori* and *Neobenedenia melleni* (Monogenea), parasites of bullseye puffer fish. *Aquaculture* 492, 361–368.

Nicholas, W.L. (1973) The biology of the acanthocephala. *Advances in Parasitology* 11, 671–706.

Noble, A.C. and Summerfelt, S.T. (1996) Diseases encountered in rainbow trout cultured in recirculating systems. *Annual Review of Fish Diseases* 6, 65–92.

Plumb, J.A. (1999) Overview of warmwater fish diseases. *Journal of Applied Aquaculture* 9(2), 1–10.

Rica, C., Marques, F., Brooks, D. and Monks, S. (1995) Five new species of Acanthobothrium Van Beneden, 1849 (Eucestoda: Tetraphyllidea: Onchobothriidae) in stingrays from the gulf of Nicoya. *The Journal of Parasitology* 81(6), 942–951.

Richardson, D. (2013) Acanthocephala. Available at: https://onlinelibrary.wiley.com/doi/abs/10.1002/9780470015902.a0001595.pub2 (accessed 20 March 2021).

Riley, J. (1983) Recent advances in our understanding of pentastomid reproductive biology. *Parasitology* 86, 59–83.

Roberts, H.E., Palmeiro, B. and Weber, E.S. (2009) Bacterial and parasitic diseases of pet fish. *Veterinary Clinics of North America: Exotic Animal Practice* 12(3), 609–638.

Rubio-Godoy, M. (2007) Fish host-monogenean parasite interactions, with special reference to Polyopisthocotylea. *Advances in the Immunobiology of Parasitic Diseases* 2007, 91–109.

Saint-Erne, N. (2010) Protozoal parasites. In: Saint-Erne, N. (ed.) *Advanced Koi Care*. 2nd edn. Erne Enterprises, Glendale, Arizona, pp. 73–79.

Santos, C.P., Mourão, E.D. and Cárdenas, M.Q. (2001) *Pseudempleurosoma gibsoni* n. sp., a new Ancyrocephalid Monogenean from *Paralonchurus brasiliensis* (Sciaenidae) from off the Southeastern Coast of Brazil. *Memórias do Instituto Oswaldo Cruz* 96(2), 215–219.

Sanz, F. (1992) Mortality of cultured seabream *(Sparus aurata [Pagrus aurata])* caused by an infection with a trematode of the genus *Microcotyle*. Available at: https://www.semanticscholar.org/paper/Mortality-of-cultured-seabream-(Sparus-aurata-by-an-Sanz/11dad79fa5d3ae314d943776babc3b3f6ff06faf (Accessed 11 March 2021).

Scholz, T. (1999) Parasites in cultured and feral fish. *Veterinary Parasitology* 84(3–4), 317–335.

Sket, B. and Trontelj, P. (2008) Global diversity of leeches (Hirudinea) in freshwater. *Hydrobiologia* 595(1), 129–137.

Soleng, A., Jansen, P. and Bakke, T. (1998) Transmission of the monogenean *Gyrodactylus salaris*. *Parasitology International* 47:319.

Whittington, I.D. (1996). *Benedeniine capsalid* monogeneans from Australian fishes: pathogenic species, site-specificity and camouflage. *Journal of Helminthology* 70(3), 177–184.

Whittington, I.D. (2004) The *Capsalidae* (Monogenea: Monopisthocotylea): a review of diversity, classification and phylogeny with a note about species complexes. *Folia Parasitologica* 51(2–3), 109–122.

Woo, P.T.K. (2006) *Fish Diseases and Disorders, Vol. 1 Protozoan and Metazoan Infections*. 2nd edn. CAB International, Wallingford, UK.

Yanong, R.P.E. (2017) *Nematode (Roundworm) Infections in Fish*. UF-IFAS Extension, Ruskin, Florida. Available at: https://edis.ifas.ufl.edu/publication/FA091 (accessed 1 August 2024).

Yanong, R.P.E. (2019) *Pentastomid Infections in Fish*. UF-IFAS Extension, Ruskin, Florida. Available at: https://edis.ifas.ufl.edu/publication/FA090 (accessed 1 August 2024).

Zhang, C., Li, D., Chi, C., Ling, F. and Wang, G. (2015) *Dactylogyrus intermedius* parasitism enhances *Flavobacterium columnare* invasion and alters immune-related gene expression in *Carassius auratus*. *Diseases of Aquatic Organisms* 116(1), 11–21.

20 Zoonotic Diseases from Fish

Nicholas Saint-Erne

Dr. Saint-Erne Consulting, PLLC, Phoenix, Arizona

Abstract

Zoonotic diseases are infections or parasitic infestations of humans that originate from animal sources. There are several microorganisms found in fish and in aquarium water that can be transmitted to humans. Zoonotic parasites can also be transmitted to humans by ingesting raw or undercooked fish.

20.1 Bacterial Infections

Bacterial infections from fish or from aquarium water can occur from contact with these common aquatic bacteria: *Aeromonas hydrophila, Clostridium botulinum, Edwardsiella tarda, Erysipelothrix rhusiopathiae, Mycobacterium, Pseudomonas, Salmonella, Streptococcus iniae,* and *Vibrio* species (Adeyemo and Foyle, 2022). These infections are most likely the result of accidental ingestion of water or material contaminated with the bacteria, from the bacteria coming into direct contact with cuts or abrasions on the person's skin, or becoming impaled by the spines of the fish's fins. People with a compromised immune system are especially susceptible to zoonotic pathogens.

20.1.1 Gram-negative bacteria

Most bacterial species that infect fish are gram-negative bacteria. *Aeromonas* are nonspore-forming, gram-negative, motile, facultative anaerobic, and rod-shaped bacteria. They are among the most prevalent bacteria in aquatic environments. They can cause diseases in aquarium fish when the fish become injured or stressed (Fig. 20.1). The most common source of infection in humans is from handling fish, and human infection can result in septicemia and gastroenteritis (Lowry and Smith, 2007).

The Enterobacteriaceae bacteria include *Edwardsiella, Escherichia, Klebsiella,* and *Salmonella* species. These are all gram-negative, facultative anaerobic rods that can live in freshwater environments. Necrotic skin lesions and gastroenteritis can occur in humans that become infected with *Edwardsiella tarda*. *Vibrio* bacteria are gram-negative, motile, facultative anaerobic, rods. They most often occur in marine environments. Infections in humans occur through puncture wounds from fish spines, or by ingestion, typically from eating raw shellfish. Clinical signs of infections in humans are necrotizing fasciitis, edema, and swelling at the puncture wound. Septicemia after ingestion of *V. vulnificus* from shellfish can sometimes cause death in clinically affected humans.

Leptospira is an aquatic bacterium that does not affect fish but can cause disease in humans and other mammals that are exposed to water contaminated with the urine of infected animals. This can occur in farm ponds that cattle drink from and urinate in, and then people swimming in the water, or handling fish from the water may become infected. It can also be transmitted to humans from rats and dogs. The *Leptospira* bacteria do not penetrate the skin but enter through ingestion, mucous membranes, or open wounds in the skin. *Leptospira* are spiral-shaped bacteria that are 6–20 μm long and 0.1 μm in diameter. These bacteria are found naturally throughout the world, except in Antarctica. A water pH of 6.9–7.4 is necessary for their survival in the environment, with rivers, shallow lakes, and ponds as well as stagnant water reservoirs being the natural habitat for the bacteria. Pathogenic *Leptospira* has been found in aquatic

Corresponding author: DrSaintErne@gmail.com

© CAB International 2025. *The Handbook of Ornamental Fish Health and Welfare* (ed. N. Saint-Erne)
DOI: 10.1079/9781789246032.0020

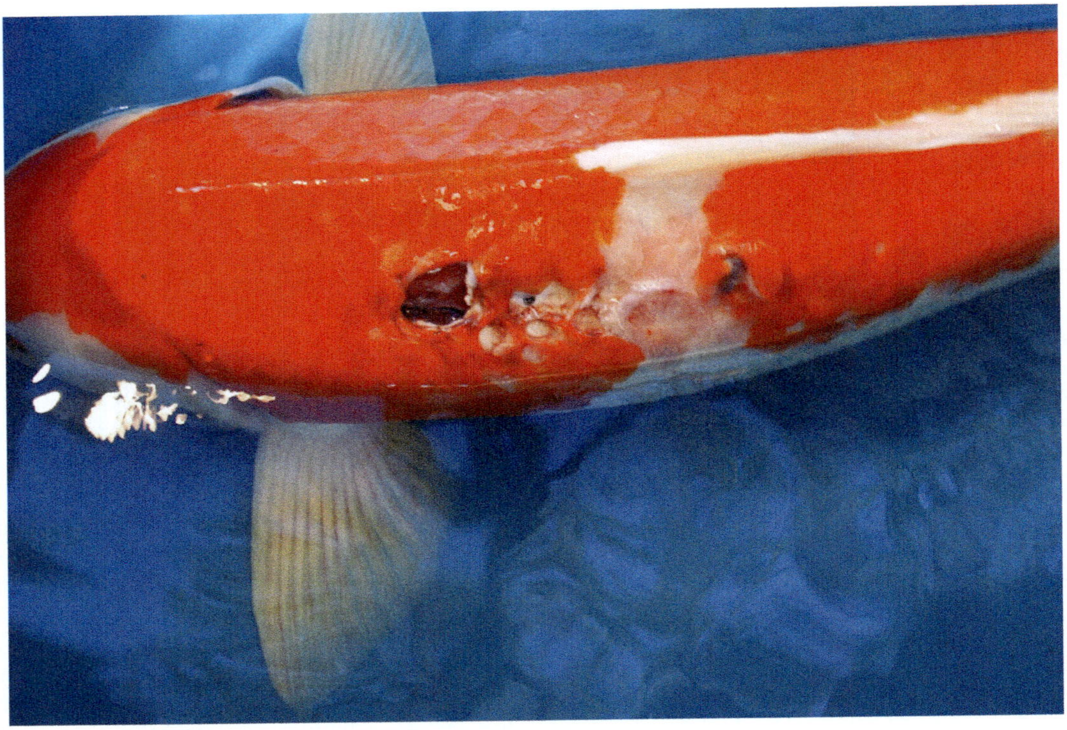

Fig. 20.1. Clinical signs of *Aeromonas* erythrodermatitis and skin ulceration in a koi (*Cyprinus rubrofuscus*). (Photograph by N. Saint-Erne.)

biofilms, which may aid survival in the environment. Occupations at risk of contracting leptospirosis include farmers, fishermen, and sewage workers.

20.1.2 Gram-positive bacteria

Clostridium species of bacteria are gram-positive rods that can be normal intestinal bacteria in many fish species and rarely cause disease in fish. Humans ingesting the clostridial toxin produced by vegetative cells can get gastroenteritis, diarrhea, and muscle paralysis that may result in death from respiratory system collapse (Lowry and Smith, 2007). *Erysipelothrix rhusiopathiae* is a gram-positive rod that is found in soil, freshwater, and marine water. Human infections with *E. rhusiopathiae* are typically obtained by punctures from the fish's fins during handling. The disease in humans can cause a localized skin infection, or a systemic infection in which the heart valves are targeted, resulting in endocarditis (Lowry and Smith, 2007).

Mycobacterium bacteria are gram-positive, aerobic, non-motile, non-spore-forming, acid-fast rods. They are slow-growing on culture media, so they are hard to diagnose through bacterial cultures. *Mycobacterium fortuitum* and *M. marinum* are recognized as the species most associated with tropical aquarium fish. Infected fish may act as reservoirs and transmit the infection to other fish in an aquarium or pond. People become infected by exposure of a cut on the hand to aquarium water or fish, hence the common name "fish handler's disease." A granulomatous nodule may form at the site of infection. *Streptococcus iniae* is a gram-positive, non-motile, coccus bacteria that can cause abdominal distention, epidermal petechiation, exophthalmia, and death in fish. Humans can develop cellulitis, arthritis, endocarditis, and fatal meningitis when infected.

20.2 Viral Zoonoses

Filter-feeding mollusks can bioaccumulate pathogenic viruses from the water. Humans can get enteric illnesses from eating virus-infected shellfish (Adeyemo and Foyle, 2022). These viral infections include hepatitis A, Norwalk-like virus, and enteroviruses. Symptoms in humans include meningitis, respiratory illnesses, myocarditis, fever, gastritis, diarrhea, rash, and nephritis. Proper sanitation when handling fish or preparing seafood can reduce the risk of viral diseases from fish and shellfish.

20.3 Parasitic Zoonoses

Humans can become infested with fish parasites from eating raw or undercooked fish. Fish-borne zoonotic digenean trematodes (*Haplorchis, Clonorchis,* and *Opisthorchis*), which are liver and intestinal flukes, can result in cholangiosarcomas in humans. The fluke, in humans, infests the common bile duct and gall bladder, feeding on bile (Wootten, 2012). *Anisakis* is a nematode of fish that uses mammals as a definitive host. Ingestion by humans of fish containing *Anisakis* larvae can lead to gastroenteritis, including vomiting and diarrhea. The larval nematode of *Angiostrongylus* (the rat lungworm) causes eosinophilic meningitis in humans. The adult worms are found in rats, and the first intermediate host is a mollusk, and both freshwater and marine fish can act as paratenic hosts. Humans are infected from eating the fish host. The tapeworms in the genus *Diphyllobothrium*, especially *D. latum,* have been found in humans from eating raw or undercooked fish that contain encysted plerocercoids (Fig. 20.2). Diphyllobothriasis can be a long-lasting infection, lasting up to 25 years. Most infections are asymptomatic, but gastrointestinal symptoms may occur in some patients. Aberrant migration of proglottids can cause cholecystitis or cholangitis. Rarely, massive infections may cause intestinal obstruction (CDC, 2019).

20.4 Preventing Zoonosis

To reduce the risk of disease spreading, remove dead fish promptly from the aquarium or pond and prevent access to other animals around fishponds (Hoole *et al.*, 2001). Wear gloves when handling fish

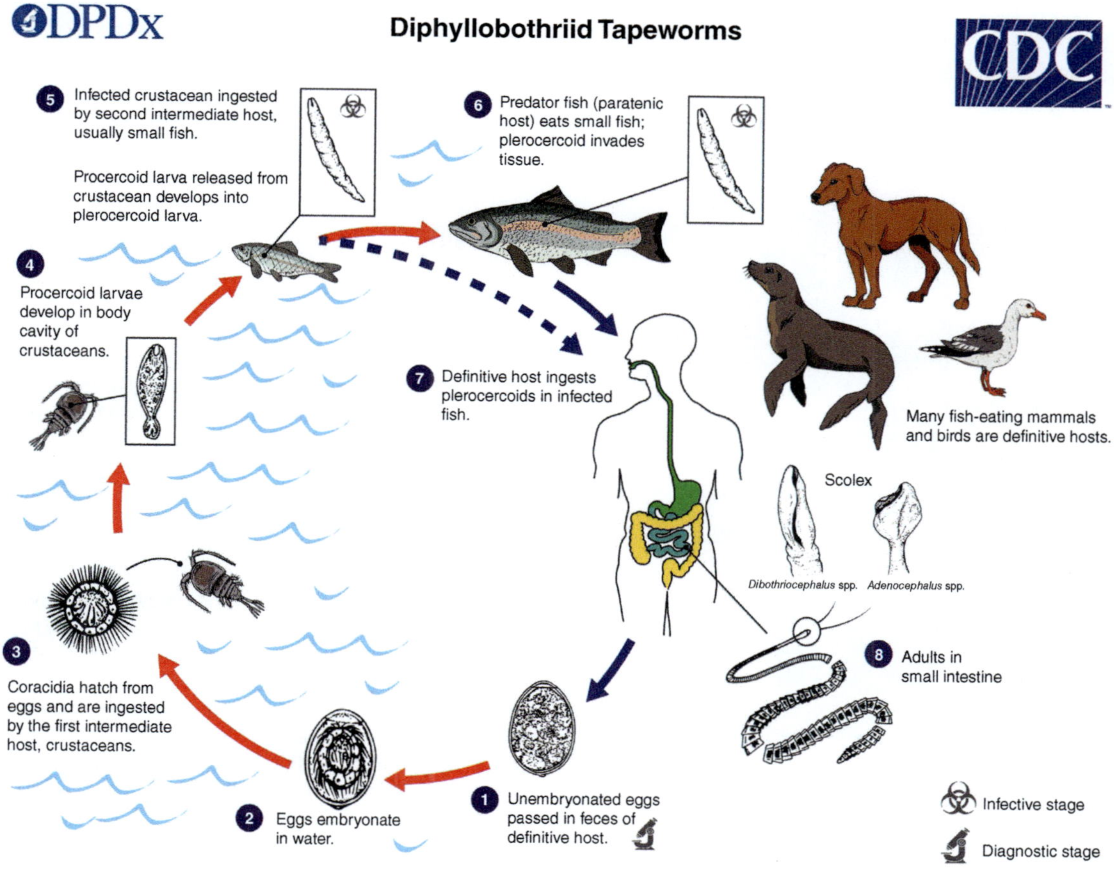

Fig. 20.2. Fish tapeworm (*Diphyllobothrium*) life cycle. (Image courtesy of the US Centers for Disease Control.)

or cleaning aquariums and equipment (Fig. 20.3). Always wash your hands thoroughly after handling fish, placing hands in aquariums, or cleaning the aquarium. Avoid contact with the aquarium if you have cuts or open sores on your hands or arms. Contact a physician if red, nonhealing sores or nodules occur on the skin and inform the doctor of the potential exposure to aquatic *Mycobacterium* or other infectious microorganisms.

It is best to not have aquariums in kitchens or food preparation areas. Avoid cleaning aquariums or dumping aquarium water in the kitchen sink or bathtub. Outdoor hoses should be used to clean aquarium filters and equipment. Children should always be supervised around aquariums. Children should be assisted with washing their hands if exposed to aquarium water.

Infants, children, pregnant women, elderly or ill adults, or persons with compromised immune systems (people with immunodeficiencies or that are receiving chemotherapy treatments) are more at risk of infectious diseases and should use caution when handling any animals.

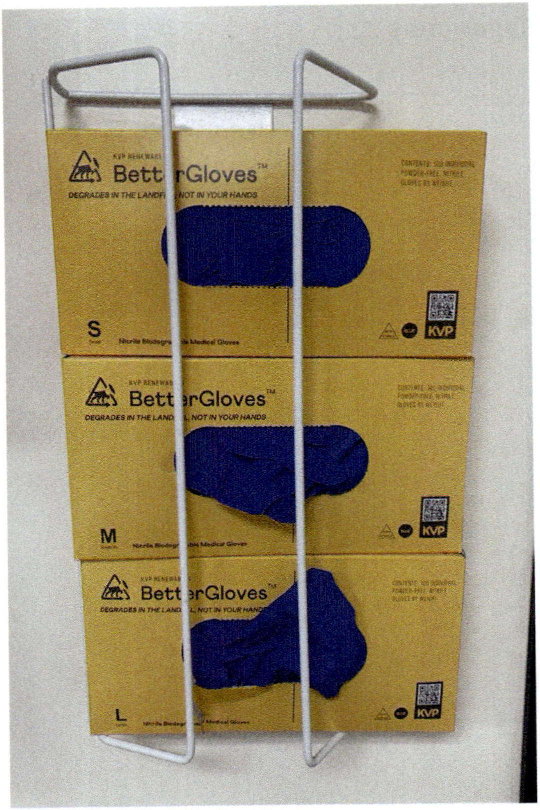

Fig. 20.3. Three sizes of gloves are available for employees to wear while working around aquariums at a fish wholesale facility. (Photograph by N. Saint-Erne.)

20.5 Conclusion

Biosecurity is important in diminishing the introduction of a pathogen into an aquarium. All new fish should be placed into a quarantine tank and examined and treated, as needed. By limiting infections and parasites entering the fish population, the risk of zoonotic diseases is also reduced. Avoiding contact with the fish and water is the prime way to prevent zoonotic infection; however, to provide proper care for fish in home aquariums, some contact with the water, or fish, will occur. Basic hygiene and thorough hand washing after contact with fish or aquarium water are good preventative protocols. Wearing gloves when working with the fish or the aquarium can prevent water contamination of cuts or scrapes, which are the entry point for aquatic pathogens (Lowry and Smith, 2007). Avoid eating raw or undercooked fish and seafood to prevent ingestion of zoonotic parasites. Flash freezing fish intended to be used as food to −20°C or below for 7 days is sufficient to kill parasites. This method is used by most Japanese restaurants to help prevent raw fish used in sushi and sashimi from spreading disease (FDA, 2017).

References

Adeyemo, O. and Foyle, L. (2022) Public health, zoonoses, and seafood safety. In: Urdes, L., Walster, C. and Tepper, J. (eds) *Fundamentals of Aquatic Veterinary Medicine*. Wiley, Hoboken, New Jersey, pp. 187–193.

CDC (2019) *Diphyllobothriasis*. Centers for Disease Control and Prevention, Atlanta, Georgia. Available at: https://www.cdc.gov/dpdx/diphyllobothriasis/ (accessed 1 August 2024).

FDA (2017) *Food Code*. US Food and Drug Administration, College Park, Maryland. Available at: https://www.fda.gov/media/110822/download (accessed 1 August 2024).

Hoole, D., Bucke, D., Burgess, P. and Wellby, I. (2001) Zoonosis. In: *Diseases of Carp and Other Cyprinid Fishes*. Blackwell Science, Oxford, p. 58.

Lowry, T. and Smith, S. (2007) Aquatic zoonoses associated with food, bait, ornamental, and tropical fish. *JAVMA* 231(6), 876–880.

Wootten, R. (2012) The parasitology of teleosts. In: Roberts, R.J. (ed.) *Fish Pathology*. 4th edn. Wiley, Oxford, pp. 337–338.

21 Non-infectious Diseases

NICHOLAS SAINT-ERNE

Dr. Saint-Erne Consulting, PLLC, Phoenix, Arizona

Abstract

Fish health can be impacted by more than infectious diseases. Trauma to the fish can be due to rough handling or netting, electrical currents running through the water, or fish jumping out of the tank. Toxins in the water, such as pollutant chemicals, heavy metals, or excess medications, can also harm the fish. Aging can contribute to neoplastic, degenerative, and metabolic diseases in fish.

21.1 Traumatic and Environmental Injuries

Fish can be injured in the aquarium by being bitten by other fish (Fig. 21.1), or from predators in an outdoor pond. Besides these attacks or damage from parasites, fish can be injured by swimming against sharp objects in the water, such as rocks, pointy driftwood, wires inside plastic plants, or décor items that have holes that the fish can swim into but then get stuck inside. This can be a problem with hollow décor in aquariums with a plecostomus that starts out small but gradually grows too large for the opening and becomes lodged inside or in the hole while trying to exit. Other items in the aquarium or pond, such as electrical equipment and water pumps can cause injuries, as described below.

21.1.1 Electrical shock

This can occur in an outdoor pond due to nearby lightning strikes or faulty electrical equipment. In an aquarium, an electrical short in a pump, or a crack in a water heater casing can result in electricity running through the aquarium. Signs of electrical shock include sudden death of some or all the fish, paralysis, erratic swimming, and curved spines. Fish that survive the electrical current passing through the water may have permanent spinal damage caused by epaxial muscle contraction that compresses the spine (Fig. 21.2). Use only electrical products approved for aquariums or ponds. All outdoor electrical outlets should have safety measures such as circuit breakers and ground fault circuit interrupter (GFCI) outlets. These will disconnect power to any pumps or electrical appliances that may become flooded or short-circuit. Contact a professional electrician for installing electrical wiring to the pond.

21.1.2 Jumping out

New fish sometimes will jump out of the aquarium or pond while exploring their new environment. In an outdoor pond, heavy rainstorms may cause the water level to rise, allowing fish to jump out of the pond. Prevent this by lowering the water level prior to rainstorms (Saint-Erne, 2010b). While spawning, koi may mate so vigorously that they swim up the side of the pond and out onto the ground. Anytime a fish leaves the water for dry land, it is an emergency! If the fish is still flopping, use a net, wet towel, or even wet hands to scoop it up and place it back into the water. If it swims away normally, chances are good that it will be fine. If it is lethargic, swims irregularly, or is not respiring, it may need artificial respiration and observation in a hospital tank.

If it is not moving when found, and even appears slightly dry on the skin, do not give up hope yet. Lift the opercula (gill covers) and see if the gills are still moist and pink. If they are, there may still be a chance, even if the fish is not moving. Place the fish

Corresponding author: DrSaintErne@gmail.com

© CAB International 2025. *The Handbook of Ornamental Fish Health and Welfare* (ed. N. Saint-Erne)
DOI: 10.1079/9781789246032.0021

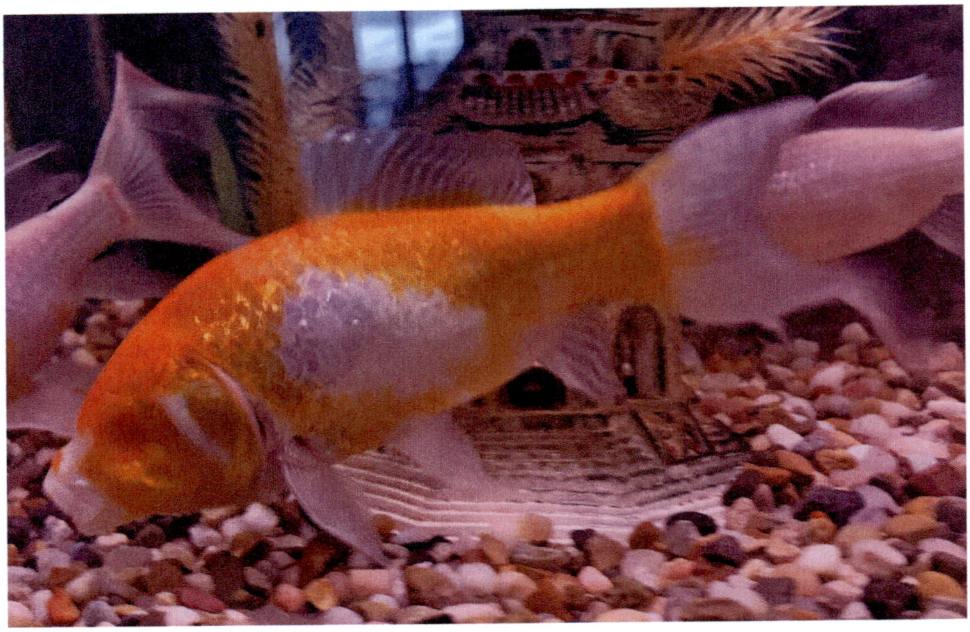

Fig. 21.1. Adult goldfish (*Carassius auratus*) missing both eyes, likely from predation by another fish when it was smaller. It lives a normal life in an aquarium with other goldfish, finding food easily with its sense of smell. (Photograph by N. Saint-Erne.)

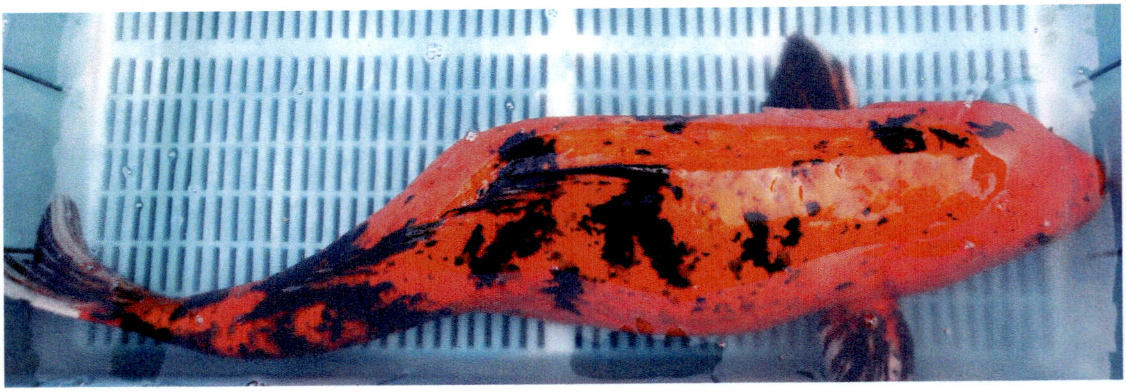

Fig. 21.2. Hi Utsuri Koi (*Cyprinus rubrofuscus*) with a curved spine due to electrical shock from lightning striking near the pond. (Photograph by N. Saint-Erne.)

in water (preferably a hospital tank) and give it artificial respiration. To provide artificial respiration, use the net or your hands to gently move the fish forward through the water. If possible, insert the thumb into the bottom of the gill slit to open the operculum, and the tip of the forefinger into the corner of the mouth to open it. Then water will flow through the mouth and across the gills. Periodically, stop moving the fish to see if it shows any gill, mouth, or fin movement on its own. If there is no movement after the tissue has had time to rehydrate, then the fish is most likely deceased. Fish that do resuscitate should be treated for topical skin wounds if present, and salt should be added to the pond or hospital tank water to 0.3% to reduce osmotic stress.

21.1.3 Supersaturation

"Gas bubble disease" occurs in fish when the water is supersaturated with dissolved gases. This is similar to the "bends" in scuba divers. The excess dissolved gases are absorbed into the fish's blood from the gills and then form bubbles inside the bloodstream, where they can cause air embolisms. The bubbles in skin capillaries can be seen in the fins and body epidermis (Fig. 21.3). Bubbles can appear within the eyes, or retro-orbital, causing the eyes to bulge out (exophthalmos). The embolisms can also occur in the internal organs, where they can produce organ damage and even death. Fin necrosis and loss has been associated with air bubbles causing embolisms in the fin capillaries.

Water pumped from a deep well may have a high level of dissolved carbon dioxide or nitrogen. If not aerated or agitated when added to the pond to release the pressurized gas, the fish will absorb the supersaturated gas from the water and get gas emboli in their gills and blood vessels. Running a garden hose submerged in the pond, which prevents gases from being released into the atmosphere, may also cause this problem, especially during warmer weather. Cold water, which holds more oxygen, can become supersaturated if quickly heated in an aquarium. Faulty water pumps can pressurize gas in the water and lead to gas emboli formation. Water agitation such as a waterfall or a fountain spraying water through the air will help to release dissolved gases and prevent supersaturation.

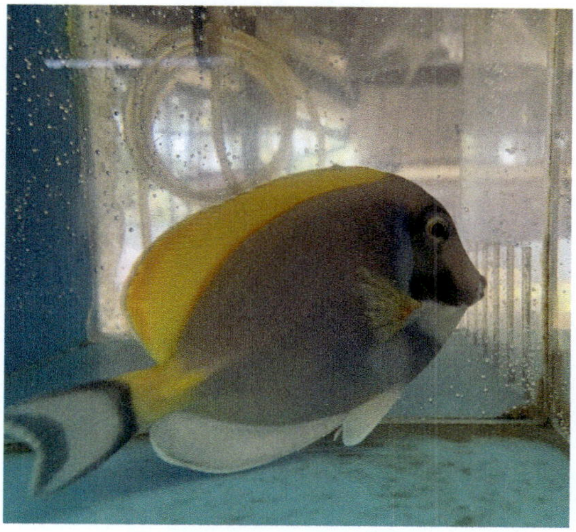

Fig. 21.3. Gas bubbles in the epithelium between the rays of the pectoral fin and on the dorsal fin of a powder blue tang (*Acanthurus leucosternon*). This aquarium also has bubbles on the wall, often a sign of supersaturation of the water. (Photograph by Nick Saint-Erne.)

Occasionally, oxygen supersaturation can be a result of excess unicellular algae in the pond water. In direct sunlight, the algae produce an abundance of dissolved oxygen, increasing the partial pressure of the gas in the water and therefore in the fish's blood. When the sunlight decreases, so does the algae's oxygen production, lowering the partial pressure of the gas in the pond water. Young fish especially have trouble equalizing the gas pressure in their blood, and the "bends" or trapped gas bubbles can occur in their bloodstream. Strong water agitation and shading of the pond will prevent this cause of supersaturation. Ponds or aquariums with water that is supersaturated often have very fine bubbles on the sides or on objects in them.

21.1.4 Thermal shock

When fish are transferred from water at one temperature to water that is significantly higher or lower in temperature, it can cause thermal shock. Gradual changes within the fish's optimum temperature range are acceptable. Ideally, water temperature differences should be no more than 5°F/3°C change per day (Saint-Erne, 2010b). If there is a large difference in temperatures, such as bringing fish inside from a cold outdoor pond, it is best to place them in a separate quarantine container and gradually warm the water before placing them into the warmer water indoors. If the water difference is not too extreme, such as bringing new fish home from a store, the best way to avoid rapid water temperature change is to place the fish in plastic bags containing their original water in the new aquarium or pond and float the bags until the water temperatures are equal. Then remove the fish from the bags and place them into the new water. It is best not to dump the old water from the bags into the aquarium or pond. Temperatures can also fluctuate widely while fish are being transported, so the bags containing the fish should be placed in sturdy cardboard or Styrofoam boxes, or in ice chests to insulate them from temperature changes. Adding ice packs to keep the fish cool in the summer or heat packs to keep them warm in the winter may be required for shipments longer than a few hours.

21.1.5 Overfeeding

In addition to making the fish fat, overfeeding can also cause hepatic lipidosis (fat infiltration of the liver) and water pollution (ammonia buildup). The best prevention is to feed good-quality fish food three or four times a day for young fish and one or two times daily for mature fish. Give only as much food as they will consume in 3–5 min. Young fish need higher protein food, around 40–60% in the diet (Urdes and Walster, 2022), but mature fish should be fed a formula with 30–38% protein (Saint-Erne, 2010b). Feeding older fish food intended for fast-growing fry (trout or catfish chow) can increase the risk of obesity and hepatic lipidosis. Adult fish may only need to eat 0.5–2% of their body weight in food volume each day, while younger fish require 4–6% of their body weight fed to them daily.

Vacation time can lead to overfeeding problems if the person in charge during the owner's absence is not used to taking care of fish. Well-meaning fish-sitters often grossly overfeed their wards, and the owner returns to dead or dying fish and toxic water conditions. The best prevention is to prepare in advance each meal in a sealed container, such as a ziplock bag. Label each container with feeding time and date and any specific instructions. Give the fish slightly less per meal than would normally be given, just to be on the safe side. Leave with the fish-sitter an emergency telephone number on which the owner or the veterinarian can be reached if a problem occurs. Commercial vacation feeders are available to use but should be tested in the aquarium prior to needing them when on a vacation (Fig. 21.4). They contain food pellets in a calcium carbonate block that dissolves in the water to release the pellets. The block may not dissolve in the water to release the food particles in the timeframe indicated on the package instructions, due to variation of water hardness in the aquarium. Vacation feeders can also be used in aquariums to provide food for bottom-feeding fish or other fish that continuously browse for food.

21.1.6 Overstocking

Large numbers of fish swimming together make a dazzling collage of colors that is hard to resist, but the aquarium or pond volume and filtration system must be adequate to handle the stocking density of all the fish. If the fish are overcrowded, oxygen content may become depleted, and ammonia toxicity can occur. Overstocked aquariums or ponds will more easily be devastated by contagious diseases, poor water quality, or problems such as pump or filter failures. In a pond that contains a stable population of young koi, as they gradually become larger, the pond may become overstocked without

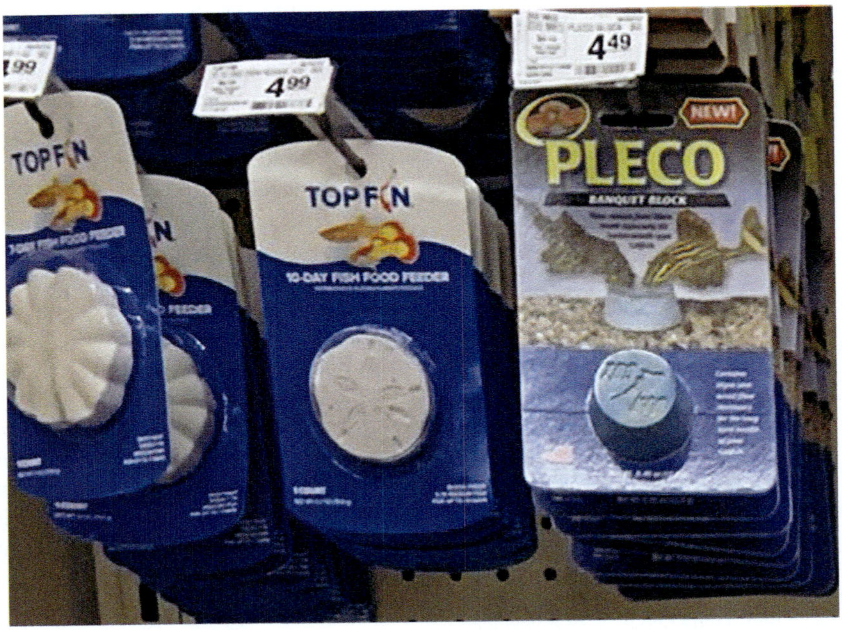

Fig. 21.4. Commercial vacation feeders are available from pet stores. The mineral block slowly dissolves to release food pellets. (Photograph by N. Saint-Erne.)

even adding more fish. Then, the pond's filtration capacity is finally overwhelmed, and catastrophe occurs suddenly in a pond that appeared to be stable. Be sure when adding fish to an aquarium or pond the adult size of the fish is known, as many fish are sold at an immature stage. Plan the stocking density based on water volume and the adult size of each fish to ensure the pond or aquarium will not be overcrowded when the fish mature.

21.1.7 Hypoxia

In stressful situations, fish require more oxygen, and their ventilation rate increases; however, hypoxia often occurs when fish are stressed. Lack of aeration, excessive water temperature, overfeeding, overstocking, and decomposing organic matter can all lead to hypoxic conditions in the aquarium or pond. Clinical signs of hypoxia include the fish open-mouth breathing and rapidly flaring its operculum, congregating at the surface (piping) or around aeration sources, anorexia, lethargy, and, in severe hypoxic cases, mortalities (Esmail *et al.*, 2015). Treatment and prevention for low oxygen levels include increasing agitation of the water and decreasing oxygen demand. Agitation and aeration can increase dissolved oxygen levels in the water by increasing the water surface contact with air and mixing the aerated water throughout the system. Using an oxygen canister attached to an air stone to bubble oxygen into the water in an aquarium, rather than just air, will rapidly increase dissolved oxygen levels. This is especially important while fish are anesthetized and have lowered respiratory rates.

21.1.8 Aggression and predation

Fish in aquariums can be attacked by other aggressive fish, with damage to the eyes, fins, and skin, including biting off scales. This damage can lead to secondary bacterial and fungal infections. Some fish species may fight for territory or bite during mating (Fig. 21.5). Male Bettas (Siamese fighting fish, *Betta splendens*) will fight with other males if placed together. Male Bettas will also attack female Bettas if placed together when the female is not ready to mate, and the male will attack the female to drive her away after mating, as only the male takes care of the bubble nest full of eggs. Female Bettas are usually more social and can be housed together in aquariums, but sometimes, one of them may become aggressive toward other female Bettas. It is important not to mix aggressive fish species (e.g. cichlids) with smaller fish (e.g. tetras and guppies),

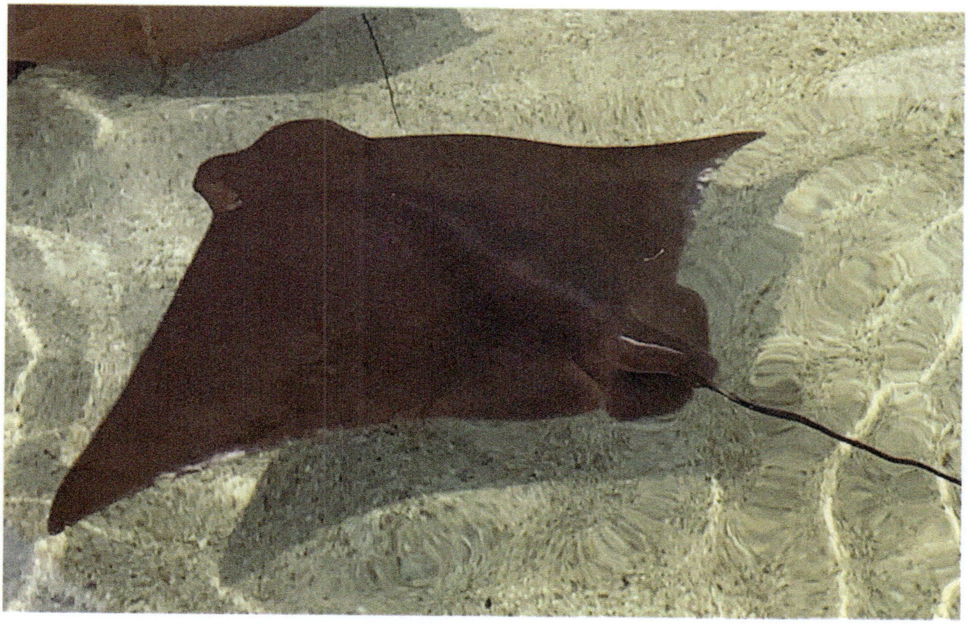

Fig. 21.5. A female cownose ray (*Rhinoptera bonasus*) with scrapes and tears (white lesions) on edge of pectoral fins from a male biting during breeding. After mating season, the fin injuries completely healed. (Photograph by N. Saint-Erne.)

as they may be eaten by the larger fish. Most retail fish stores will have labels on the aquariums, indicating which fish species can be housed together.

In outdoor ponds, goldfish, koi, or other fish can be preyed upon by cats, raccoons, otters, mink, fish-eating birds, and even bears in some areas (Fig. 21.6). Fry and small fish can be eaten by frogs, snakes, water turtles, crayfish, and insects, such as diving beetles and dragonfly nymphs. Proper pond construction, with straight sides and deep water around the edges, limits some predation, but fencing around or strings strung above the pond may be necessary to deter predators (Fig. 21.7).

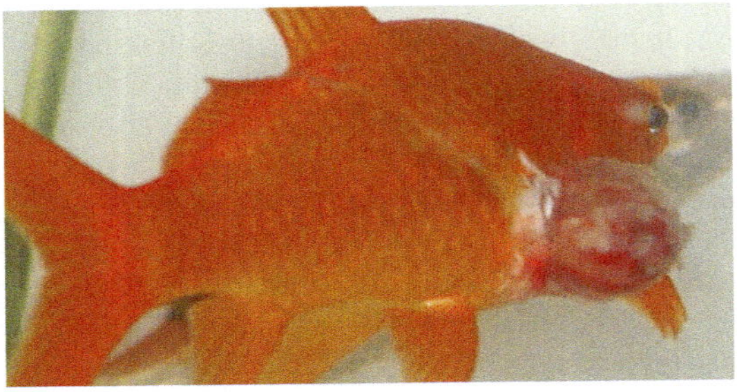

Fig. 21.6. Goldfish (*C. auratus*) with torn dorsal fin and wound into coelom from a heron strike. This fish was treated and fully recovered. (Photograph by N. Saint-Erne.)

21.1.9 Head and lateral line erosion

Head and lateral line erosion (HLLE) syndrome is also called "hole-in-the-head" disease or Lateral Line Depigmentation Syndrome (LLDS). It was originally thought to be caused by a protozoan infestation of *Spironucleus* (formerly identified as *Hexamita*), because they were present at the site of lesions in some fish. It now appears protozoa may have been secondary pathogens, and stress, such as from water quality problems, poor nutrition, or overcrowding, may be the primary problem. The exact etiology is unknown, but a combination of parasites, bacteria, viruses, nutritional deficiencies, high nitrate, poor water quality, stray electrical currents, and carbon in the filter system has been implicated (Roberts, 2012). HLLE is seen mostly in oscars, discus, and other large South American cichlids (Fig. 21.8). African cichlids, such as tilapia, also have been affected by HLLE, as have ornamental marine fish species (Fig. 21.9), primarily Acanthuridae (surgeon fishes and tangs) and Pomacanthidae angelfishes (Yanong and Lewbart, 2024). Suggested treatments include feeding medicated fish food that contains antibiotics and metronidazole, improving water quality, checking the water for electrical currents, removing carbon from the filter, and increasing vitamin C in the diet. For treating HLLE in *Uaru* cichlids, lowering

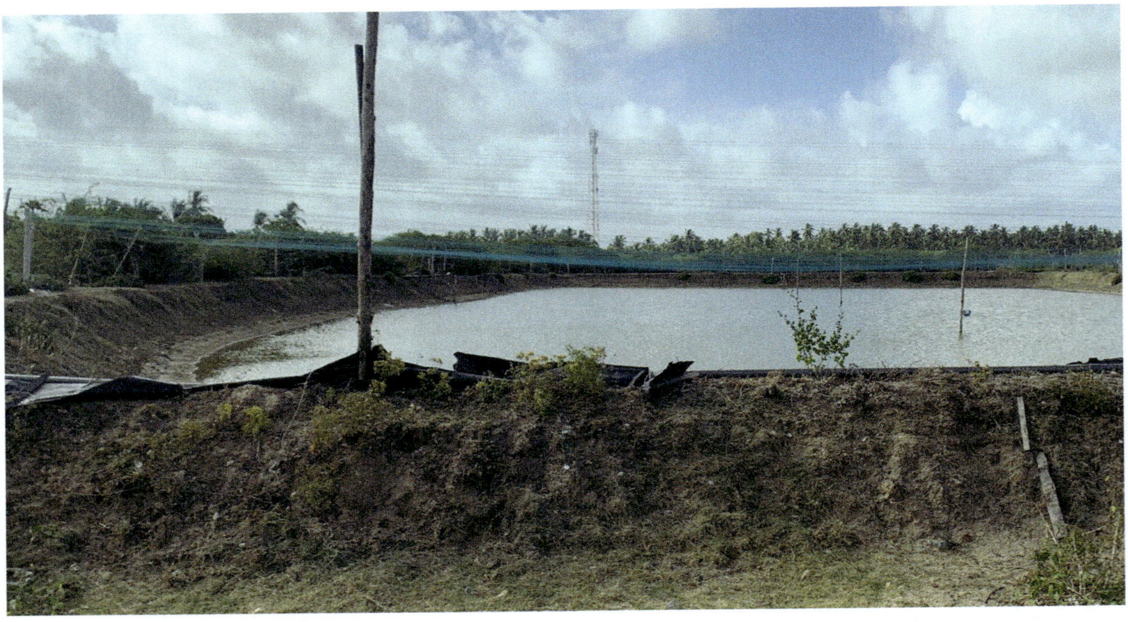

Fig. 21.7. Fishpond in Sri Lanka with wires over it to reduce predation from birds. (Photograph by N. Saint-Erne.)

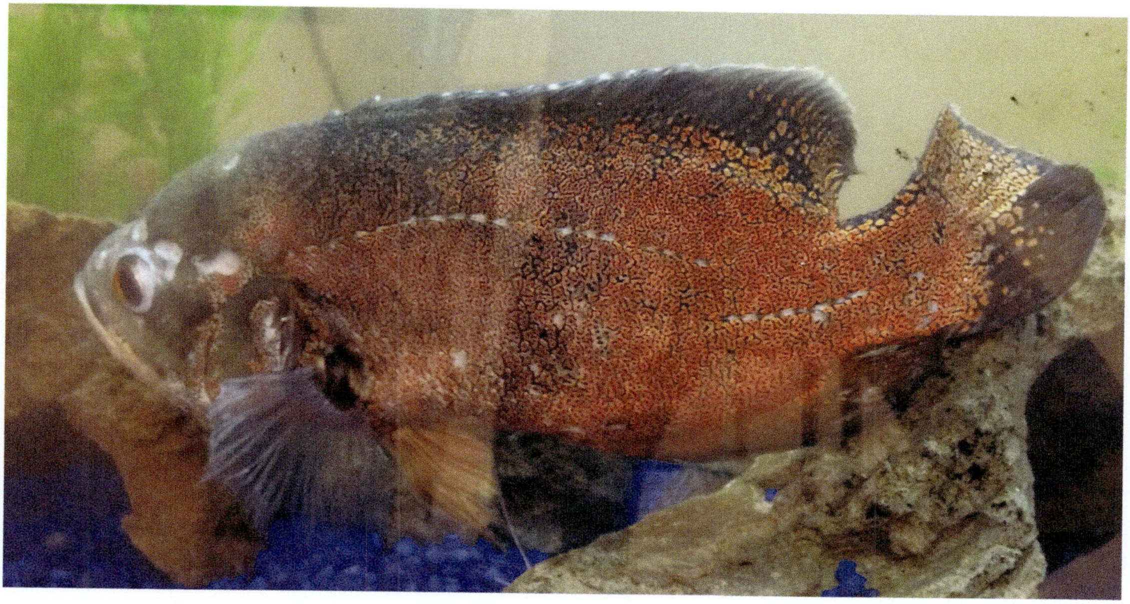

Fig. 21.8. Oscar (*Astronotus ocellatus*) fish with head and lateral line erosion that was being kept in a small aquarium with poor water quality. (Photograph by N. Saint-Erne.)

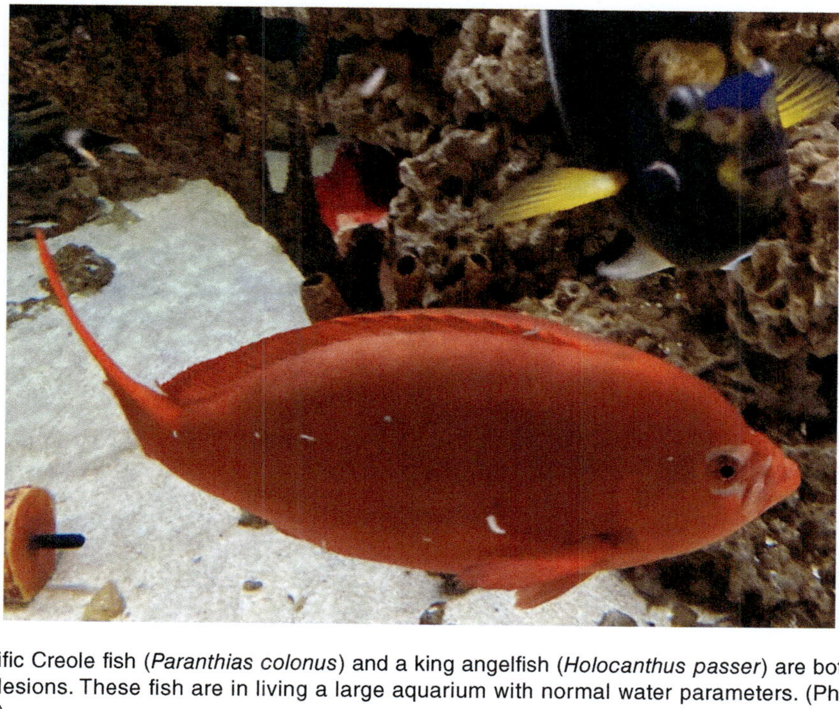

Fig. 21.9. Pacific Creole fish (*Paranthias colonus*) and a king angelfish (*Holocanthus passer*) are both showing head erosion lesions. These fish are in living a large aquarium with normal water parameters. (Photograph by N. Saint-Erne.)

the water pH below 7.0 has been reported to be beneficial (Bagnall, 2023).

21.1.10 Solar radiation

Koi in shallow water that are in direct sunlight for an extended time each day with no shade may suffer from sunburn. The lesions appear as hyperemia (redness) of the skin, usually the white parts, and blistering along the margins of the scales on the back. Severe cases may result in ulceration of the skin. Treat with topical antibiotic ointment to prevent secondary infections and provide shade over the pond or floating structures on the water's surface to provide shelter.

21.2 Toxicity

Good water quality is the key to good fish health and welfare. Normal water quality parameters have been discussed in previous chapters. Excess levels of ammonia, nitrite, nitrate, or chlorine can occur in aquariums or ponds and cause fish deaths. Other factors listed below can also contribute to toxic water conditions for fish.

21.2.1 Pond construction material

When constructing a rubber-liner fishpond, be sure to use appropriate and safe materials. Swimming pool liners may be coated with algicides. Roofing rubber liners may also be coated with toxic chemicals. Be sure to use only liners that are labeled as safe for fish. The best liners currently are made from ethylene-propylene-diene-monomer (EPDM) rubber.

Concrete ponds must be coated with a non-toxic sealing agent to prevent the gradual leaching of toxic lime into the water. After the concrete has hardened, scrub and rinse it several times, fill it with water, and let it sit for a few days. Then drain, rinse again, and let air-dry. Then apply a non-toxic pond sealant to the concrete surface. Refill the pond after the sealant is completely dry.

Cement blocks repurposed to build structures in a pond may contain chemicals that affect the water quality and harm the fish. Pressure-treated wood designed for marine applications may have toxic chemicals in the wood and should not be used for building docks or bridges in ornamental fishponds.

21.2.2 Toxic chemicals in the pond

Garden fertilizers, weed killers, and insecticides are toxic if sprayed where they can land on the water or run into the pond when it rains or when the lawn is watered. Use caution when spraying chemicals in a garden near the pond, especially on windy days. Be sure neighbors are not spraying in a manner that could blow toxins into the pond.

Oil, gasoline, and antifreeze can poison ponds near areas where automobiles are parked. The carbon monoxide exhaust is also toxic if sucked into air pumps and then released into the pond aerators. Constructing ponds away from garages or driveways will avoid these hazards.

Wood preservatives used for outdoor decking can be toxic, and chemically treated lumber should not be used around the pond. Rainwater running off the wood and into the pond can leach out the chemicals and poison the fish. Creosote used as preservative on telephone poles and railroad ties is very toxic, so chemically treated wood should not be used around ponds. Consult an experienced lumber dealer about suitability of available wood when doing construction around ponds.

21.2.3 Heavy metals

Heavy metals (e.g. aluminum, copper, iron, lead, mercury, and zinc) can be dissolved in tap water sources and cause toxicity to the fish. Knowing if heavy metals are in the water is an important part of diagnosing slow growth and acute mortalities in young fish and decreased reproductive health in mature fish (Kasper *et al.*, 2022). A low pH increases the solubility of metal ions in the water, increasing toxicity. Hard water helps reduce the toxic effects by causing the metal to precipitate out of the solution. Copper containers or pipes and galvanized tubs should not be used for fishponds, as copper and zinc metal poisonings may occur. Do not use wire mesh screens in the ponds or filters because of possible metal poisoning. Use only a plastic mesh screen if needed for the filtration system. Water test kits are available for checking for heavy metals, or local agriculture laboratories may be able to perform testing. Check the tap water as well to see if that is the source of the heavy metals.

21.2.4 Oil in the water

Many submersible water pumps used in aquarium filters have oil within their housings. Sometimes, cracks in the housing or leaks around gaskets will allow oil to leak into the water. It will form an oil film on the surface. Immediately turn off and remove the faulty pump. Let the water surface calm and then remove the surface water with the oil slick using a waterproof shop vacuum. If that is not available, a clean plastic bucket can be carefully pushed into the water so that the surface water overflows into it, skimming the oil into the bucket. Dump the bucket before it is full and repeat until the oil slick has been removed. Paper towels can be used to wipe off the aquarium edge. In a small aquarium, paper towels can be carefully laid on the water surface to absorb the oil, then gently removed (Meyer, 1999).

Where feasible without risk to the environment, an outdoor pond can be overfilled so that the surface water with the oil slick overflows out of the pond. After extracting the oil, do a 50% water change in the pond, adding dechlorinator to the new water. Replace the pump immediately to provide oxygen to the fish and to maintain biological filtration.

21.2.5 Inappropriate material

Using inappropriate materials as filter media is an often-overlooked cause of toxicity. Fiber mats used in air filters or evaporative coolers can have antifungal agents added to them, so they should not be used as filter materials.

Gravel for the bottom of the aquarium should be specific for use in aquariums. Materials collected outdoors may contain toxic chemicals or organic debris. If using collected rocks or driftwood in an aquarium, be sure to clean it first, then disinfect it in a bleach solution soak. Afterward, rinse it thoroughly and let it air-dry, or use an aquarium water dechlorinator in a bucket with the gravel to remove the chlorine before adding the gravel into an aquarium. Using sharp-edged gravel can cause abrasions to the ventral surface of bottom-dwelling fish, as well as to the barbels of fish that forage for food among the substrate, such as *Corydoras* catfish. This can lead to lesions on the skin and secondary bacterial or fungal infections.

Goldfish are prone to taking gravel into their mouth when feeding on the bottom, and many cases have occurred where gravel has become lodged in their oral cavity. Removal of the foreign body may require anesthesia and using blunt forceps gently inserted into the mouth to extract the stone (Hoole *et al.*, 2001).

21.2.6 Medication overdosage

Overdosage of fish medications such as trichlorfon, formalin, potassium permanganate, and copper sulfate can be highly toxic to fish. Trichlorfon or other organophosphate chemicals can cause seizures, muscle spasms, and even spinal injury when overdosed. Atropine sulfate injections will counteract the toxicity if given soon after the overdosage occurs. For overdosage of medications, water changes should be performed. UV lights, protein skimmers, and activated carbon in the filter can be used to remove medications from the water.

To reduce the risk of overdosage, be sure to always follow medication label directions carefully, measure the medication accurately, and correctly calculate the water volume in aquariums and ponds. Do not guess—it may cost the lives of the fish! Use a flowmeter on the garden hose when initially filling a fishpond, or use the readings on the domestic water meter, making sure all other water uses (sinks, toilets, baths, sprinklers) are not being used at the same time. Write down the exact gallon volume for future reference. When estimating gallons in a filled pond, make accurate measurements of the pond dimensions and water depths. Draw the pond to scale with the dimensions indicated. Then use a calculator to make an accurate calculation of the total volume of water in the pond. The water volume contained in the filter and connecting pipes must also be considered if the filtration system will be used during treatments.

21.2.7 Molds

Feeding moldy fish foods containing mycotoxins produced by the fungus *Aspergillus flavus* can cause neoplastic changes. The tumor consists of an invasive malignant trabecular hepatocarcinoma (Hardy, 2012). Mycotoxin also induces hepatic necrosis, branchial edema, and generalized hemorrhages. Death occurs from liver failure and hemorrhaging. Diagnosis can be made by examining the food and by microscopic examination of the histopathological changes in the liver cells. Always keep foods cool and dry in airtight containers. Do not use old, rancid, or moldy fish food.

21.2.8 Algae

Algal blooms that can occur in ponds may lower the oxygen level in the water, causing hypoxic conditions, or produce toxins directly that kill the fish. Blue-green algae (cyanobacteria) can quickly overgrow in an aquarium with high nitrate and phosphate levels. Barbed diatoms can lodge in gills of fish, causing damage if accumulated in large numbers (Kasper *et al.*, 2022). In addition to problems caused by living algae, use of algicides can contribute to fish loss. The algicide is not directly toxic to the fish, but the chemical as well as the dead and decomposing algae will lower the dissolved oxygen in the water. The resulting hypoxia can affect the fish. It is important to remove as much algae as possible before treatment with an algicide, add extra aeration during treatment, and then monitor water quality for 1–2 weeks after treatment.

21.2.9 Hydrogen sulfide

Hydrogen sulfide, which can form in pond bottom sediment, deep aquarium gravel, or anaerobic areas of filtration systems, is toxic to fish because it interferes with reoxidation of cytochrome a_3 in respiration (Boyd, 2014). Under anaerobic conditions, heterotrophic bacteria reduce sulfates in decaying organic matter to produce hydrogen sulfide gas, which is very soluble in water. Exposure of fish to hydrogen sulfide results in hyperpnea, followed by apnea, and finally respiratory arrest (Torrans and Clemens, 1982). Unionized hydrogen sulfide (H_2S) is extremely toxic to fish, even at concentrations as low as 0.002 mg/l, and any detectable level should be prevented.

Hydrogen sulfide (H_2S) produces black sediment in the pond gravel, the soil of potted water plants, or filter beds with lack of water flow. It has a foul rotten-egg odor and is toxic to humans as well as to fish. At high levels, hydrogen sulfide quickly deadens the sense of smell, and lethal levels may still exist but go unnoticed. When strong rotten-egg odors appear while working in the pond, take frequent breaks to areas away from the smell to be sure to not become overwhelmed.

Like ammonia, hydrogen sulfide is toxic to fish in its unionized state. Its ionized form is non-toxic. The water temperature and pH levels will control how much will be ionized. Low pH and low temperatures increase the toxic unionized state. High pH or high temperatures increase the ionized state. However, due to the extreme toxicity of H_2S to fish, even at higher pH or temperatures, the small percentage of unionized H_2S present may still cause fish deaths. Do frequent water changes when H_2S is detected, aerate the water, and stir the gravel beds frequently to prevent anaerobic production of H_2S gas. Ensure there are no areas of ponds or filtration systems where water stagnates, and debris accumulates. Potassium permanganate added to the water at 2–6 mg/l removes hydrogen sulfide and reverses its toxicity to fish.

21.3 Tumors

Tumors have been reported from many species of bony fishes. Neoplasia in Chondrichthyes fish (sharks, skates, rays) and primitive fishes, including lungfish, bowfin, sturgeons, and paddlefish, are less commonly reported. While the word "tumor" is often interpreted to mean neoplasia, it actually refers to any abnormal swelling of tissues and could be due to infections (such as *Mycobacterium* granulomas, or oncogenic viruses) or trauma, as well as neoplasia. When a tumor is a result of neoplasia, it may be benign (does not spread), malignant (spreads aggressively to surrounding tissues, often called a *cancer*), or metastatic (spreads via blood or lymph to other organs of the body). In fish, most tumors are focal and benign, although they can grow large locally. Some are malignant and invade other surrounding tissues, but metastasis is an uncommon phenomenon in fishes (Groff, 2004). Neoplasia can result from exposure to an environmental chemical (carcinogen), radiation, or an infectious agent or be due to a genetic component. Neoplasia is classified according to its histogenesis, or the tissues from which the growth is derived (Groff, 2004).

21.3.1 Cutaneous neoplasia

These are the most common neoplasms of fishes. They are generally benign and can be surgically removed, although recurrence is common without complete surgical excision, which is difficult to accomplish due to the inelastic nature of fish skin (Fig. 21.10). Papilloma is the most common cutaneous neoplasm of fish and appears as a raised irregular growth on the integument. The main cell type involved is squamous epithelial cells that are growing outward in folds, rather than lying flat along the surface of the basement membrane. Squamous cell carcinoma is a malignant cutaneous neoplasia that is invasive into the hypodermis and has a prominent blood supply.

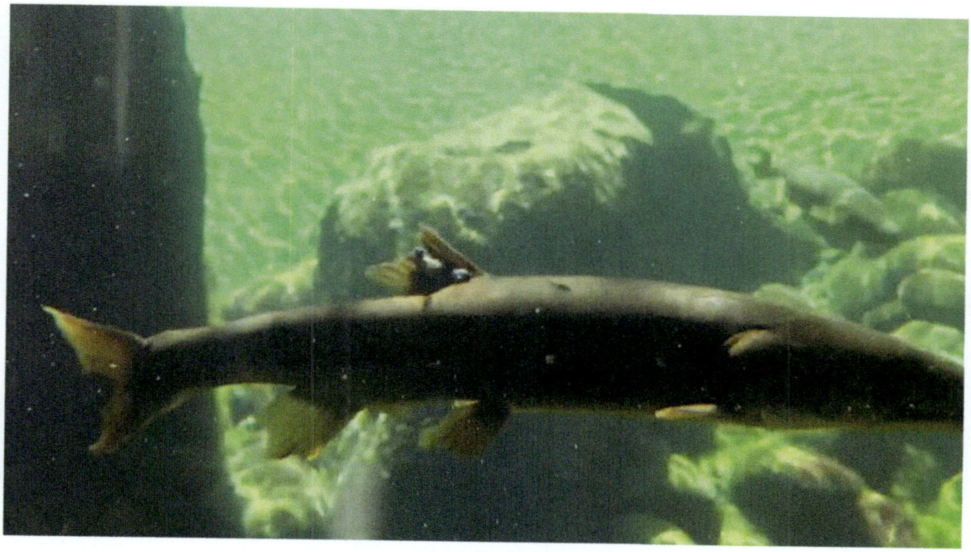

Fig. 21.10. Epithelial tumor on the dorsal fin of a Colorado pikeminnow (*Ptychocheilus lucius*). (Photograph by N. Saint-Erne.)

Hikkui disease is a hyperplastic skin disease in koi (*C. rubrofuscus*), now believed to be a form of epithelial neoplasia, from either perivascular cells (hemangiopericytoma) or spindle cells in the skin (Sirri *et al.*, 2016). Originally called "Hi Kui Wa-mu" (literal translation is "red eating worm") by the Japanese koi breeders because the red color on the fish was degenerating, and it was suspected to be due to a parasite. It was shortened to one word: Hikkui, with an extra "k" added in, as Hikui spelled with one "k" is a different word and means "short" in Japanese. The disease causes hyperplasia and erosion of the fish's epithelium, especially on red-pigmented skin (Fig. 21.11). The skin becomes thickened, sometimes hemorrhagic, and then sloughs off. Skin can become discolored and scarred at the site of the degeneration. Lesions may clear spontaneously and recur periodically in the same fish. Hikkui is seen primarily in Kohaku, Sanke, and Showa (Go-Sanke) koi varieties. Ogon, chagoi, karasu, and other darker-colored koi varieties in the same pond with koi having Hikkui lesions are often not affected. Treatment consists of topical skin disinfection with antibiotic application. This debrides the hyperplastic skin to remove the affected tissue, which seems to increase the rate of healing of the lesion. Topical antibiotics also kill bacteria that could produce a secondary infection. Lesions may still recur regardless of the treatment used.

21.3.2 Adenomas

Neoplasia involving glandular tissue is called an adenoma. Thyroid adenomas have been reported in some cyprinid fish, with swelling of the thyroid tissues between the first and second gill arches in the pharynx. This may be hyperplasia, though, rather than neoplasia, as it can occur secondarily to iodine deficiency (Hoole *et al.*, 2001). Renal adenomas can result in ascites and polycystic kidneys, although similar lesions can occur from *Sphaerospora* protozoan infestations. Malignant adenomas that spread to other tissues are referred to as adenocarcinomas. Renal adenocarcinomas have been reported in tilapia, oscars, and guppies.

21.3.3 Mesenchymal tumors

Neoplasms that are classified as spindle cell tumors are common in fish and are identified by the fusiform shape of the neoplastic cells. These are a mesenchymal tumor that includes fibroma and fibrosarcoma, and the peripheral nerve tumors, neurofibromas, and neurilemmomas (derived from Schwann cells). These tumors consist of whorls of mesenchymal cells. Lipomas are mesenchymal tumors of fat cells, with some interspersed fibrous cells. Neoplasms of cartilage have been reported, including chondromas of the gill arch and fin rays (Fig. 21.12). Calcification of fibrous connective

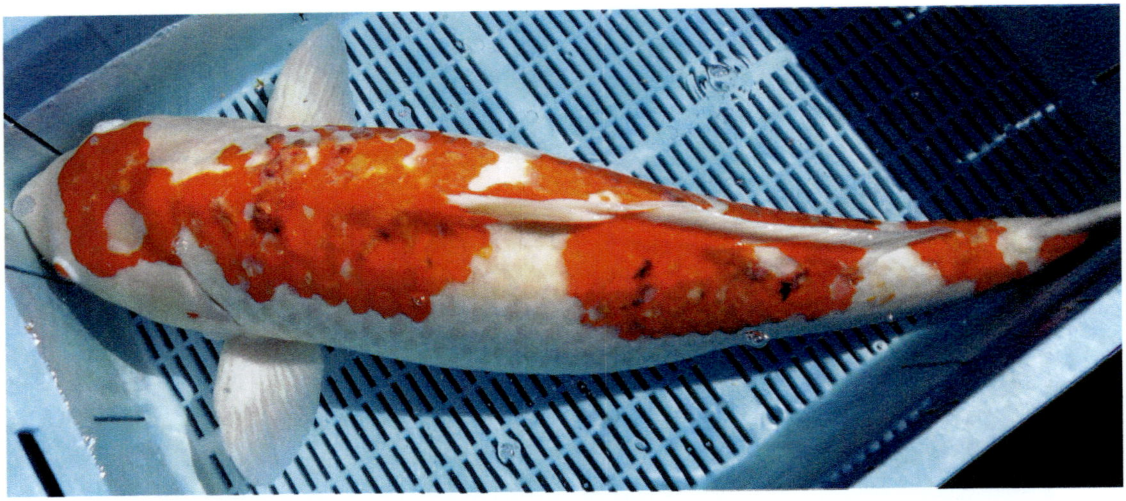

Fig. 21.11. Kohaku koi (*C. rubrofuscus*) with Hikkui lesion of hemorrhages and epithelial hyperplasia on the red-pigmented areas of the skin. (Photograph by N. Saint-Erne.)

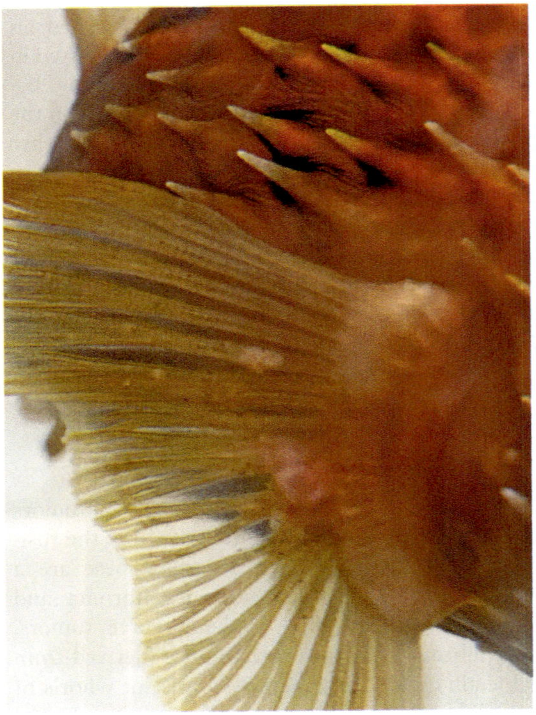

Fig. 21.12. Spiny puffer (*Diodon holocanthus*) with chondrosarcoma on the pectoral fin. (Photograph by N. Saint-Erne.)

tissue tumors is not uncommon and should not be confused with chondromas or osteomas (Groff, 2004).

21.3.4 Hematopoietic tumors

These are referred to as lymphoma or lymphosarcoma and occur in the lymphohematopoietic tissues of fish: the mesonephros part of the kidney, the spleen, thymus, and submucosa of the gut. Because the kidney is the primary site of lymphohematopoiesis in fishes, these tumors often originate in the kidney, or spread to the kidney (Groff, 2004). These tumors are composed of hemocytoblasts and lymphoblasts and are frequently associated with a leukemic condition.

21.3.5 Pigment cell tumors

Melanomas and melanosarcomas are the most common pigment cell tumors (chromatophoromas) reported in fish species (Hoole *et al.*, 2001). Hybrids of platys (*Xiphophorus maculatus*) and swordtails (*X. helleri*) have commonly developed skin melanomas, and this is associated with a sex-linked gene. Goldfish are prone to erythrophoromas, which are raised, tan- to orange-colored, nodular, or papillomatous growths on the fish's skin (Fig. 21.13). They are generally benign but may be locally invasive.

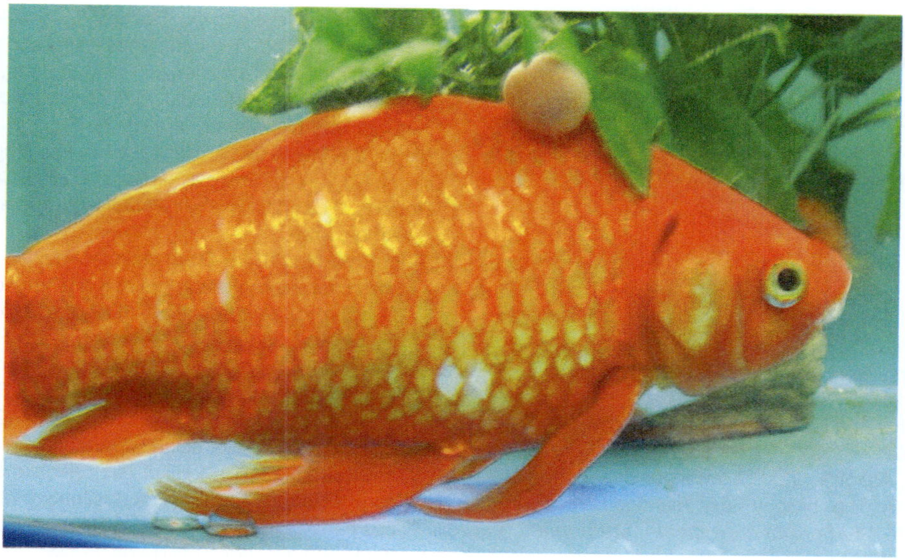

Fig. 21.13. Goldfish (*C. auratus*) with a benign erythrophoroma skin tumor on its dorsum anterior to the dorsal fin. (Photo by N. Saint-Erne.)

Chromatophoromas have also been reported in Corydoras catfish, Hawaiian butterflyfish, and Pacific rockfish (Groff, 2004).

21.3.6 Gonadal neoplasms

These include ovarian and testicular leiomyomas and fibroleiomyomas of yellow perch, Sertoli cell neoplasms in cyprinids, seminomas in African lungfish and sea bass, and ovarian adenocarcinomas. Gonadal neoplasms are often seen in koi and can be surgically removed if encountered early, when coelomic swelling is first observed (Fig. 21.14). In advanced cases, the neoplasm has local invasion and affects the liver and intestines and can cause compression and organ damage, internal bleeding, ascites, and anorexia. Tumors can become so large that they cause pressure necrosis and even rupture of the body wall. Surgical removal is often successful, but early intervention is important to prevent secondary complications (e.g. tissue necrosis, intestinal compression, bacterial infection) that will lead to a poor prognosis. (Saint-Erne, 2010a). Radiography, ultrasonography, CT imaging, and laparoscopy are useful in diagnosing abdominal (coelomic) neoplasia. These methods can also provide guidance for excisional or aspiration biopsy. Surgical removal can provide a significant improvement in the quality of life for the fish.

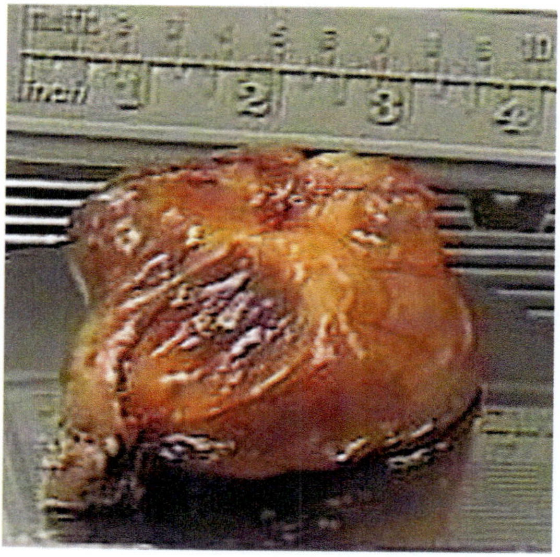

Fig. 21.14. Ovarian tumor surgically removed from a koi (*C. rubrofuscus*). (Photograph by N. Saint-Erne.)

21.5 Conclusion

Many possible health issues can occur due to stressful handling and transportation of fish in the commercial pet industry. Traumatic and toxicity problems can occur in home aquariums and ponds as well. Maintaining proper water quality by routine testing of the water will avoid many toxic situations. Paying attention to everything that goes into the pond or aquarium, from the source water to gravel, rocks, and décor items, will help reduce losses from trauma and toxicity. Proper monitoring of fish, especially as they age, will help identify tumors and neoplasia.

References

Bagnall, G. (2023) Personal Communication. ZooMed Laboratory, San Luis Obispo, California.

Boyd, C.E. (2014) Hydrogen sulfide toxic, but manageable. *Global Aquaculture Advocate*, March/April 2014, pp. 34–36.

Esmail, M.Y., Astrofsky, K.M., Lawrence, C. and Serluca, F.C. (2015) The biology and management of the Zebrafish. *Laboratory Animal Medicine* 3, 1015–1062.

Groff, J.M. (2004) Neoplasia in fishes. In: Vassallo, J. (ed.) *Veterinary Clinics of North America: Exotic Animal Practice*. Vol. 7, No. 3. Elsevier Saunders, Philadelphia, Pennsylvania, pp. pp. 705–756.

Hardy, R.W. (2012) Mycotoxins. In: Roberts, R.J. (ed.) *Fish Pathology*. 4th edn. Wiley, West Sussex, UK, pp. 419–421.

Hoole, D., Bucke, D., Burgess, P. and Wellby, I. (2001) Noninfectious diseases. In: Hoole, D., Bucke, D., Burgess, P. and Wellby, I. (eds) *Diseases of Carp and Other Cyprinid Fishes*. Blackwell Science, Oxford, pp. 125–146.

Kasper, S., Adeyemo, O., Becker, T., Scarfe, D. and Tepper, J. (2022) Environmental toxins and pollutants. In: Urdes, L., Walster, C. and Tepper, J. (eds) *Fundamentals of Aquatic Veterinary Medicine*. Wiley, Hoboken, New Jersey, pp. 22–29.

Meyer, S.A. (1999) Oil slick. In: *Aquarium Fish Magazine*. Vol. 11, No. 1. Fancy Publications, Mission Viejo, California.

Roberts, R.J. (2012) *Fish Pathology*. 4th edn. Wiley, Ames, Iowa.

Saint-Erne N. (2010a) Diagnostic techniques and treatments for internal disorders of Koi (*Cyprinus carpio*). *Veterinary Clinics of North America: Exotic Animal Practice* 13, 333–347.

Saint-Erne, N. (2010b) Traumatic injuries and toxicity. In: Saint-Erne, N. (ed.) *Advance Koi Care*. Erne Enterprises, Glendale, Arizona, pp. 121–126.

Sirri, R., Pretto, T., Montesi, F., Berton, V., Mandrioli, L. and Barbé, T. (2016) Hikui (sic) disease in nine koi carp (*Cyprinus carpio*): first description of a cutaneous perivascular wall tumour. *Veterinary Dermatology* 27(4), 301.e74. doi:10.1111/vde.12338.

Torrans, E.L. and Clemens, H.P. (1982) Physiological and biochemical effects of acute exposure of fish to hydrogen sulfide. *Comparative Biochemistry and Physiology. C: Comparative pharmacology* 71(2), 183–190. doi:10.1016/0306-4492(82)90034-x.

Urdes, L. and Walster, C. (2022) Freedom from thirst, hunger and malnutrition. In: Urdes, L., Walster, C. and Tepper, J. (eds) *Fundamentals of Aquatic Veterinary Medicine*. Wiley, Hoboken, New Jersey, pp. 223–224.

Yanong, R.P.E. and Lewbart, G.A. (2024) *The Aquarium Fish Medicine Handbook*. CRC Press, Boca Raton, Florida.

22 Fish Facility Husbandry and Biosecurity

NICHOLAS SAINT-ERNE

Dr. Saint-Erne Consulting, PLLC, Phoenix, Arizona

Abstract

This chapter will describe the best husbandry methods for keeping fish healthy during the handling and shipping processes necessary for moving them from the fish farm to the fish keeper. Following these processes will help the fish wholesalers and retail stores maintain the health of the fish in the best manner possible.

22.1 Fish Health in a Global Industry

Saltwater and freshwater aquarium fish are both collected from the wild and commercially cultured around the world. The fish go through stresses due to changes in water quality, netting and bagging for shipment, transportation from the collector or farmer to the exporter and wholesaler, then to the retailer, and finally to the aquarium keeper. If the fish are kept in good water quality, handled carefully, and treated to reduce parasites, they will arrive at the final destination in a healthy state. Unfortunately, the fish may come into the fish stores, and ultimately home aquariums, with health concerns. Proper observation, handling, feeding, water quality, disease diagnosis, and treatments at the fish farm, wholesale facilities, and retail stores will improve the quality of the fish prior to sending them home with customers.

22.1.1 Facility disinfection

Disinfectants and soaps typically used to clean animal facilities are not used in aquatic facilities as they may be toxic to the fish. In aquatic facilities, disinfectants that are safe for use around fish should be used for cleaning equipment and floor surfaces. There are a few commercial products that are recommended for use in aquaculture facilities (Sanders, 2020). Table 22.1 lists the commonly available fish-safe disinfectants and how to use them. Bleach and other disinfectant solutions can be corrosive and irritate the eyes, skin, and respiratory tract. Wear personal protective equipment (PPE) when using disinfecting chemicals.

Bleach is usually diluted in water at 1:10 to make a concentration between 5200–7500 mg/l of chlorine bleach for disinfection, or 1:100 to make a lower concentration of 525–750 mg/l for sanitizing surfaces. Bleach solutions used for disinfecting must remain wet on the surface for an adequate amount of time to be effective. The higher the concentration, the shorter time the bleach will need to be in contact with surfaces to kill microorganisms. A 10-min contact time with the 1:10 dilution is recommended by the Centers for Disease Control (CDC) for disinfection. This concentration will kill *Mycobacterium*. Approximate dilutions are 13 ounces (377 ml) of 6% bleach in a gallon (3.8 l) of water for a 1:10 dilution (equals 5400 mg/l if using 6% bleach solution), or 1.3 ounces (38 ml) of 6% bleach in a gallon (3.8 l) of water for a 1:100 dilution (600 mg/l). Always add the bleach solution to the water when preparing the solution. Do not premix the water and bleach solution, as it loses potency over time.

22.1.2 Facility maintenance

Facilities should always be kept in a clean and orderly manner (Saint-Erne, 2023). Aquatic facilities must

Corresponding author: DrSaintErne@gmail.com

© CAB International 2025. *The Handbook of Ornamental Fish Health and Welfare* (ed. N. Saint-Erne)
DOI: 10.1079/9781789246032.0022

Table 22.1. Aquaculture-safe disinfectants. Author's own table.

Benzalkonium chloride (e.g. Lysol®) is a quaternary ammonium compound that dissolves the outer lipid layer of cell membranes. Benzalkonium chloride is more effective against *Mycobacterium* than bleach. It does produce suds that may make it harder to rinse away. Soak equipment in benzalkonium chloride mixed with water to make a 1% solution for effective disinfection. Leave the equipment in the benzalkonium solution for at least 5 min, or spray the surface and let it air-dry. Benzalkonium chloride is often used as a net disinfectant. Rinse all surfaces with water after use. Not recommended for use on brass, copper, or aluminum surfaces.

Peroxymonosulfate-sodium chlorine (e.g. Virkon® Aquatic) is designated for use in aquaculture and is safe for fish. It is useful for the treatment of *Aeromonas* and most other aquatic bacteria and viruses, such as Koi Herpes Virus and Spring Viremia of Carp, but it is not effective against *Mycobacterium* bacteria. Use a 1% solution to disinfect surfaces and equipment.

Potassium permanganate ($KMnO_4$) acts as a strong oxidizing agent to destroy many pathogens. The concentration used for bath treatment with fish is 2 mg/l, but for disinfection of equipment, 20 mg/l for an hour is recommended (Herwig, 1979). Typical application will turn the water purple to pink in color for several hours. The purple or pink color will turn brown as the chemical oxidizes organic matter in the water. More potassium permanganate needs to be added when the color turns to brown to continue using the solution as a disinfectant. Never apply potassium permanganate directly to the fish's skin!

Sodium hypochlorite (NaOCl) is the active ingredient in liquid bleach. It destroys pathogens by denaturing proteins. Liquid bleach may come in 5.25%, 6.0%, 7.5%, or even higher concentrations of sodium hypochlorite, so it is important to determine the concentration of sodium hypochlorite in the bleach solution being used. While bleach can be an effective disinfectant, it is a poor cleaner, and it rapidly loses activity in the presence of organic matter. Since a solution of bleach in water will provide only disinfection, a two-step process is needed, where cleaning is performed prior to disinfection. After sufficient contact time, the surface should be rinsed with clean water to remove any bleach residue (3M, 2011). Bleach is also reactive and can form toxic compounds when mixed with other cleaning chemicals, such as ammonia.

have a written schedule for maintenance and cleaning to keep up an acceptable appearance and preserve the health of the fish. The maintenance schedule should be posted for review by personnel to ensure they are aware of the cleaning processes. Below are examples of cleaning processes that should be completed on a schedule:

22.1.2.1 Floor maintenance

Trash and debris, including dead fish, should be picked up off the floor each day. On a weekly basis, the floor should be swept, including removing debris from under the tanks and filters. Any debris that accumulates in the floor drain should be removed during weekly cleaning.

22.1.2.2 Aquarium maintenance

To maintain a healthy and clean environment for the fish, staff members should wipe algae from tanks using an algae pad or scraper and siphon debris off the bottom of the aquariums. Record which aquariums are being cleaned each day on the maintenance schedule. Cleaning some of the aquariums each day should be done so that they are each cleaned weekly, or more often as necessary, to keep sediment off the bottom and the walls cleaned of algae and biofilm. Table 22.2 lists the process for cleaning individual aquariums.

22.1.2.3 Filter system maintenance

Each fish system may be fitted with a filter containing a water pump, fluidized bed chamber, cartridge filters, foam pads or filter sock, an ultraviolet sterilizer, a heater or chiller for temperature regulation, and an aerating biological filter (Fig. 22.1). In addition, saltwater systems are fitted with a foam fractionator (protein skimmer). The fluidized bed should be observed daily to ensure the sand or beads are freely moving and the water is not channeling around any compaction. The cartridge or canister filters should be backflushed or cleaned once weekly. Any foam pads or filter bags (Fig. 22.2) that trap particulate matter should be rinsed off or replaced daily. Clean deposits and debris from the filter components when performing weekly maintenance tasks on the systems. Keep the outside of the filter housing clean.

22.1.2.4 Water pump maintenance

If the flow of a pump is reduced, check the filter basket (if present) to be sure it is not full of debris that is obstructing the water flow. There may also be an obstruction in the water line blocking water flow.

Table 22.2. General cleaning procedure for aquariums. Author's own table.

A. Daily cleaning: Aquariums scheduled for maintenance should be siphoned to remove sediment, but any dirty tanks should be siphoned daily, especially if heavily stocked with fish. Siphoning is to be done after feeding to remove any uneaten food.
  1. Ensure there is enough water in the filter sump to perform the siphoning without running the sump too low to pump water back into the tanks.
  2. UNPLUG ANY AQUARIUM HEATER THAT WILL BE ABOVE WATER DURING SIPHONING.
  3. Use a designated cleaning pad or brush to scrub algae from aquarium walls.
  4. Use a siphon hose with a piece of netting attached over the end to prevent fish from being accidentally siphoned out.
  5. Place the other end of the hose directly into a floor drain (if available) when siphoning.
  6. Siphon under sponge filters and air stones to remove waste and residual food.
  7. Once siphoning is complete, ensure all required valves are open, heaters are plugged back in, and the filter sump is filled to the required level.

B. Tank Disinfecting:
  1. This should be prior to any new fish being added to an empty tank. Scrub the tank and disinfect it with benzalkonium chloride or potassium permanganate solution ($KMnO_4$), especially if there were sick fish in the tank. Shut off water flow from the filter if cleaning one tank in a connected recirculating filtration system.
    (a) Rinse filter sponges and netting on the drains, if applicable.
    (b) Add potassium permanganate to the tank at 2 mg/l.
    (c) Leave the potassium permanganate solution in the water for 15 min.
    (d) Drain the tank, then refill and drain it again using a pump or siphon hose.
    (e) Wipe out any remaining disinfectant solution (wear gloves).
    (f) Fill the tank and ensure all required valves are open to the proper levels.
  2. New fish should only be added into an empty aquarium, not to one that still has fish remaining from a previous shipment.

Water pumps should not blow air bubbles into the water, as that can lead to supersaturation. For variable speed pumps, ensure they are at the proper setting.

22.1.2.5 *Fluidized bed tower maintenance*

Very little maintenance is required for the fluidized bed towers. If a large quantity of the sand in a fluidized bed aggregates at the bottom of the tower causing reduced sand suspension, these aggregates need to be broken apart using a spray from a water hose inserted down into the fluidized bed tower. Alternatively, a hose can also be used to siphon the aggregated sand out of the tower if necessary.

The only other maintenance required is the periodic addition of sand to replenish the bed. When collapsed, the depth of the sand should be 25–35% of the height of the tower. Use only the appropriate grain-size sand to top off the beds. The sand should be the same size as any remaining sand in the tower to prevent stratification. Rinse the sand off if necessary to remove dust, then pour the sand into the top of the tower.

22.1.2.6 *Protein skimmer maintenance*

The collection cup at the top of the protein skimmer should be rinsed and drained daily. On a weekly basis, thoroughly wash out the collection cup and drain line. The body of the skimmer tower needs no maintenance. The venturis likewise should not need any maintenance, although depending on water chemistry in the systems, they may need occasional disassembly and cleaning.

22.1.2.7 *Aerating (Bioball) tower maintenance*

The bioball gas-exchange tower needs no maintenance other than the occasional removal of mineral or salt accumulation from the outside of the container. Wipe this surface using a wet sponge. Ensure that water is flowing freely through all the bioballs in the tower and not just down one side. For effective bacterial nitrification, water should be flowing downward continuously through the bioballs, but they should be exposed to the air and not submerged in water.

22.1.2.8 *Ultraviolet light unit maintenance*

Ultraviolet (UV) lights can be used to kill free-floating algae and some microorganisms in the water. They also will break down ozone and many chemicals or medications added to the water. The recommended dose of ultraviolet radiation to kill bacteria

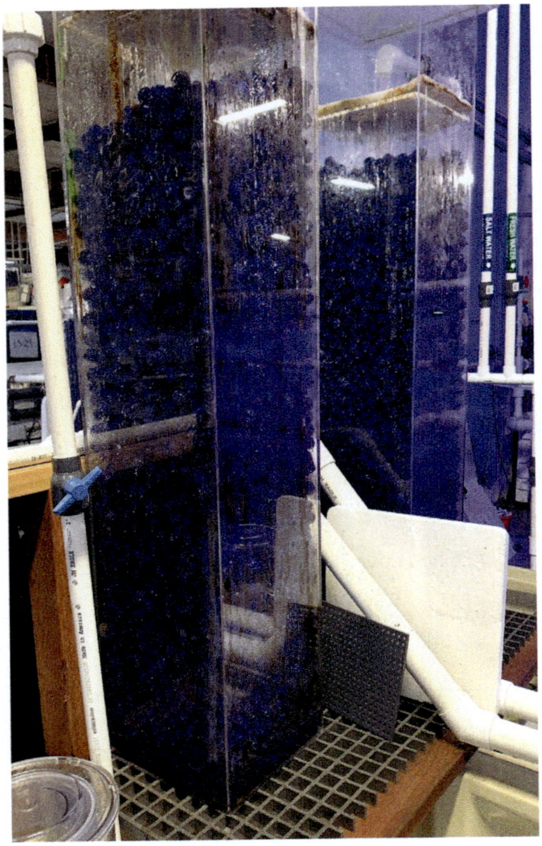

Fig. 22.1. Example of an aeration filter (Bioball tower) that provides biological filtration for the removal of ammonia, nitrite, and carbon dioxide from the water. These also supply oxygen to the water. (Photograph by N. Saint-Erne.)

is 10–25 mJ/cm^2 (OIE, 2006). To kill some viruses requires 125–200 mJ/cm^2, while small parasites may require 1000 mJ/cm^2. UV is an effective killer of pathogens in clear water but is ineffective if the water is heavily contaminated with suspended material or some dissolved minerals which prevent light penetration, or if the bulbs have exceeded their recommended working life. The UV bulbs will last about 12 months and need to be replaced on a regular schedule. It is helpful to label the UV light units with the dates of bulb changes to monitor when they were last changed. UV light is harmful to the eyes, so one should never look at an illuminated UV source.

22.1.2.9 Sump maintenance

The sumps will occasionally need to have detritus and sand removed from them. Large amounts of

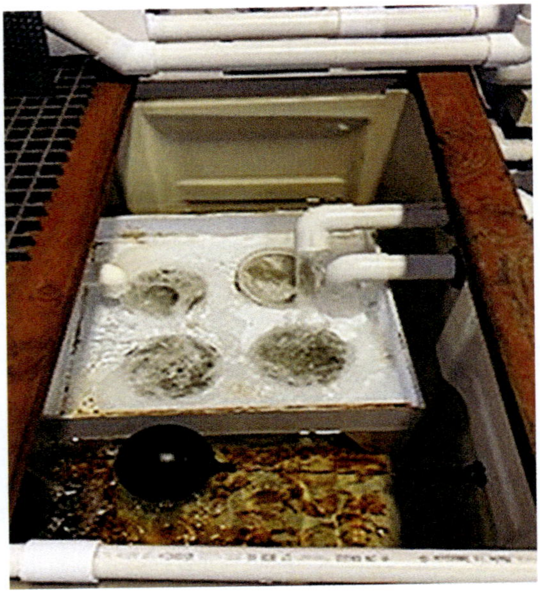

Fig. 22.2. When debris accumulates in the filter bags, the water will back up in the filter bag tray. Clean or exchange the filter bags daily to keep water flowing through them easily. (Photograph by N. Saint-Erne.)

the sand can be removed using a small cup or similar apparatus. Detritus and any remaining sand can be vacuumed out using a canister filter. Do not install a filter cartridge or element in the canister filter. Use the intake line as a vacuum and place the return line into a bucket. Be careful when vacuuming sand to go slowly, as attempting to vacuum sand too quickly into the canister filter will jam the impeller. Discard the collected sand into the trash.

22.1.2.10 Replenishment line maintenance

The water replenishment lines, valves, and flowmeters that supply the systems should be checked regularly (Fig. 22.3). On a weekly basis, the flowmeters should be cleaned by opening the associated valve fully and then closing it completely. Repeat this cycle several times. If the flowmeters and/or water lines become clogged, the pump valve feeding the system replenishment line can be shut off; the flowmeter removed, disassembled, thoroughly cleaned, and then reassembled; and the valve reopened.

22.1.3 Fish disposal

Remove dead fish from tanks and off the floor daily and record them on the appropriate inventory

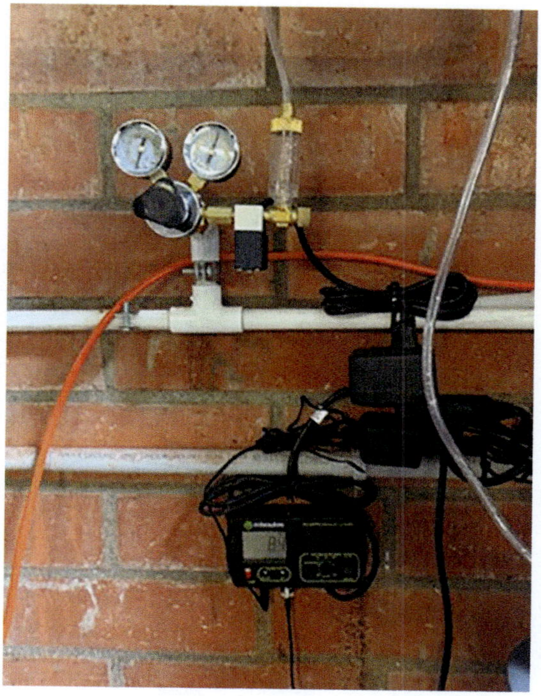

Fig. 22.3. Water valves and flowmeters should be checked and cleaned weekly. (Photograph by N. Saint-Erne.)

form. If more than 5% of fish are removed from a tank as dead, then the tank should be put on hold until the fish can be evaluated. Dead fish must be sealed in a plastic bag after being accounted and must be placed into a trash container. If trash collection is more than a day away, freeze bags of dead fish and dispose of them right before the trash is collected.

Dead fish also accumulate under the aquariums from fish jumping out. Remove the fish from under the tanks and record the losses on the appropriate inventory form. Do not allow fish to accumulate under the aquariums or on the floor. Use lids on tanks containing fish prone to jumping.

22.1.4 Isolating sick or injured fish

Fish that have been isolated due to a disease need to be diagnosed and treated with the appropriate medications and can only be returned to the original tanks after being cured. Aquariums containing isolated or quarantined fish should be separated from the main aquariums and clearly marked as "Fish Hospital" or "Quarantine Tank" (Fig. 22.4). Severely injured or dying fish should be euthanized after examination, using an overdose of anesthetic in a small volume of water. If any wrong species of fish arrive from a supplier mixed in with another species, move them into the appropriate tank after being quarantined if they are healthy. If it is a species not normally carried, it must be separated into a tank in the Hospital area and can be adopted out.

22.1.5 Facility conditions

Access to the facility should be secured to prevent entry by unauthorized persons. The facility should have a Maintenance Schedule and a Daily Inspection form to ensure all required tasks are being completed (Fig. 22.5). Equipment, such as hoses, vacuums, brooms, and other maintenance supplies, should be properly stored for easy access (Fig. 22.6). The facility needs to be maintained in a clean manner with appropriate conditions for workers and fish.

The central area of the facility should have a digital thermometer and hygrometer that records the minimum and maximum temperatures and humidity for reference (Fig. 22.7). Each workday, record the minimum and maximum readings for temperature and humidity on the maintenance schedule and then reset the meter. The appropriate temperature for tropical fish health is 70–78°F/21–26°C for facilities that have aquarium temperatures at ambient air temperature. Humidity in the facility should be maintained in the range of 40–70%. In addition, there should be an aquarium thermometer to measure the water temperature in each fish system. Any abnormal temperature variations should be addressed to determine the cause and prevent future temperature variations.

Generators or other emergency power sources should be available to support vital functions during power shortages and should be tested regularly. Main system water pumps, filters, and other essential life support components should have a reserve supply so that they may be replaced without affecting the operation of the system. Facilities must be checked within 2 h of a power outage to ensure the filtration systems are functioning to prevent fish loss from lack of water circulation.

During the day, bright lighting is important to carefully examine the fish for health and when netting the fish for shipping. However, fish need a dark period to rest, so the lights over the fish systems should be turned off at night. Fish are easily startled when lights are suddenly turned on at night.

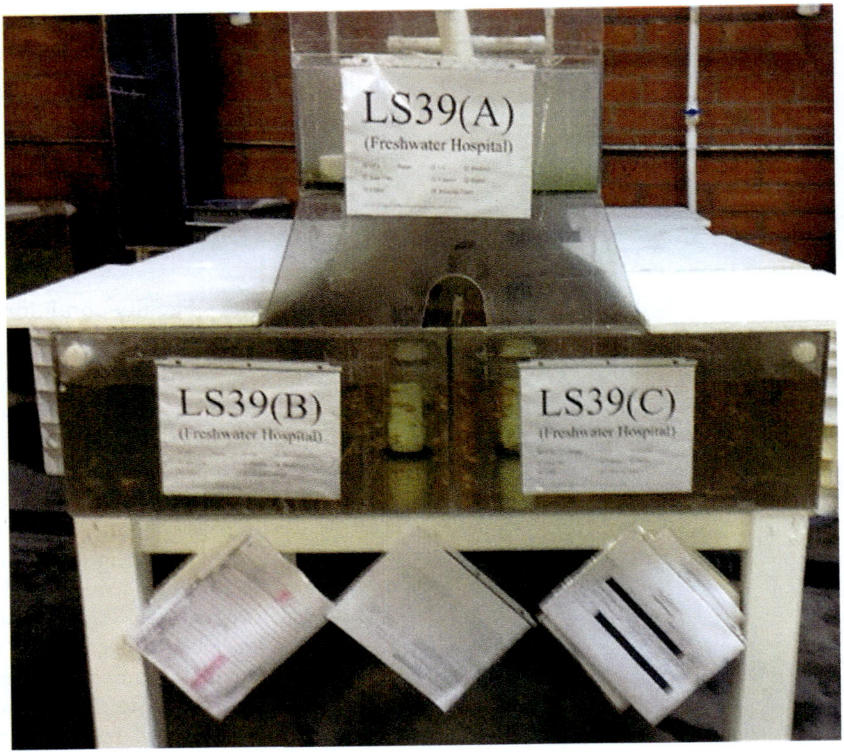

Fig. 22.4. Separate fish system for isolating and treating sick and injured fish. (Photograph by N. Saint-Erne.)

Having exterior windows in the facility will allow natural daylight into the room at sunrise to gradually increase the light, before turning on the overhead lighting. Where bright task lighting is needed for people working in the room at night, it should be restricted to the area where needed, without excessively lighting the aquariums. Care should be taken to ensure that fish are not disturbed by nighttime security lighting. Emergency lighting in the facility should be in the area by the offices and by the exits, but not directly over the fish tanks.

Safety issues are an important consideration. Everyone should be aware of potential hazards and alert the facility management of any unsafe conditions or practices. All chemicals should be stored in locked cabinets, and appropriate Personal Protective Equipment (PPE) used when needed. Persons using any chemicals should be trained in their use and be authorized to use them. An eyewash Station should be available for use by all employees. All exterior exits should be marked for visibility. Fire extinguishers should be placed around the facility, especially near the exits. Appropriate smoke and fire monitors should be in place around the facility. All large oxygen tanks should be secured to a wall to prevent them from falling over (Fig. 22.8). Fish species that pose dangers to handlers (sharp teeth or venomous spines) should have the tanks appropriately labeled (Fig. 22.9).

Pest control is necessary to prevent insects, rodents, or other animals from entering the facility. The exterior of the building must have pest control measures in place around entryways. Rodent bait stations are placed around the building perimeter (Fig. 22.10). Interior pest control measures include rodent traps along any exterior walls and on either side of any exterior doorway. Electric flytraps may be used if flying insects are a concern but should be placed in an area away from personnel, and not over the fish tanks. Bait stations and traps need to be inspected and replaced periodically.

22.1.6 Record keeping

There are several functions that should be recorded for future review. Previous records mentioned were a maintenance schedule and log for monitoring filters or aquariums that need to be cleaned or

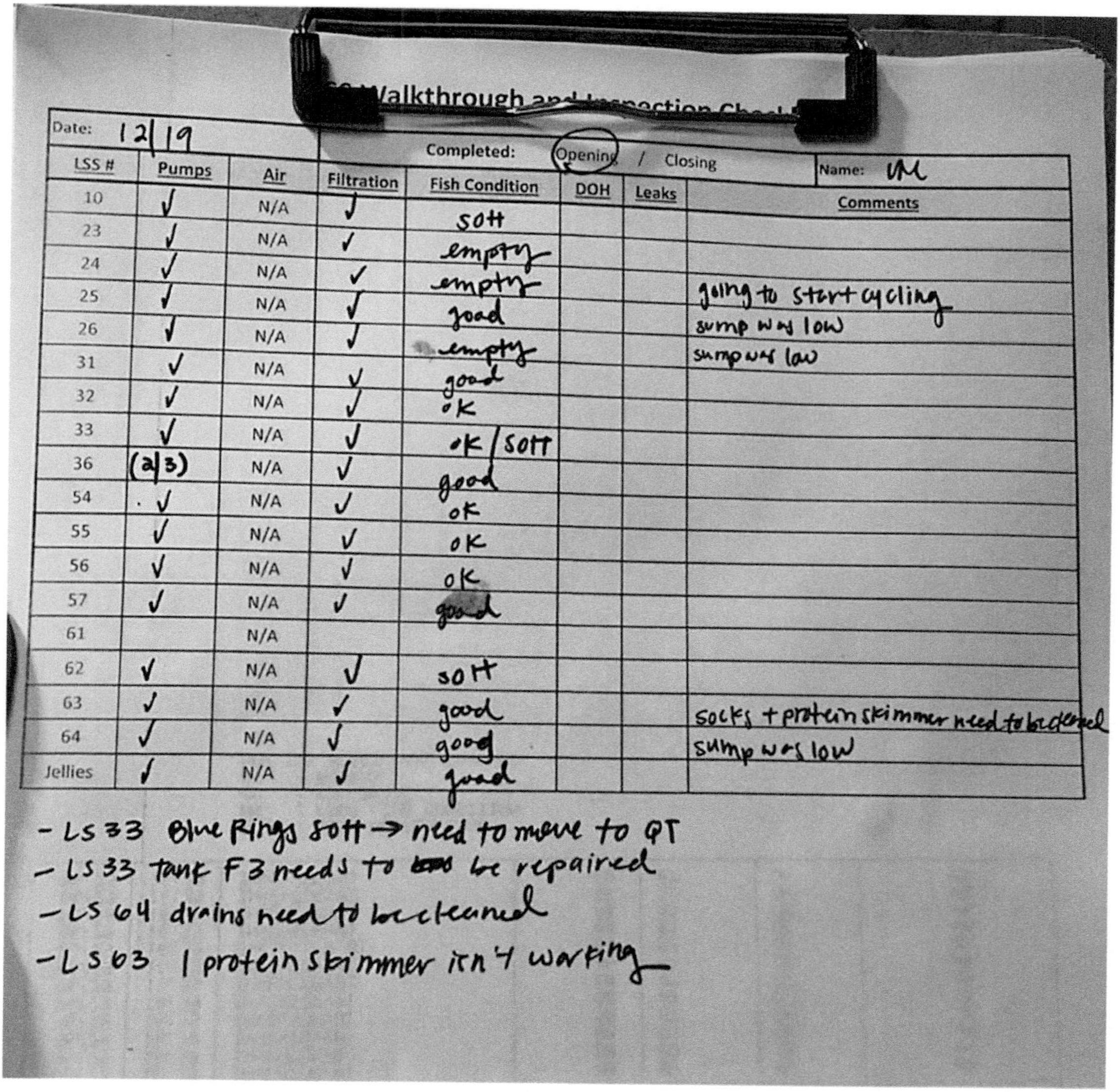

Date: 12/19 | Completed: Opening / Closing | Name: [illegible]

LSS #	Pumps	Air	Filtration	Fish Condition	DOH	Leaks	Comments
10	✓	N/A	✓	soft			
23	✓	N/A	✓	empty			
24	✓	N/A	✓	empty			
25	✓	N/A	✓	good			going to start cycling
26	✓	N/A	✓	empty			sump was low
31	✓	N/A	✓	good			sump was low
32	✓	N/A	✓	ok			
33	✓	N/A	✓	ok / soft			
36	(2/3)	N/A	✓	good			
54	✓	N/A	✓	ok			
55	✓	N/A	✓	ok			
56	✓	N/A	✓	ok			
57	✓	N/A	✓	good			
61		N/A					
62	✓	N/A	✓	soft			
63	✓	N/A	✓	good			socks + protein skimmer need to be cleaned
64	✓	N/A	✓	good			sump was low
Jellies	✓	N/A	✓	good			

- LS 33 Blue Rings soft → need to move to QT
- LS 33 tank F3 needs to be repaired
- LS 64 drains need to be cleaned
- LS 63 1 protein skimmer isn't working

Fig. 22.5. Daily Inspection Checklist. (Photograph by N. Saint-Erne.)

repaired, and an inspection checklist to record the health of the fish in each aquarium system and if there is any problem in that system. Other helpful records include:

Water Chemistry Log: This spreadsheet shows the results of water chemistry analysis. This should include data for all water tests conducted on the fish systems in the facility. When abnormal water tests are reported for a fish system, the system should be examined to ensure that all the filtration equipment is working properly. Water changes should be made as needed to return the water to the correct parameters.

Fish Health Record: This spreadsheet shows results from various diagnostic tests (mucus scrapings, biopsies, necropsies) performed on fish. The spreadsheet indicates the source of the fish, date tested, fish tested, date of receipt, results of the test, and any action taken based on the results, including medications. Testing should occur on fish that appear unhealthy, and results of tests should be recorded in the Fish Health Record. Suppliers of

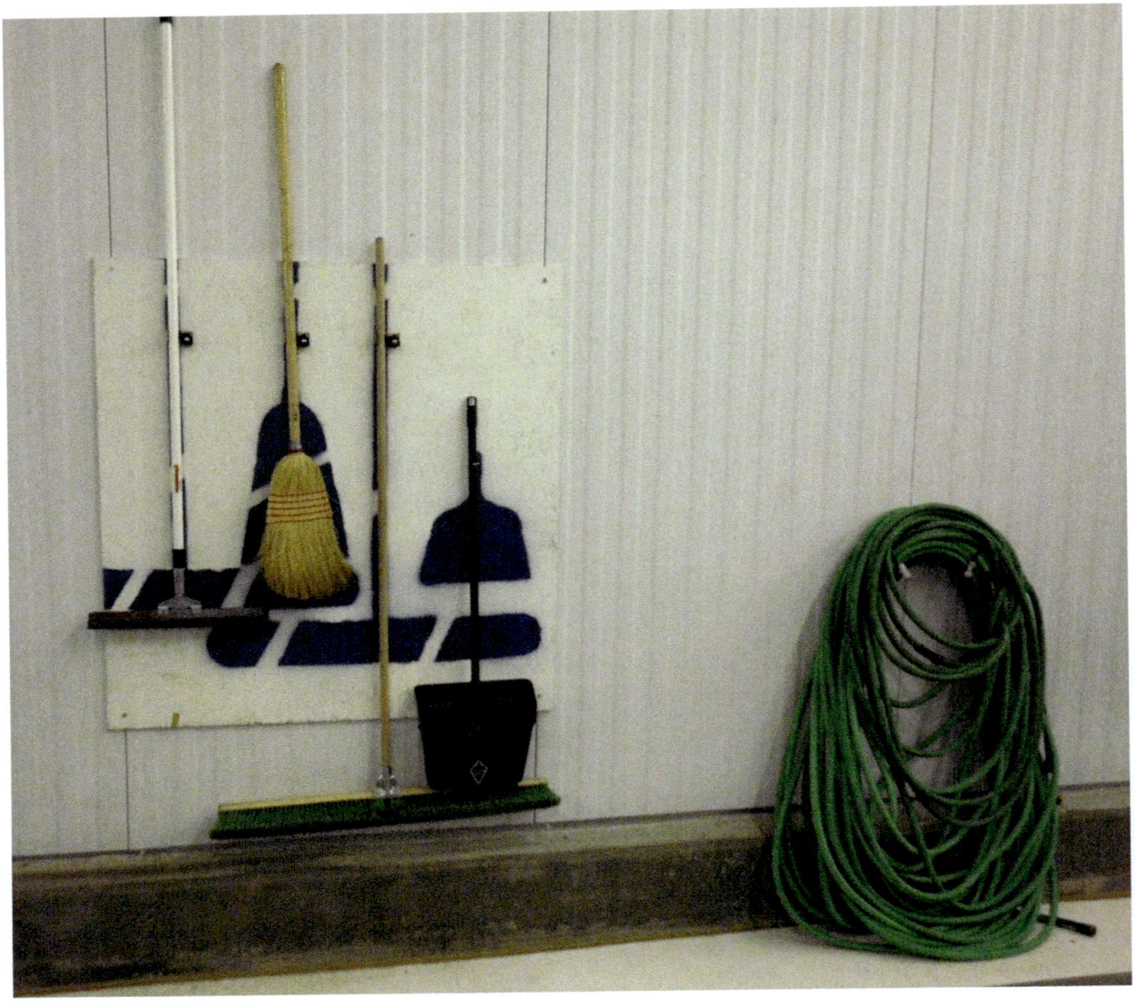

Fig. 22.6. Proper storage of cleaning equipment. (Photograph by N. Saint-Erne.)

fish with health issues should be notified of the results of diagnostic testing.

Chemical Receipt Log: This includes an inventory of any potentially dangerous chemicals that are used in the facility. When a delivery of a chemical arrives, it should be recorded on the Chemical Receipt Log, and the products kept in the chemical storage room or cabinet. Each record in the database should correspond to a single container and not merely the chemical itself. All records should be maintained for at least 6 months. Listing the received dates and expiration dates ensures that unstable chemicals are not kept beyond their useful life. Information fields for each record in the Chemical Receipt Log should contain at a minimum:

- Chemical name
- Size of container and quantity received
- Date of receipt
- Storage location
- Expiration date
- Initials of person entering the information into the log

Most commercially packaged chemical containers will have adequate labels that include hazard information. However, the commercial container should be labeled using an indelible pen with the date received. Any chemicals that are transferred or repackaged into secondary containers need to be marked with their contents and all the essential information as on the original container label.

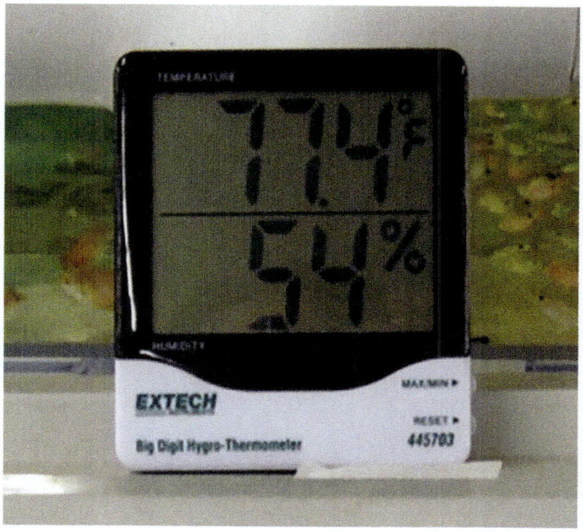

Fig. 22.7. A digital thermometer/hygrometer that also records minimum and maximum temperature and humidity levels should be used in the facility to monitor conditions in the building. (Photograph by N. Saint-Erne.)

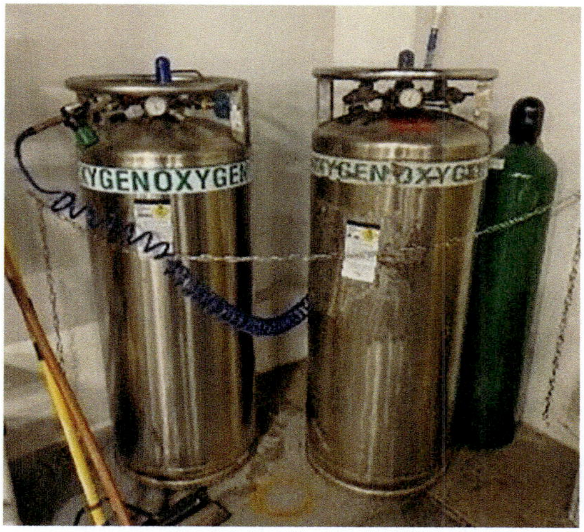

Fig. 22.8. Oxygen cylinders are secured to the wall with a chain to prevent tipping. (Photograph by N. Saint-Erne.)

Fish Treatment Log: As medications are used in the facility, the Fish Treatment Log will be updated with the date, name of the medication being used, dosage, actual amount used, which fish tanks were treated, how the chemical was dispensed, and the user's initials. Water treatment chemicals (e.g. sodium thiosulfate dechlorinator or sodium bicarbonate) are not considered medications and do not need to be listed in the Fish Treatment Log. Referring to the Fish Treatment Log will enable users to determine if treatments were provided to the fish and if the treatments were successful.

22.2 Receiving New Fish Shipments

The first step in preparing to receive fish is to determine the time of arrival for the shipments expected that day. Knowing when the air shipment will land and be delivered to the fish facility by truck will help manage labor for the day. After the truck arrives at the facility, the pallets of fish are removed from the truck and placed in an appropriate area where the fish can be unpacked, acclimatized, and put away into designated aquariums. When the shipments arrive, the pallets should be arranged near the receiving table, and the receiving crew assembled. Once all boxes have been unloaded, the boxes are counted to ensure they are all present (Fig. 22.11). The box or pallet count should match the courier and airway bill information supplied with each shipment. If these numbers do not match, it must be noted on the paperwork for the individual shipment. Once this is done, begin unpacking the fish.

22.2.1 Unpacking fish

One person will be needed to check the incoming fish bags off the appropriate invoices. This is usually a member of the management team. Two people will unpack the boxes of fish. These people should be familiar with identifying all the fish, as not all the boxes will be labeled as to their contents. The unpackers will place the bags onto receiving carts, along with the appropriate bag labels. Two unpackers will move the fish to the acclimatization area. These individuals will also be responsible for placing the labels supplied by the invoice checker onto the appropriate bags. Once their cart is full of bags, they will take the cart to the first empty acclimatization table, place one bag into an empty acclimatization tote, and remove the label from the bag, placing it on the front of the tote. When all bags are offloaded, the driver should return to the receiving area to load the cart again if necessary. One associate will cut open the bags of fish, pour the contents of the bag into the acclimatization tote, and then dispose of the bag into the trash.

Prior to the fish arriving, they should be assigned to be placed in appropriate tanks in the fish systems. That tank location should be indicated on the label placed on the fish bag, based on the following criteria:

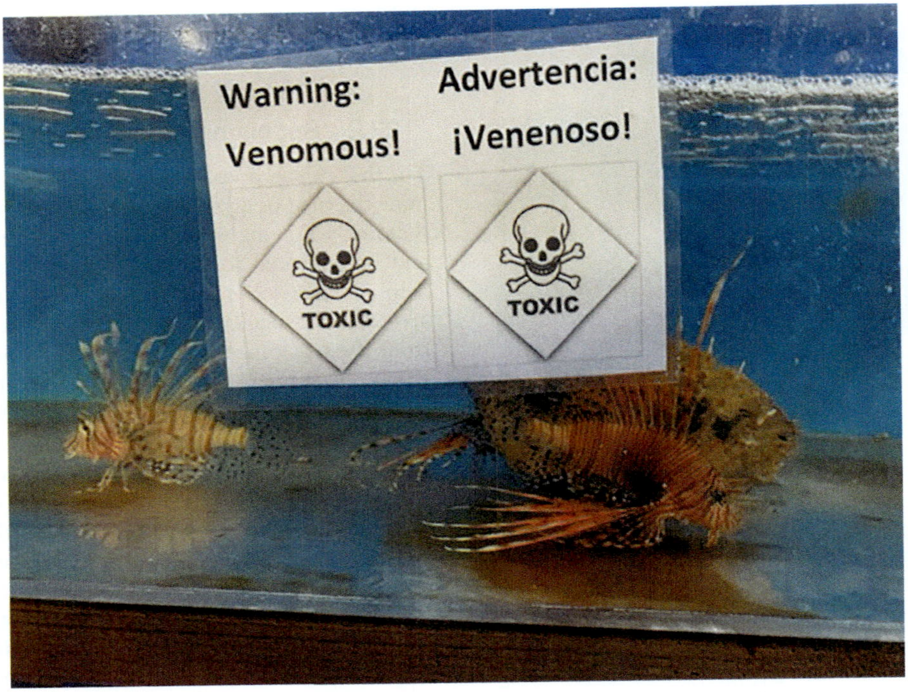

Fig. 22.9. Red Lionfish (*Pterois volitans*) with venomous spines are labeled with a warning sign. (Photograph by N. Saint-Erne.)

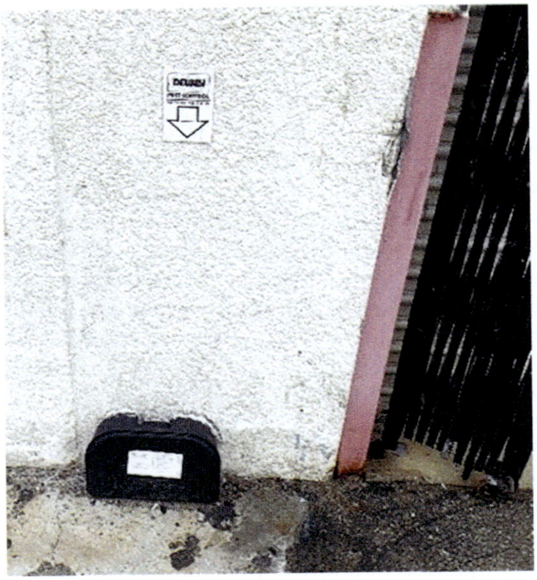

Fig. 22.10. Outside rodent bait station by doorway. (Photograph by N. Saint-Erne.)

1. Identify the fish that are arriving regarding their size and required water chemistry.

  A. Size: Verify the capacity of the different systems depending on the size of the incoming fish. Always avoid a high density in the aquariums so that the filtration system will be able to support the fish in healthy water conditions.

  B. Water chemistry: Verify the specific water conditions needed for the incoming fresh and saltwater fish and make sure those are available in the system.

2. Assign the fish system where the fish will be placed. Make sure that the criteria of size and water chemistry for the incoming livestock are followed correctly.

3. Assign the appropriate acclimatization procedure.

  A. Select the proper acclimatization procedure for each species. Acclimatization procedure can vary depending on the type of fish/invertebrate.

  B. Always handle the livestock with care.

Once all the bags are on the acclimatization tables, invoices checked in, and bags opened, the acclimatization process can begin. Associates can begin removing dead fish from the acclimatization totes. The number of dead fish should be written on the label for the tote.

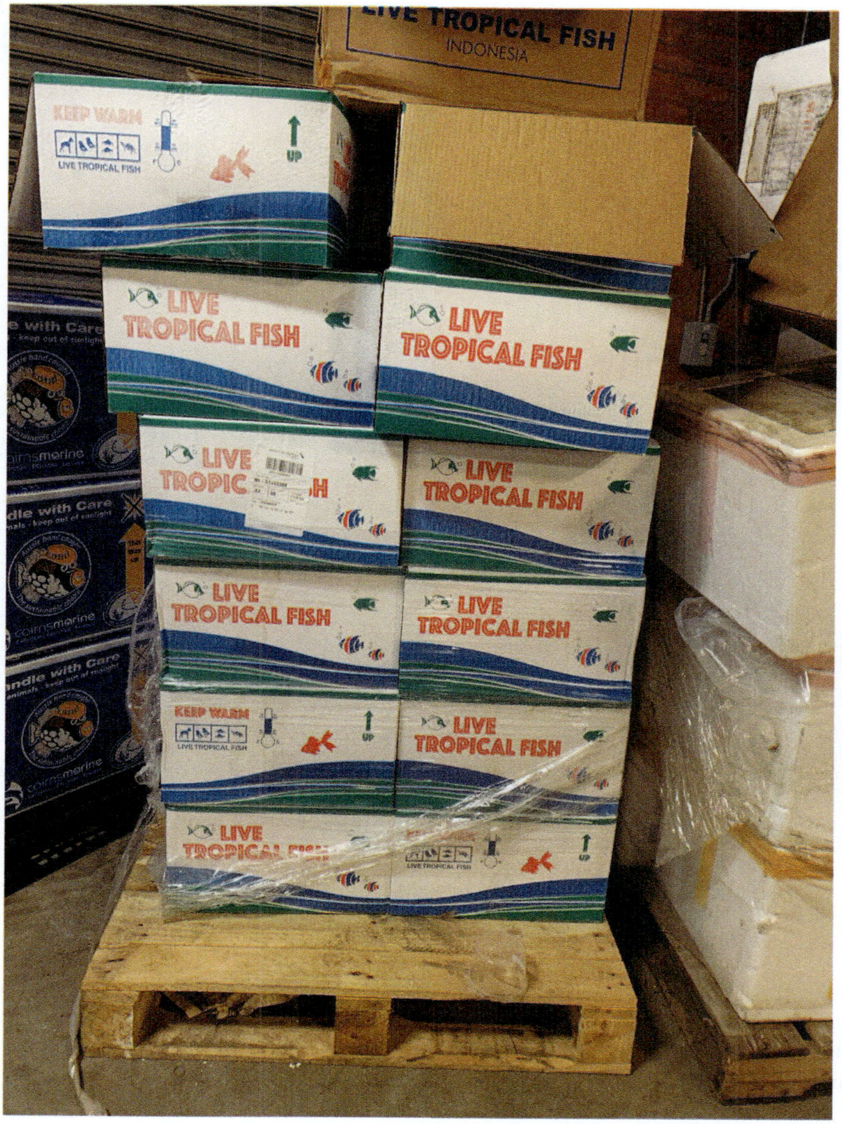

Fig. 22.11. Boxes of fish delivered to a fish wholesale facility. (Photograph by N. Saint-Erne.)

22.2.2 Acclimatization procedures

Acclimatization may include gradual water change by dripping water into the totes containing fish, or temperature acclimatization only by floating bags of fish in a tank, and then releasing the fish into the tank once temperatures have equilibrated. When the fish bags are unpacked, they must be checked for dead fish. If there are dead fish in a bag, or the water is dirty from fish waste, the fish should be acclimated by the drip method (Fig. 22.12).

After opening the bag, place the fish into an acclimatization tote, and remove any dead fish from the acclimatization tote. Ensure proper water and air are turned on in the lines going into the totes. Add the freshwater or saltwater hoses and airlines into the acclimatization tote. Add bags of fish into the acclimatization container, using only as much water from the bag as needed for covering the fish. It may be helpful to add an ammonia neutralizer into the water in the tote while the fish are

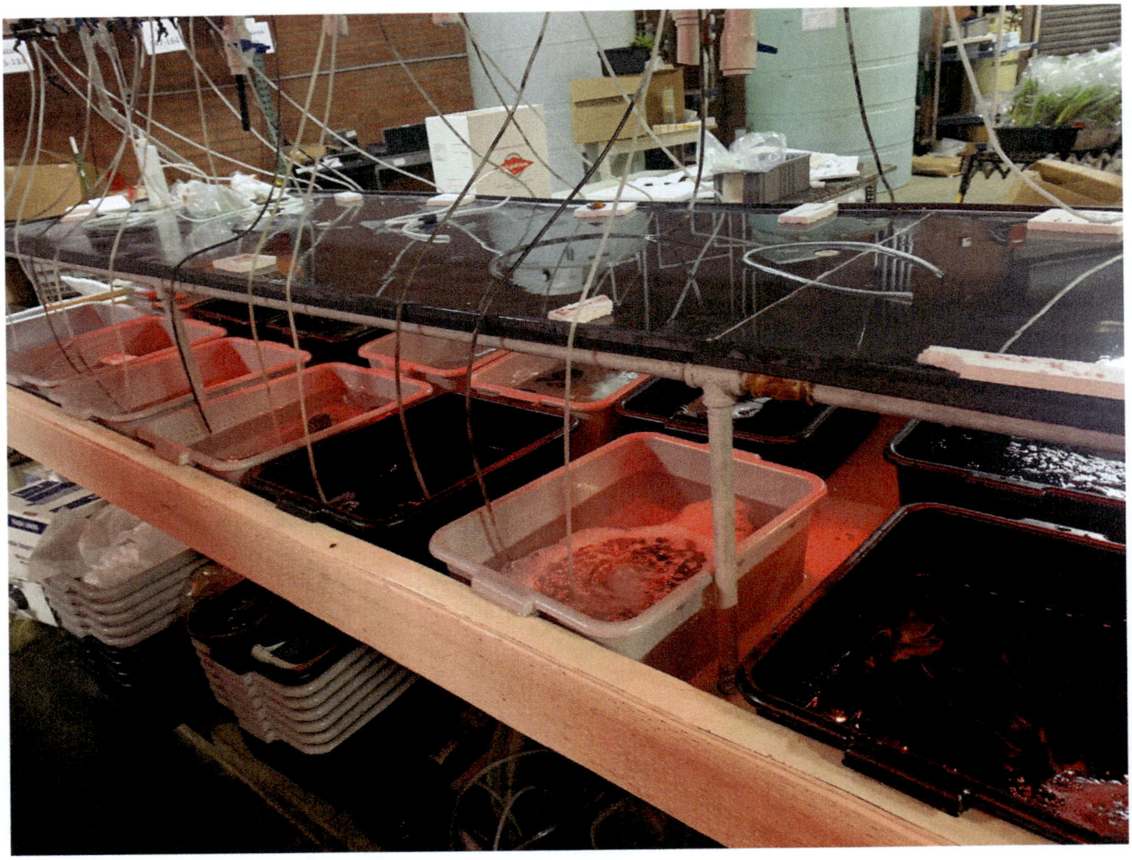

Fig. 22.12. Drip acclimatization table and totes for incoming fish at a wholesale facility. Different hoses contain air attached to air stones, fresh water, and salt water. (Photograph by N. Saint-Erne.)

being acclimated to prevent the accumulated ammonia in the shipping water from becoming toxic as the pH of the water is raised during drip acclimatization. Add the bag label onto the tote. Run the system water into the acclimatization container for specified time, then the tote containing the fish can be moved to the designated tank in a fish system and the label placed onto that tank. Turn off the water flowing through the hoses to that table once all the totes have been emptied.

If the water in the bags is not excessively dirty and the bags do not have dead fish in them, the unopened bags may be floated for 15 min or more in an aquarium in the fish system to equalize the temperature, and then the bag is opened, and the fish removed from the bag and placed into that tank. Some species of fish that may do better with drip acclimatization include catfish, loaches, algae eaters, bala, and rainbow sharks. The manager should make the decision in each shipment on which fish to acclimate based on inspection of each bag of fish. All newly arrived fish should be placed on hold until examined for health. If the fish are not healthy, they should be diagnosed and treated. The fish should stay on hold until healed.

22.2.3 Tank covers

Use covers on acclimatization totes and tanks for fish that are known to jump out of containers. If the fish are to remain overnight in the acclimatization totes, all totes must have a cover. The following species need to have their acclimatization totes and tanks always covered:

- Bala Sharks, Red Tail Sharks, Rainbow Sharks (regular and albino)
- Koi (all sizes)

- Gouramis (all species)
- Clown Loach
- Barbs (most species)
- Australian Rainbow Fish
- Danios (most species)
- African Cichlids
- South American Cichlids
- Angelicus Botia
- Hatchetfish

22.3 Feeding

Nutritionally balanced diets and appropriate feeding regimens are critical in ensuring that fish remain healthy. Once the fish are placed in the assigned aquariums, feed them following the established schedule. The type of food varies depending on the fish species (Table 22.3). Do not feed fish before preparing for shipment so the fish that will be shipped that day can be identified. After all the fish being shipped for the day have been packed, the remaining fish should be fed.

Common foods for feeding fish in wholesale/retail facilities include:

Commercial flake food
Pelleted food (large and small sizes)
Algae wafers: For algae-eating fish and herbivores
Brine shrimp (live and/or frozen)
Blood worms (frozen)
Mysis shrimp (frozen): Can be fed to all fish
Krill (frozen): For larger fish/predatory fish
Clams on half shell (frozen): For puffers/triggerfish
Silversides (frozen): For predatory fish

22.3.1 Feeding frequency

Fish need to be fed at least once per day, and young fish should be fed three to four times per day. For facilities that are not open every day, feed fish at least once per weekend or a 3-day holiday. When practical, the fish should not be fed the day they are going to be shipped. This reduces food in the intestinal tract when packing fish. Fish that are scheduled to be shipped out that day are not fed in the morning, but then if they are not picked to ship, they should be fed at the end of the day.

22.3.2 Types of food

The type of food being used varies depending on the fish species. Refer to Table 22.3 feeding chart for identifying the type of food required by each species. All small tropical fish (tetras, danios, rasboras, rainbowfish, barbs) and livebearers should be fed appropriately sized flake food or pellets at least once daily. They should be supplemented with frozen

Table 22.3. Feeding chart. Author's own table.

Fish feeding chart	Dry foods		Frozen food
	Flake food	Pellets	Brine shrimp or blood worms
Schooling Tropical Fish	D		W (optional)
Livebearers	D		W (optional)
Goldfish		D	
Koi		D	
South American Cichlids	D	D (optional)	W
Angelfish	D		2W
Large Oscars		D	W
African Cichlids Carnivores—Peacocks, Auratus, Electric Yellow or Blue Labidochromis	D	D	W
African Cichlids Herbivores—Kenyi, Zebras, and other Mbuna cichlids	D	D	W
Catfish, Loaches, Botias	D	D	W
Algae Eaters, Plecos	D	D	W
Eels, Knifefish, Bichir		D	2W
Bettas (can be fed flakes or small pellets)	D	D	

D = Feed Daily
W = Feed Weekly
2W = Feed Twice Weekly

food at least once a week. Goldfish with normal body shapes are fed flakes or pellets, but the fancy egg-shaped goldfish should be fed sinking pellets, so they do not ingest air from feeding at the surface, or flake food that has been placed under the water rather than floating on the surface. Koi can be fed sinking pellets as well as flakes. Cichlids are fed pellets or flake food, along with weekly supplements of frozen food. Angelfish are fed flake food plus twice-weekly supplements of frozen food. Corydoras catfish, loaches, botias, and other bottom-feeders need to be fed sinking pellets and frozen brine shrimp. Plecos and algae eaters are fed sinking pellets or wafers and frozen foods. Peacock eels, dragon gobies, knife fish, and other “picky” eaters should be fed frozen brine shrimp.

22.3.3 Food storage

Feed should be stored in dedicated areas that are dark, temperature and humidity controlled, and pest-free to ensure its nutritional quality. Keep sealed, bulk containers of food in the refrigerator or freezer for prolonged storage. Food for immediate daily use in smaller quantities should be in resealable containers and can be kept in the refrigerator or freezer or at room temperature. Feed used for daily feeding should be of a quantity that is used up frequently and then replaced with feed from bulk storage. No personal food or drink should be stored in the refrigerator or freezer used for storing fish food.

22.4 Disease Diagnosis

The primary function of the aquatic veterinarian and the husbandry team is to ensure that healthy fish are shipped to customers. Each morning, the fish health team members should view every tank in the facility and check for signs of illness or other contraindications for shipping. Each tank should be inspected for fish quality and health, unusual behavior, color changes, injury, and other factors that would indicate possible disease. Any fish that show signs of illness should be examined to determine their health and then treated appropriately.

22.4.1 Newly arrived fish

All incoming populations of fish should be put on hold for 24 h. Fish that remain on hold after 24 h due to losses or poor health should be sampled to diagnose any disease. To determine the cause of a fish disease, the fish should be visually examined for any signs of disease, and then appropriate numbers of fish from the population are tested to diagnose any pathogens. This will help determine the appropriate treatment for the fish. The fish should be checked for diseases or parasites and treated as necessary. If any of the fish are positive for a disease, then the entire population in that tank should be treated. A new sample should then be tested after treatment. The process should continue until all sampled fish from the batch were negative for the disease.

22.4.2 Placing fish on hold

Fish should not be released for shipping on the day they arrive. Any newly arrived fish that are obviously sick, or that are not eating or active, or appear ill should remain on hold until they recover. The fish system or tank should be labeled to indicate the tanks are on hold for diagnosis and treatment (Fig. 22.13). Members of the husbandry team should place any tank on hold that has a significant loss in it (more than 5%). Additionally, any fish that were available for sale, but which now appear unhealthy, should be placed on hold. Any fish that have a history

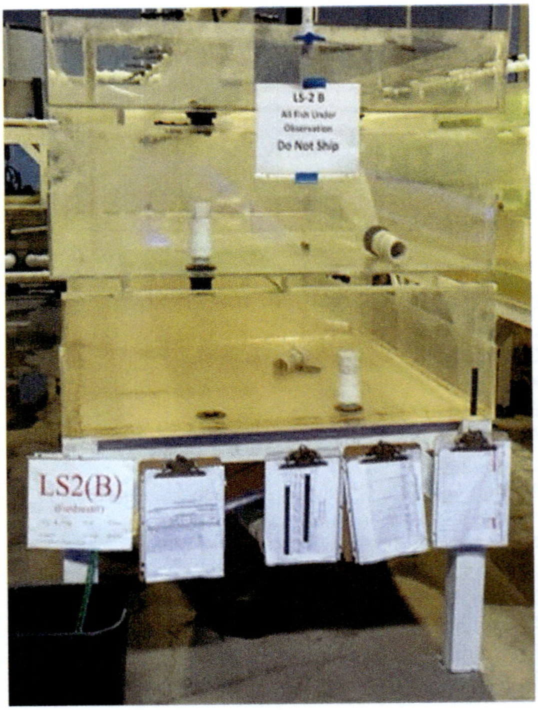

Fig. 22.13. Fish system with Hold notice on tanks. (Photograph by N. Saint-Erne.)

of proving problematic after arrival should be left on hold until it is reasonably certain there are no problems. The fish husbandry manager is responsible for determining the hold status of any tank. Any associate should bring to the attention of the fish husbandry manager a tank of fish that are acting abnormally or that contain dead fish. Fish should never be picked for shipping from a tank that is put on hold. Simultaneously with this process, notes should be made on the health report indicating which fish need further diagnosis. Later in the day, these fish can be biopsied or otherwise examined to determine their ailments and course of treatment.

22.4.3 Releasing fish from hold

Before releasing any fish from being on hold, the fish must be acting normally and eating, after they have been treated, and have negative diagnostic tests for any parasites that had been previously found on the fish.

22.5 Safe Chemical Storage and Handling

Personal Protective Equipment should be worn when handling chemicals, as indicated in 22.5.2 Chemical Safety Guidelines. A copy of the Chemical Safety Guidelines should be posted in the chemical storage area. Chemical products should be safely stored in a Chemical Room or locked storage cabinets, away from the aquarium systems and the water supply, and the storage area labeled with signage (Fig. 22.14). Access to medications and chemicals should be limited to the husbandry team only, using locking cabinets and doors to restrict entry. A list of associates with keys needs to be maintained by the fish health manager. A log of chemicals and medications used should be maintained and updated as new products arrive [See 22.1.6 Record Keeping]. Personal Protective Equipment (PPE) should be stored in the Chemical Room and used as appropriate by people handling chemicals. Chemicals used in the diagnostic laboratory may be stored in locking cabinets in the lab or in the Chemical Room.

Material safety data sheets (SDS) provide essential information on specific chemical substances. Included are data on the physical, chemical, and toxicological properties of the substance along with concise information on handling, storage, and disposal, and appropriate PPE. The SDS for the products used at the facility should be obtained from the manufacturer's websites and downloaded and stored in a computer file. Printed copies can be stored in a 3-ring binder where the chemicals are stored or used.

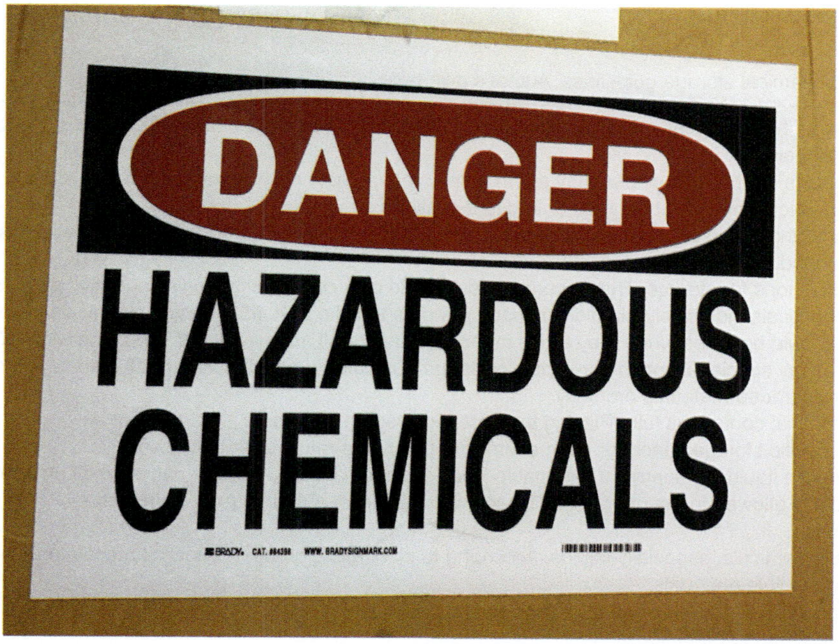

Fig. 22.14. Sign on the door to the Chemical Storage Room. (Photograph by N. Saint-Erne.)

Several medications and water treatments used with fish are considered hazardous to humans. Appropriate PPEs, which may include gloves, mask, chemical apron, and goggles, should be worn when handling chemicals. When a chemical spill occurs, see the SDS for information on proper clean-up precautions. Follow the cleaning guidelines on the product SDS for PPE required and proper disposal of the product. Wear the appropriate gloves when handling medications or sick fish. This will reduce the risk of disease transmission or drug exposure. Eyewash stations should be available, located near the chemical storage or the lab. Each team member should become familiar with the use of these safety features, and specifically where they are in the facility. Eyewash stations should be tested monthly.

22.5.1 General guidelines for chemical storage

Safely storing chemicals in laboratories requires considering many health and safety factors. Proper use of containers and lab equipment is critical. Listed below (Table 22.4) are some general guidelines for safe chemical storage. Spend a few minutes going through the laboratory with this list on a regular basis, and you should avoid any major incidents with chemical storage.

22.5.2 Chemical safety guidelines

Medications, disinfectants, and other chemicals used in fish facilities can be highly toxic to fish and humans (e.g. formalin, hypochlorite, peroxide) and must be handled and applied with due care using the PPE appropriate to the individual chemical being applied and the specific application. The recommendations and safety advice on the use of individual chemicals supplied by the manufacturer and on the SDS should be strictly followed. Below is a list of safe handling recommendations for commonly used chemicals:

Benzalkonium chloride: Protective gloves should be worn when transferring concentrated benzalkonium chloride to vessels for the preparation of disinfectant or net dip.

Disinfectants/floor cleaning solutions: Gloves should be worn. Wash skin if contacted.

Formalin: Wear chemical-resistant gloves when handling formalin. Use in well-ventilated areas. Wear goggles to prevent splashes into the eyes.

Formalin/malachite green solution: Wear chemical-resistant gloves when handling formalin/malachite green solution. These chemicals must be used in well-ventilated areas. Goggles must be worn to prevent splashes into the eyes when pouring from bulk containers. Wearing a chemical apron will prevent staining of clothing. It is recommended to wear a dust mask when mixing malachite green crystals into formalin to avoid inhalation of dust.

Table 22.4. Safe chemical storage guidelines. Author's own table.

- Do not store large, heavy containers or liquids on high shelves or in high cabinets. A good rule is to store these at shoulder level or below.
- Do not store bottles on the floor unless they are in some type of secondary containment.
- Do not store chemicals near heat sources or in direct sunlight.
- Avoid storing anything on top of cabinets. This can interfere with the fire suppression system. Ensure at least 18 inches of clearance around all sprinkler heads.
- Do not use bench tops for storage. These workspaces should only contain chemicals currently being used.
- Do not store chemicals indefinitely. Humidity causes powders to cake or harden. Liquid chemicals evaporate. All containers should be dated when they arrive in the lab. Ensure all manufacturers' expiration dates are strictly followed. Pay special attention to reactive or dangerous compounds. Dispose of all outdated, hardened, evaporated, or degraded materials promptly.
- Do label all chemical containers fully. Placing the date received on each one.
- Do provide a specific storage space for each chemical and ensure return after each use.
- Do store flammable liquids in approved flammable liquid storage cabinets. Usually, only a small amount of flammable liquid is allowed in the open room. Check with your local authority (e.g. fire marshal) for allowable limits.
- Do separate all chemicals, especially liquids, according to compatible groups. Follow all precautions regarding storage of incompatible materials.
- Do use appropriate resistant secondary containers for corrosive materials. This protects the cabinets and catches any leaks or spills due to breakage.
- Do seal containers tightly to prevent the escape of vapors.

Hydrogen peroxide: Wear protective gloves when handling peroxide. Use in well-ventilated areas. Wearing a chemical apron will prevent staining of clothing.

Malachite green crystals: Wear a dust mask, as well as protective gloves when using this chemical. Wearing a chemical apron will prevent staining of clothing.

Methylene blue crystals: Wear a dust mask as well as protective gloves when using this chemical. Wearing a chemical apron will prevent staining of clothing.

MS-222 or other tranquilizers: No protective wear is required. Wash hands after handling. Wash skin if it gets on exposed skin. Wear goggles if risk of splashing into the eyes is present.

Potassium Permanganate: Wear a dust mask and protective gloves when mixing this compound into a solution. Wear protective gloves when using the solution. Potassium permanganate is a strong oxidizer and will stain anything it comes in contact with. Wearing a chemical apron will prevent staining of clothing. Hazardous in case of skin contact (irritant), eye contact (corrosive), ingestion or inhalation.

Praziquantel: A dust mask is worn when dispensing this drug from the bulk container to individual dosing containers.

Water test reagents: No protective equipment needed. Wash hands after use.

22.6 Biosecurity

One highly effective way to reduce the risk of infection and disease at a fish breeding or a wholesale facility is the development of a biosecurity plan (OATA, 2006). The principles of biosecurity include:

- Risk Assessment: Making a written plan on disease risks and their prevention.
- Disease Surveillance/Diagnostic Testing: Appropriate diagnostic assays are used to determine the presence or absence of diseases.
- Control of Movement:
  - People: Minimize access/wear PPE
  - Animals: "All in/all out"
  - Quarantine: Evaluate critical points where disease can enter and leave an aquaculture facility
  - Equipment: Clean, then disinfect
  - Water quality and flow: Source and outflow
- Emergency Preparedness:
  - Diseases: Develop contingency plans should a disease occur
  - Contingency plans for emergencies (power outages, fire, flood, earthquake, storms)

Quarantine is an important risk management measure that should be considered when developing strategies for aquatic animal health management. It can also be used effectively to increase biosecurity at the farm production level (Arthur *et al.*, 2008). The World Organisation for Animal Health (formerly the Office International des Épizooties, OIE), provides a definition of quarantine in the Aquatic Animal Health Code (OIE, 2006): "Quarantine means maintaining a group of aquatic animals in isolation with no direct or indirect contact with other aquatic animals, in order to undergo observation for a specified length of time and, if appropriate, testing and treatment, including proper treatment of the effluent waters."

The Food and Agriculture Organization of the United Nations (Arthur *et al.*, 2008) defines three levels of risk in biosecurity: (i) the quarantine of "high-risk" species, such as aquatic animals being moved either internationally or domestically between regions of different health status that are destined for use in aquaculture, capture fishery development, or other applications where release or escape of animals or the pathogens they may be carrying into the natural environment is likely to occur; (ii) the quarantine of "lower-risk" species, such as aquatic animals destined for the ornamental trade; and (iii) the routine quarantine of aquatic animals at production facilities. The stringency of quarantine applied should be commensurate with the estimated level of risk, which is a function of the source and destination of the aquatic animal movement. Importations of exotic species for aquaculture development and those originating from wild populations will often require stringent quarantine measures.

Proper biosecurity requires newly arrived fish to be isolated and acclimatized. If the incoming fish are carrying any pathogens, then quarantine and appropriate treatments will prevent the diseases from transferring to the existing fish in the facility. Associates should start work with the species and areas that are "cleanest," that is, those likely to have the least pathogens, such as previously treated fish, and the most vulnerable, young, or stressed fish. Newly arrived fish may need to be treated with caution, and care should be taken to ensure diseases are not transferred to or from them. Deal with the fish requiring disease treatment last. Working in this way reduces the potential for pathogen transfer to "clean" fish (OATA, 2006).

All staff entering the quarantine facility must be adequately trained in the husbandry of the species being held in quarantine and be familiar with the biosecurity protocols. Waterproof boots and protective clothing should be worn into the quarantine area, and personnel should walk through a foot bath to disinfect the footwear on entering and leaving quarantine areas (Fig. 22.15). The hands should be washed before work, and when leaving the quarantine or treatment area. Protective gloves and other PPE should be worn when mixing chemicals or adding medications into aquarium systems.

For home aquariums and pond keepers, biosecurity can be provided by setting up a separate quarantine aquarium or holding pond (Fig. 22.16). In this manner, new fish can be kept in a clean tank that has an established biofilter, or has sponge filters added into it, and be isolated from existing fish. After observation and treatment for a period of at least two and preferably 4 weeks or more. If the fish are healthy, they can then be transferred to the main aquarium or pond.

22.7 Conclusion

Every step in the transfer of fish from the producer to the wholesaler, then the retail store, and finally the home aquarist can cause stress and illness in the fish. Fish that are healthy at the farm, and carrying a low parasite load, may never show signs of disease. But once those fish are netted, transported, and then unbagged and placed into a new environment with possibly different water parameters, the stress can weaken the fish and allow pathogens to multiply on the fish, causing diseases. Proper handling, shipping methods, and water quality will keep the fish healthier. Quarantine and biosecurity measures at each step of the process will reduce the risk of spreading the diseases not only to other fish in the facilities but also to the environment and, with zoonotic diseases, to the fish handlers.

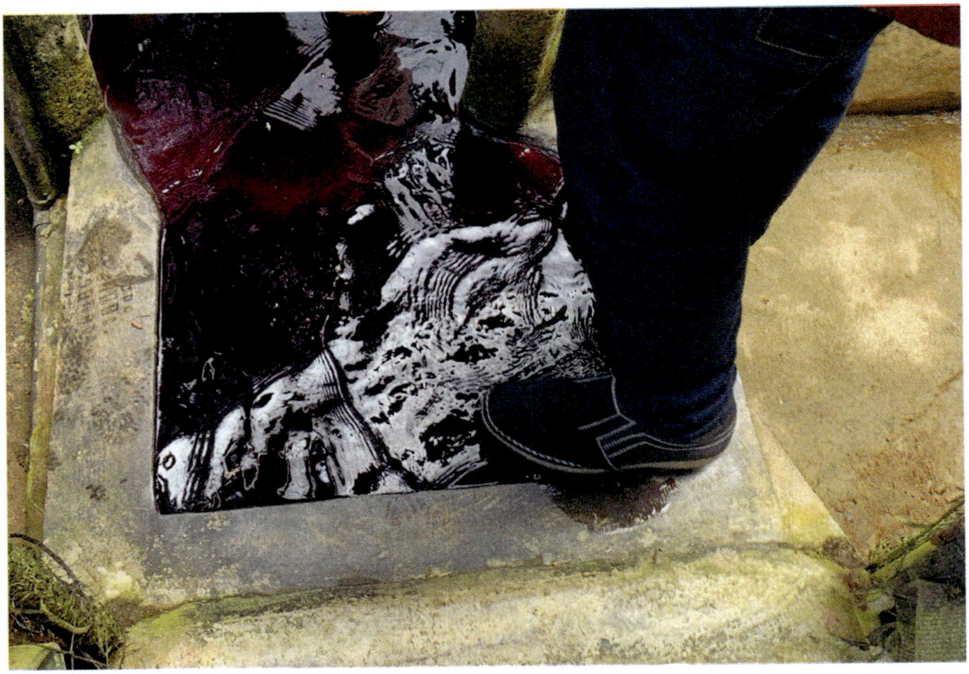

Fig. 22.15. Footbath containing Potassium Permanganate solution at a tropical fish farm. (Photograph by N. Saint-Erne.)

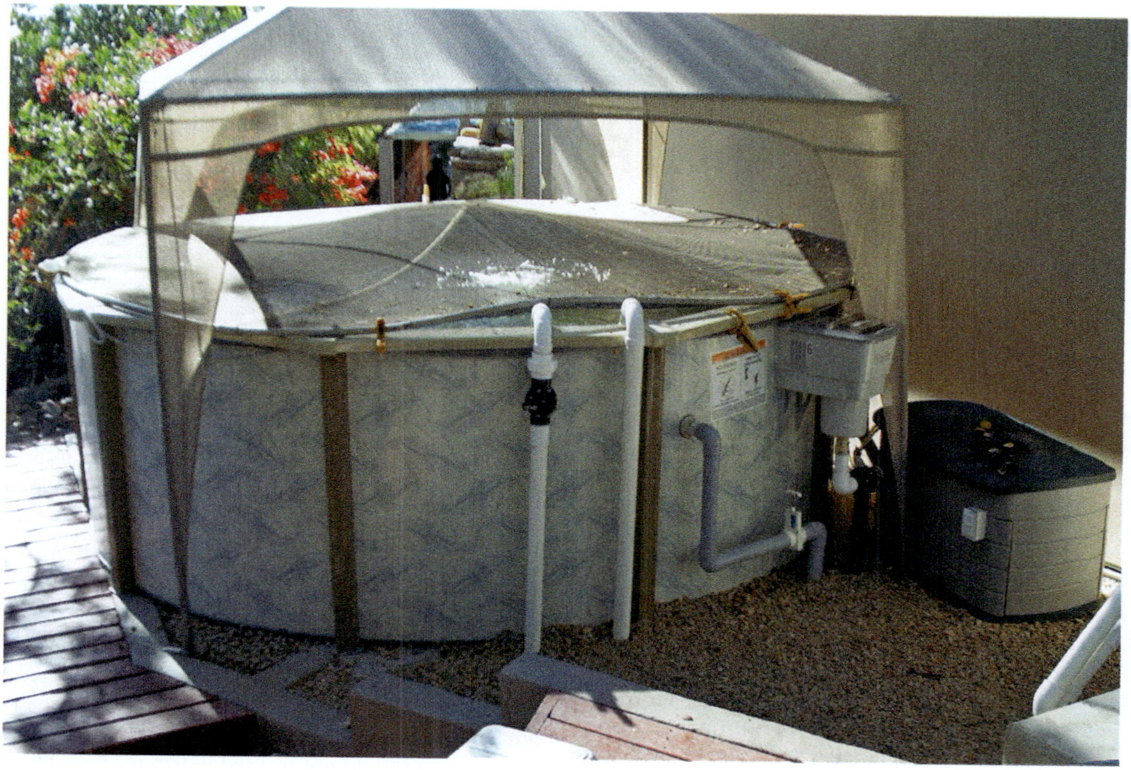

Fig. 22.16. An above-ground swimming pool with filtration, screen top, and a shade tent over it, being used as a quarantine tank by a koi pond owner. (Photograph by N. Saint-Erne.)

References

3M (2011) *Disinfection with Bleach*. Building and Commercial Services Division, 3M Company, St. Paul, Minnesota.

Arthur, J.R., Bondad-Reantaso, M.G. and Subasinghe, R.P. (2008) *Procedures for the Quarantine of Live Aquatic Animals: A Manual*. FAO Fisheries and Aquaculture Department, Rome.

Herwig, N. (1979) *Handbook of Drugs and Chemicals Used in the Treatment of Fish Diseases*. Charles C. Thomas Publisher, Springfield, Illinois.

OATA (2006) *Biosecurity and the Ornamental Fish Industry*. Ornamental Aquatic Trade Association, Wiltshire, UK.

OIE (2006) *International Aquatic Animal Health Code*. 9th edn. Office International des Épizooties, Paris, France.

Saint-Erne, N. (2023) *Fish Husbandry Operations Manual*. Tropical Fish International, Gardena, CA.

Sanders, J. (2020) *How to Disinfect Fish Equipment*. Aquatic Veterinary Services, Soquel, California. Available at: https://cafishvet.com/fish-ponds/how-to-disinfect-fish-equipment/ (accessed 1 August 2024).

23 Administering Medications to Ornamental Fish

NICHOLAS SAINT-ERNE

Dr. Saint-Erne Consulting, PLLC, Phoenix, Arizona

Abstract

When used appropriately after making an accurate diagnosis, medications can help to treat or cure diseases in fish but must be used with care to ensure they are not underdosed to be ineffective in the treatment or overdosed to potentially harm the fish. Medications can be administered in the water, in the diet, applied topically to the fish, or given by injections.

23.1 Ornamental Fish Drugs

United States Federal Law (the US Federal Food, Drug and Cosmetic Act) defines the term "drug" to include "articles intended for use in the diagnosis, cure, mitigation, treatment, or prevention of disease in man or other animals" and "articles (other than food) intended to affect the structure or any function of the body of man or other animals" (FDA, 2022). Of the medications used to treat animals in the USA, chemical treatments (drugs) are approved by the US Food and Drug Administration (FDA), and biological treatments (vaccines) are approved by the US Department of Agriculture (USDA).

Medications used for treating fish are often the same as those used in our other veterinary patients, but some are unique to treating fish and not available through the normal pharmacy distribution network. Veterinarians can choose any approved drugs to use on patients, even if the approved drug is not labeled for the species or purpose for which it will be used. This is extra-label use of FDA-approved drugs, and it allows access to medications that otherwise would not be available for the species seen in aquatic veterinary medicine. Extra-label use is permitted only by, or on the order of, a licensed veterinarian when a valid veterinarian-client-patient relationship exists. Extra-label use of a drug may not be administered via feed and must not result in a residue that may present a risk to public health (FDA, 2020).

Treating aquarium and pond fish has also utilized many chemicals that are not approved for veterinary use by the FDA. Unapproved drugs for use in any species do not qualify as extra-label drug use. These drugs should not be used in fish produced for food. Historically, these unapproved drugs have been marketed through pet stores and pond supply companies. There are some approved medication options used in treating aquaculture (food fish) species, and some of these have application for treatment of ornamental fish diseases. Many of these approved medications are safer not only for the fish but also for the person using the medication.

23.2 Administering Drugs to Ornamental Fish

When administering drugs to ornamental fish, it is important to assess the quality of the water in which they live. It is difficult to control or prevent infectious and parasitic diseases of fish when the water quality is less than optimum. By improving the water quality, stress on the fish is reduced, and its immune system can keep many diseases in check.

Ornamental fish can succumb to a variety of viral, bacterial, fungal, and parasitic diseases (Table 23.1), as well as from poor water quality, toxins in the

Corresponding author: DrSaintErne@gmail.com

 © CAB International 2025. *The Handbook of Ornamental Fish Health and Welfare* (ed. N. Saint-Erne)
DOI: 10.1079/9781789246032.0023

Table 23.1. Common ornamental fish diseases and their treatments.

Causative organism	Disease signs	Treatments
Virus		
Lymphocystis	White irregular growths extending from fins or skin	• Formalin • Surgical excision and topical skin disinfection
Cyprinid Herpesvirus-1 (Carp Pox)	Raised smooth bumps on fins or skin of Koi	
Cyprinid Herpesvirus-3 (Koi Herpes Virus)	Gill hyperplasia and erosion, skin hyperplasia, kidney failure in Koi	• Vaccine to prevent infection
Fungus		
Saprolegnia (Water mold)	Long whitish cotton-like filaments on fins or skin, also can occur on fish eggs, uneaten food, or fish	• Methylene Blue • Hydrogen Peroxide • Pimafix (Mars Fishcare/Aquarium Pharmaceuticals Inc.)
BACTERIA		
Aeromonas, Pseudomonas, Edwardsiella	Fin and tail rot, skin ulcers, dropsy (ascites), pop-eye, red fins, and skin	• Antibiotic injections, based on sensitivity testing results • Melafix (Mars Fishcare/Aquarium Pharmaceuticals Inc.) • Pimafix (Mars Fishcare/Aquarium Pharmaceuticals Inc.) • *Edwardsiella* vaccine (Intervet Inc.)
Flavobacterium columnaris	Fuzzy skin or lip lesions	
NOTE:	Bacterial infections often occur with poor water quality or when fish have parasite problems	
PROTOZOA		
Skin Parasites		
Ichthyophthirius multifiliis *Costia (Ichthyobodo)* *Chilodonella* *Trichodina* *Tetrahymena* *Epistylis*	White spots on body and fins, scraping body on rocks (flashing); increased slime coat (white or grayish cast on skin) Increased gill movements, fins clamped to sides, lying on bottom	• Formalin • Minn Finn (AquaSolver) • ProtoPro (LiveAquaria)
Oodinium (Velvet Disease)	Golden speckled cast on skin	• Copper Sulfate
Internal Parasites		
Spironucleus (Hexamita)	Lesions in Cichlids along head and lateral line (Hole-in-Head)	• Metronidazole in food
Worms		
Camallanus	Red worms protrude from vent	• Fenbendazole • Praziquantel • Minn Finn (AquaSolver)
Capillaria	Poor growth, weight loss	
Skin and gill flukes	Inflamed gills, excess mucus on skin, scraping body on rocks (flashing)	
Encysted digenean flukes		
Leeches and other worms	Worms on outside of fish or in tank	
Crustacea		
Fish Lice *(Argulus)*	Small discs that move across the skin of the fish, or swim through the water	• Dimilin • Trichlorfon
Anchor Worms *(Lernaea)*	Gray to white worm-like parasites attached to the fish's skin; the head is embedded under the skin	

Note: Follow label dosage instructions for using each product.

water, predation, interspecies aggression, and neoplastic, traumatic, and metabolic diseases. It is important to assess all these factors and perform good diagnostic testing to ensure that the correct treatments are being given. Also, there can often be more than one problem occurring. For example, an obvious bacterial lesion might actually be secondary to damage of the epithelium caused by microscopic skin flukes (monogenean trematodes). Both pathogens must be treated to provide relief for the fish.

It may be possible to separate diseased fish into an isolation tank for treatment, versus treating the whole aquarium or pond. The isolation tank can be of a known volume of water, and smaller than the main habitat, which makes dosing of medications for a water bath easier to calculate and requires less medication. If a fish is being treated for a contagious pathogen, then even fish that are not currently showing signs of infection should be treated. Also consider the effects of medications on the biological filter in an aquarium or pond. If the drug affects the nitrifying bacteria, then daily water testing and water changes may be required.

Aeromonas and other bacteria species are almost always present in water and even on the fish itself. Bacteria are often opportunistic pathogens that proliferate when the fish is weakened or injured. Maintain the water temperature in the treatment tank at the fish's optimum temperature (68°F/20°C to 73°F/23°C for koi and goldfish; 75°F/24°C to 78°F/26°C for tropical fish) to increase the fish's immune response and aid healing. Some fish diseases (such as Cyprinid Herpes Virus-3 and Ich) are best treated at even higher water temperatures. Prevent osmotic stress due to skin lesions by adding salt to the water (0.1–0.3% solution) for freshwater fish species.

Maintaining good nutrition during treatment of fish is also critical to proper treatment. However, some fish, when severely affected, will stop eating and may even need to be force-fed or tube-fed. Feeding frozen brine shrimp or freeze-dried tubifex worms may entice reluctant eaters more than flake fish food. Frozen brine shrimp can be used to mix with medication for feeding tropical fish. Nutritional deficiencies, especially of amino acids, fatty acids, and vitamins A, C, and E, have been shown to reduce the amount of globulin and antibody an animal can produce in response to an infection. This would reduce the animal's resistance to the disease. Proper nutrition, with adequate vitamin, mineral, and fatty acid supplementation, is essential in maintaining optimum fish health (Saint-Erne, 2010).

23.3 Routes of Drug Administration

Medications are administered to ornamental fish most commonly by adding them directly to the aquarium or pond water. Medication can also be topically applied directly to the skin of the fish while it is briefly held out of the water (Fig. 23.1). Some medications can be incorporated into the food and given orally or administered using a rubber tube placed through the mouth into the stomach or intestines. Larger-sized fish can be injected with medications intramuscularly, intraperitoneally (intracoelomically in fish), and intravenously (Loh, 2012).

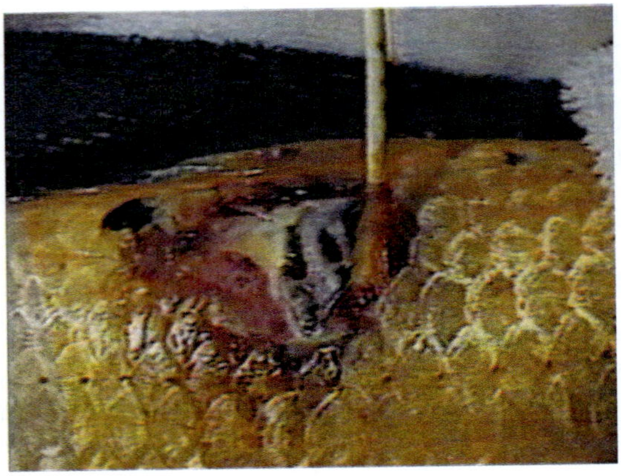

Fig. 23.1. Topical treatment of an ulcer on a koi (*Cyprinus rubrofuscus*) with povidone-iodine solution. (Photograph by N. Saint-Erne.)

In any treatment method, water quality must be considered, as even with the best medication, fish in poor-quality water are less likely to recover. Water changes must also be made between dosages of medications given via bath applications. Follow label directions on all medications and be sure of accurately measuring water volume to ensure the correct dose is administered.

23.3.1 Baths and dips

Treating fish by prolonged immersion in a medication added to the water is often termed a "bath." A short immersion in a medicated solution, followed by returning the fish to the normal aquarium water, is termed a "dip." Using a separate bare aquarium with a known volume of water and a sponge filter for a hospital tank makes treating fish easier than trying to treat in the main aquarium (Fig. 23.2). Some medications can be removed from the water after treating the aquarium by adding activated carbon into the filter media. Some medications (Fig. 23.3) can be neutralized, so the water does not need to be filtered or exchanged after treatment.

For better mixing of drugs in the aquarium water, add the measured dose of a powdered medication to a small volume of warm water and shake vigorously in a tightly closed container and then pour the solution

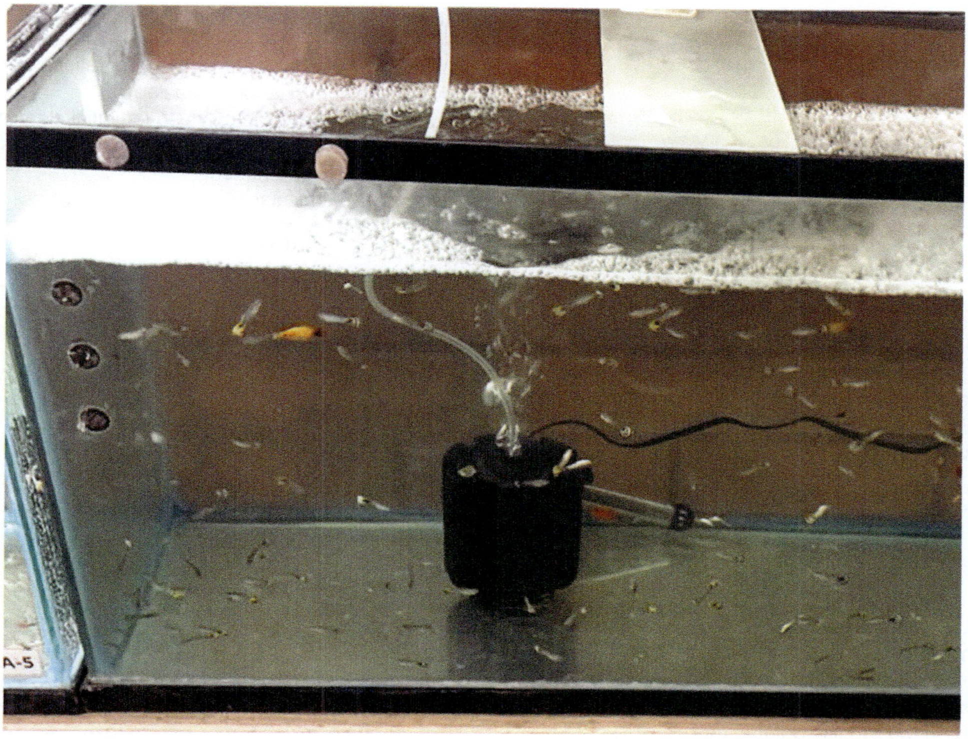

Fig. 23.2. Bare aquarium with a sponge filter and heater used for an isolation, quarantine, or treatment tank. (Photograph by N. Saint-Erne.)

into the water. For liquid medications, measure the required dose into a syringe and spray it through a 25-gauge needle under the water while mixing to better disperse the solution. Commonly used fish medications that are added to the aquarium of pond water are listed in Table 23.2.

23.3.2 Topical medications

In situations where it is not too stressful to handle the fish, it is helpful to debride open wounds and then gently swab or spray the lesions daily with povidone-iodine solution or similar skin disinfectant and then apply an antibiotic ointment. This will remove necrotic tissue and reduce bacterial and fungal growth. Be sure not to damage new skin growth on subsequent days of topical treatments.

23.3.3 Injectable drugs

Intramuscular (IM) injections are given in the epaxial muscles along the back, next to or immediately behind the dorsal fin (Fig. 23.4). The needle is pointed anteriorly at a shallow angle, and it is advanced forward along the surface of the scale and under the anterior scale. In many species of fish, there is an area immediately behind the dorsal fin where the skin does not have scales so that the needle can be inserted without penetrating or damaging any scales. When removing the needle, if it has passed through any scales, push down on the scales, as the needle is extracted to avoid removing scales impaled on the hypodermic needle. Fish skin is not elastic, so some drug may flow out of the hole if large volumes are injected in one area. Apply digital pressure over the injection site to help diffuse the medication and to seal the puncture.

Intraperitoneal (intracoelomic, ICoe) injections are given on the abdomen, above and behind the pelvic fin. In some fish species, there may be an area caudal to the pelvic fin devoid of scales which facilitates needle entry into the coelom (Fig. 23.5). The hypodermic needle is inserted anteriorly at a shallow angle to avoid deep penetration and entry into the intestines or other organs. The drug is injected just inside the internal body wall into the space between the body wall and the organs.

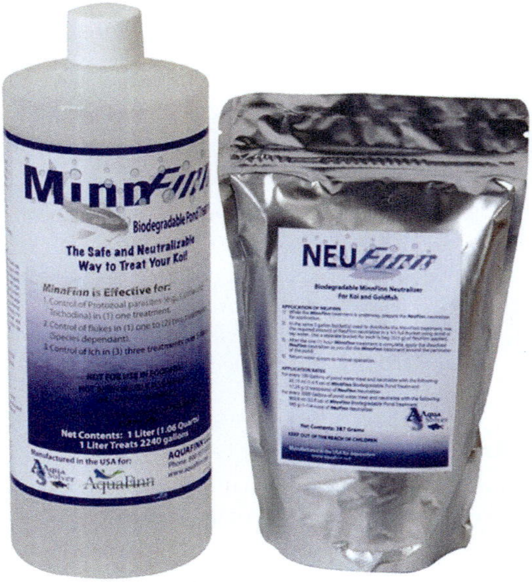

Fig. 23.3. Short-term dip treatments can be done with Minn Finn in the aquarium because it includes a neutralizing agent, Neu Finn, which is added to the water at a designated time to neutralize the Minn Finn treatment. (Photo by Nick Saint-Erne.)

Table 23.2. Medications added to the aquarium or pond water.

Prolonged Baths:
Chloramine-T
Copper Sulfate
Dimilin
Formalin
Fenbendazole
Levamisole
Malachite Green
Methylene Blue
Praziquantel
ProtoPro (LiveAquaria)
Salt (sodium chloride): 0.1–0.5%
Trichlorfon
Medications used for short-term dips:
Formalin
Hydrogen Peroxide
Minn Finn (AquaSolver)
Salt (sodium chloride): 1.0–3.0%
Tricide-Neo (Molecular Therapeutics LLC)

Intravenous (IV) injections can be given in the caudal vein below the spine in the caudal peduncle (Fig. 23.6). Access to the vein can be done either through a lateral or a ventral approach in the caudal peduncle—the body area posterior to the vent

Table 23.3. Medications used topically on fish skin.

Antibiotic Ointments (ophthalmic preparations work well)
Povidone-iodine Solution (Betadine)
Hydrogen Peroxide 3% (only use for initial cleaning, as prolonged use will delay new skin growth)
Silver Sulfadiazine ointment
Tricide-Neo (Molecular Therapeutics LLC)

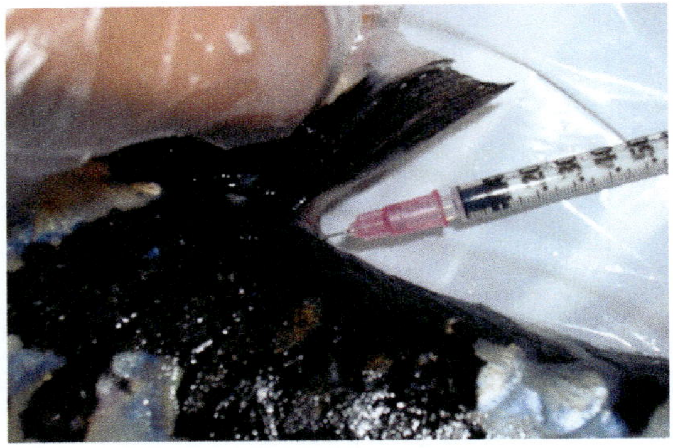

Fig. 23.4. Intramuscular injection in a koi fish (*C. rubrofuscus*) with needle inserted behind dorsal fin into the epaxial muscles. (Photograph by N. Saint-Erne.)

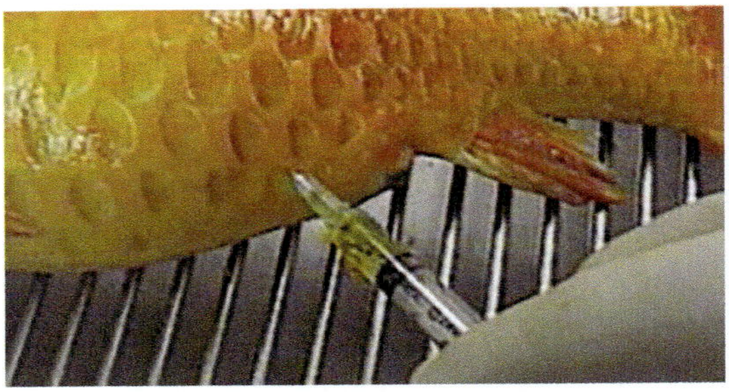

Fig. 23.5. Intracoelomic injection in a koi fish (*C. rubrofuscus*) anterior to the vent and the anal fin. (Photograph by N. Saint-Erne.)

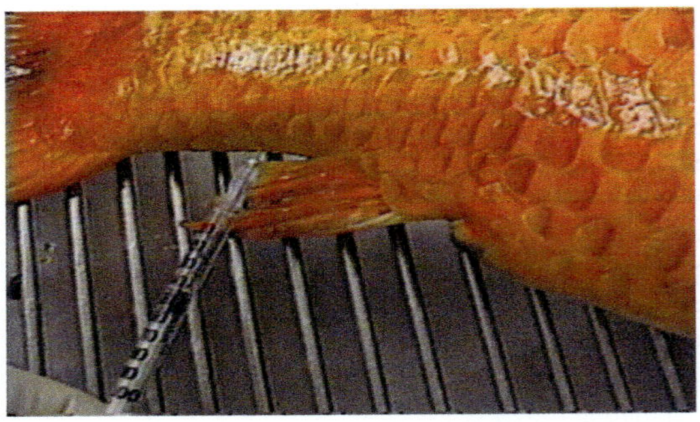

Fig. 23.6. Intravenous injection in a koi fish (*C. rubrofuscus*) with the needle inserted into the caudal vein ventral to the vertebrae in the caudal peduncle. (Photograph by N. Saint-Erne.)

Table 23.4. Aquatic veterinary medicine formulary.

Drug	Category	Dosage
Alfaxalone	Anesthetic	12–24 mg/kg IM; 1–6 mg/l bath
Amikacin	Antibiotic	5 mg/kg IM, repeat in 1–3 days
Ammonium chloride	Fishless Tank Cycling	12 mg/l to start bacterial nitrification
Antibiotic ointment	Antibiotic	Apply topically to skin wounds
Atropine	Antitoxin	0.1 mg/kg IM, ICoe
Aztreonam (Azactam)	Antibiotic	100 mg/kg IM, ICoe every 2–5 days
Benzalkonium chloride	Disinfectant	10 mg/l solution for cleaning nets
Butorphanol	Analgesic	0.1 mg/kg IM for post-surgical pain control
Carprofen	Analgesic	1–5 mg/kg IM
Ceftazidime	Antibiotic	22 mg/kg IM every 2–3 days (q2-3d)
Chloramine-T	Antibacterial	2.5–20 mg/l dip for 1–4 h
Chlorhexidine	Antibacterial	1–2 mg/l for a 1-h dip
Copper Sulfate	Antiparasitic	0.2 mg/l in marine aquariums
Dexamethasone	Anti-inflammatory	1–2 mg/kg IM, ICoe
Diazepam	Anesthetic	0.1–0.5 mg/kg IM, ICoe
Diflubenzuron (Dimilin)	Antiparasitic	0.06–0.10 mg/l q7d
Doxycycline	Antibiotic	2 g/kg of food PO daily
Enrofloxacin	Antibiotic	5–14 mg/kg IM, ICoe q2-3d
Epinephrine (1:1000)	Hormone	0.2–0.5 ml IM, ICoe, IC
Epoetin (Epogen)	Erythropoiesis	200 mg/kg IM
Eugenol (clove oil)	Anesthetic	10–100 mg/l dip
Fenbendazole	Antiparasitic	25–50 mg/kg BW PO; 2–10 mg/l bath
Florfenicol	Antibiotic	10–50 mg/kg IM, ICoe; 40–50 mg/kg PO daily
Formalin (37% formaldehyde)	Antiparasitic	25 mg/l (=1 ml/10 gallons) bath q2d
Furosemide	Diuretic	1–5 mg/kg IM, ICoe
Gentamicin	Antibiotic	1–3 mg/kg IM one time
Hydrogen peroxide 3%	Antifungal	5 mg/l bath; 20 mg/l for 1-h dip
Isoflurane or Sevoflurane	Anesthetic	0.5–2.0 ml/l dip
Kanamycin	Antibiotic	20 mg/kg ICoe, 50–100 mg/l bath
Ketamine	Anesthetic	5–20 mg/kg IM; 1 g/l dip
Levamisole	Antiparasitic	10 mg/l bath; 50 mg/l for 2-h dip
Lidocaine 2%	Anesthetic	0.1–2 mg/kg IM
Lufenuron	Antiparasitic	0.13 mg/l bath
Meloxicam	Analgesia	0.1 mg/kg IM SID
Metomidate	Anesthetic	1–10 mg/l dip
Metronidazole	Antiparasitic	2–10 mg/g of food PO; 25 mg/l bath q48h
MS-222	Anesthetic	25–100 mg/l dip
Nitrofurazone	Antibacterial	1–2 mg/l bath
Ovaprim	Spawning Hormone	0.5 ml/kg IM, ICoe
Oxytetracycline	Antibiotic	50–75 mg/kg BW, added to food for 10 days
Potassium permanganate	Antiparasitic	0.5–2 mg/l bath
Povidone-iodine solution	Skin Disinfectant	Apply topically to skin lesions
Praziquantel	Antiparasitic	5–25 mg/kg IM, ICoe; 2–10 mg/l bath
Prednisolone	Anti-inflammatory	1 mg/kg IM, ICoe
Propofol	Anesthetic	1–7 mg/l dip
Robenocoxib	Anti-inflammatory	2 mg/kg IM q3-4d
Sea Salt/non-iodized salt	Osmoregulation	1–5 g/l bath for freshwater fish
Silver sulfadiazine cream	Antibacterial	Apply topically to skin lesions
Sodium bicarbonate (baking soda)	Buffer	25–100 mg/l
Sodium thiosulfate	Dechlorinator	10 mg/l
Sulfadimethoxine/ormetoprim	Antibacterial	50 mg/kg IM, PO

Continued

Table 23.4. Continued.

Drug	Category	Dosage
Trichlorfon	Organophosphate Insecticide	0.25–0.50 mg/l
Trimethoprim/sulfamethoxazole	Antibacterial	30 mg/kg IM, ICoe; 20 mg/l bath
Vitamin B complex injectable	Nutritional	4 mg/kg IM
Vitamin C injectable	Nutritional	5–12 mg/kg IM, PO q24-48h

Key: IC = Intracardial; ICoe = Intracoelomic; IM = Intramuscular; PO = per os (by mouth).
The doses listed as mg/l refer to adding the drug into the water (milligrams of drug per liter of water); mg/kg refers to milligrams of drug per kilogram fish body weight (BW), unless stated as mg/kg of food, when it is added to the food based on the weight of the food.
Bath refers to continuous duration of immersion, whereas dip is a limited-time immersion in the medication.

and anterior to the tail fin. In larger fish species, there may be veins in the mouth or inside the operculum (gill cover) that are large enough to use for IV injections.

23.3.4 Medicated food

Clients need a veterinary feed directive issued by a veterinarian within a valid veterinarian-client-patient relationship before prescription medications can be mixed in food to be used with food animals. Livestock producers must obtain a veterinary feed directive from a veterinarian before using antibiotics considered necessary for treating human diseases in livestock feed and drinking water.

Medicated food can be made in the clinic by mixing the medication in with the appropriate amount of fish food pellets, then adding some egg whites, fish oil, or vegetable oil as a binding agent, stirring together, and then spreading out in a pan and letting dry. Store medicated food in an airtight container in the refrigerator. Tube-feeding a mixture of antibiotics and soaked, mashed fish pellets can be used in the treatment of larger fish, such as cichlids and koi.

23.4 Aquatic Veterinary Medicine Formulary

Table 23.4 lists the most frequently used medications in aquatic veterinary medicine (Lewbart and Yanong, 2022). However, there are many other drugs (Herwig, 1979) that have been used in the past that are not currently utilized. Table 23.4 contains the commonly recommended dosage ranges, but not all drugs are suitable for use in all fish species. When working with unfamiliar fish species or medications, start with the lower dosages (Loh, 2012). Most medications used in ornamental fish species are not approved for use in fish by the US FDA. Using drugs approved for humans or other animal species in fish is considered "extra-label" drug usage and must be discussed with the client in a valid veterinarian-client-patient relationship. Many of the drugs used in the ornamental fish industry are not approved drugs for use in any species. It is illegal to use non-approved drugs in food fish species.

This formulary is intended for use in ornamental fish species only. Before using any medications in an aquarium or pond, ensure an accurate measurement of the water volume has been made (Saint-Erne, 2010). Underdosage of medications will reduce the effectiveness of the treatment and overdosage can cause additional stress to the fish, or even death.

23.5 Conclusion

When used appropriately after making an accurate diagnosis, medications can help to treat or cure diseases in fish but must be used with care to ensure they are not underdosed to be ineffective in the treatment or overdosed to potentially harm the fish. Follow label directions on all medications and be sure of accurately measuring aquarium water volume to ensure the correct dose is administered. Water quality must also be taken into consideration when adding medications. A valid veterinarian-client-patient relationship is required for extra-label use of drugs in aquaculture, as well as for use of veterinary feed directive drugs.

References

FDA (2020) *The Ins and Outs of Extra-Label Drug Use in Animals: A Resource for Veterinarians*. Available at: https://www.fda.gov/animal-veterinary/resources-you/ins-and-outs-extra-label-drug-use-animals-resource-veterinarians (accessed 16 January 2020).

FDA (2022) *FDA Regulation of Animal Drugs*. https://www.fda.gov/animal-veterinary/resources-you/fda-regulation-animal-drugs (accessed 16 August 2022).

Herwig, N. (1979) *Handbook of Drugs and Chemicals Used in the Treatment of Fish Diseases*. Charles C. Thomas, Springfield, Illinois.

Lewbart, G.A. and Yanong, R.P.E. (2022) Fish. In: Carpenter, J.W. and Harms, C. (eds) *Exotic Animal Formulary*. 6th edn. Elsevier, St. Louis, Missouri, pp. 16–52.

Loh, R. (2012) *Fish Vetting Medicines*. Richmond Loh Publishing, Perth, Australia.

Saint-Erne, N. (2010) Application of chemicals to the pond. In: Saint-Erne, N. (ed.) *Advanced Koi Care*. 2nd edn. Erne Enterprises, Glendale, Arizona, pp. 147–164.

24 Ornamental Fish Welfare

Chris Walster

C&J Walster Ltd., Stafford, UK

Abstract

Until recently, the welfare of ornamental fish kept in aquariums has been taken for granted by fish keepers, the ornamental fish industry, and sometimes even animal welfare organizations. This is attributed to the low cost of many ornamental fish, lack of reliable information about their health care, or a perceived lack of veterinarians with skills in aquatic animal health. Veterinarians and veterinary organizations are increasingly becoming involved in aquatic veterinary medicine to help improve the welfare of pet fish (Walster *et al.*, 2015).

24.1 Fish Welfare

When discussing fish welfare, we need to differentiate between "welfare" and "animal rights." Many people believe that animal rights and animal welfare are identical, but they are not. Animal rights refer to animals having all the same rights as humans do and advocate that they should not be used by humans for food, entertainment, companionship, research, or any other use and should only be allowed to live in their natural environment. People concerned with animal welfare believe that while humans should not abuse or exploit animals, if we make the animals' lives comfortable, physically and psychologically, we are respecting their welfare (Bekoff, 2007). Animal welfarists believe that if animals experience comfort and normal activities, appear happy, and are free from prolonged or intense pain, fear, hunger, and other unpleasant states, then we are fulfilling our obligations to them. If individuals show normal growth and reproduction and are free from disease, injury, malnutrition, pain, and suffering, they are doing well. For ornamental fish kept as pets, if we provide appropriately sized aquariums with proper filtration and water quality, adequate nutrition, and husbandry, then we can maintain them in comfort for longer than they would survive in their natural environment (Fig. 24.1). They can even be allowed to reproduce in home aquariums, just as they are bred in commercial tropical fish farms around the world and have been for over a century.

Fish are diverse with over 35,100 species described (FishBase, 2023) occupying numerous habitats and ecosystems. Fish may be pelagic (live near the surface) or benthic (live on the bottom), and may shoal together or live solitary lives. The majority of fish species are prey for bigger fish or other animals and are oviparous with high fecundity, producing numerous eggs due to the high rate of attrition that offspring incur. In considering the welfare needs of over 35,000 fish species, it is not surprising that although much progress has been made in the last 20–30 years, often driven by economic imperatives, there are severe limitations to our knowledge, particularly of species behavioral needs, although our ability to provide good general welfare should match that of other species. The Companion Animal Welfare Council (CAWC) recognizes ornamental fish as companion animals, which means society expects owners and producers to provide suitable care, but equally recognizes the benefits that keeping companion animals brings to society. In the CAWC "Report on the Welfare of Non-domesticated Animals Kept for Companionship," the definition of companion animal used was "all animals kept by private individuals or private groups for companionship, interest or hobby, together with those kept for related purposes such as breeding, supply, or education"

Corresponding author: chris.walster@btconnect.com

© CAB International 2025. *The Handbook of Ornamental Fish Health and Welfare* (ed. N. Saint-Erne)
DOI: 10.1079/9781789246032.0024

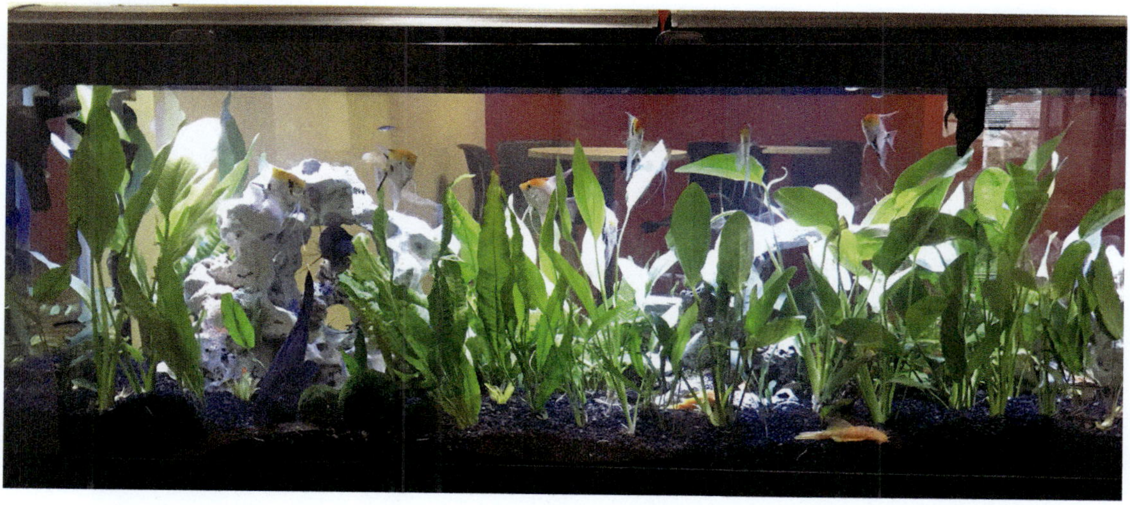

Fig. 24.1. A filtered and uncrowded aquarium with live plants and a healthy environment for the fish. (Photograph by N. Saint-Erne.)

(CAWC, 2003). This definition of companion animals is useful as it provides the reasons why people keep ornamental fish.

24.2 Production

Farming ornamental fish raises a variety of welfare concerns, varying from health issues such as the levels of fish mycobacteriosis in farmed fish (notably *Mycobacterium marinum*) to processes used in wild collection versus captive breeding. There are five major welfare concerns encountered in the ornamental fish industry: (i) selective breeding and culling, (ii) collecting from the wild, (iii) cosmetic manipulation, (iv) withholding food, and (v) transportation.

24.2.1 Selective breeding and culling

Ornamental fish need to be of a suitable quality to sell. This means they should have the "desired" body shape and coloration (note that many domesticated ornamental fish are selectively bred for features that deviate from the wild type, as is indeed the case for most, and probably all, other domesticated animals). For farmed fish, the quality can be controlled by selective breeding programs and choosing the most suitable individuals to continue breeding for a desired characteristic, such as color or fin and body shape (Fig. 24.2). However, in species that do not breed true, regardless of how selective the breeding program, a large percentage of the offspring will be culled due to undesirable characteristics. This is particularly of concern with goldfish (*Carassius auratus*) and koi (*Cyprinus rubrofuscus*); only a small percentage of the offspring will have the correct coloration or body conformation. Indeed, culling rates of over 90% can occur at some koi farms in Japan. This dramatic figure is somewhat ameliorated by the fact that under natural conditions, it is likely that only a few percentage of offspring will reach maturity. Fish farmers are thus applying a similar level of selective pressure, albeit in a different direction to that which occurs naturally. From a welfare perspective, this still leaves the questions: is it right to spawn fish knowing that many of the offspring will be killed due to human whim, and how can we ensure culled fish are humanely handled during their final disposition?

24.2.2 Collecting wild fish

Wild collection probably evokes the most controversy concerning ornamental fish and is the most complex issue regarding production, since it involves more than just ornamental fish welfare, impinging on environmental and human welfare issues. The industry and the hobby worldwide would not condone indiscriminate and inappropriate capture methods. Indeed, standards setting bodies such as the Marine Aquarium Council (MAC) provide guidelines for marine fish collection that

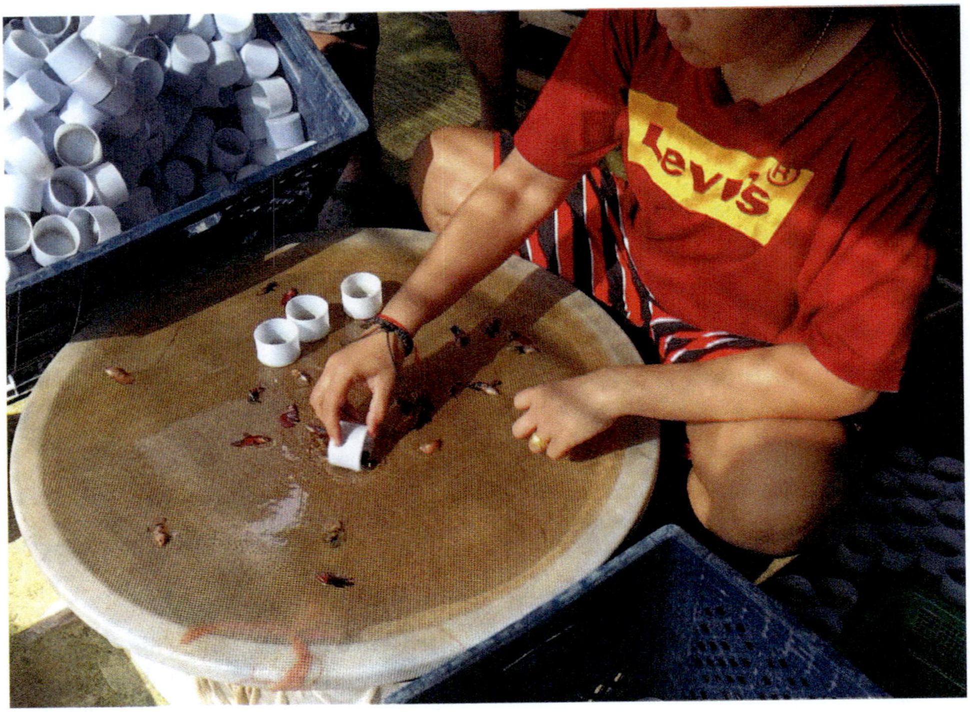

Fig. 24.2. Separating *Betta splendens* fish by color variety at breeding farm in Thailand. (Photograph by N. Saint-Erne.)

are audited to ensure compliance by certified companies. Methods of capture such as the use of sodium cyanide are condemned by all the trade bodies, such as the Ornamental Fish International (OFI), the Pet Industry Joint Advisory Council (PIJAC), and the Ornamental Aquatic Trade Association (OATA). Other unwelcome capture practices include physically invasive capture methods, such as the use of a two-pronged stabbing pole to spear the Mandarin dragonet fish in the Philippines (Sadovy, 2001). Overfishing for the ornamental trade is reported to have occurred in many areas of Asia and South America. This is reported to have led to steep declines in fish stocks and to the local demise of certain species of ornamental value, as is well documented for some Asian freshwater fish, such as the Harlequin rasbora (*Trigonostigma heteromorpha*) and Bala shark (*Balantiocheilos melanopterus*) (Ng and Lim, 1997). These declines led to concomitant increase in prices, with the increased price giving the incentive for the species to be commercially farmed.

However, wild collection of fishes can be done sustainably and with good fish welfare practices. The point is perhaps best illustrated by Project Piaba (Fig. 24.3). This project, which has run for over 30 years, is based on the Rio Negro, a tributary of the Amazon River. The main fish species (by number) captured here is the Cardinal Tetra (*Paracheirodon axelrodi*). The project carries out scientific research but also educates the fishermen on appropriate methods of catching, improving holding facilities, and how best to forward the fish on to Manaus, Brazil, for export. The project has seen dramatic decreases in losses sustained during transportation to Manaus; shown that the fishery is sustainable; improved the income of the local peoples; and taught them that they need to protect the environment. The slogan of Project Piaba is "Buy a fish, save a tree," which is very apt (Chao, 2001). It would seem clear that where a fishery is properly managed, then there is no detriment to fish welfare or the environment. By contrast, if the fish collectors were not allowed to continue, and had to resort to farming, lumbering, or cattle ranching to make a living, the environment in the Amazon where they live would suffer great damage, whereas the collection of fish preserves the forest environment.

There are also some fish species that only persist due to their being bred by the ornamental fish

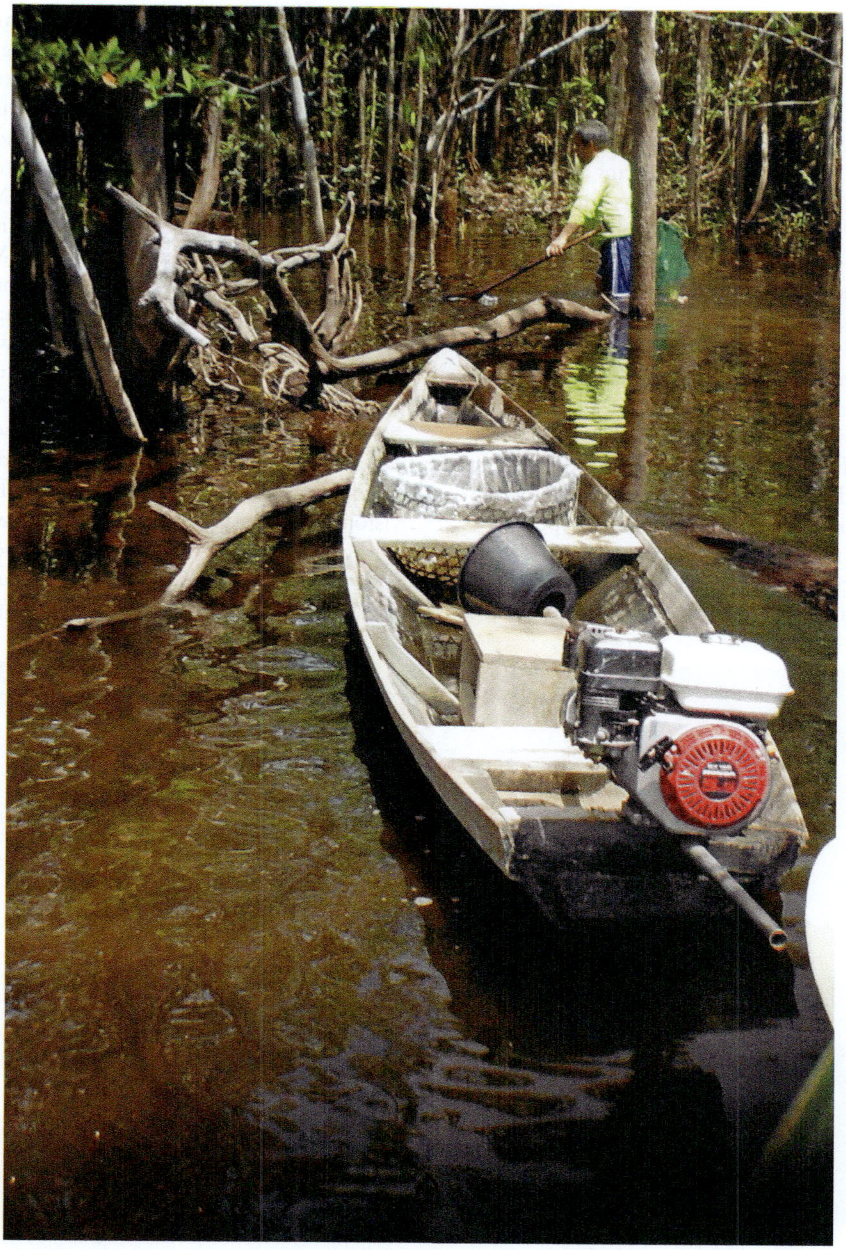

Fig. 24.3. Piabeiro in the Rio Negro collecting tropical fish using his canoe paddle to herd the fish into his hand net. The fish are then placed in a plastic-lined wicker basket in the canoe. (Photograph by N. Saint-Erne.)

industry, their saving grace from habitat destruction. Such species include the White Cloud Mountain Minnow (*Tanichthys albonubes*) and Endler's Livebearer (*Poecilia wingei*), which breed readily in ornamental fish farms but may be extinct in the wild due to habitat destruction. Fishes selected for the ornamental aquarium trade tend to be small and have a limited natural home range, allowing them to be perfect candidates for home aquariums.

24.2.3 Cosmetic manipulation

In previous years, some ornamental fish species such as glassfish (*Chanda* sp.) and Corydoras catfishes (*Corydoras* sp.) have been injected with various colored dyes to make them more vibrant and increase their commercial value. Injecting glassfish has been condemned by trade bodies and also by hobbyists. It has also been shown that glassfish that have been injected with these dyes show increased infection with lymphocystis virus, which produces cellular hypertrophy, causing raised wart-like lesions on the skin of the fish. Also, "tattooing" has been practiced whereby fish have their skin scarified and then placed in dyes, or manually tattooed (Fig. 24.4). These practices, which confer no benefit to the fish, should be condemned on welfare grounds. OATA has recommended that its members do not trade in dyed fish of any type.

Genetically modified (GM) fish species (*Danio rerio*, *Gymnocorymbus ternetzi*, *Puntius tetrazona*, and others) have been produced in Singapore and the USA (Fig. 24.5a,b). These fish are modified with fluorescing-colored genes during embryonic development and those fish that incorporate the fluorescing genes into their own DNA will be colored and can pass that coloration on to their own offspring. Currently, legislation (EU Directive 2001/18/EC) prevents the importation of GM fish into Europe and the UK. This is similar in Australia, although Canada has now allowed GM fish to be imported. However, the commercial reproduction of the originally GM fish has produced many fish species in five vibrant colors that are now among the most popular-selling aquarium fishes in the USA.

Some fish species, especially goldfish varieties and balloon mollies, are intentionally bred with physical deformities, similar to what dog breeders do with bulldog species. Oranda goldfish may suffer impaired vision due to excessive growth of the wen. Bubble-eyed goldfish (Fig. 24.6) have upward-faced eyes and propensity to damage their "bubbles," and telescope-eyed goldfish are also predisposed to eye

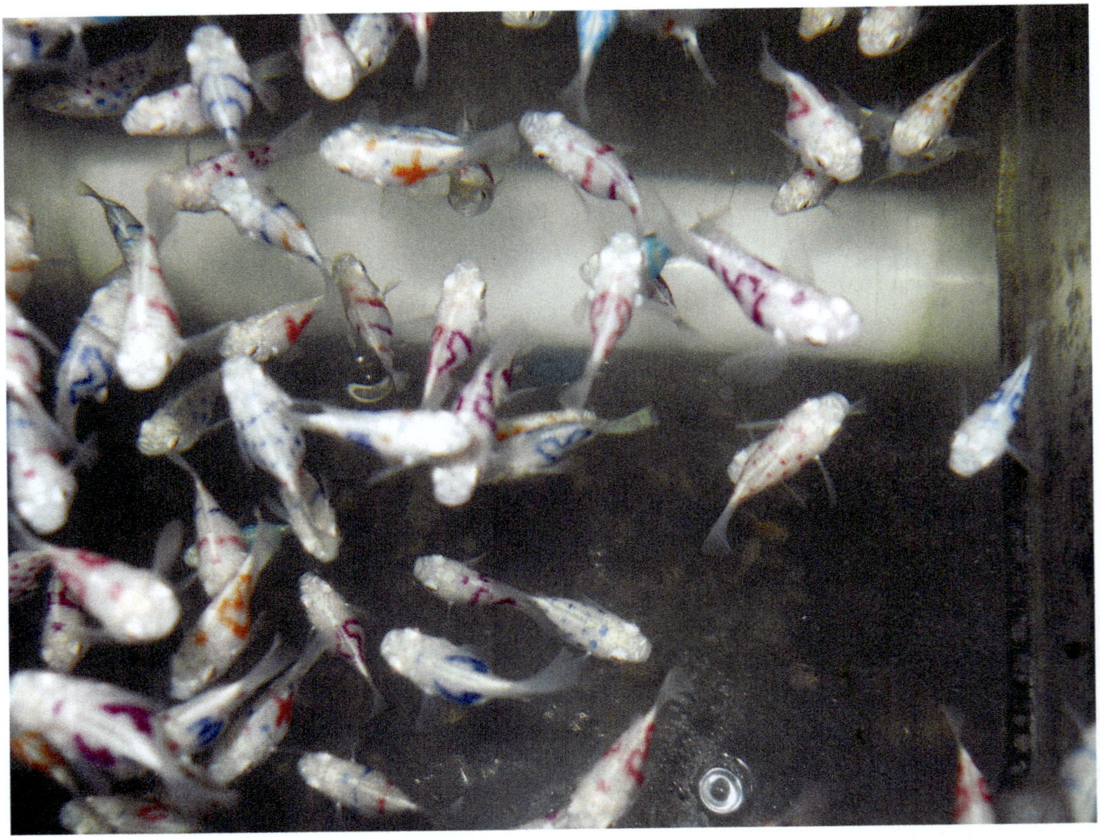

Fig. 24.4. Tattooed balloon-belly mollies. (Photograph by N. Saint-Erne.)

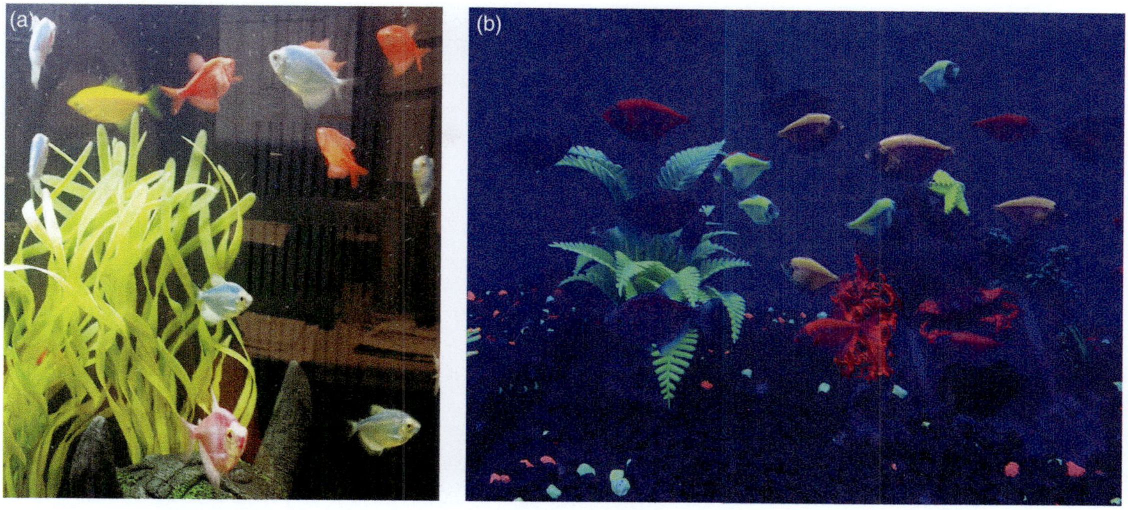

Fig. 24.5a,b. Genetically modified fluorescing tetra fish under normal lighting and with blue lighting. (Photograph by N. Saint-Erne.)

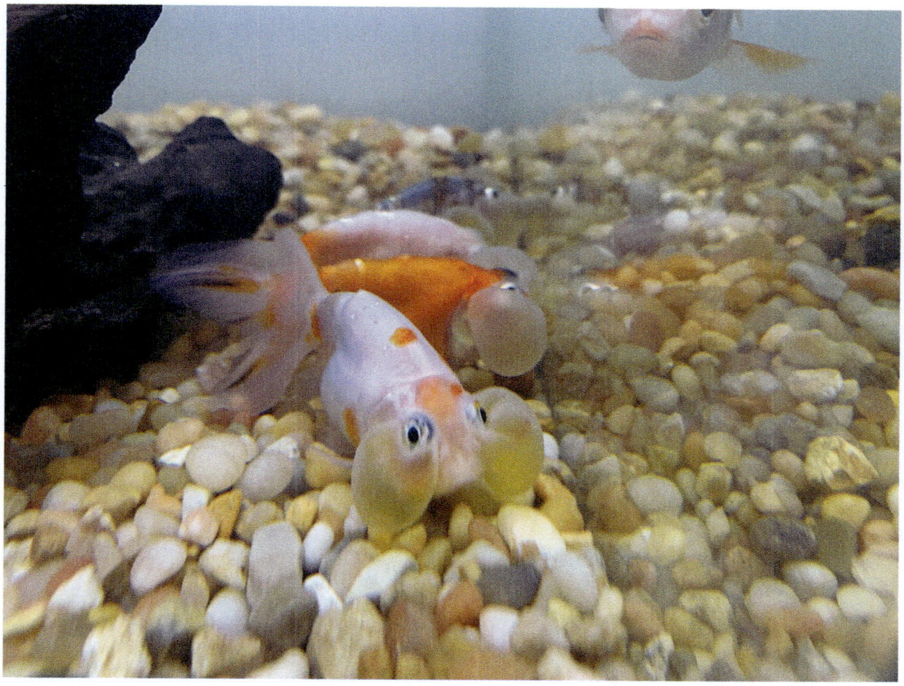

Fig. 24.6. Bubble-eyed goldfish variety (*Carassius auratus*). (Photograph by N. Saint-Erne.)

trauma. The rotund-bodied goldfish have impaired swimming ability and are prone to swim bladder problems that can cause them to float upside-down at the surface, which can prove fatal. This is one of the most common reasons a fish hobbyist will contact a veterinarian. Other issues include excessively long fins that are found in longfin varieties of many fish species; and the enlarged "horn" seen on flower horn cichlids (Fig. 24.7), which is an abnormality created by crossbreeding several species of cichlid fish. Shortened bodies are due to spinal deformities and are seen in parrot cichlids (Fig. 24.8)

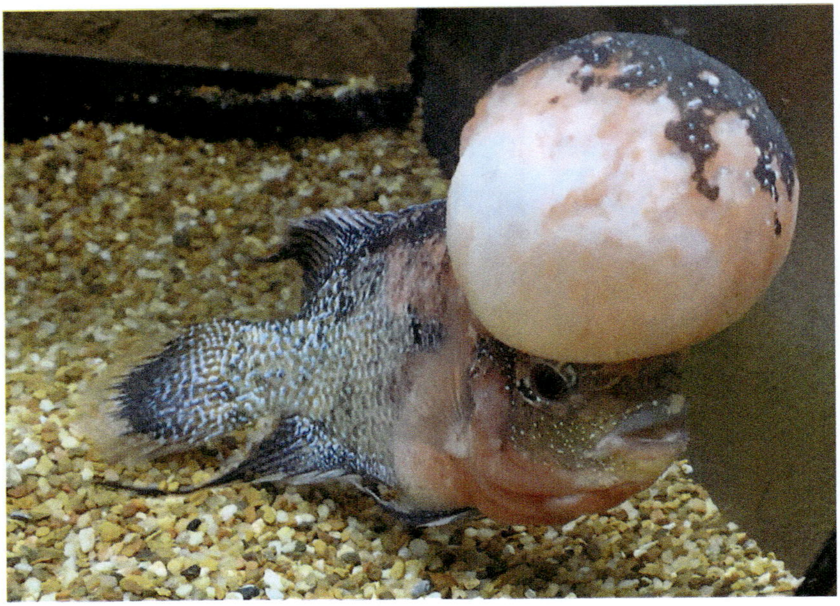

Fig. 24.7. Excessively large "horn" on a flower horn cichlid hybrid. (Photograph by N. Saint-Erne.)

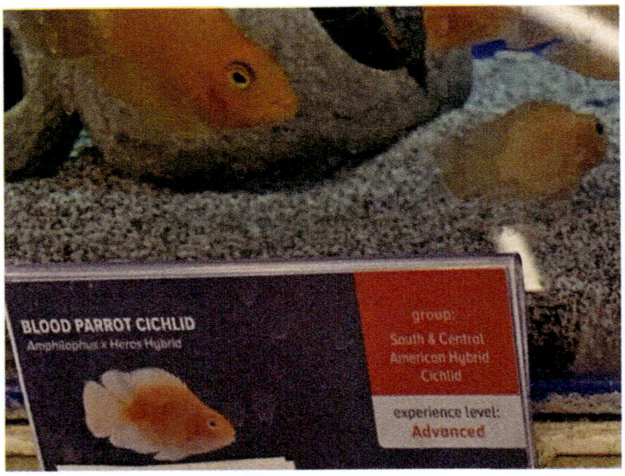
BLOOD PARROT CICHLID
group:
South & Central
American Hybrid
Cichlid
experience level:
Advanced

Fig. 24.8. Parrot cichlids are hybrid fish that have shortened bodies and smaller than normal mouths. (Photograph by N. Saint-Erne.)

and balloon-belly mollies. All these issues can be related to breeding for specific conformation.

24.2.4 Withholding food

For cold-water fish, such as goldfish, which are sold based on a specific size, there is a slight issue over how producers maintain batches of fish at the correct market size throughout the year, when breeding only occurs during one season. This is achieved by slowing growth rates by decreasing food availability. Although this is an accepted management practice, it can lead to "weaker" fish with decreased health or greater susceptibility to pathogens as they get older with limited nutrition available. This is particularly relevant in smaller sizes of koi and goldfish. However, if this management technique is applied correctly (providing minimally adequate nutrition for sustenance with all the necessary nutrients, vitamins, and minerals), it need not result in compromised welfare and is a technique widely used in the management of many other farmed fish species.

24.2.5 Transportation

The transportation of fish, just like other animals, is covered by extensive national, regional, and international laws and codes of practice. There are few published figures for percentage mortalities while the fish are transported. This is a potential welfare issue that warrants further research. However, economic losses that would occur if there were high mortality rates during transportation would lessen the profitability of the fish retail industry, so maintaining minimal shipping losses is important to the success of the ornamental fish industry. Improving the welfare of the fish includes proper handling of the fish during stops between transportation points, making water changes, removing sick or dead fish, and medicating the shipping water (Fig. 24.9).

24.3 Advocating Fish Welfare

If fish welfare needs fall short of that afforded to higher vertebrates, it is not by lack of evidence but by societal opinion and engrained behaviors toward fish (Fig. 24.10). While referring to stockmanship and good welfare, it was stated that "Instead of focusing solely on improving knowledge, it is normally necessary to target underlying beliefs and attitudes towards specific behaviours" (Hemsworth *et al.*, 2009). This is very relevant to all areas of fish utilization by humans.

As veterinary professionals, we can improve fish welfare by becoming involved in:

1. Educating hobbyists, farmers, industry, and other veterinarians using university outreach programs or information provided by the Food and Agricultural Organization of the United Nations, FAO Document Repository fish technical papers, or resources provided by veterinary societies such as The Fish Veterinary Society (FVS) or The World Aquatic Veterinary Medical Association (WAVMA).
2. Ensuring fish are fully included and recognized in welfare and veterinary legislation.
3. Developing welfare codes for more fish species, such as the Royal Society for the Prevention of Cruelty to Animals (RSPCA) welfare standards for farmed Atlantic salmon, and in particular for non-farmed species.
4. Developing standards such as the OATA Code of Conduct aimed at improving welfare at all levels of the ornamental fish industry: breeders, exporters, wholesalers, retail stores, and fish keepers.

24.4 Conclusion

Greater involvement of the veterinary profession in fish welfare should be encouraged. At present, many veterinary colleges provide little information on fish health, although there is a requirement under OIE Day One Competencies to include aquaculture teaching in those regions where aquaculture

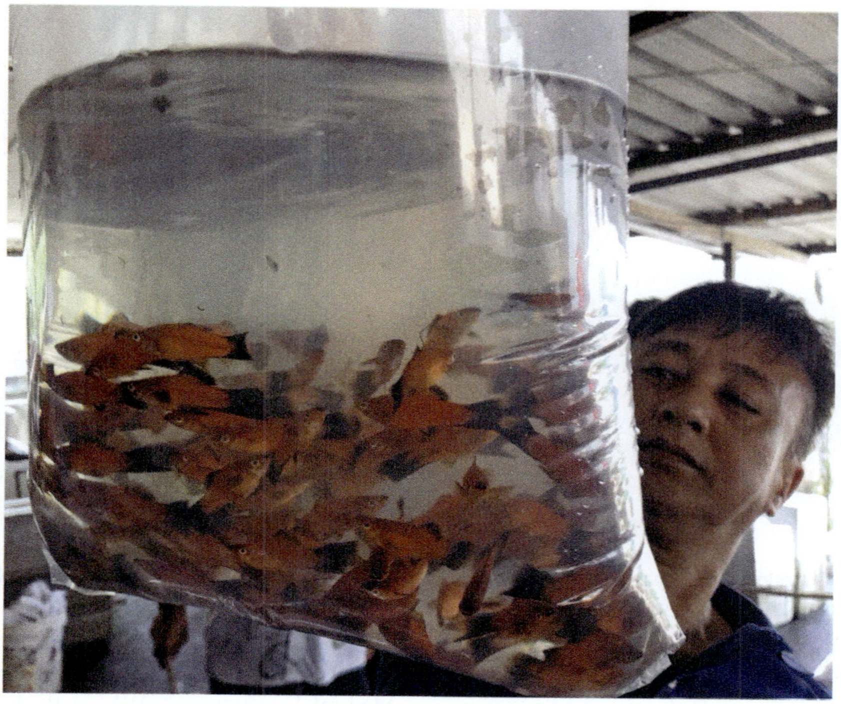

Fig. 24.9. Inspecting the fish during transportation from the farm in Malaysia to the wholesale distributor. (Photograph by N. Saint-Erne.)

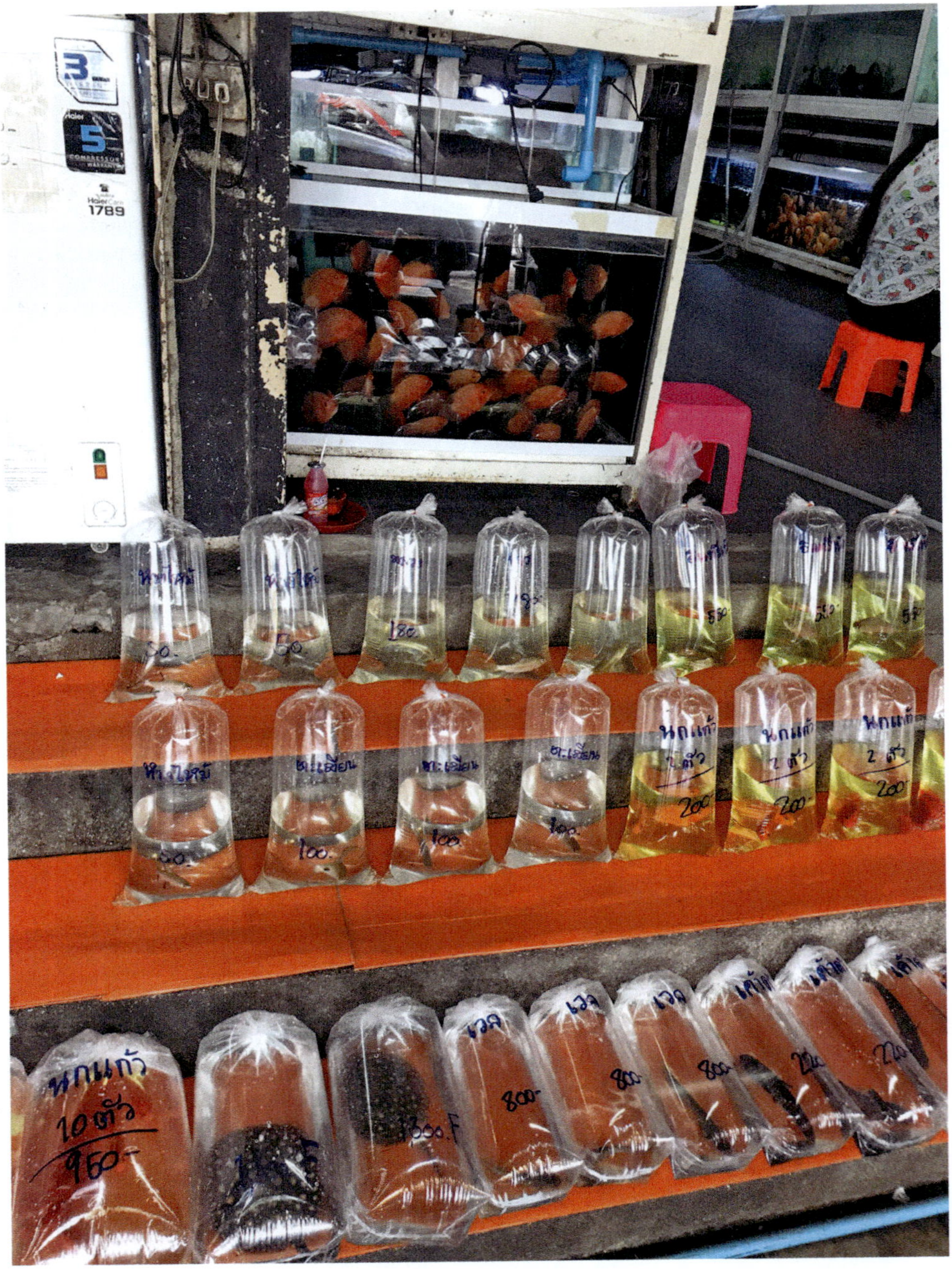

Fig. 24.10. Street vendors selling bags of fish at the Chatuchak Weekend Market in Bangkok, Thailand. (Photograph by N. Saint-Erne.)

is important economically. However, for demand to develop, the veterinary profession must first ensure that active practitioners are equipped with the skills necessary to provide a creditable service. Veterinary organizations such as the World Aquatic Veterinary Medical Association (WAVMA), the Fish Veterinary Society (FVS), the Australian New Zealand College of Veterinary Scientists Aquatic Animal Health

Chapter (ANZCVS), and the American Association of Fish Veterinarians (AAFV) provide educational materials for veterinarians to achieve this.

The improvement of fish welfare depends on many factors, of which a key one is that the public perception of the welfare of fish needs to improve. Currently, they are often seen from an economic perspective; that is, it is cheaper to buy a new fish than pay for treatment even when treatment is available, or simply they are not worth the effort. Fish need to achieve the same status as other companion animals, whereby veterinary intervention is sought on emotional grounds rather than economic. Issues of how to change societal attitudes and educate aquarists are discussed at length in Sullivan (2014). She concludes, "There is now sufficient research into fish behaviour to conclude that fish are intelligent animals and can suffer, making them a priority for welfare protection. The main barrier to providing good welfare for ornamental fish is a lack of knowledge."

References

Bekoff, M. (2007) Aquatic animals, cognitive ethology, and ethics: questions about sentience and other troubling issues that lurk in turbid water. *Diseases of Aquatic Organisms* 75, 87–98.

CAWC (2003) *Report on the Welfare of Non-domesticated Animals Kept for Companionship*. Companion Animal Welfare Council, Devon, UK.

Chao, N.L. (2001) The fishery, diversity, and conservation of ornamental fishes in the Rio Negro Basin, Brazil—A review of Project Piaba (1989–99). In: Chao, N.L. (ed.) *Conservation and Management of Ornamental Fish Resources of the Rio Negro Basin, Amazonia*. Universidade do Amazonas, Manaus, Brazil, pp. 161–204.

FishBase (2023) Available at: https://www.fishbase.se/search.php; https://www.fishbase.se/home.php (accessed 8 May 2023).

Hemsworth, P., Barnett, J. and Coleman, G. (2009) The integration of human-animal relations into animal welfare monitoring schemes. *Animal Welfare* 18(4), 335–345.

Ng, P.K.L. and Lim, K.K.P. (1997) The diversity and conservation status of fishes in the nature reserves of Singapore. *Proceedings of the Nature Reserves Survey Seminar. Gardens' Bulletin Singapore* 49, 245–265.

Sadovy, Y. (2001) The threat of fishing to highly fecund fishes. *Journal of Fish Biology* 59, 90–108.

Sullivan, M.E. (2014) *Fishing for Answers: Improving Welfare for Aquarium Fish*. The University of Western Australia, Perth, Australia.

Walster, C., Rasidi, E., Saint-Erne, N. and Loh, R. (2015) The welfare of ornamental fish in the home aquarium. *Companion Animal* 20(5), 303–306.

25 Welfare of Fish in Public Aquariums

Sharmie Johnson

Wildlife World Zoo & Aquarium, Veterinary Medical Department, Litchfield Park, Arizona

Abstract

As with zoological parks, public aquariums are under the scrutiny of the public and have an obligation to provide optimum health and welfare for the fish in their care. Supplying proper water quality, nutrition, space, compatible species, and environmental enrichment helps to ensure good fish health. Trained staff members, including aquarists, curators, and veterinarians, oversee the design, construction, and maintenance of aquarium exhibits and monitor the fish to prevent or treat injuries and diseases.

25.1 The Pursuit of Well-Being

The topic of fish welfare has been debated for more than a century. There are differing points of view regarding the capacity for fish to feel pain and have conscious awareness of that pain. The past two decades have seen changes made in research and aquaculture regarding the care and welfare aspects of keeping fish and aquatic invertebrates in captivity (Mather, 2019). Zoological institutions improve welfare through positive environmental enrichment, development of realistic exhibits replicating a natural environment, providing up-to-date medical care, and offering a variety of dietary items for the animals in their care. Public aquariums in general follow the same principles regarding ever-changing improvements in welfare for fish as do their zoo counterparts. Two core concepts form the foundation of public aquariums: conservation and education. The mission of zoos and aquariums worldwide is to promote awareness of the plight of animals that are displayed and their natural environments, in order to protect these species for generations to come.

It is beyond the scope of this chapter to end the debate. Everyone has a different view as to what should be done and to what capacity and cost; however, the most current information will be presented with the hope of encouraging readers to continue their own education on this important topic. The focus of the chapter will concentrate on the provision of well-being of freshwater fish and aquatic invertebrates in public aquariums.

25.2 Historical Basis

Fish have been purposefully held in captivity for millennia. The earliest records date to the Sumerians in 2500 BC. Several early civilizations developed ways of confining fish in ponds for the purpose of food production. In 500 BC, the ancient Egyptians were successful in advancing aquaculture practices with Nile perch (*Lates niloticus*) for religious purposes, and in 1000 BC, the Chinese began breeding carp (*Cyprinus carpio*). Since 1100–1200 AD, the ancient Hawaiians have created massive ocean-side ponds (loko i'a) adjacent to natural stream runoffs from the terraced garden plots maintained above (Fig. 25.1). The ponds were used to cultivate algae to feed the fish. The brackish water attracted many native fish to the ponds. A system of wooden grates with various size openings was strategically placed at the pond's opening to the sea so that the fish would swim in when small and be conditioned to feeding. Over a short time, the fish would grow to sizes that were too large to return to the ocean and hence be trapped in the pond. Whole communities

Corresponding author: vetdept@wildlifeworld.com

© CAB International 2025. *The Handbook of Ornamental Fish Health and Welfare* (ed. N. Saint-Erne)
DOI: 10.1079/9781789246032.0025

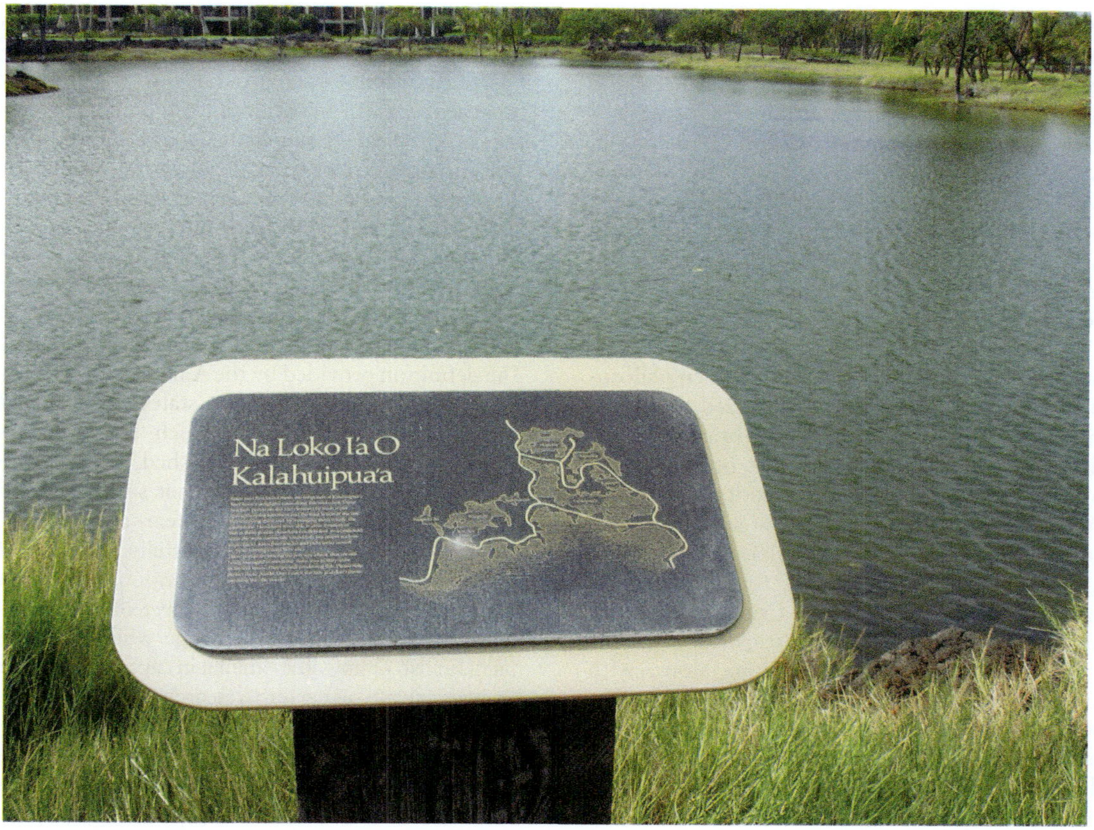

Fig. 25.1. Restored ancient Hawaiian fishponds (Loko i'a) on the Big Island, Hawaii. (Photograph by Sharmie Johnson.)

were fed using this system (McDaniel, 2018). When Captain James Cook arrived on the Hawaiian Islands in 1778, there were approximately 360 fishponds producing two million pounds of fish annually (Wikipedia, 2020).

Goldfish kept as pets appeared in Japan around 1500 AD and became disseminated throughout Europe by the end of the 17th century. Fish were brought indoors for display once the technique of water-cycling with plants was introduced in 1805, and in 1853, the first two public aquariums opened simultaneously at the London Zoo and in New York City (Grier, 2008). The term "aquarium" was coined by the English naturalist Henry Gosse, the unofficial first aquarium curator of the London Zoo. The term combines the Latin root *aqua* meaning "water" with the suffix *-arium* meaning "a place for" or "relating to" (Merriam-Webster Online, 2007). The fish hobby soon emerged afterward, and the first fish breeding facility was built in Florida (USA) in the 1920s. Improved air transportation made it possible to provide aquarium fish to faraway regions in the 1950s. Hobbyists in the 1960s saw improvements in electrical equipment and tank design, further launching the ornamental fish market into its present state, valued globally to be approximately US$5 billion. Currently, this market consists of 125 countries in trade with more than 2500 species of ornamental fish, and 60% of the aquarium industry involves trade in freshwater species. Public aquariums procure 1% of that industry (Dey, 2016). To date, there are more than 400 commercial public aquariums worldwide (Corwin, 2012). In the private sector, there are estimated to be approximately 151.1 million freshwater fish and 8.61 million saltwater fish in homes and private businesses. The success of this industry is attributed to the development of sophisticated equipment, advancements in tank design, husbandry practices, medical care expertise, and availability (History of fishkeeping, undated; Grier, 2008).

Captive breeding programs have reduced the pressure on wild populations, and the concern for the welfare of captive fish has paralleled the growth of the industry. The concept of animal welfare saw its beginnings in Victorian England in the late 1800s with the birth of the Animal Protection Movement, which sought to bring about proper care for working horses and stray animals (Wrenn, 2012). In modern times, animal welfare programs have evolved to protect many species of animals.

The concept of animals as conscious beings was commonplace until the 17th century when philosophers such as Rene Descartes theorized that there was a separation of mind and body (brain), that the mind was unique to human beings only, and that animals lacked feelings and emotions (Volpato, 2009). The following century saw a shift in philosophy supporting the concept that animals could experience pain and suffering. Social reform in England and the passing of the Cruelty to Animals Act in 1876 (AAVA, 2020) in response to public outcry against animal vivisection, along with Darwin's theory that emotion is an adaptation that species use for survival, gained momentum for animal welfare. In 1928, the pendulum again shifted when animal behavioralists stated that there was no acceptance for feelings or emotions displayed by animals in research. Changes in thinking occurred again in the late 20th century with the rebirth of philosophies regarding the consideration of emotions in animals. This has led to the present controversy over whether animals like fish are sentient beings, capable of feeling pain and suffering as a result of that pain (Volpato, 2009). The welfare of fish in private and public settings is not the sole concern for the times. Fish and aquatic invertebrates used in aquaculture, sport/recreational fishing, and research have also come under scrutiny. As of 2000, 8% of the 2.9 million animal-based research procedures used fish. They are the third-largest group of animals maintained for research, and countless articles have been devoted to the care of these animals in a research setting (Williams *et al.*, 2009).

25.3 Animal Welfare Versus Animal Rights

Animal welfare, and specifically the welfare of captive fish, is a much-debated topic among scholars, veterinarians, researchers, public zoos and aquariums, animal rights groups, and laypersons, to name a few. It is possible that the debate will never be settled. Confusion exists around this topic partly because the terms animal welfare and animal rights are inappropriately interchanged with one another. This incorrect use of terms is partly responsible for the "fueling of the fire" between groups or individuals that find themselves with opposite viewpoints. What is animal welfare, and how does it differ from animal rights? A simple definition that most agree with is one that asks the question, "How is an animal coping with the condition in which it lives?" The definition provided by the American Veterinary Medical Association (AVMA) states that "animal welfare is the condition in which an animal is healthy, comfortable, well-nourished, safe, able to express innate behavior, and is not suffering from unpleasant states such as pain, fear, and distress" (AVMA, 2020). This is a thoughtfully constructed statement with which any conscientious individual would agree. Achieving every aspect of that statement can be a daunting challenge when trying to maintain fish or any other animal in captivity, whether through private ownership, research, or aquaculture, or in a public aquarium.

Animal rights, by definition, take the animal's welfare to an elevated plane in which the animal is in charge of its own existence and is granted the same rights as a human being and is not subjected to any conditions imposed by human beings. Welfare advocates believe that animals can be utilized by humans if moral guidelines are adhered to, while rights supporters believe it to be morally unjust to use an animal in any way. The cause and awareness of suffering by the animal is the core concept (BBC, 2014).

Differences between cultures as to what is deemed appropriate welfare for fish have led to the categorization of welfare-based concepts (Robertson, 1936; Näslund and Johnsson, 2016). Currently, four basic concepts have evolved concerning fish and aquatic invertebrate welfare: feeling based, physiology based/function based, behavioral based, and preference based (Volpato, 2009). The feeling-based approach uses science to prove or disprove that fish are sentient creatures. The evaluation of the emotional state of the fish in captivity and its response to negative and positive stimuli is the focus. Fish are presumed to experience pain, fear, and anxiety and have the awareness of suffering as a direct result (Näslund and Johnsson, 2016). This concept forms the core thinking of animal rights activism (History of fishkeeping, undated). Public aquariums are diligent in preventing misinterpretation of behavior by the fish as a negative feelings-based welfare issue through education of the aquarium visitors. Placards are placed adjacent to tanks explaining the behavior, or docents or staff members are present to answer any questions.

The physiology-based or function-based concept explores morphological and physiological changes in an animal subjected to noxious stimuli, resulting in a measurable amount of pain and subsequent suffering. This involves the application of certain toxins, like bee venom or acetic acid, with post-toxin observation of effects on the animals' systems, such as increased opercular rate or aversion, and abolishment of these changes with the pre-administration of narcotic antagonists.

Observation of behavioral changes is the basis for the third concept. Specific conditions are imposed on the animals that result in particular behaviors. Manipulation of the nervous and endocrine systems with hormones and anatomical ablation are often used.

The preference-based concept attempts to identify the optimal state of fish welfare by providing a condition that the fish freely chooses to remain in. These studies use choice and preference to determine the cognition state of the animal. Choice tests provide the fish with a few variables to choose from, which through evolution possibly determine survival. Preference tests show consistent choices for a specific condition and are probably genetically determined (Volpato, 2009). Using the choice/preference-based approach to keeping fish in a public aquarium setting through knowledge of the natural environment for the species to be kept is paramount to success. Specific studies with Nile tilapia (*Oreochromis niloticus*) identified the preference for these fish to consistently choose a particular substrate, shelter, light intensity and color, and water temperature. Providing optimal welfare conditions specific for each species exhibited is based on studies such as this.

A fifth concept, referred to as nature-based, has evolved and mandates that the fish reside in an environment where natural behaviors can occur. This approach can conflict with the other concepts as stress is permitted to occur as it would in the natural environment. This approach is used commonly to acclimatize fish for release back into the wild (Williams *et al.*, 2009).

25.4 Life in the Spotlight: Public Aquariums

The goal of an attending veterinarian in a public aquarium is the procurement of the health and welfare of its occupants. It is a team approach comprising veterinarians, veterinary technicians, curators, directors, assistant directors, aquarists, volunteers, and a plethora of veterinary and possibly human medical field specialists. It is because of the expertise, experience, and guidance from these individuals that improvements in welfare are possible. When considering fish welfare based on environmental aspects, tank design and size are customized for the species to be displayed (Fig. 25.2). Every attempt is made to create a realistic natural exhibit. The strategic placement of objects in the tank promotes natural behaviors, including reproduction, shoaling, and sheltering. In contrast to private ownership, public aquariums have the benefit of displaying fish and invertebrates in large systems that can be millions of gallons in some facilities.

Many aquariums have tanks with confluent pools attached. This feature allows for the segregation of animals for examination, target feeding, medical treatment, diagnostic testing, reproductive concerns, nursery, injury, and non-infectious diseases. The added benefit is a reduction in handling stress, and the fish can be kept in the same system with the same water parameters. This is beneficial for large specimens such as arowana, arapaima, payara, pacu, large catfish, paddlefish, freshwater stingrays, and gar. In small and large systems, isolation of individuals can be accomplished using floating cages (Fig. 25.3) suspended within the main tank (Hibbitt *et al.*, 2017). This is especially helpful with gravid fish and fry, depending on the diameter of the netting.

If disease necessitates removal of animals from the main display tank, this can be accomplished by maintaining hospital or quarantine tanks where the fish can be relocated. These tanks are usually found in the employee service areas behind the public side of the exhibits or in a separate building (Figs 25.4 and 25.5). The best option is a quarantine building that is separate from the public aquarium. New arrivals are quarantined and treated for appropriate diseases and parasites when indicated. Diseased or injured fish are also maintained in quarantine until the conditions are resolved.

These tanks are kept as separate systems to prevent the spread of disease, and all equipment is specific

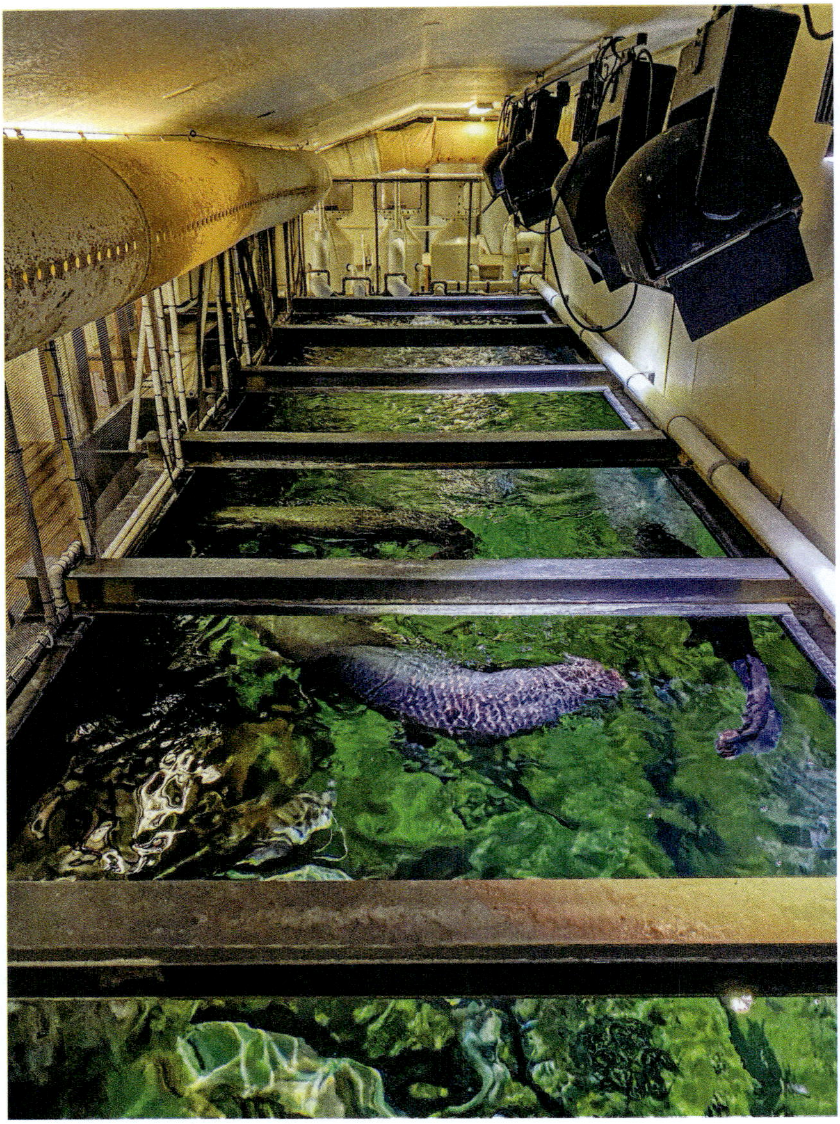

Fig. 25.2. The service side of a large, 227,124-l (60,000-gallon) display tank. (Photograph by Lorenzo Fuentes.)

to an individual tank. Disinfection of equipment, nets, aquarists' clothing, and dive gear is an ongoing process. Fish can be easily treated in hospital systems either through food, injections, or bath treatments. The ability to segregate animals in attached pools or alcoves and large hospital systems is not practical for the private aquarist. Private collections typically do not have the space and tanks available for proper medical treatment or quarantine. This results in a large degree of morbidity and mortality through introduction of disease and improper acclimatization of new fish. Public aquariums improve the welfare of the inhabitants as a direct result of this ability to isolate animals. The ability to maintain large and separate life support and emergency backup systems combined with

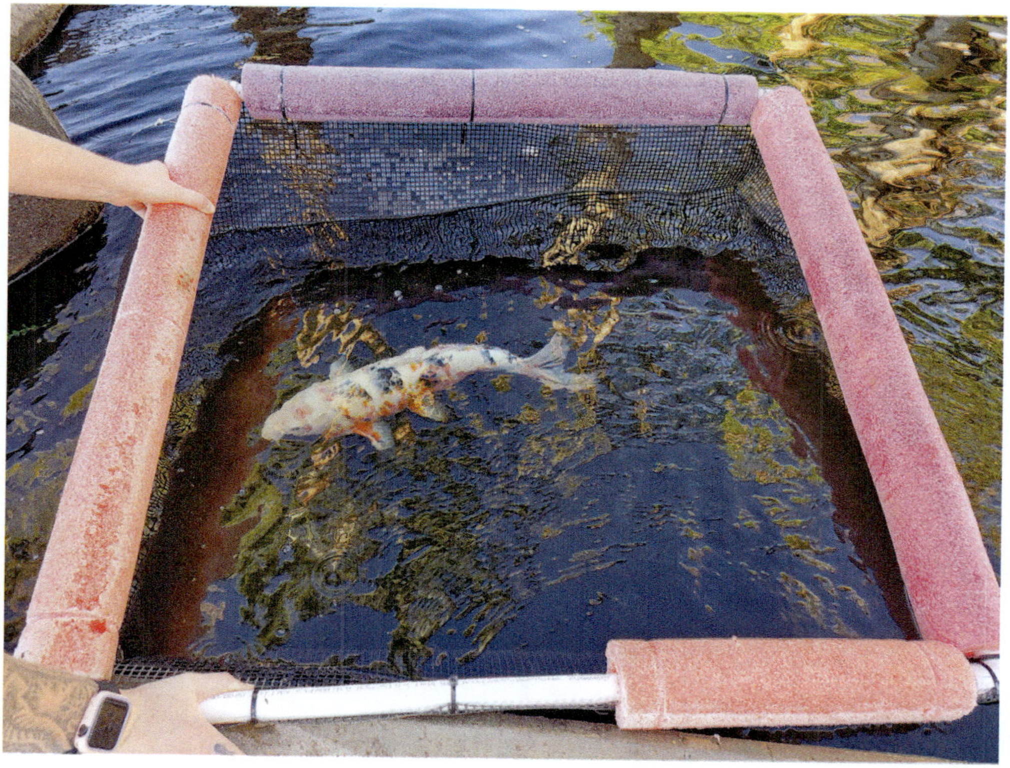

Fig. 25.3. Floating isolation unit for injured fish or those requiring treatment for non-infectious conditions and used for acclimatization in a koi pond exhibit. (Photo by Sharmie Johnson.)

large reserves of conditioned water (Fig. 25.6a,b) allow the public aquarium to prepare and resolve most crises without incident (J. Beals, Arizona, 2020, personal communication).

Maintaining water quality is paramount to the successful operation of an aquarium, whether private or public. It is the most important aspect of fish health. Fish can adjust to sub-optimal conditions, but this leads to chronic stress due to increased energy use (Johansen *et al.*, 2006). State-of-the-art water quality testing and sophisticated monitoring equipment and warning systems are available to public institutions due to financial ability. The aquarists can measure exact levels for a wide number of water parameters with over-the-counter test kits (Fig. 25.7) available to the home aquarist that measure ranges and display results as a color change (J. Beals, Arizona, 2020, personal communication). Results are quickly available. This allows for the acute detection of problems while at a low toxicity level before the fish start experiencing stress. Also, public aquariums can utilize the services of outside laboratories for testing that cannot be performed in-house. A second positive attribute to having access to advanced water quality testing is that parameters can be matched more readily to the natural environment from which the fish come, thus reducing stress and disease.

Maintaining fish in a water exhibit that duplicates their natural environment, along with housing them with species native to that same environment, promotes positive welfare. Aquarium curators and staff are knowledgeable regarding the biology of the species kept. They have years of education and experience providing the expertise required to thoughtfully plan exhibits, considering water requirements specific to the species housed, the social nature of the species, dietary requirements, reproduction, strategic

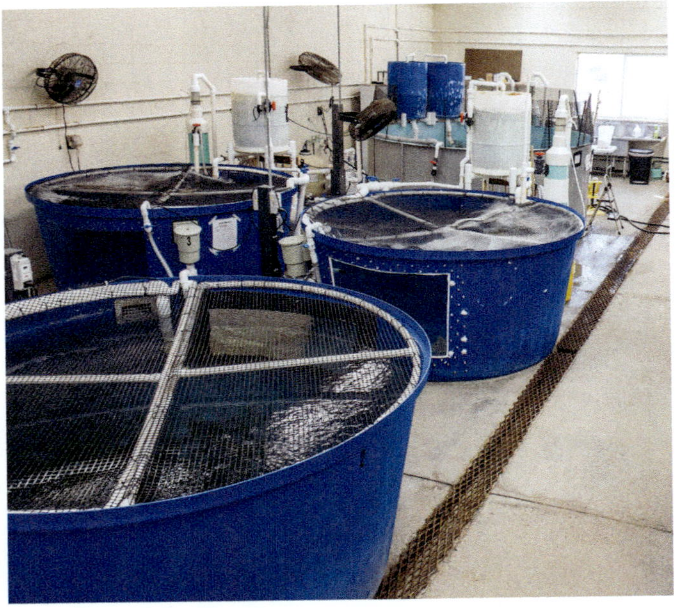

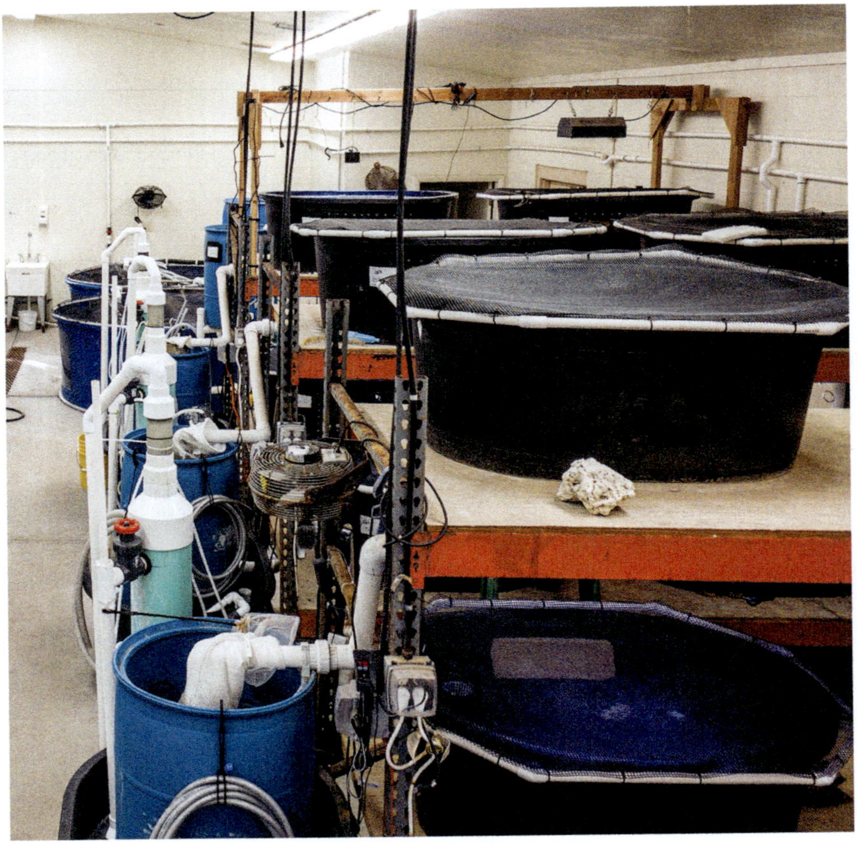

Figs. 25.4 and 25.5. The quarantine tanks used at Wildlife World Zoo & Aquarium. (Photograph by L. Fuentes.)

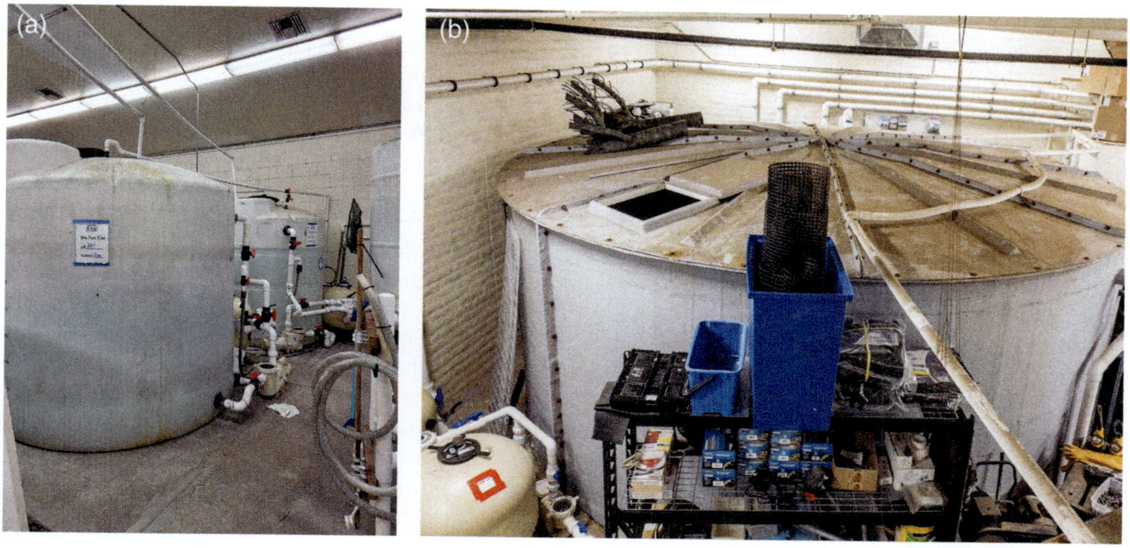

Fig. 25.6a,b. Reserve marine and freshwater tanks used for water exchange and top-off due to evaporation. (Photograph by L. Fuentes.)

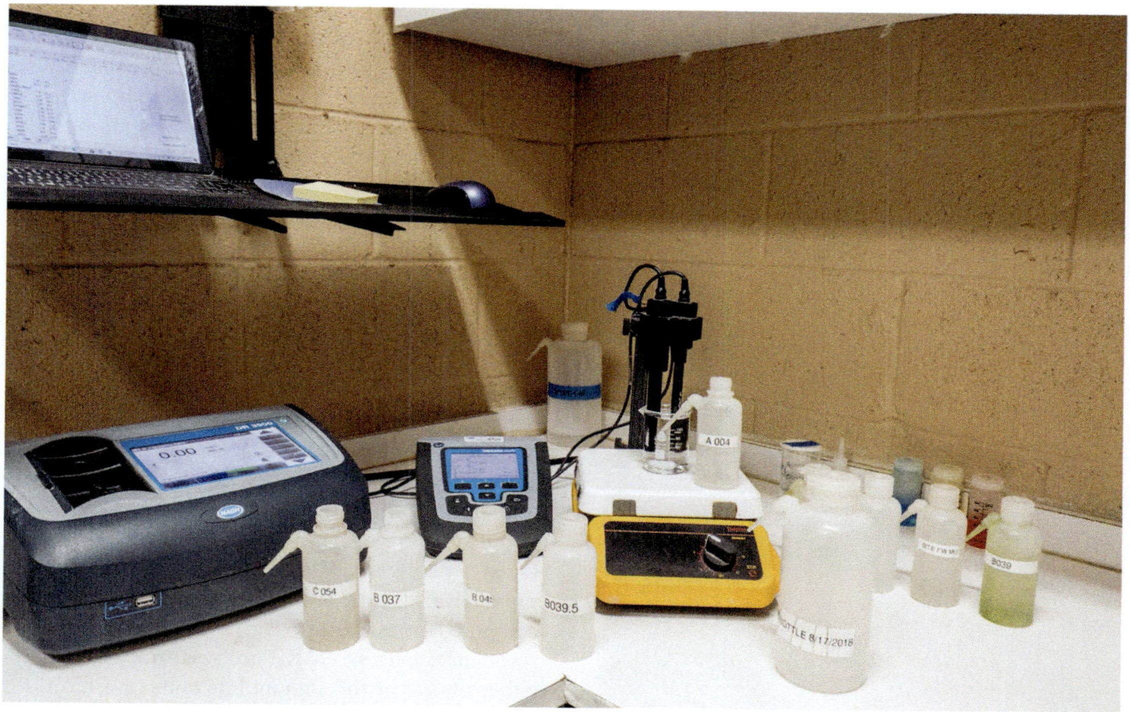

Fig. 25.7. On-site water quality laboratory. (Photograph by L. Fuentes.)

placement of natural or artificial rockwork, logs, plants, substrate, photoperiod, luminal intensity, simulation of seasonal changes typical of the regional native environment and climate (FAO, 2019). Sadly, the home aquarist typically keeps species together that are not compatible since they originate from different continents with differing water condition requirements, or have aggressive behaviors that can lead to trauma, malnutrition, disease, and death. Most of these fish are put together because they are "pretty" without any regard for their biological and water quality needs. Thoughtful consideration must be done while selecting fish species to cohabitate. Choosing species that are non-aggressive and display natural behaviors determines the success of an exhibit through better coping abilities in a captive environment.

Public aquariums experience morbidity and mortality in their collection, as does the hobbyist fish keeper. The large collection size and financial capabilities enable public aquariums to employ an aquatic veterinarian, or have contracted a private veterinarian who specializes in aquatic animals, for regular rounds and emergency treatments. The welfare benefit to the collection is immense. Animals are provided with experienced veterinary care in a timely manner. The fish and invertebrates undergo diagnostic testing (Fig. 25.8) in a humane manner

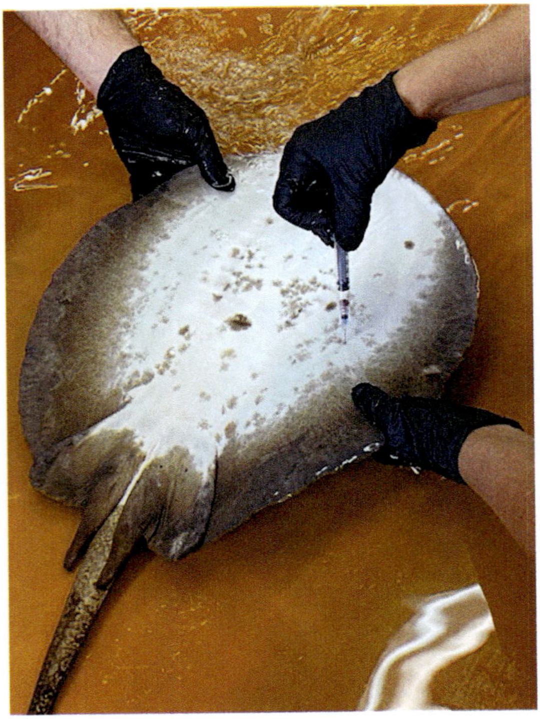

Fig. 25.8. Dr Johnson obtaining a blood sample from an anesthetized freshwater stingray (*Potamotrygon motoro*). (Photograph by Marie Dillon.)

using anesthetics when indicated, minimizing stress of handling.

Treatment is evidence-based and individualized to the patient or specific tank inhabitants (Figs 25.9a and b). Generally, the aquarists perform rounds on the animals in their charge at the start and close of each day. The fish are observed throughout the day as the staff perform their duties. Concerns are reported to the curator, who then informs the veterinarian. The fish or invertebrates are assessed by the veterinarian visually initially; then a physical examination, diagnostic tests, and treatments are initiated if indicated.

Scheduled veterinary rounds with the curatorial and senior staff are also performed regularly. Hobbyists usually are not able to observe their fish continuously and are fraught with the handicap of either not recognizing illness in their fish or not acting on time to procure professional guidance. Commonly, they are faced with providing their own medical care after spending countless time on the internet, consulting with pet shop owners or employees, or their inexperienced but well-meaning neighbors, friends, and family members. They purchase over-the-counter medications that may be inappropriate or possibly ineffective due to lack of proper diagnostic testing and knowledge regarding the pharmacology of such medications. Financial constraints or lack of concern for the welfare of the fish are also considerations. The dedicated veterinary hospitals in large public aquariums are state-of-the-art. Diagnostic and therapeutic procedures that were once limited to terrestrial animals and humans are available for aquatic animals as well. Specialized water tables for anesthesia during examination and surgery (Fig. 25.10a,b), and advances in anesthetic techniques make surgical procedures commonplace.

Removal of skin masses, ocular surgery, and intracoelomic procedures such as a salpingohysterectomy, as well as removal of enlarged egg masses, tumors, or granulomas, and fin, skin, and gill biopsies are frequently performed on fish under anesthesia (Fig. 25.11). Diagnostic digital radiography (Fig. 25.12), sonography (Fig. 25.13), and advanced imaging such as computed tomography (Fig. 25.14) and magnetic resonance imaging (MRI) are performed routinely either on-site or through mobile units or referral to a hospital. Financial constraints are not a concern in most public aquariums, as they might be with hobbyists' aquariums.

Public aquariums have a plethora of veterinary and human-side medical professionals available for assistance. Consultations with aquarium staff and

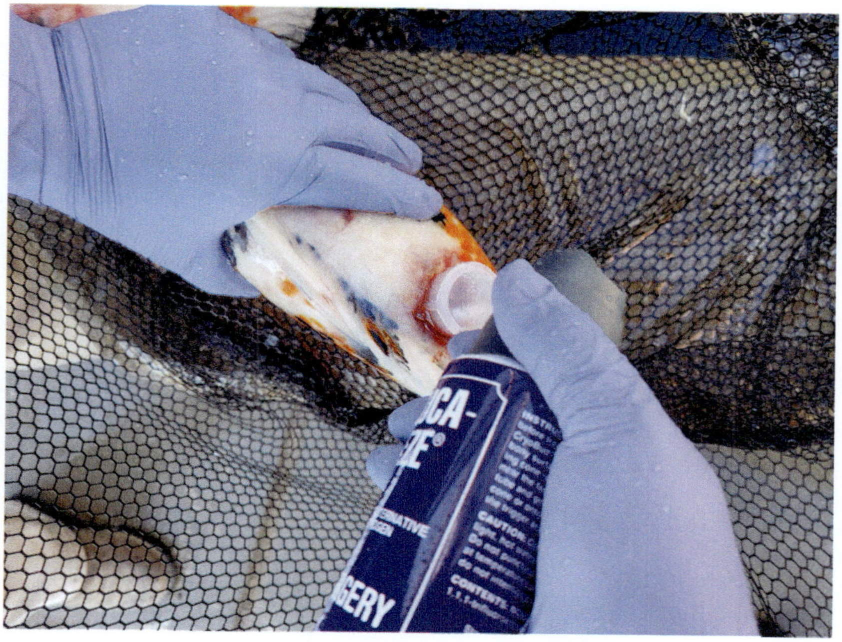

Fig. 25.9a Marie Dillon, BS, CVT, treating a skin tumor on a koi using a cryogenic unit (Verruca-Freeze, CryoSurgery, Inc., Nashville, TN, 37205, USA). (Photograph by S. Johnson.)

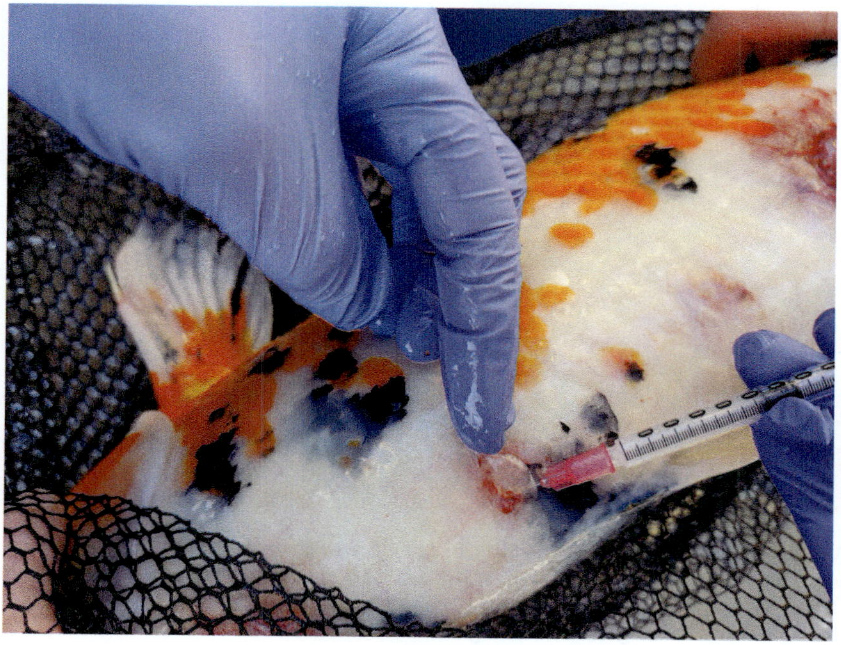

Fig. 25.9b. The same koi receiving an injection of an immunostimulant (Amplimune, Crystal Creek Natural, LLC, Spooner, WI. 54801, USA). (Photograph by S. Johnson.)

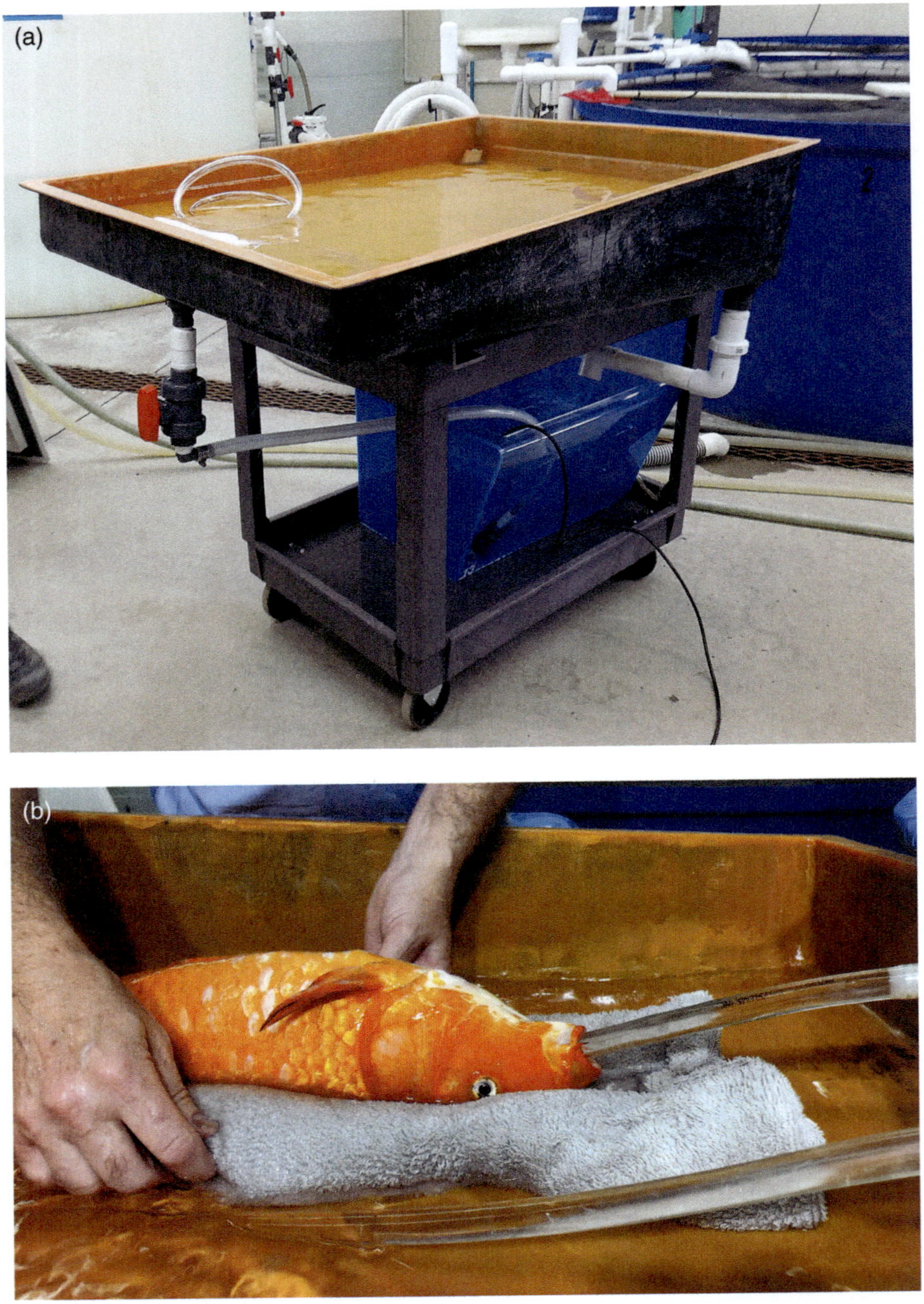

Fig. 25.10a,b. Anesthesia and surgical table. The fish can be induced with an appropriate anesthetic agent and then examination, treatments, or surgery can be performed. The table is a modified utility cart with a recirculating system set up between the main tank (top) and the smaller tank (below). Water containing the anesthetic agent is pumped into the oral cavity of the patient, exits the gills, flows through a drain into the tank below, and is returned through tubing by another pump back to the patient. The concentration of the anesthetic agent is adjusted as needed by either diluting or increasing the concentration of the agent. Recovery from anesthesia is done by providing 100% dechlorinated water without an anesthetic agent through the system or in a separate container. (Photo by Sharmie Johnson.)

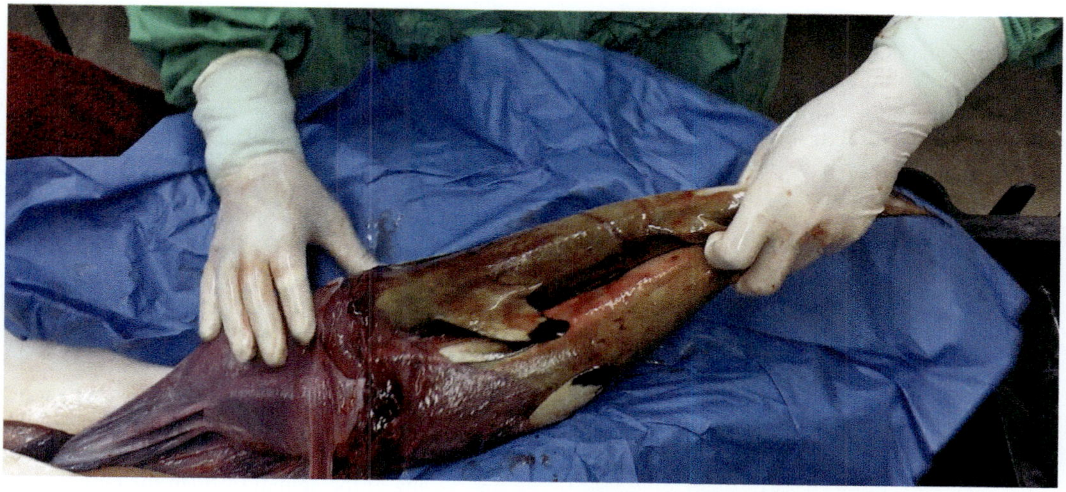

Fig. 25.11. Dr Johnson performing a cesarean section and hysterectomy on a black-tipped reef shark (*Carcharhinus melanopterus*). (Photograph by L. Fuentes.)

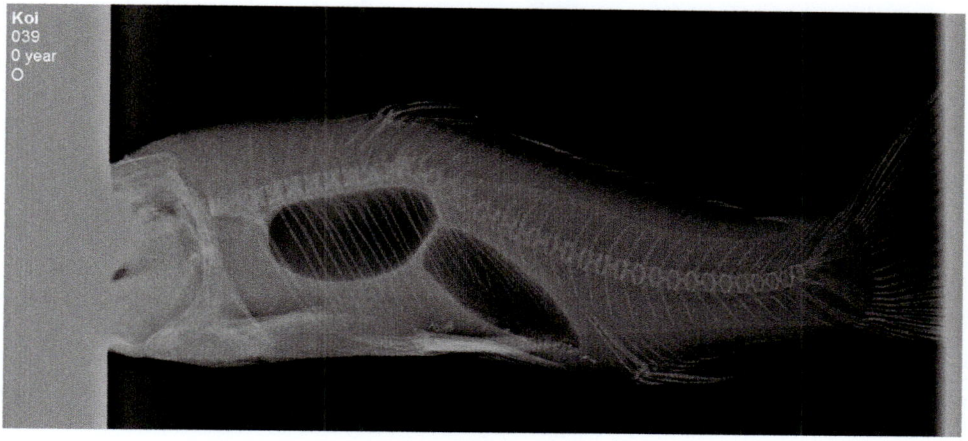

Fig. 25.12. Radiograph of an adult koi (*Cyprinus rubrofuscus*) with scoliosis associated with damaged vertebrae. (Photograph by S. Johnson.)

veterinarians around the world are also done with regularity. Direct access to manufacturers, food suppliers, fish breeders, and wholesalers also benefits the public aquarium industry (J. Beals, Arizona, 2020, personal communication). Databases are maintained through professional organizations, such as the Association of Zoos & Aquariums (AZA). Scientific journals and professional veterinary associations are dedicated to the medical and surgical care of aquatic animals. Such groups include the World Aquatic Veterinary Medical Association (WAVMA), the American Association of Fish Veterinarians (AAFV), the International Association of Aquatic Animal Medicine (IAAAM), and the American Association of Zoo Veterinarians (AAZV). These are just a few resources available to aquatic veterinarians. Veterinary teaching hospitals also contribute to the medical care of aquatic animals, and many offer programs that educate and train future aquatic veterinarians. A veterinarian in a zoo or aquarium does not face some of the challenges that a private practitioner does. Diseases associated with human interference with genetic manipulation do not contribute to negative welfare issues in public aquariums. Health concerns associated with the breeding for specific traits such as ocular, fin, and body conformation abnormalities observed with fancy goldfish (Walster *et al.*, 2015) are not encountered in public aquarium exhibits.

Another positive aspect of public aquariums is the utilization of behavioral training. Individual fish are target trained for specific medical procedures and treatments. Animals are trained to station at specific sites and are rewarded with tactile stimulation or food reinforcement. This is similar to the training done with terrestrial animals, marine mammals, and elasmobranchs. Physical examination, ultrasound procedures, blood collection, skin scrapings, injections, oral medications, and morphometrics can be performed easily and in a non-stressful, non-dangerous setting for both the animals and personnel. Movement of large fish to different tanks or for medical procedures at a remote site can be trained by conditioning the fish to swim over stretchers or through open-sided nets (Fig. 25.15).

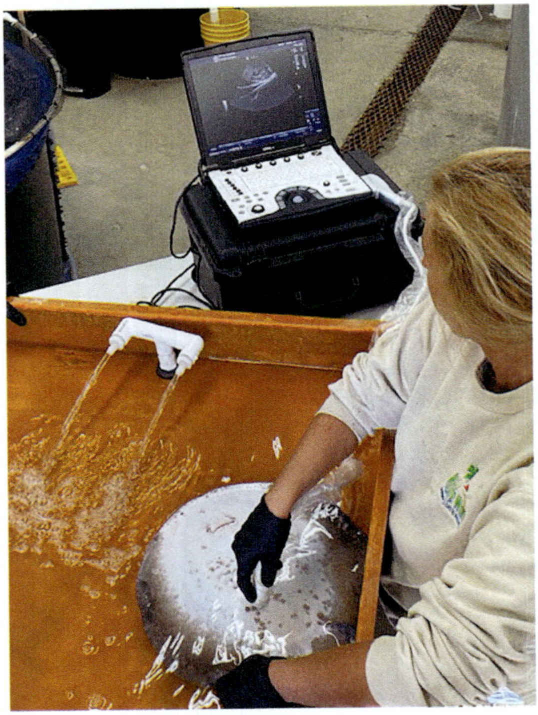

Fig. 25.13. Dr Johnson performing a coelomic ultrasound on an anesthetized freshwater stingray. (Photograph by Marie Dillon, CVT.)

Gradually, the stretcher depth is reduced, and the fish is lifted from the tank, or in the case of the open-sided net, the sides are closed. This alleviates the chasing of the animal through the tank, reducing stress and struggling once the fish is captured. Operant training is also important for behavioral observation that can potentially lead to earlier medical intervention if an abnormal behavior is observed or the animal is not feeding properly (Fig. 25.16). Conditioning aggressive fish to feed at specific targets allows for the more submissive ones to feed completely without harassment or injury. This prevents starvation in the less gregarious species and overfeeding in the more aggressive ones in a multi-species system (Corwin, 2012).

Studies with Chinook salmon (*Oncorhynchus tshawytscha*) showed a reduction in adverse behavior to handling and transport when the fish were positively reinforced by feeding prior to direct human contact (Galhardo and Oliveira, 2009). Minimalization of stress in any animal is paramount to survival. Research in fish has demonstrated that they

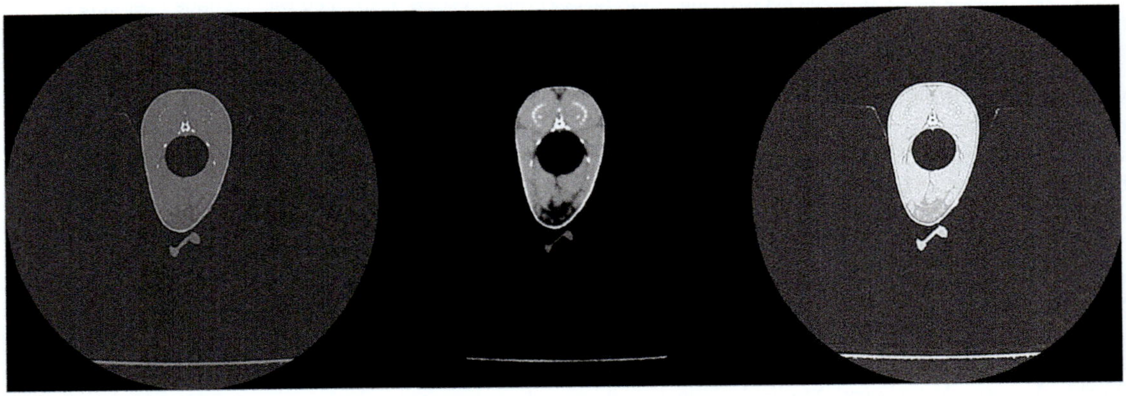

Fig. 25.14. A computed tomography (CT) performed on a spotted pike characin (*Boulengerella maculata*). (Photograph courtesy of Martin Haulena, DVM, Vancouver Aquarium.)

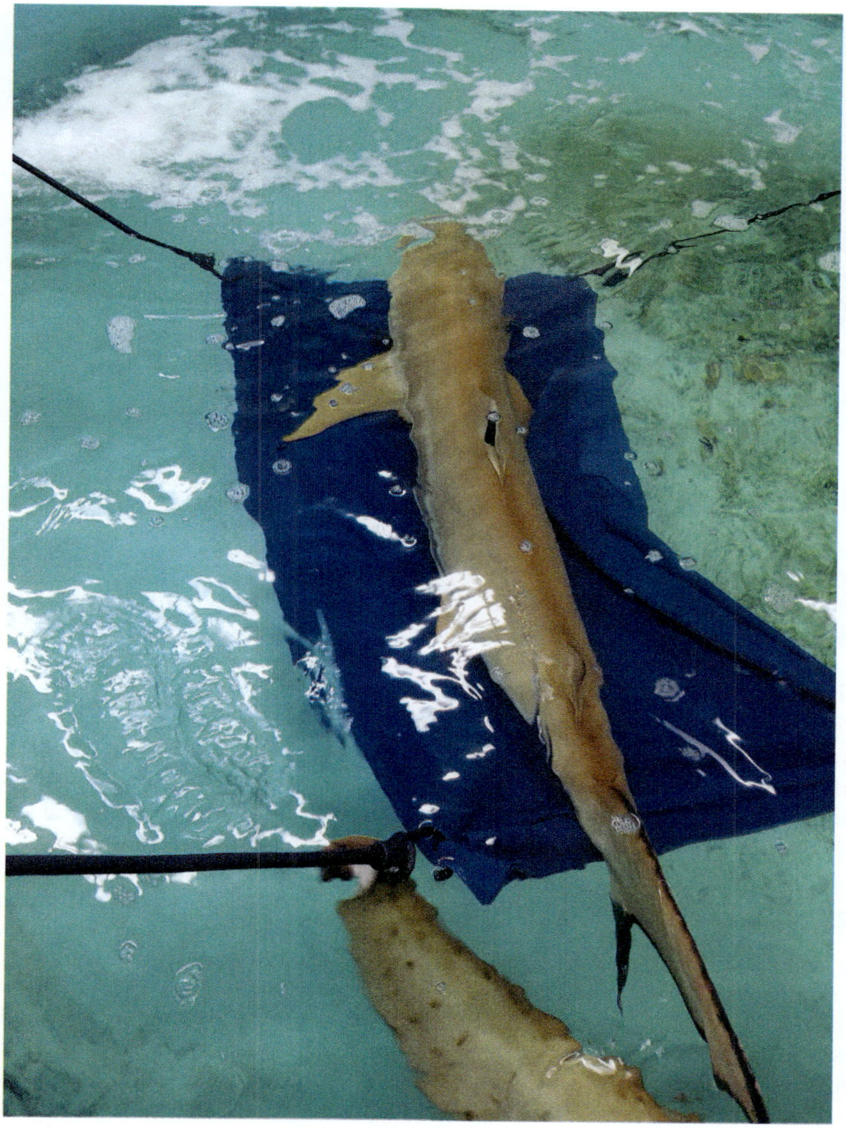

Fig. 25.15. A black-tipped reef shark is recovering from anesthesia on a stretcher fabricated from shade cloth. This will also be used to move the shark to a transfer tank and then back to its exhibit. (Photograph by S. Johnson.)

respond physiologically in a manner like other higher forms of vertebrates. Chronic stress can potentiate disease conditions due to immunosuppression (Braithwaite and Huntingford, 2004; Håstein *et al.*, 2005).

Disease and injuries can manifest in such extreme forms as to warrant a humane end point in the form of euthanasia. This occurs when treatment modalities have failed or are considered impractical and unlikely to improve the condition of the patient. Under most circumstances, a collective decision is made by the attending veterinarian, curator, and aquarists responsible for that animal. Guidelines established by the AVMA are strictly followed to ensure that the fish is euthanized in the least stressed and pain-free manner (AVMA, 2020).

Post-mortem examinations are conducted on all deceased fish to determine a cause of death if possible. This is done to ensure that proper diagnostic testing and treatments are performed for all surviving

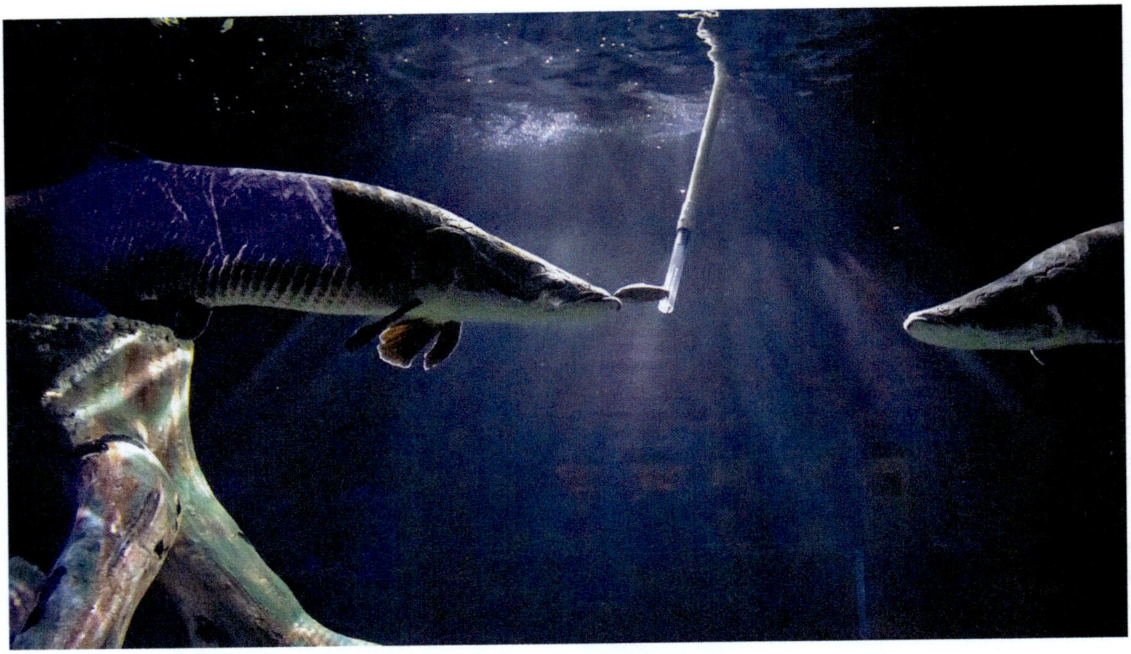

Fig. 25.16. Target feeding of a large arapaima (*Arapaima gigas*). (Photograph by L. Fuentes.)

fish exposed to the deceased animal, if indicated. Time is critical in the prevention of disease outbreaks and post-mortem examinations are instrumental in thwarting further morbidity and mortality.

25.5 Stress in Fish

Research has demonstrated that fish manifest physiological and behavioral responses to stress and that they do possess complex mental processes that can be described as awareness of their circumstances. It is this awareness or mental capacity that defines welfare (Galhardo and Oliveira, 2009). Fish respond to stress in three stages, similar to other vertebrates. The primary response is the activation of the hypothalamus-sympathetic-chromaffin (HSC) cell axis, which produces the catecholamines adrenaline and noradrenaline from the chromaffin cells that are analogous to the adrenal medulla in tetrapods. This is the "fight-or-flight" response period where the fish's cardiac and respiratory rates, blood pressure, and blood flow to the muscles are increased. Glucose is also released into the blood. In response to the increase in metabolic needs, the hypothalamic-pituitary-interrenal (HPI) tissue axis is also stimulated to produce cortisol from the interrenal tissue, which is equivalent to the adrenal cortex in other animals. The HPI response is involved with the regulation of energy metabolism through cortisol production and mineralocorticoid balance. It is also responsible for the production of β-endorphins from the pituitary gland. Anatomically the dorsal posterior cardinal veins of the anterior kidney contain the chromaffin cells and the interrenal tissue surrounds it (Galhardo and Oliveira, 2009).

The secondary response to stress brings about the physiological and behavioral changes observed, including abnormal blood parameters, acid-base abnormalities leading to ion loss across the gills, and changes in respiratory rate and character, hydrothermal balance, cellular response, and immune function (Galhardo and Oliveira, 2009).

The tertiary or prolonged stress response leads to a reduction in reproduction and growth potential. Eventually, immune suppression leads to disease and death (Galhardo and Oliveira, 2009).

The behavioral response to acute stress reflects cessation of immediate activities in order to focus on the perceived threat. Fish manifest either a freezing posture where they rest on the bottom without fin movement or display a fight-flight response by confrontation or avoidance through hiding, swimming away, or shoaling. Body rocking and flashing have also been observed in response to noxious stimuli (Galhardo and Oliveira, 2009). Continual exposure to a stressor results in changes in feeding response, swimming patterns, and territorial or sheltering behaviors.

25.6 Can Fish Experience Pain, and Does It Cause Them to Suffer?

Pain perception in fish and aquatic invertebrates and their ability to experience suffering is a much-debated issue. Before delving into the topic, one must first define pain. The definition of pain is taken in two parts. First, there must be the detection of pain itself, then there is the conscious perception or awareness of the pain. The controversy exists over the second part (Ross and Ross, 2008). In a survey sent to listservs for the AAZV and WAVMA, veterinarians, veterinary students, researchers, veterinary technicians, and animal care staff were questioned regarding their belief about pain sensation and pain awareness in aquatic invertebrates. Sixty percent of the 112 responders stated that they believed invertebrates could feel pain. Another 33% somewhat agreed. Eighty-seven percent of those surveyed were veterinarians (Wahltinez *et al.*, 2020). Many of the responders are individuals who diagnose and treat pain for many species of animals daily. Even among this group, there is uncertainty.

What is the reasoning for this? The answer to this lies partly in the anatomy of the central nervous system of teleosts and invertebrates and partly in the social conditioning of human beings. The simple behaviors and limited learning abilities observed in the past were thought to be regulated at the brainstem (Galhardo and Oliveira, 2009). Fish lack a neocortex and have poorly developed prefrontal cortical lobes. These sites in higher vertebrates are responsible for the conscious perception of pain and suffering in humans and non-human primates. Because of this, some researchers speculate that they do not consciously experience the awareness of pain. Recent research on fish behavior, neuroanatomy, and cognitive abilities has shown that fish are capable of complex behaviors and learning capacity. Fish possess nociceptive nerves and are capable of responding to noxious stimuli with aversion, decreased feed response, increased opercular and cardiac rates, and weight changes (Braithwaite and Huntingford, 2004; Chatigny *et al.*, 2018). Invertebrates also possess nociceptors and axons that respond to noxious stimuli (Ross and Ross, 2008). Both sides of the debate agree that fish and invertebrates respond to noxious stimuli through nociceptive behavior. Because of this, it is prudent to minimize this response when performing procedures that could be construed as painful to a human being (Chatigny *et al.*, 2018).

Pain scales exist for several species of terrestrial vertebrates, notably rabbits, cats, dogs, ruminants, and horses. These are graded scales based on posture, facial grimace, and movement. Fish and aquatic invertebrates are not able to grimace due to lack of facial expression. They lack the ability to form postural changes like other animals do when in a state of pain, and they do not communicate verbally or attempt to bite due to lack of flexibility when manipulated. Researchers are left with aversion behavior and other behaviors that deviate from that normally displayed by that species. Behavioral studies in rainbow trout (*Oncorhynchus mykiss*) revealed that the fish displayed fear abatement to novel objects when treated with a narcotic. The fear response returned with the addition of a narcotic antagonist. Studies on Atlantic salmon (*Salmo salar*) and zebrafish (*Danio rerio*) demonstrated similar findings (Chatigny *et al.*, 2018). Arguments can be made that narcotic-induced sedation was the cause for the behavioral changes. Because fish do not communicate in a way that we can understand, the subjective state of the emotions of pain and fear can only be studied based on the physiological and behavioral aspects demonstrated by humans experiencing pain or fear (Galhardo and Oliveira, 2009).

25.7 Anatomical Dissection of Pain Perception

Nociception, or pain perception, occurs no further than the level of the spinal cord. A noxious stimulus travels via nerve endings on the skin to the spinal cord eliciting a rapid withdrawal response through reflexive reactivity without conscious brain involvement. Cognitive pain perception occurs in the same neuroanatomical structures but involves further transmission of impulses from the spinal cord to the brain with the recognition of the stimulus being a negative experience to be recorded in memory as a means to avoid the stimulus in the future (Gerber *et al.*, 2015).

The telencephalon of the fish is structurally similar to the limbic system in terrestrial animals. This is the site responsible for emotion, memory, and pain perception in humans. Rainbow trout (*Oncorhynchus mykiss*) possess 22 nociceptors in their head, and these are morphologically and functionally like those in humans. Information travels from these receptors via the trigeminal nerve to the brain. A-delta and C fibers have been identified in higher vertebrates and teleosts. These fibers are responsible for conveying somatosensory and nociceptive impulses to the brain (Sneddon, 2002, 2003). This demonstrates that fish possess the proper neuroanatomical equipment to send information to the telencephalon (Gerber *et al.*, 2015) further supporting the potential for cognition. Additional studies supporting this were observed in rainbow trout described earlier when subjected to a noxious stimulus to nociceptors in their head. The fish responded adversely in the absence of morphine compared with no reaction when the fish were pretreated with an opioid. In a similar study with rats, morphine acts on the trigeminal nerve. Conclusions were that results from both studies showed that the animals' reactions could not be reflex based alone and that the higher centers of the brain were involved with awareness of the stimulus (Gerber *et al.*, 2015).

Other studies in rainbow trout and goldfish identified neuronal activity from nociceptors to the spinal cord, cerebellum, tectum, and telencephalon when the fish were subjected to noxious stimuli and displayed aversive behavior. These findings provide further evidence that teleosts do not act on reflex alone at the level of the spinal cord and brainstem (Davie and Kopf, 2006). The central nervous systems of fish and mammals have many homologous neuronal structures, neurotransmitters, and mechanisms of action. Consciousness in mammals is not the product of one particular site in the brain but is attributed to the intricate neuronal connections with specific characteristics that work together in producing conscious thoughts and in keeping the allostasis of the central nervous system. These interconnections occur in fish as well (Galhardo and Oliveira, 2009).

Similar neuroanatomical structures can be found in both teleosts and terrestrial mammals. The pertinent regions of the brain and part of the spinal cord are represented in an arapaima (*Arapaima gigas*) and a red kangaroo (*Macropus rufus*), seen below in Figs 25.17a and b. Nociceptors are present in many areas of the body, but for simplicity, only those present in the head are illustrated and are represented by lightning bolts. These are the sites that convey information to the trigeminal nerve following mechanical, thermal, or chemical stimulation.

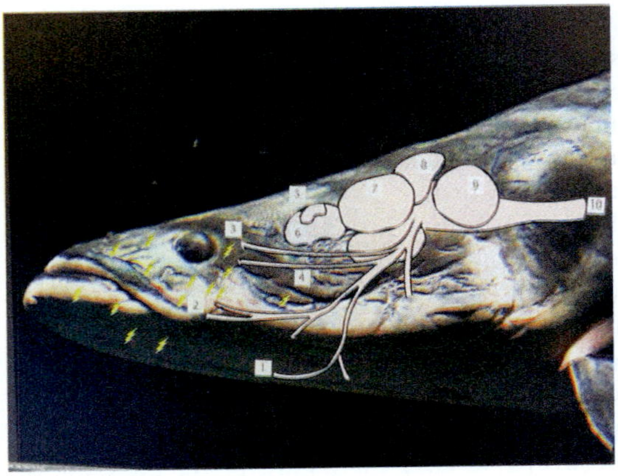

Fig. 25.17a. (*Arapaima gigas*). (1) Mandibular branch of the trigeminal nerve (V). (2) Maxillary branch of the trigeminal nerve. (3) Ophthalmic branch of the trigeminal nerve. (4) Facial nerve (VII) exiting the trigeminofacial ganglionic complex. (5) Amygdala and hippocampus contained within the telencephalon. (6) Telencephalon or cerebrum. (7) Optic lobe. (8) Cerebellum. (9) Medulla oblongata. (10) Cranial aspect of the spinal cord. (Illustrations and graphic interpretation courtesy of Warren Johnson, PhD, MD.)

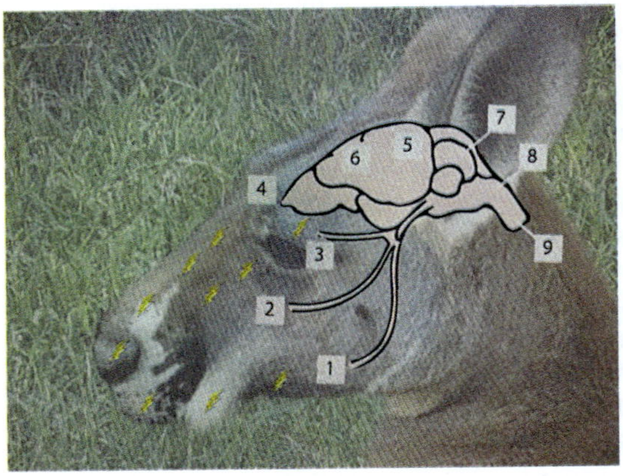

Fig. 25.17b. (red kangaroo, *Macropus rufus*). (1) Mandibular branch of the trigeminal nerve (V). (2) Maxillary branch of the trigeminal nerve. (3) Ophthalmic branch of the trigeminal nerve. (4) Olfactory bulb. (5) Cerebrum (neocortex). (6) The location of the amygdala and hippocampus contained within the deeper structures of the cerebrum. (7) Cerebellum. (8) Medulla oblongata. (9) Cranial aspect of the spinal cord. (Graphic interpretation courtesy of L. Fuentes.)

Recent evidence has also identified corticosteroid receptors in the lateral pallium of the forebrain of fish. This suggests that this site, like the hippocampus in mammals, is the region of the brain responsible for interpretation and reaction to stress and most likely a site of cognition in the fish as has been shown in mammals. Cortisol receptors, found mainly in the hippocampus, bind cortisol during acute stress response and enhance cognition through improved memory. Chronic stress has the opposite effect by decreasing the learning and memory ability as a direct result of reducing hippocampus volume (Galhardo and Oliveira, 2009).

The detection, interpretation, and resulting action of a stimulus in mammals occurs in the prefrontal cortex, amygdala, and hippocampus. Research in goldfish (*Carassius auratus*) has shown that spatial memory is processed in the forebrain by the medial and lateral pallium, which are homologous to the mammalian amygdala and hippocampus, respectively. The goldfish were capable of reactions that reflected a complex memory ability (Galhardo and Oliveira, 2009). Koi have also been trained to target and retrieve objects, swim through hoops, and pick cards in a poker game! The author has observed koi that demonstrate aversion behavior by hiding under rockwork when staff approach with nets still held out of the water. A few affected fish were regularly netted for treatment of skin neoplasms. Of interest, it was only the targeted fish that hid. The same fish behaved in a food-seeking behavior when the same staff approached for rounds without nets (Fig. 25.18).

The amygdala in higher vertebrates has been identified as the neuroanatomical structure involved with the processing of information regarding fear and pain and is responsible for the behavioral responses associated with them (Veinante *et al.*, 2013). The medial pallium in teleosts is homologous to the amygdala, further supporting the view that fish can process information that is fear or pain based. The identification of dopaminergic activity in fish subjected to a fearful state with associated avoidance behavior is also characteristic of higher vertebrates (Davie and Kopf, 2006).

Determination of sentience and cognition in all species is based on comparison with human neuroanatomy. This may be an unfair and unrealistic assumption that human beings are the center of the universe neuroanatomically and cognitively and that other species are derivations of that. Evaluation of the research into the subject for the past two decades supports the theory that ontogeny recapitulates phylogeny and that the same information can be processed to the central nervous system in distinctly different but similar ways. Other research findings concluded that fish have consciousness and display a variety of sophisticated behaviors that indicate complex mental capabilities demonstrated through extended associative learning and that pain perception is possible. The presence of nociceptors and opioid receptors, ability to produce endogenous opioids, presence of a central nervous system, blunting of nociceptive responses by analgesics (especially morphine), and avoidance learning that is also observed in humans in response to painful stimuli are all indicators of probable awareness or pain perception in fish (Huntingford *et al.*, 2006; Ross and Ross, 2008).

A common ground regarding fish welfare can possibly be found between the philosophers who support fish and aquatic invertebrates as sentient beings and the scientists who do not, based on the collection of objective information that is species and situation specific for indicators of stress, health status, and behavior and not on the presence of pain, sentience, and suffering as a result of the lack of specific neuroanatomical and neurophysiology as it compares to humans (Browman *et al.*, 2019). After all, the objective of any aquarium curator, veterinarian, or aquarist is to provide optimal husbandry for the fish and minimize any cause for visible discomfort. Decreasing the discrepancy between the adaptations that an animal makes to its environment enhances its welfare (Håstein *et al.*, 2005).

A function-based approach to fish welfare in a public aquarium can be adapted from the operational welfare indicators (OWI) that were developed for aquaculture practices in Europe. The concept advocates the proper training of aquarists and veterinarians in recognizing stress and health issues based on knowledge of normal behavior, including swimming and shoaling, reproduction, and foraging behaviors (Martins *et al.*, 2012). Evaluation of the water quality parameters, both physical and chemical, using the most up-to-date technology available is important in fish welfare. Daily evaluation of the physical appearance of the fish for body condition scoring (BCS), ventilatory rate, and body color changes such as darkening or pallor that can be indicative of stress, disease, reproduction, aggression, or submissiveness all are useful in the assessment of health and overall welfare (Martins *et al.*, 2012; FAO, 2019). Stereotypic and abnormal behaviors are commonly observed with acute or chronic stress and are indicators of poor welfare. Positive welfare indicators are seen in fish that display exploratory, food-anticipatory, and reward-related operant behaviors (Martins

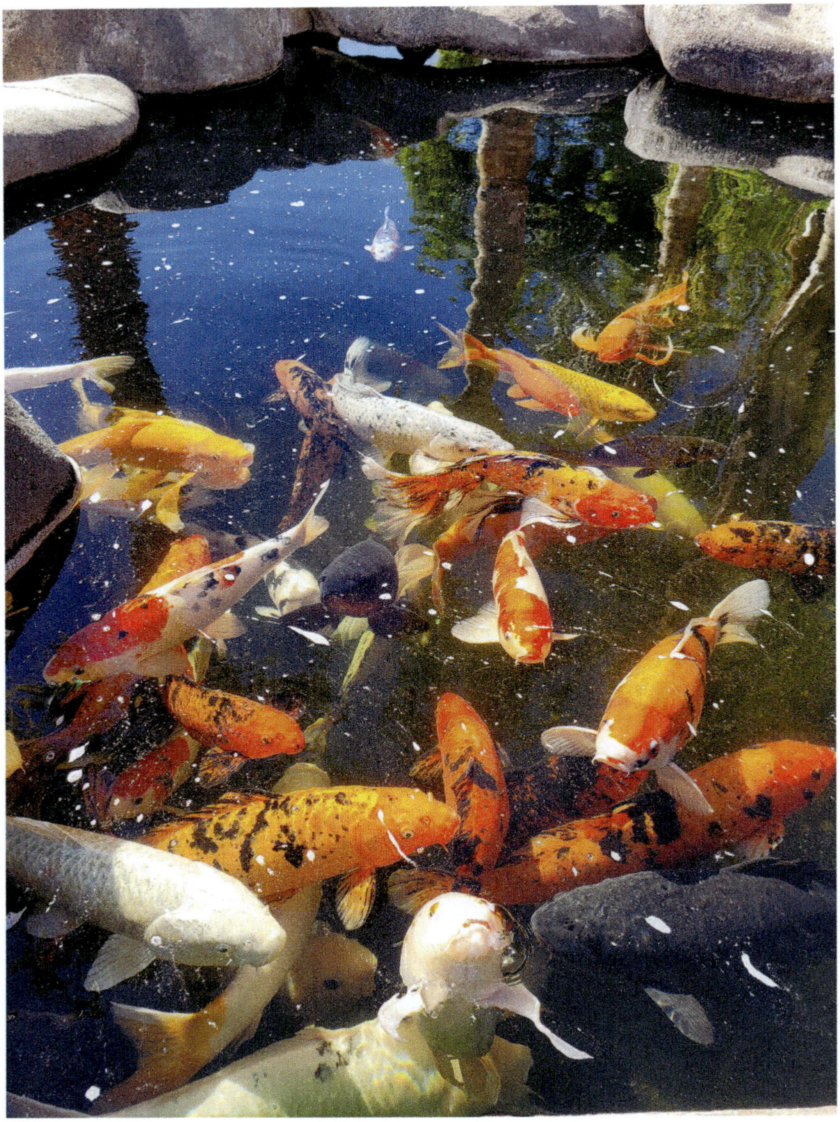

Fig. 25.18. These koi are food motivated and conditioned to feed at one side of the pond. They react in a positive manner by congregating at the surface when the staff approach without nets. (Photograph by S. Johnson.)

et al., 2012). Operational welfare indicators should be as science-based as possible.

It is important to recognize that some members of the scientific community, zoo and aquarium professionals, and the general public consider a "feelings-based" approach to animal welfare as important as a "functional-based" one. Controversy will exist until it can be scientifically proven that fish are sentient beings. There is not a clear-cut right or wrong approach to this welfare concept. What is important is to be considerate of all viewpoints presented and apply any method possible for the individual circumstances that will have a positive impact on the welfare of the fish and aquatic invertebrates in the collection.

25.8 Welfare Indicators

25.8.1 Foraging behavior

For large multi-species exhibits, fish are chosen from the same part of the world that also occupy different strata of the water column. This encourages normal foraging behavior without competition between species that are bottom, mid-water, or surface feeders. Competition can also be reduced by choosing some species that are nocturnal feeders while the others are diurnal in their foraging behavior (Martins *et al.*, 2012; FAO, 2019).

Use of floating or sinking food, or food that suspends within the water column, ensures that all the fish receive the appropriate amounts of food and minimizes the potential for starvation from food competition, or over-nutrition leading to obesity and other health and water quality problems. Foraging behavior is one of the most important OWI that aquarists and veterinarians can use to determine the presence of a stressor or disease-induced welfare issue. Any change in food intake, including the timeliness of foraging resumption following a perceived stress, can be used to assess welfare (Martins *et al.*, 2012; FAO, 2019).

25.8.2 Ventilatory rate

The opercular rate of fish is a commonly used indicator of stress and poor welfare (Martins *et al.*, 2012). The rate and character of the ventilatory activity are tightly regulated to maintain the proper oxygenation of the tissues and the acid-base balance. Chemoreceptors in the buccal mucosa or in the vasculature of the gills can respond to changes in the oxygen and carbon dioxide content of the aquatic environment and correspondingly change the ventilatory rate within a matter of seconds. Ventilatory activity is inversely related to the oxygen content of the water (Martins *et al.*, 2012; FAO, 2019). Evaluation of hyper-ventilatory rate within an individual can be a sign to the veterinarian to assess hematocrit, glucose, and blood lactate levels if possible. If many individuals are affected, that should prompt the aquarists to immediately check water parameters including temperature, pH, ammonia, nitrite, nitrate, oxygen saturation, salinity, water hardness, and efficacy of the pumps and filters. Analysis for water toxins and chemicals, electrical current, parasites, and harmful algae should also be considered (FAO, 2019).

Light and noise levels also affect welfare. Evaluation should be done in both the employee service areas and the public side of the exhibits (Johansen *et al.*, 2006). Biotechnical indicators of welfare include hematology and biochemical assessment, cortisol measurements in the fish or in the water or feces, up- and down-regulation of targeted genes, and expression of the stress protein metallothionein in the gills and gastrointestinal system (Johansen *et al.*, 2006; Martins *et al.*, 2012). Evaluation of the character of the skin and mucous layer can be an indication of stress or disease. Stress alone can cause ulcerations in the skin without the presence of inciting pathogens. In the future, evaluation of stress-induced gene expression may become an important tool in determining the welfare of fish (Johansen *et al.*, 2006).

25.8.3 Temperature

Fish are poikilothermic, with a few exceptions. The standard environmental temperature (SET) or preferred optimal temperature zone (POTZ) should be maintained based on the temperature preference for the species exhibited. An increase for every single degree above SET results in decreased feed conversion, and each decrease below SET results in a reduction in metabolic rate and can result in shifts in ionic balance leading to hypo-salinity in freshwater fish. Oxygen saturation is also temperature dependent, with warmer water holding less oxygen. Aquarium staff must calculate the oxygen saturation required for exhibits based on fish density and water flow as well (Johansen *et al.*, 2006).

25.8.4 Nitrogenous compounds and pH

Continuous surveillance of nitrogenous compounds such as ammonia (NH_3), nitrite (NO_2), and nitrate (NO_3) is critical, as ammonia and nitrite are especially toxic to fish. Aquarists are careful not to overstock tanks, to provide water flow in stagnant areas and to maintain the proper water temperature, pH, and salinity in order to minimize toxic levels of these compounds. Deviation of pH from optimal mandates a thorough evaluation of feeding techniques, water flow rates, stocking density, carbon dioxide (CO_2) levels, and water source. Changes in pH create metabolic stress in the fish and can increase the toxicity of chemicals that might be present in the environment, particularly heavy metals (Johansen *et al.*, 2006).

25.8.5 Light and noise

Photoperiod affects behavior and physiology of fish and invertebrates (Johansen *et al.*, 2006).

Most fish avoid bright light, necessitating provisions for shelter. One-way glass can be used to reduce outside light exposure through the public access doors. A gradual transition of light intensity from dawn to dusk can reduce the startle response. The use of lighting to simulate cloud cover and moonlight is also an option for emulating the natural environment (Fig. 25.19) and triggering spawning behaviors.

Fish possess highly developed detection systems for noise and vibration. Because levels vary during the time of day and season associated with visitor attendance, fish may need to be conditioned to these changes when anticipated. Aquarium staff, volunteers, or docents may need to be stationed adjacent to exhibits that house sensitive and reactive species of fish to prevent injury from tapping on the glass or excessive noise in the public walkways.

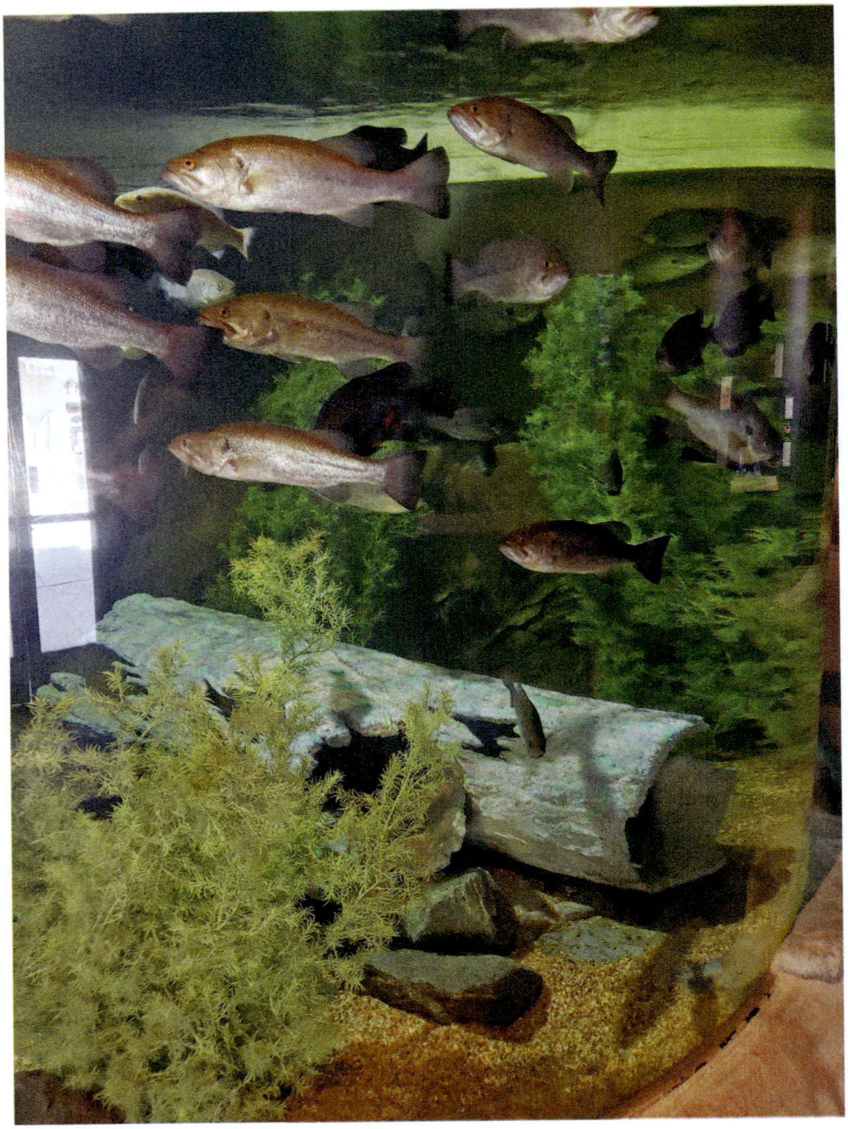

Fig. 25.19. Changes in photoperiod are used in this exhibit to simulate natural light rhythms for the bluegill (*Lepomis macrochirus*) and largemouth bass (*Micropterus salmoides*). (Photograph by S. Johnson.)

25.8.6 Flow rates

Flow rates within a system should emulate the currents found in the natural environment. Trout and salmon prefer fast water flow rates compared with other species, such as the cyprinid fish that prefer slow-moving or static waterways. Oxygen uptake is also influenced by flow rates. Some fish species have improved their ability for increased oxygen uptake through adaptation of absorbing oxygen from the air (Johansen *et al.*, 2006). Examples of this are arowana (*Osteoglossum bicirrhosum, Scleropages formosus*), arapaima (*Arapaima gigas*), lungfish (*Neoceratodus forsteri, Protopterus aethiopicus, Lepidosiren paradoxa*), and electric eels (*Electrophorus electricus*). Anabantids, such as *Betta splendens*, have a labyrinth organ in the pharynx that can hold a bubble of air gulped at the surface and act like a lung to extract oxygen from the air. These fish evolved in areas of warm, stagnant water with low flow and therefore low dissolved oxygen levels.

25.8.7 Stocking density

The number of fish that can be safely kept in an aquarium is determined by the species to be kept. Low stocking densities in small aquariums favor good water quality but can increase stress in species that normally form large shoals. In smaller fish, the stocking density is determined by the length of fish per volume of water in the tank. While the old rule for tropical fish aquariums is usually 1–2 gallons of water per inch of fish body length, in public aquariums, much more water volume than this is needed for good fish welfare. Larger fish need considerably more space and water volume than a similar weight of smaller fish.

25.8.8 Swimming behavior

Fish display one of three types of normal swimming behaviors. Territorial swimming behaviors are observed in aggressive species, like trout and salmon that fin nip (Fig. 25.20). Schooling (shoaling) behavior is

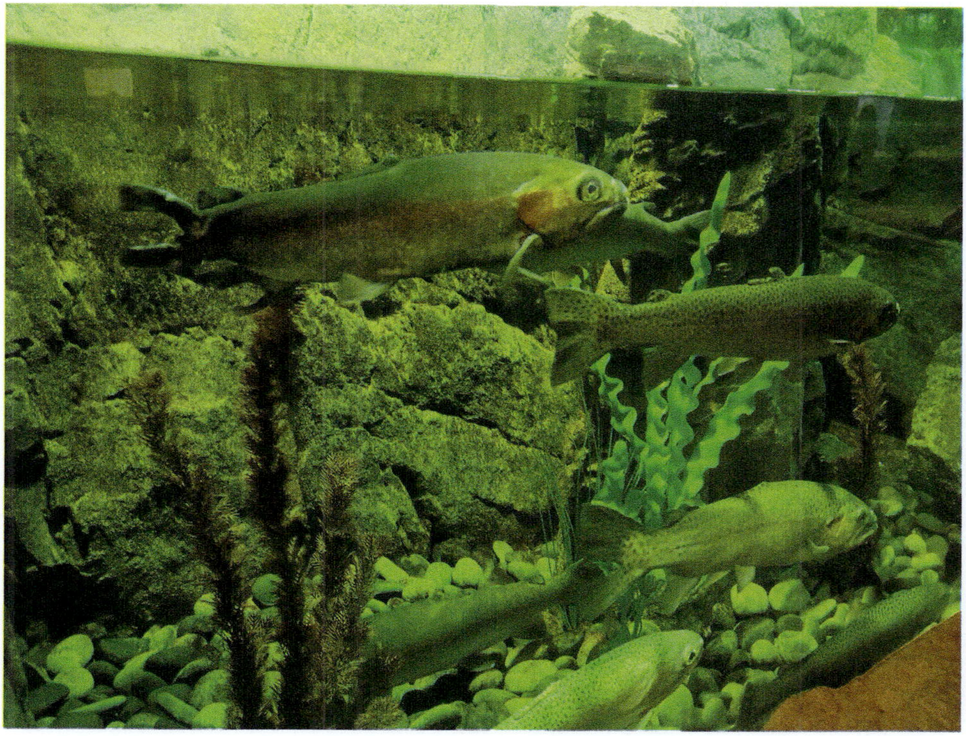

Fig. 25.20. These territorial rainbow trout (*Oncorhynchus mykiss*) have mutilated each other's fins. (Photograph by S. Johnson.)

observed in groups of fish that maintain close contact with each other and are dependent on one another for protection, foraging, and reproduction. The third group of fish prefers a solitary existence and will be seen to swim independently of other fish (Johansen *et al.*, 2006).

Changes in swimming behavior, including aversion, hiding, and postural defects, are also useful indicators of stress and should cue the staff to evaluate the environment for the presence of potentially aggressive tank-mates, poor water quality, pathogens, or toxins (Martins *et al.*, 2012). Knowledge of normal swimming activity of an individual or the group is important when assessing changes associated with swimming rate or maneuverability, and can be used as an indicator of poor welfare. When in question, cameras can be used to observe the fish remotely without influencing their behavior (Williams *et al.*, 2009). A positive indicator of good health is the observation of fish swimming at normal speed and with normal opercular rate, and not darting to the bottom or back of the tank. Monitor for fin or skin lesions suggestive of fin-nipping and aggression, and observe normal feed anticipatory response, whether individually or within the group (Martins *et al.*, 2012; FAO, 2019). Stereotypic behavior, such as compulsive circling and vertical swimming, can be a coping mechanism associated with stress. These abnormal behaviors have been witnessed in African catfish (*Clarias gariepinus*) and Atlantic halibut (*Hippoglossus hippoglossus*) when subjected to high stocking density. Research into this behavior has shown the coping mechanism to be endogenous opioid production (FAO, 2019).

25.8.9 Physical appearance

Increases or decreases in growth rate are indications of welfare that are associated with changes in food conversion. Body condition scoring (BCS) and measurement of length-weight data can also provide insight to the overall health of the population. A positive indicator of health and welfare in aquacultured species is evaluation of the length of fish to its weight. Positive welfare is directly proportional to the weight of the fish. This may not be comparable in exhibited species. Increased weight can be an indicator of poor health because of obesity (Fig. 25.21), egg coelomitis, ascites, organomegaly, and neoplasia.

25.9 Quarantine

New fish are purchased from commercial distributors, breeders or from other institutions. The current emphasis is to obtain fish that are captive bred if possible. All new fish and invertebrates should be

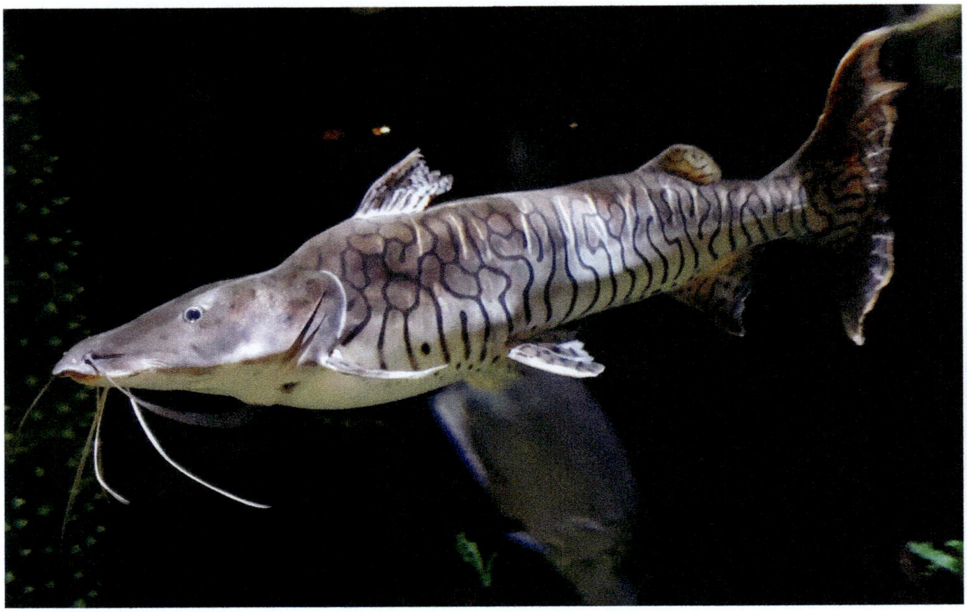

Fig. 25.21. Obesity, seen as an enlarged belly, in a tiger shovelnose catfish (*Pseudoplatystoma fasciatum*). (Photograph by S. Johnson.)

quarantined for a period consistent with the life cycles of the pathogens common for that species. Quarantine tanks (Fig. 25.22) should be "all in and all out" with disinfection in between new shipments. They should have separate water and plumbing systems, individual cleaning equipment and nets, or disinfection between use if equipment must be shared. Footbaths at entryways and protective clothing should be available. Reseeding of beneficial bacteria for biofiltration should be done prior to subsequent use. Ultraviolet sterilizers on the filtration systems should be used, when possible, to destroy harmful bacteria, fungi, parasites, and pathogenic algae.

During the acclimatization process, fish should be handled only when necessary to reduce stress. To prevent anxiety, new fish can be placed adjacent to tanks containing dither fish. These are well-acclimatized, calm fish that help to reduce nervousness in the new arrivals that can observe them. Calm fish do not display flashing behavior, which can be indicative of a predator-prey response (Williams *et al.*, 2009).

25.10 Filtration

Multi-species exhibits containing fish, reptiles (Fig. 25.23), and birds can produce a large volume of waste. Adequate filtration, water flow, regular cleaning, and appropriate water changes are important in maintaining positive welfare for aquarium occupants. Coliform bacterial counts or total cell counts (TCC) for bacteria are also considerations for sustaining health and water quality.

Public aquariums produce large volumes of discharge water following tank maintenance and water changes. Local regulations must be followed regarding the recycling or disposal of wastewater. Wastewater may need to be disinfected prior to discharge in sewers or natural waterways.

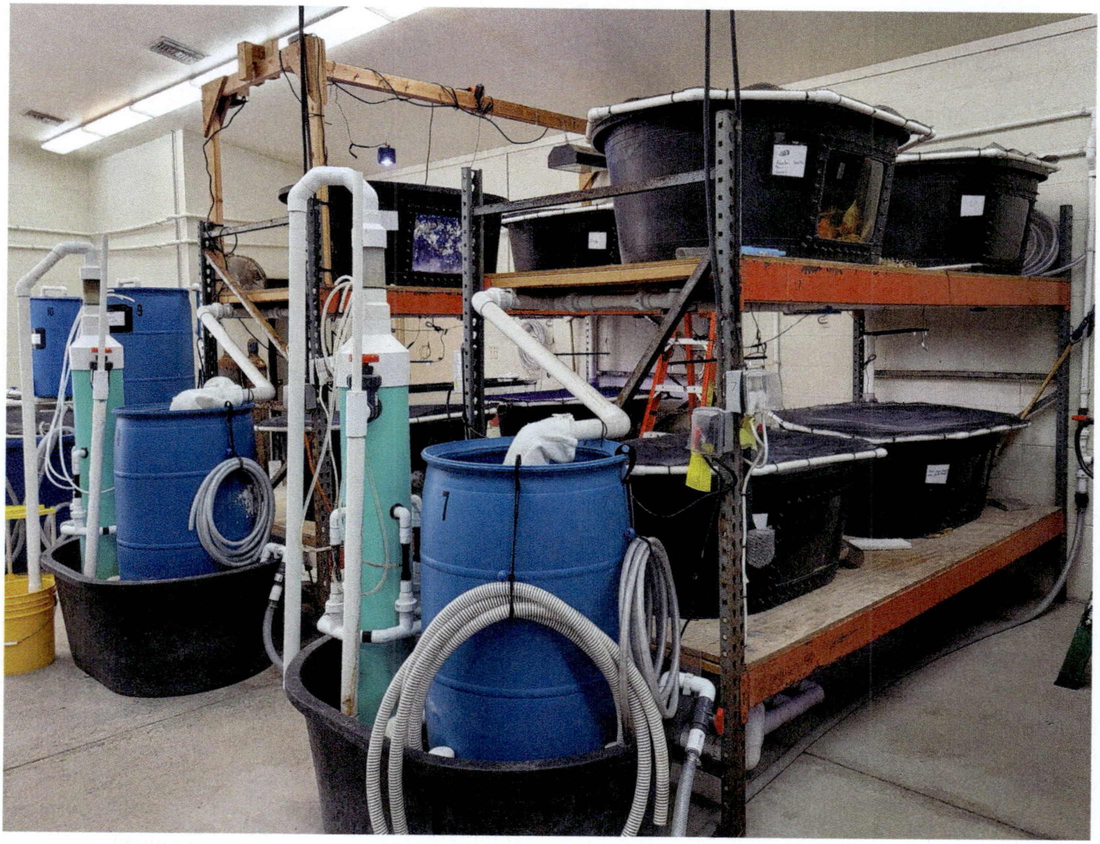

Fig. 25.22. Separate isolation tanks for fish quarantine or treatment. (Photograph by S. Johnson.)

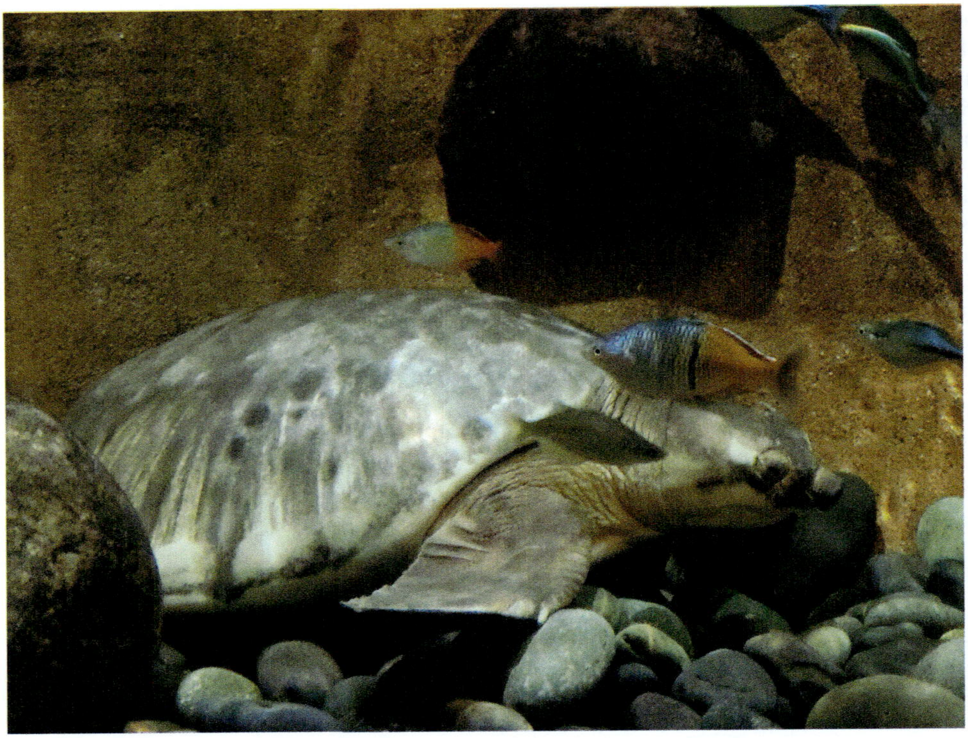

Fig. 25.23. A male fly river turtle (*Carettochelys insculpta*) housed with rainbow fish (*Melanotaenia boesemani*). (Photograph by S. Johnson.)

25.11 Environmental Enrichment

Discussions on fish welfare are not complete without the consideration of environmental enrichment. This concept is well integrated in zoological institutions and provides complexity to the environment for reducing abnormal behaviors in animals in captivity that may occur when kept in stimuli-deprived conditions. Maladaptation to captive life could manifest as psychological, physiological, morphological, or behavioral dysfunction leading to disturbances in health, reproduction, and survival (Näslund and Johnsson, 2016). Even though difficult to measure scientifically, there is a consensus that enrichment for a captive population of fish does improve its welfare (Williams *et al.*, 2009).

Historically, the first report of enrichment for fish was in 1919 when positive effects pertaining to improved health were observed in fish kept in troughs that were given substrate and sheltering sites (Robertson, 1936). The benefits of food and husbandry enrichment for captive animals were described in 1925 by Yerkes. Zoo design in the 1960s reflected a shift from cement floors and bars to exhibit designs based on the species' natural history and behavior. During this same time, forage behaviour-based research demonstrated that animals displayed more inquisitive and exploratory behavior and overall interest in their food if they had to work for it, versus being fed *ad libitum*. This suggested that the animals had a biological need to forage or hunt, and that deprivation of this natural behavior was a cause of stress or frustration (Mellan and Sevenich MacPhee, 2001).

In the past several decades, environmental enrichment programs have been defined by the natural history of a species and the exhibit. The goals of any enrichment program are to enhance animal welfare through psychological and physiological well-being, successful reproduction, and parental rearing of offspring; identify and reduce chronic stressors that can lead to poor health and promote the animals' ability to cope with acute stressors; reduce and eliminate aberrant behaviors; provide opportunities for expression of normal species-specific behaviors;

and lastly provide for successful reintroduction (Mellan and Sevenich MacPhee, 2001).

The purpose of enrichment for fish in a public aquarium is to promote and stimulate the natural behavior that would occur in a healthy wild fish. The natural behaviors exhibited by fish are foraging, reproduction, territorial (Figs 25.24a and b), and schooling. These behaviors can all be stimulated by changes within the natural environment.

Seasonal enrichment changes can be reproduced by varying light intensity, wavelength, and photoperiod. Adding or removing leaves on branches, tree roots, and logs and adding new rocks or shells and substrate can simulate the engorgement of a river during the monsoons. This creates the opportunity for a nursery and promotes exploration, foraging, and sheltering.

25.11.1 Structural complexity within an exhibit

Adding structural complexity to an aquatic environment provides physical enrichment for its occupants (See Table 25.1). Adding and varying objects and substrates within the aquarium is a means to achieve this. The primary goals of physical enrichment in the aquarium are to provide shelter from aggressive species or predatory fish (Fig. 25.25) and to allow fish to escape strong currents (Näslund and Johnsson, 2016). Studies have shown that the addition of shelters can reduce aggression and provide a refuge for subordinate animals. By supplying a visual barrier and by allowing dominant fish to become territorial over the added structure, the aggressiveness to other fish may be reduced.

By claiming the structure as its territory, aggressive fish are less likely to leave the structure undefended to pursue other animals. Aggression appears to be inversely proportional to the degree of complexity and number of added structures within the tank.

25.11.2 Types of environmental enrichment

Currently, there are five categories of environmental enrichment: physical, sensory, dietary, social, and occupational. By supplying environmental enrichment in an aquarium, the fish will be better suited to express the five freedoms of welfare that

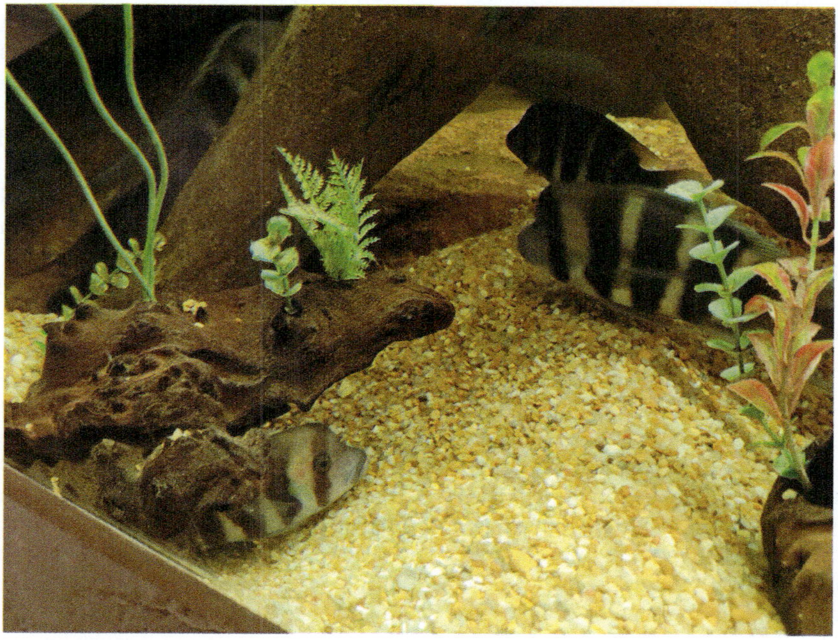

Fig. 25.24a. The left frontosa cichlid (*Cyphotilapia frontosa*) is defending a nest site that it has excavated in the substrate. (Photograph by S. Johnson.)

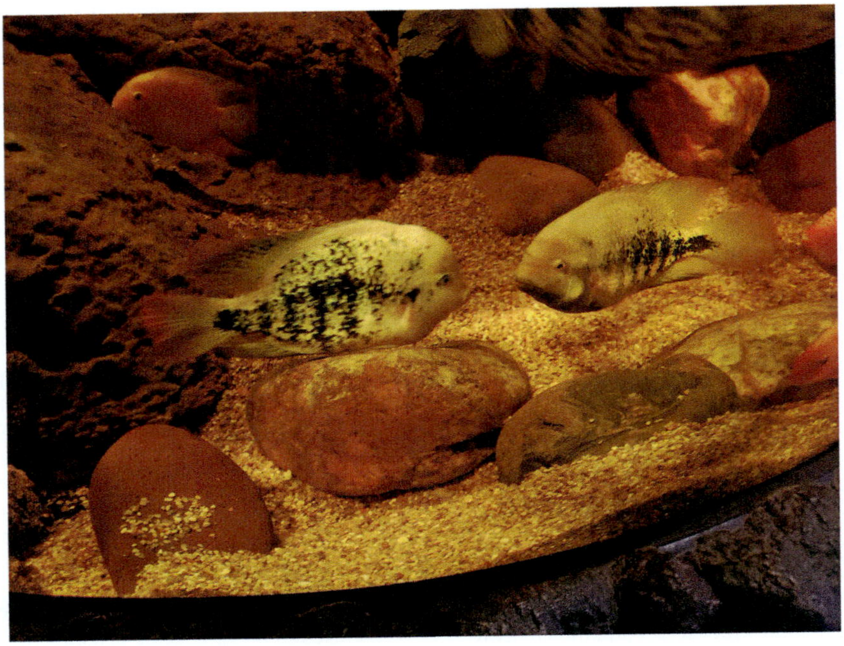

Fig. 25.24b. These male zebra mbuna (*Pseudotropheus zebra*) cichlids are sparring for territorial and breeding rights. (Photograph by S. Johnson.)

are used in designing programs for terrestrial animals in captivity. These components of good welfare include:

- Freedom from hunger and thirst
- Freedom from discomfort
- Freedom from pain, injury, or disease
- Freedom to express normal behavior
- Freedom from fear and distress

The integration of environmental enrichment into aquatic animal habitats will promote good husbandry practices including special attention to nutrition, housing, temperature, lighting, and water quality (Garcia, 2015).

25.11.3 Physical

Environmental enrichment through aquarium design should accommodate animal behavior so that the visitors observe real fish doing real things. The movement toward realistic natural habitats reflects the change in public attitude toward conservation, the environment, and the confinement of animals in general. The goal of the public aquarium is to educate people about the occupants and the environment from which they originate to promote conservation through appreciation and awareness. Allowing fish to be fish without preconceived misconception, bias, or by incorrectly assigning human-like traits is important in planning their aquariums. The goal of modern-day aquariums is to construct easy-to-manage exhibits that balance the needs of the fish with the space available while ensuring at least 90% visibility for the visitors. Maintaining the welfare of its occupants is ensured through careful consideration by the designers and staff. Exhibits are designed to be environmentally appropriate and provide the micro niche for the species displayed (Seidensticker and Doherty, 1996).

Furnishings and décor within the aquarium should be naturalistic and typical of the native environment for that species (Fig. 25.26a,b). If natural rockwork, logs, and plants are not available, they can be fabricated. These structures allow for social activity, breeding, and safety and serve as a potential nursery for fry (Maple and Perkins, 1996). Several fish species, including pike and zebrafish, reduce swimming activity with the addition of plants to the tank. This reduces stress through less energy expenditure. Artificial or natural vegetation has also reduced the startle response in some studies. The plants also

Table 25.1. Environmental enrichment options that can be used in a public or home aquarium, adapted from Williams *et al.* (2009), used with permission granted by Sage Publishing.

Enrichment	Potential advantages	Potential disadvantages
Substrate	• Additional biological filtration • Simulates the natural environment • Provides sites for spawning, territory claims • Nesting sites and foraging • Variety of sizes and colors offer choice	• Additional bio load on system • Additional maintenance • Media for parasite reproduction • Difficulty identifying decayed animals, plants, eggs, and fry • Can decrease available swimming space • Potential water chemistry alteration
Artificial rock, caves, and pipes	• Provides shelter • Available spawning site • Mark territorial sites and provides a static object to aid navigation • Provides an optical barrier	• Aggressive territorial behavior • May absorb test chemicals altering laboratory values • Entrapment/collapse hazard • Release of toxic chemicals • Obscure view of fish, delaying medical help if diseased or injured
Plants	• Provides shelter and spawning substrate • Easy to clean if plastic and contributes to natural look	• Entanglement risk • Can obscure view of fish, delaying medical treatment • Real plants can be a fomite for pathogens • Plastic plants could leach toxic substances • Broken or frayed pieces of artificial plants could be consumed by fish
Recirculation instead of flow-through	• Consistent water quality, slower rate of change in water chemistry parameters • Lower water usage • Can sterilize water before reuse • Easy to change water • Temperature regulation to induce spawning	• Requires more maintenance than flow-through systems • Can cause long-term stress associated with noise from filtration system • Diseased organisms and added medications can be difficult to remove • Nitrogenous waste must be diluted
Water movement	• A requirement for specific species and life stages • Pulsing flows and currents are more realistic	• High water usage if flow-through may be detrimental to some species and life stages • Additional noise and vibration may cause chronic stress • Increased pump maintenance
Artificial light	• Simulates natural light to species-specific levels • Defines night and day and gives fish the required cue by which to set diurnal and seasonal cycles physiologically and behaviorally • Day-length, dawn, dusk and moonlight phases are a cue for spawning in many species • Gradual increase and decrease may reduce startle response to lights turning on/off	• Can simulate perpetual long summer day-length if not coordinated properly with ambient lighting
Conspecifics	• Housing in groups of appropriate species • Appropriate stocking densities relevant to ontology • Appropriate stocking densities may reduce aggression • More natural and realistic • Reduce stress by providing security in numbers	• Species-specific aggression • Some group sizes of densely shoaling species may be too small to obtain benefit in even the largest systems • Group size may be inappropriate to species or life stage, or the scientific intention

Continued

Table 25.1. Continued.

Enrichment	Potential advantages	Potential disadvantages
Dither fish	• Small shoals of small species may be used as companions to large nervous species serving as sentinels • Multiple life stages of a single species may be important for social interaction and learning • Dither fish may be housed in adjacent aquariums in full view of the subject fish	• Risk of piscivory • Multi-species aquariums may complicate research for test conditions • Species combinations may not be regionally relevant increasing the risk of disease in naïve species • Intraspecies interactions may not be benign and behavioral and even chemical signals between the species may not have the intended result
Live food	• Active hunting/foraging instincts invoked • Variation in food target • Enriched live foods promote improved nutrition and chemosensory stimulus	• Pathogen introduction • Continuously varying the diet can reduce the overall feeding of some species that have evolved to specific prey types and, in some cases, limited size ranges • Not consumed naturally in herbivorous and some omnivorous diets
Fish–human interaction	• Training of fish to respond to the presence of a human can facilitate examination, diagnostic, and medical procedures • Familiarization with nets and equipment can reduce the stress for future events	• May not be desirable if the scientific intention is to observe a behavior • Reinforcement of a behavior with a food reward may not be desirable or safe

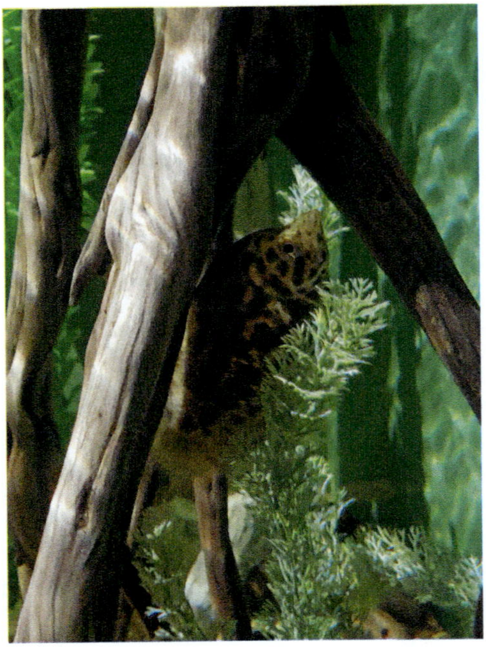

Fig. 25.25. This Leopard Ctenopoma (*Ctenopoma acutirostre*) is displaying natural behavior by mimicking a leaf under an artificial tree root. This site is defended by this fish and is used to ambush prey. (Photograph by S. Johnson.)

provide a biome for beneficial bacteria and algae to grow on, referred to as periphyton. These organisms serve as a food source and biological filter. Sugarcane and bamboo are commonly used for this (Näslund and Johnsson, 2016). Cichlids and cyprinids especially enjoy this type of enrichment (Gerber *et al.*, 2015).

25.11.4 Sensory

Providing substrate and complex furnishings to a tank increases the cognitive ability of fish through promotion of brain cell proliferation within the forebrain, as shown by proliferating nuclear cell antigen immunohistochemistry and an increase in neurogenic differentiation 1-a biomarker for neurogenesis. When Atlantic salmon were provided with environmental enrichment, their brain size increased; however, it decreased following removal of the stimulus. The importance of proper tank bottom substrate cannot be over-emphasized. Salmon and trout had less fin damage and displayed less aggression with substrate added into their aquarium, as opposed to those fish raised in a tank with a clear bottom. The substrate also provides shelter for bottom-dwelling species, foraging behavior, and security through camouflage. Skin lesions in Dover

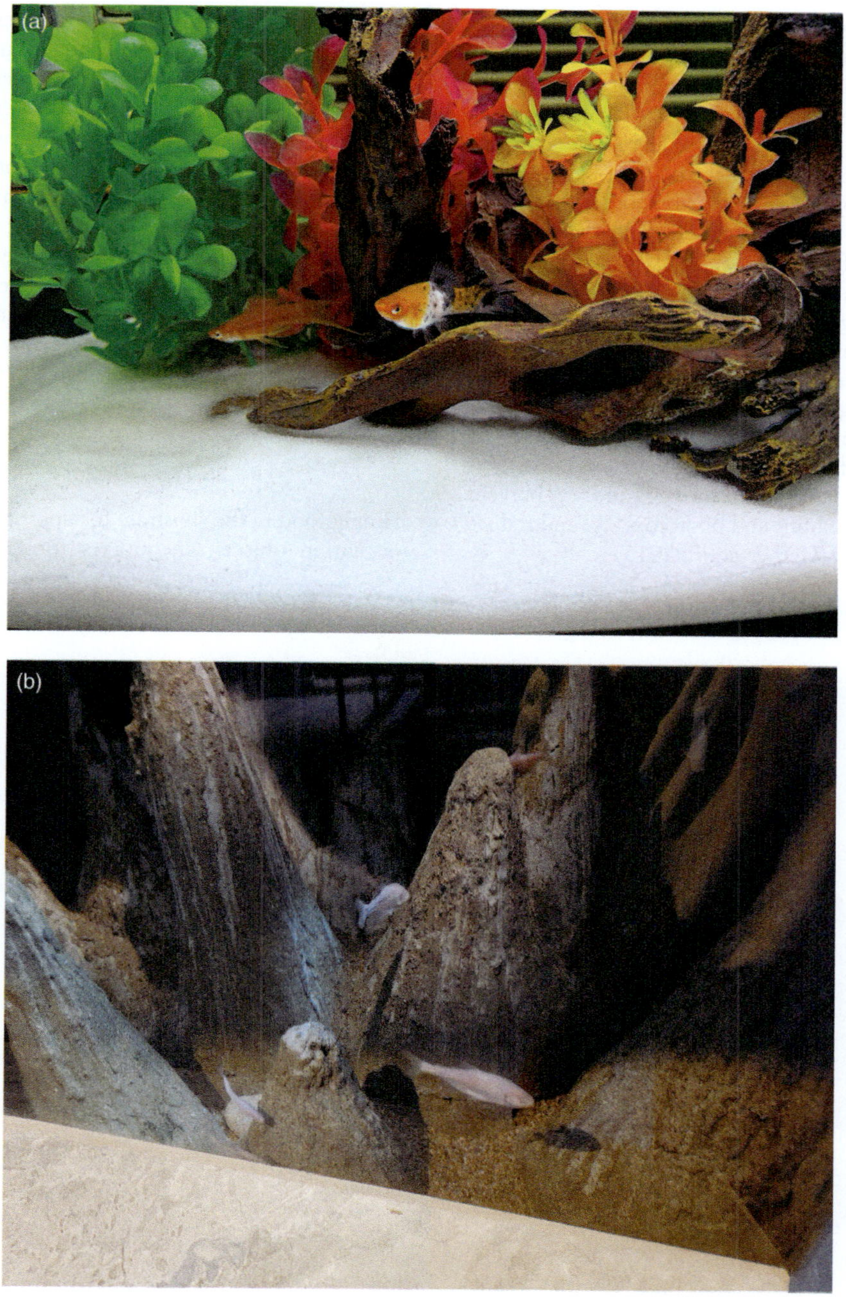

Fig. 25.26a,b. Artificial plants, logs, and rockwork in an aquarium create a realistic-looking environment. (Photographs by S. Johnson.)

sole (*Solea solea*) were eliminated when placed in a tank with a sand substrate. The natural exfoliative nature of the sand removed dead skin and associated bacteria within the devitalized tissue (Gerber *et al.*, 2015).

Studies have shown that catfish and salmon grow better in aquaculture settings if overhead covers are provided. Catfish are a nocturnal species that inhabit dark water environments. Decreasing light intensity through the addition of covers and dark tank colors has been shown to reduce cortisol levels. Salmon without shelter had a 30% increase in basal metabolic rate (BMR) compared with conspecifics with shelter. These fish also showed 2–3 times increase in basal cortisol levels. Some examples of covers are camouflage netting, baskets with small stones, floating objects (driftwood, plant leaves), branches (Fig. 25.27) or treetops submerged just below the surface of the water. Plastic containers with slits cut into them to allow water flow can be used as a refuge for fry. In outside exhibits, partial shelters are created by using boulders, artificial rockwork overhangs, trees, branches, and water turbulence (Fig. 25.28) with currents or sprinklers. A reduction in sunlight intensity can reduce the temperature of the water in summer months; prevent ultraviolet damage to the eggs and fry; prevent sunburn of dorsal fins and phototoxicity; and reduce oxidative stress (Gerber *et al.*, 2015).

Environmental enrichment provides fish with behavioral choices associated with changes in their environment. Reducing the stress from constant human interaction, either through tank maintenance in the service area or visitors on the public side, can be achieved through positive reinforcement via feeding strategies. Varying the type, amount, and administration times that coincide with public viewing can reduce the fear and anxiety associated with this. Keeping tanks at or slightly above eye level along with providing a solid backdrop on the non-public side provides a reduction in stress for the aquatic animals (Seidensticker and Doherty, 1996).

25.11.5 Dietary

Hiding food in the substrate for appropriate species, or within objects, encourages foraging, provides

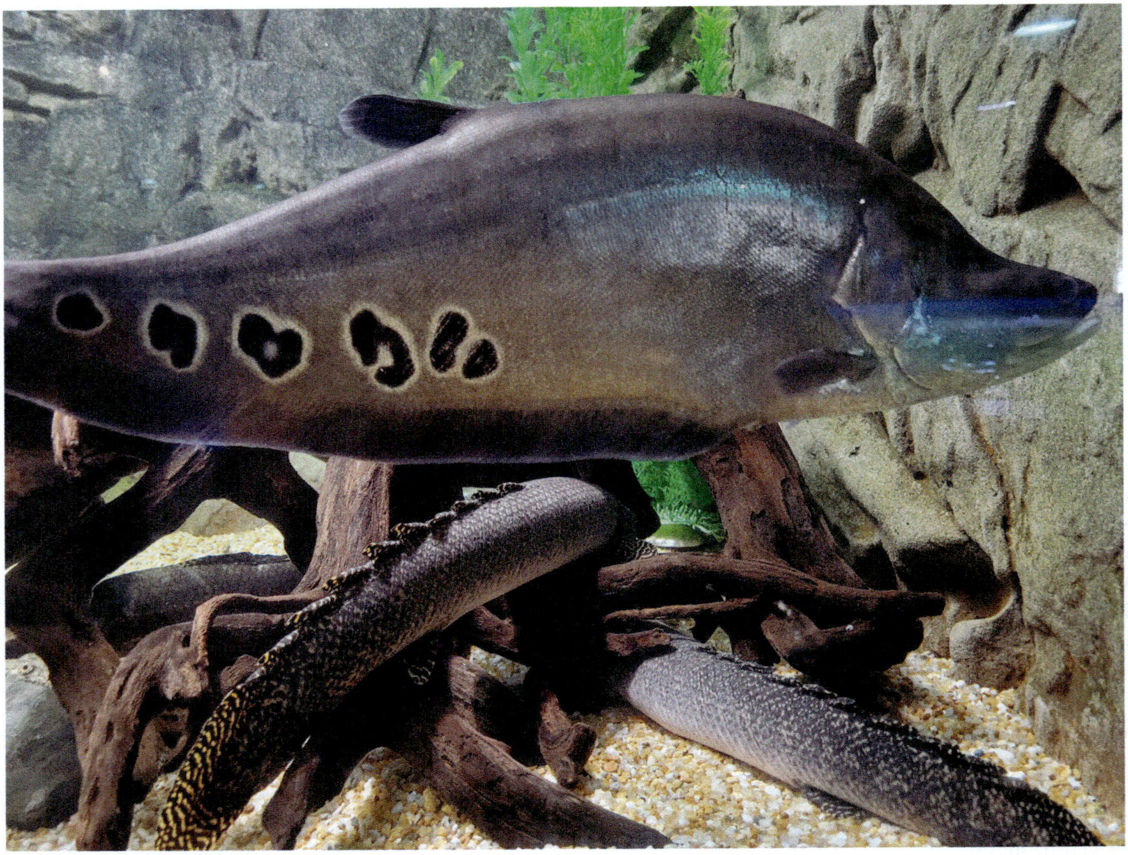

Fig. 25.27. The bichir (*Polypterus ornatipinnis*) hides from the clown knifefish (*Chitala ornata*) and blends with the color of the branches. These two species occupy different waters of the world. The fish coexist peacefully, but problems could arise from disease that is novel to each species. (Photograph by S. Johnson.)

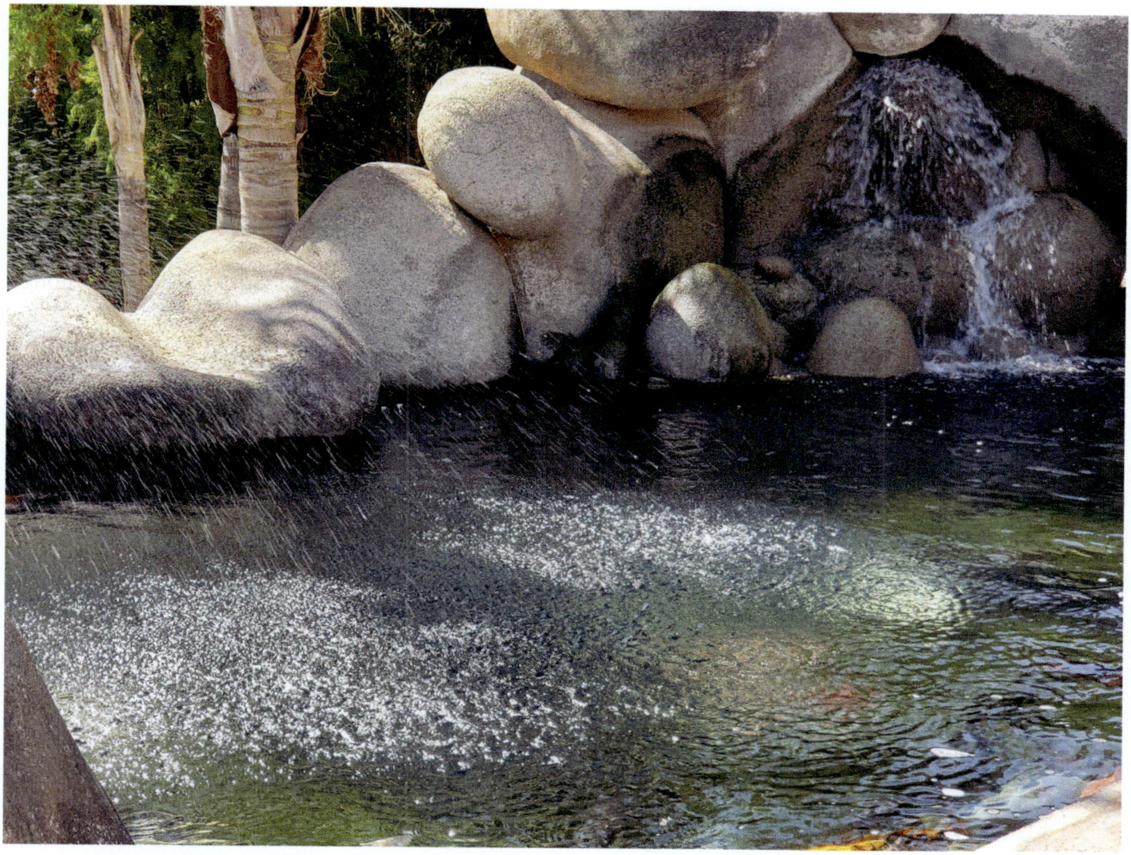

Fig. 25.28. A waterfall provides surface agitation, increasing gas exchange. The sprinkler also does this and reduces the water temperature. Artificial boulders form an overhang creating a niche for the fish that provides shade and security. (Photograph by S. Johnson.)

exercise, and improves cognitive ability through tactile stimulation. This is commonly done with marine invertebrates such as the octopus. Food is placed in sealed containers and the animal must open the container to receive the food reward. Algae are placed in plastic balls with slits cut into them for tangs and other grazers. Parrotfish are offered chalk blocks for wearing down their teeth, as are snail shells for pufferfish. Fruit, vegetables, insects, algae, and pieces of fish can be frozen in small ice cubes that require the fish to swim after and manipulate the cubes to get the food (Fig. 25.29a,b). Live insects and worms can be offered, which promotes hunting activity and valuable invertebrate-derived proteins, fats, and fatty acids. Care must be exercised when feeding live food due to an increased risk of parasitism. The source of the food should be thoroughly evaluated.

Manipulation of thawed, frozen food using submersible pumps to create a water current can give the impression of movement of the food, encouraging feeding behavior in difficult-to-feed species. This is commonly done with seahorses that are fed thawed mysis shrimp in a clear bowl at the bottom of the tank (Fig. 25.30). A current is passed over the bowl, causing the shrimp to move about, creating a feeding response in the sea horses. Using gentle water currents can also encourage newly acquired, submissive, or ill fish to eat.

When using any thawed food, particularly from frozen fish, appropriate vitamin supplementation with B vitamins, especially thiamine (vitamin B1), should be considered due to the potential presence of any thiaminases in the food. The addition of any structures to the tank used for enrichment must not interfere with water quality or foraging (Gerber *et al.*, 2015).

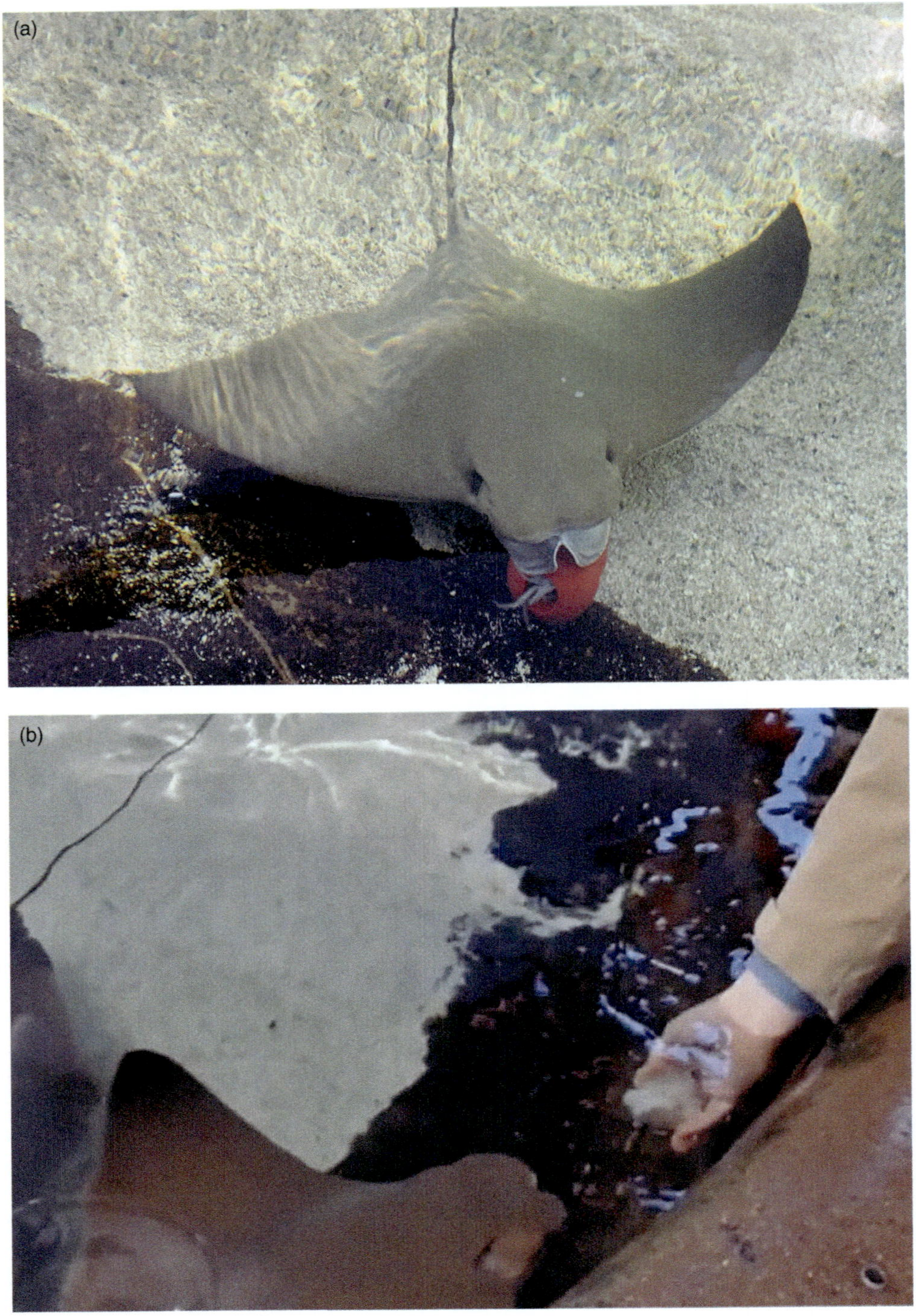

Fig. 25.29a,b. Cownose rays (*Rhinoptera bonasus*) being fed squid in a Kong brand dog chew toy and shrimp in an ice ball. (Photographs by N. Saint-Erne.)

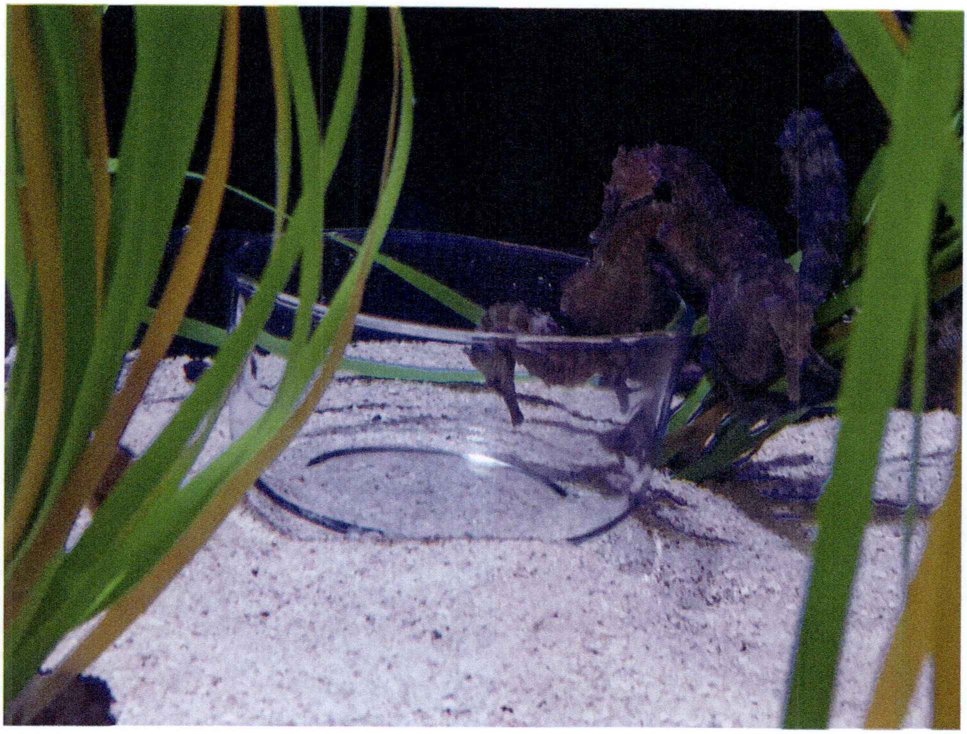

Fig. 25.30. Lined seahorses (*Hippocampus erectus*) are shown foraging frozen food in a glass bowl to illustrate a feeding technique that makes prepared food look alive. (Photograph by S. Johnson.)

25.11.6 Social

Social support through the formation of shoals (Figs 25.31a and b) encourages positive welfare by reducing stress due to protection from predators and enhancing foraging success and breeding opportunities (Galhardo and Oliveira, 2009). Creating a community or mixed-species exhibit displaying fish from the same natural habitat allows the fish to perform normal interspecies behaviors such as territory procurement and different foraging opportunities (AAZK, undated).

Choose species for display that are exhibitable. Gregarious fish that are very social possess a high holding attendance factor. This is defined as the amount of time that a visitor stops and looks at the aquarium. The fish should appear comfortable without evidence of stress and behave in a normal manner. This contrasts with displaying secretive, submissive fish that hide much of the time. This type of species would be one that would give the impression of negative welfare. If the aquarium deems it necessary to possess such species for conservation reasons, then the fish should be maintained off-exhibit.

Some fish are so aggressive or predatorial that they need to be housed singly or in same species groups only (Gerber *et al.*, 2015). Avoiding housing fish of different species with the same body shape or color pattern in the same aquarium helps to prevent aggression.

25.11.7 Occupational

Occupational enrichment serves to reduce physical and psychological monotony by introducing variation within the tank, exercise, and performance of preferred behaviors. Allowing fish to choose their options increases their control over the environment (Gerber *et al.*, 2015).

25.11.8 Negative impact of enrichment

Not all enrichment has a beneficial impact on fish. Choice of enrichment must take into careful consideration the species and life cycle influences.

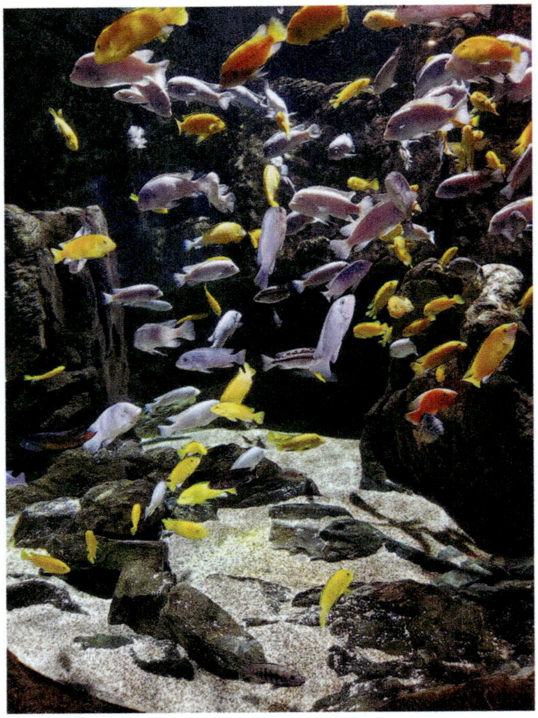

Fig. 25.31a. This variety of African cichlids provides a "Wow" factor due to the highly social nature and coloration variability of the fish. (Photograph by S. Johnson.)

An example of a negative enrichment involves the use of visual separation of pairs of flathead minnows (*Pimephales promelas*). When the males could observe one another, territorial behaviors were displayed. When the males were deprived of this, they turned their aggressive tendencies toward their mates, which led to trauma and death (Williams *et al.*, 2009).

25.12 Conclusions

Environmental enrichment promotes positive welfare by encouraging exploration, foraging behaviors, and exercise. Aquarists are encouraged to provide visual stimuli by changing the structures within an exhibit and seasonal and auditory stimuli through changes in light intensity simulating dawn, sunlight, dusk, moonlighting, cloud cover (Fig. 25.32), water currents, and sound (thunder and rain simulators). In this way, public aquariums take into consideration fish welfare and the aquatic sciences: "Showing the animals respect and care due to the species seems both the ethically correct and scientifically valid course of action" (Williams *et al.*, 2009).

Changes in diet promote growth and can be a stimulus for reproduction. Operant conditioning during feeding times and the predictability of feeding

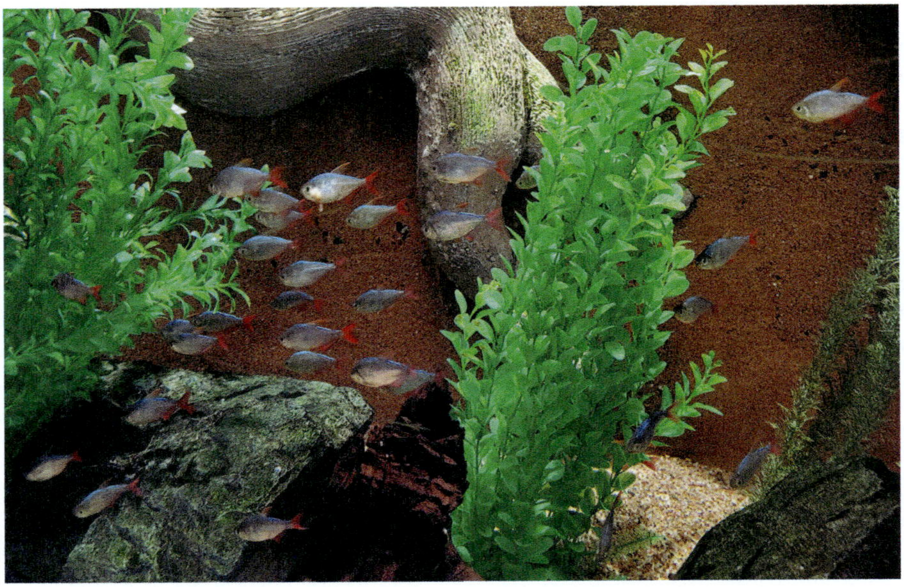

Fig. 25.31b. A school of Columbian tetras (*Hyphessobrycon columbianus*) are a species that peacefully coexist. (Photograph by S. Johnson.)

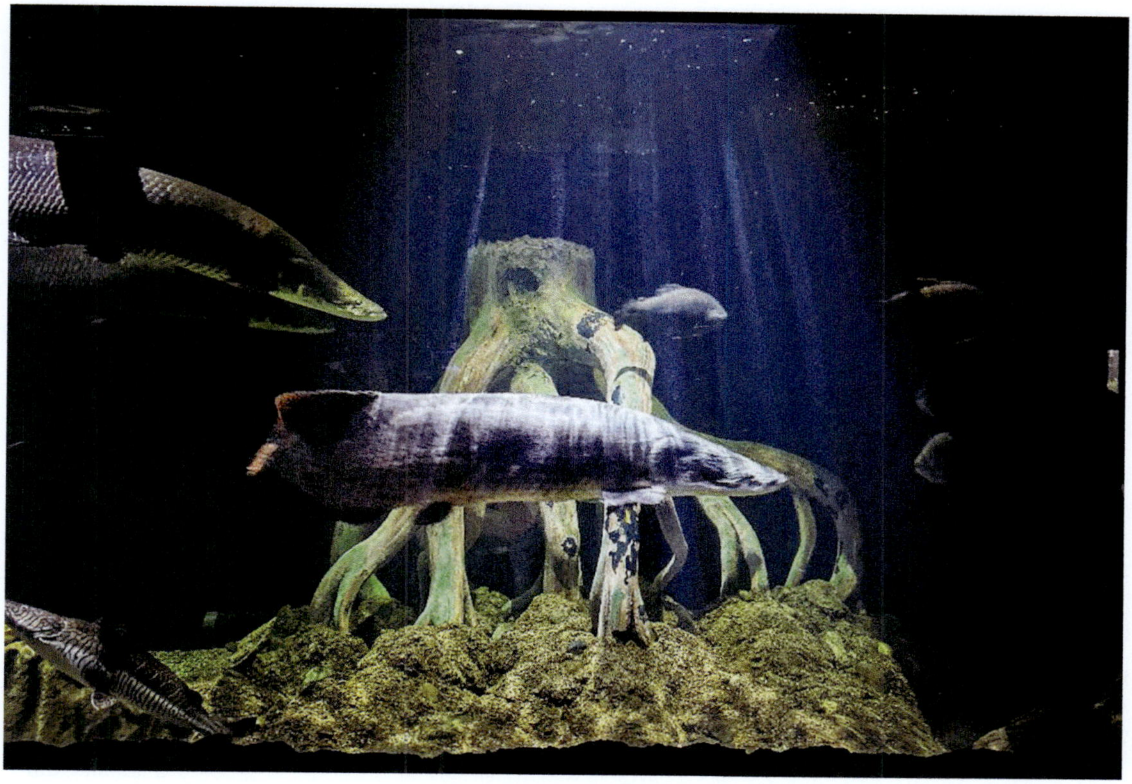

Fig. 25.32. Arapaima (*Arapaima gigas*) swims through artificial sun rays created by lighting. (Photograph by L. Fuentes.)

are also important in stress reduction. A food reward can coincide during times of stress such as public attendance and noise, and internal and external tank maintenance.

Public aquariums should be promoters of good welfare in the captive collection by encouraging behaviors through OWI and enrichment. Examples are positive feed response and attraction to the front of the tank through reward; and prevention of negative behaviors, such as aversion and hiding through elimination of acute or chronic stress. Prevention of tank-mate aggression, maintaining proper water quality, and promotion of an appropriate realistic natural exhibit for the species exhibited all promote good welfare.

Environmental enrichment can provide many beneficial effects for fish and aquatic invertebrates in a captive setting. Further research needs to be done to determine the proper type and amount of enrichment for a given species, and life cycle of that species, in order to not negatively impact growth, reproduction, and survival. Promoting species-specific behavior through enrichment, as observed in wild counterparts, allows fish to cope with captivity (Gerber *et al.*, 2015). Enrichment needs to be evaluated on a case-by-case basis. Not all enrichment is positive for fish welfare. In some instances, an increase in aggression is observed if too few furnishings are added. Too many furnishings lead to maintenance concerns through poor water quality associated with difficulty in proper cleaning, formation of anaerobic dead spots, and decreased swimming ability.

Welfare should always be evaluated in any circumstances where animals are captive. They are completely dependent on their human keepers and aquarists. Fish and aquatic invertebrates are complex, beautiful creatures and they deserve the absolute best care that we can offer. When we place them in a tank, we are obligated to them to know their natural history, preferred habitat, food, and feeding preferences. We must maintain a pristine environment free of contaminants and pollutants and provide a safe environment free from aggression. We must guard against outside influences that

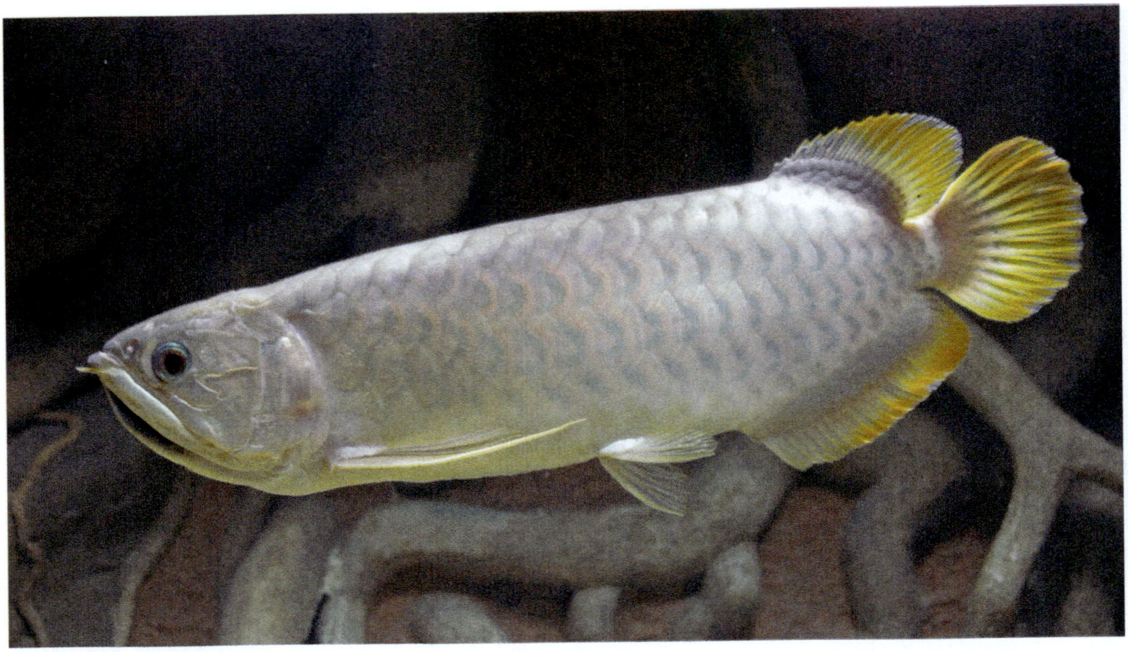

Fig. 25.33. Asian arowana (*Scleropages formosus*). Chinese fish keepers believe that the red and gold scales of the Asian arowana are reminiscent of coins, and the bearer of such a magnificent fish will be blessed with prosperity and good fortune. My good fortune is that a fish such as this is in my charge. My prosperity is measured by the company that I keep. (Photograph by S. Johnson.)

produce stress and potential disease. Further, we must promote education of our colleagues and aquarium visitors to ensure that these wonderful creatures do not pass quietly into the night and that their natural habitats are protected until the end of time. Lastly, remember the Golden Rule:

"Do unto others as you would have them do unto you" (Leviticus 19:18).

Acknowledgments

I would like to thank Jeff Beals, aquarium curator of Wildlife World Zoo & Aquarium, for his contribution to this chapter. I would also like to acknowledge Lorenzo Fuentes, senior aquarist, for photography and graphic interpretation. I am grateful to Warren Johnson, PhD, MD for illustrations and Cameron Johnson for information technology (IT). I am also grateful to Mickey Ollson, director of Wildlife World Zoo & Aquarium, his wife Connie, and their family for providing me the opportunity to be their veterinarian. Finally, I would like to thank Nick Saint-Erne, DVM, Martin Haulena, DVM, the aquarists and veterinary technical staff (Marie Dillon, BS, CVT) from Wildlife World Zoo & Aquarium for providing consulting services and back-up support, respectively. It is my good fortune to work with these people and with the wonderful animals, including fish (Fig. 25.33). And last but not least, thanks to Taz the red kangaroo for his patience while modeling!

References

AAVA (American Anti-Vivisection Society) (2020) Our history. Available at: https://aavs.org/about/our-history/ (accessed 13 June 2020).

AAZK (undated) Suggested guidelines for fishes enrichment. Available at: https://www.aazk.org/wp-content/uploads/Suggested-Guidelines-for-Fishes-Enrichment.pdf (accessed 7 June 2020).

AVMA (American Veterinary Medical Association) (2020) *Guidelines for the Euthanasia of Animals: 2020 Edition*. Available at: https://www.avma.org/sites/default/files/2020-02/Guidelines-on-Euthanasia-2020.pdf (accessed 3 March 2023).

BBC (2014) Introduction to animal rights. Available at: https://www.bbc.co.uk/ethics/animals/rights/introduction.shtml (accessed 19 July 2020).

Braithwaite, V.A. and Huntingford, F.A. (2004) Fish welfare: do fish have the capacity for pain perception and suffering? *Animal Welfare* 13, 587–592.

Browman, H.I., Cooke, S.J., Key, B., Rose, J.D., Derbyshire, S.W.G. *et al* (2019) Welfare of aquatic animals: where things are, where they are going, and what it means for research, aquaculture, recreational angling, and commercial fishing. *Journal of Marine Science* 76(1), 82–92.

Chatigny, F., Creighton, C.M. and Stevens, E.D. (2018) Updated review of fish analgesia. *Journal of the American Association for Laboratory Animal Science* 57(1), 5–12.

Corwin, A.L. (2012) Training fish and aquatic invertebrates for husbandry and medical behaviors. In: Heidenreich, B. (ed.) *Veterinary Clinics of North America: Exotic Animal Practice*. Elsevier, Philadelphia, Pennsylvania, pp. 455–467.

Davie, P.S. and Kopf, R.K. (2006) Physiology, behaviour and welfare of fish during recreational fishing and after release. *New Zealand Veterinary Journal* 54(4), 161–172.

Dey, V.K. (2016) The global trade in ornamental fish. Available at https://www.bassleer.com/ornamental fishexporters/wp-content/uploads/sites/3/2016/12/GLOBAL-TRADE-IN-ORNAMENTAL-FISH.pdf (accessed 15 May 2020).

FAO (2019) Welfare of fishes in aquaculture. Available at: https://www.researchgate.net/publication/335219925_Welfare_of_Fishes_in_Aquaculture (accessed 2 June 2020).

Galhardo, L. and Oliveira, R.F. (2009) Psychological stress and welfare in fish. *Annual Review of Biomedical Sciences* 11:1–20. Available at: https://www.researchgate.net/publication/282368816_Psychological_Stress_and_Welfare_in_Fish (accessed 6 July 2020).

Garcia, J.L. (2015) Helping fish flourish: environmental enrichment for aquatic species. Available at: https://www.dvm360.com/view/helping-fish-flourish-environ mental-enrichment-aquatic-species (accessed 6 July 2020).

Gerber, B., Stamer, A. and Stadtlander, T. (2015) Environmental enrichment and its effects on welfare in fish. Available at: https://www.researchgate.net/publication/285523279_Environmental_Enrichment_and_its_effects_on_Welfare_in_fish (accessed 2 June 2020).

Grier, K.C. (2008) Pets in America: a history. Available at: https://en.wikipedia.org/wiki/Aquarium#History_and_popularization (accessed 11 May 2020).

Håstein, T., Scarfe A.D. and Lund, V.L. (2005) Science-based assessment of welfare: aquatic Animals. *Revue Scientifique et Technique-Office des Epizooties* 24(2), 529–547.

Hibbitt, J.D., Rees, E. and Brown, C. (2017) Black-tip reef shark reproduction and neonate survivorship in public aquariums. In: Smith, M., Waqrmolts, D., Thoney, D., Hueter, R., Murray, M. and Ezcurra, J. (eds) *Elasmobranch Husbandry Manual II: Recent Advances in the Care of Sharks, Rays and their Relatives*. Ohio Biological Survey, Columbus, Ohio, pp. 443–450.

History of fishkeeping (undated) Available at: www.goldfish-as-pets.com/history_of_fishkeeping.html (accessed 11 May 2020).

Huntingford, F.A., Adams, C., Braithwaite, V.A., Kadri, S., Pottinger, T.G. *et al.* (2006) Current issues in fish welfare. *Journal of Fish Biology* 68, 332–372.

Johansen, R., Needham, J.R., Colquhoun, D.J., Poppe, T.T. and Smith, A.J. (2006) Guidelines for health and welfare monitoring of fish used in research. *Laboratory Animals* 40, 323–340.

Maple, T.L. and Perkins, L.A. (1996) Enclosure furnishings and structural environmental enrichment. In: Kleiman, D.G., Allen, M.E., Thompson, K.V., Lumpkin, S. and Harris, H. (eds) *Wild Mammals in Captivity, Principles and Techniques*. University of Chicago Press, Chicago, Illinois, pp. 212–222.

Martins, C.I.M., Galhardo, L., Noble, C., Damsgård, B., Spedicato, M.T. *et al.* (2012) Behavioural indicators of welfare in farmed fish. *Fish Physiology and Biochemistry* 38(1), 17–41.

Mather, J.A. (2019) Ethics and care: for animals, not just mammals. *Animals* 9(12): 1018. doi:10.3390/ani9121018.

McDaniel, J. (2018) The return of Kū'ula restoration of Hawaiian fishponds. Available at: https://seagrant.soest.hawaii.edu/the-return-of-kuula/ (accessed 15 July 2020).

Mellan, J. and Sevenich MacPhee, M. (2001) Philosophy of environmental enrichment: past, present, and future. In: Krebs, B.L. (ed.) *Zoo Biology*. Wiley-Liss, Hoboken, New Jersey, pp. 211–226.

Merriam-Webster Online (2007) Definition of aquarium. Available at: http://www.m-w.com/dictionary/aquarium (accessed 11 May 2020).

Näslund, J. and Johnsson, J. (2016) Environmental enrichment for fish in captive environments: effects of physical structures and substrates. *Fish and Fisheries* 17, 1–30.

Robertson, A. (1936) Hatching fry in gravel (No. 2). *American Fisheries Society* 3(23), 146–156. doi:10.1577/1548-8640(1936)323[19:HFIGNJ2.0.Co;2.

Ross, L.G. and Ross, B. (2008) *Anaesthetic and Sedative Techniques for Aquatic Animals*. 3rd edn. Blackwell, Oxford.

Seidensticker, J. and Doherty, J.G. (1996) Integrating animal behaviour and exhibit design. In: Kleiman, D.G., Allen, M.E., Thompson, K.V., Lumpkin, S. and Harris, H. (eds) *Wild Mammals in Captivity, Principles and Techniques*. University of Chicago Press, Chicago, Illinois, pp. 180–190.

Sneddon, L. (2002) Anatomical and electrophysiological analysis of the trigeminal nerve in a teleost fish, *Oncorhynchus mykiss*. *Neuroscience Letters* 319(3), 167–171.

Sneddon, L. (2003) Trigeminal somatosensory innervation of the head of a teleost fish with particular reference to nociception. *The Humane Society Institute for*

Science and Policy 972(1–2), 44–52. doi:10.1016/S0006-8993(3)02483-1.

Veinante, P., Yalcin, I. and Barrot, M. (2013) The amygdala between sensation and affect: a role in pain. *Journal of Molecular Psychiatry* 1(1): 9. doi:10.1186/2049-9256-1-9.

Volpato, G.L. (2009) Challenges in assessing fish welfare. *Institute for Laboratory Animal Research* 50(4), 329–337.

Wahltinez, S.J., Harms, C.A., Lewbart, G.A., Stacy, N.I. and Nunmaker, E. A. (2020) Animal welfare in aquatic invertebrates: current status and the role of veterinarians in advancing welfare efforts. In: *Proceedings of the International Association of Aquatic Animal Medicine (IAAAM)*. IAAAM, Tampa, Florida.

Walster, C., Rasidi, E., Saint-Erne, N. and Loh, R. (2015) The welfare of ornamental fish in the home aquarium. *Companion Animal* 20(5), 302–306.

Wikipedia (2020) *Ancient Hawaiian Aquaculture*. Available at: https://en.wikipedia.org/wiki/Ancient_Hawaiian_aquaculture (accessed 15 July 2020).

Williams, T.D., Readman, G.D. and Owen, S.F. (2009) Key issues concerning environmental enrichment for laboratory-held fish species. *Laboratory Animals* 43(2), 107–120.

Wrenn, C.L. (2012) Applying social movement theory to nonhuman rights mobilization and the importance of faction hierarchies. *The Peace Studies Journal* 5(3), 27–44.

26 Quarantine Protocol

AZUREEN ERDMAN

New River, Arizona

Abstract

A fundamental precept in maintaining healthy fish is to quarantine new species on arrival and not mix them with other fish until they are designated as healthy. Proper isolation, disease diagnosis, and treatments are necessary to ensure healthy fish at the end of a quarantine period. Appropriate handling, isolation, and treatment procedures should be used during the quarantine period.

26.1 Quarantine Procedures

The period to hold fish in quarantine depends on the results of observation and testing performed on intake and throughout the quarantine period. It is recommended that the fish undergo quarantine for a minimum of 2–4 weeks. During this time, they are examined, tested, and appropriately treated (Hadfield and Clayton, 2011). After completing treatment, the fish should be retested and examined again. If a pathogen or infectious disease is detected after the initial treatment, the fish will require further treatment and retesting. If the disease is of a serious and/or untreatable nature, destruction of all infected aquatic animals within that tank and any with exposure in the facility should be considered. Complete disinfection of the building, water, and all equipment will need to be performed before restocking (Arthur *et al.*, 2008).

The quarantine facility should comply with the following specific construction and equipment requirements (OATA, 2023):

1. Windows should be screened to prevent the entry of insects and pests.
2. Floor and walls should be constructed of concrete, tiles, or other impervious material to enable hose down and disinfection. The floor should be smooth and of sufficient grade to drain to an enclosed holding tank.
3. Floor-to-wall junctions and all gaps and cracks in the walls, floor, and ceiling should be effectively sealed so that the quarantine area can contain all leaks and floods that might occur.
4. Lighting should be of sufficient intensity to allow proper inspection of all aquatic animals.
5. Floor drainage with an insertable plug or other mechanism to prevent the accidental escape of aquatic animals or uncontrolled release of water should be installed. Drainage should be to an approved holding tank. The holding tank should be of a suitable size to contain the total volume of all tanks used for the holding of aquatic animals.
6. Doors should be equipped with self-closing mechanisms to ensure that they remain shut after entry, or there should be a self-closing insect-proof screen door installed.
7. The quarantine facility should provide facilities for staff to wash their hands and change outer clothing prior to entering or leaving the quarantine area.
8. There should be an area just outside the entrance for dedicated footwear along with a set of slip-resistant waterproof boots in a variety of sizes. Individuals should wear this footwear only within the quarantine facility. Slip-resistant rubber shoe covers should be maintained in this area for visitors who do not wish to change from their street shoes (Fig. 26.1).
9. A footbath containing disinfectant (hypochlorite, potassium permanganate, Betadine®, or another approved disinfectant) should be placed at the entrance door of the quarantine facility (Fig. 26.2). The foot bath solution should be routinely replenished for

Corresponding author: az.erdman@gmail.com

© CAB International 2025. *The Handbook of Ornamental Fish Health and Welfare* (ed. N. Saint-Erne)
DOI: 10.1079/9781789246032.0026

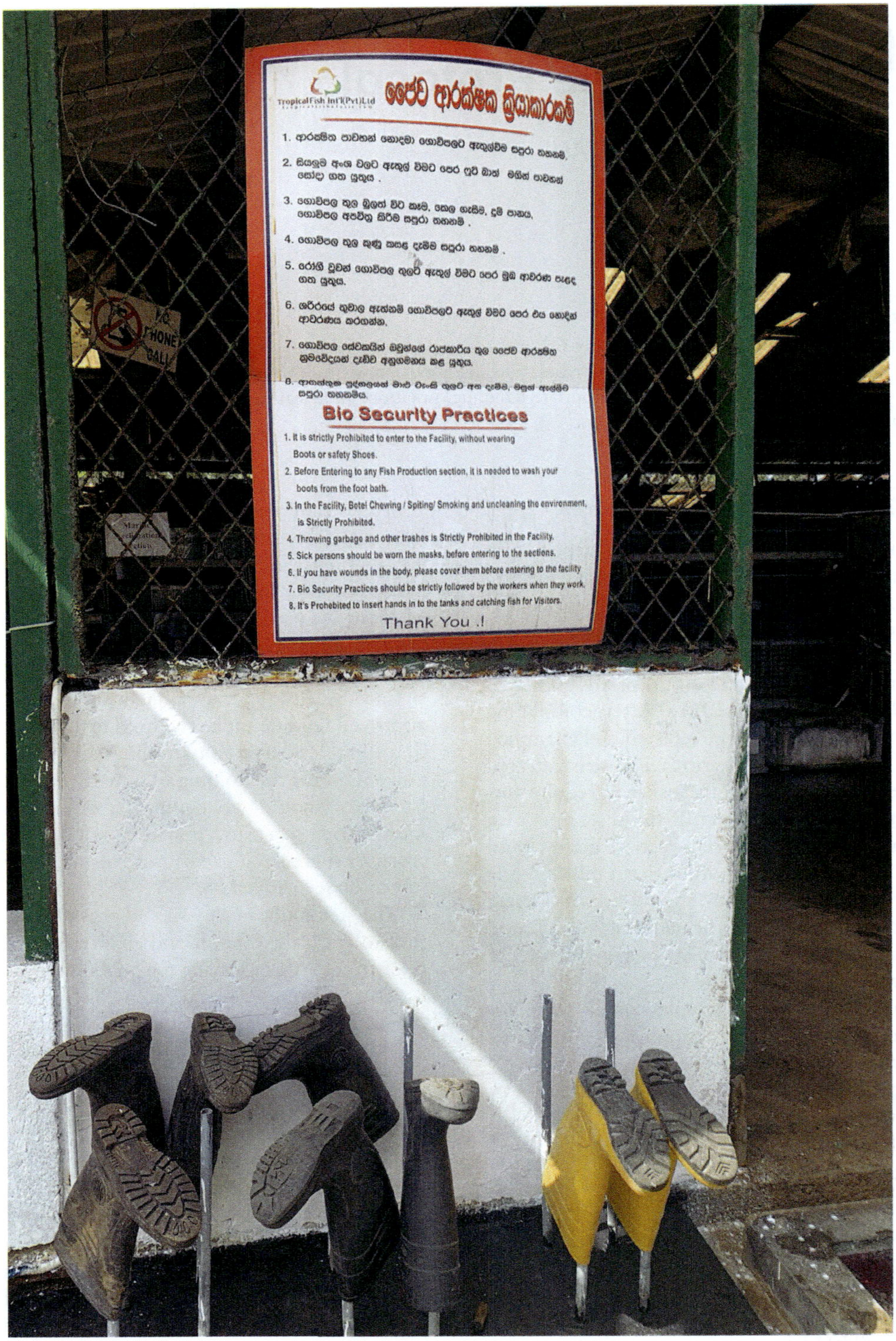
Bio Security Practices
1. It is strictly Prohibited to enter to the Facility, without wearing Boots or safety Shoes.
2. Before Entering to any Fish Production section, it is needed to wash your boots from the foot bath.
3. In the Facility, Betel Chewing / Spiting/ Smoking and uncleaning the environment, is Strictly Prohibited.
4. Throwing garbage and other trashes is Strictly Prohibited in the Facility.
5. Sick persons should be worn the masks, before entering to the sections.
6. If you have wounds in the body, please cover them before entering to the facility
7. Bio Security Practices should be strictly followed by the workers when they work.
8. It's Prohebited to insert hands in to the tanks and catching fish for Visitors.
Thank You .!

Fig. 26.1. Boots, stored next to the foot bath, to be worn on entering the fish farm in Sri Lanka. (Photograph by N. Saint-Erne.)

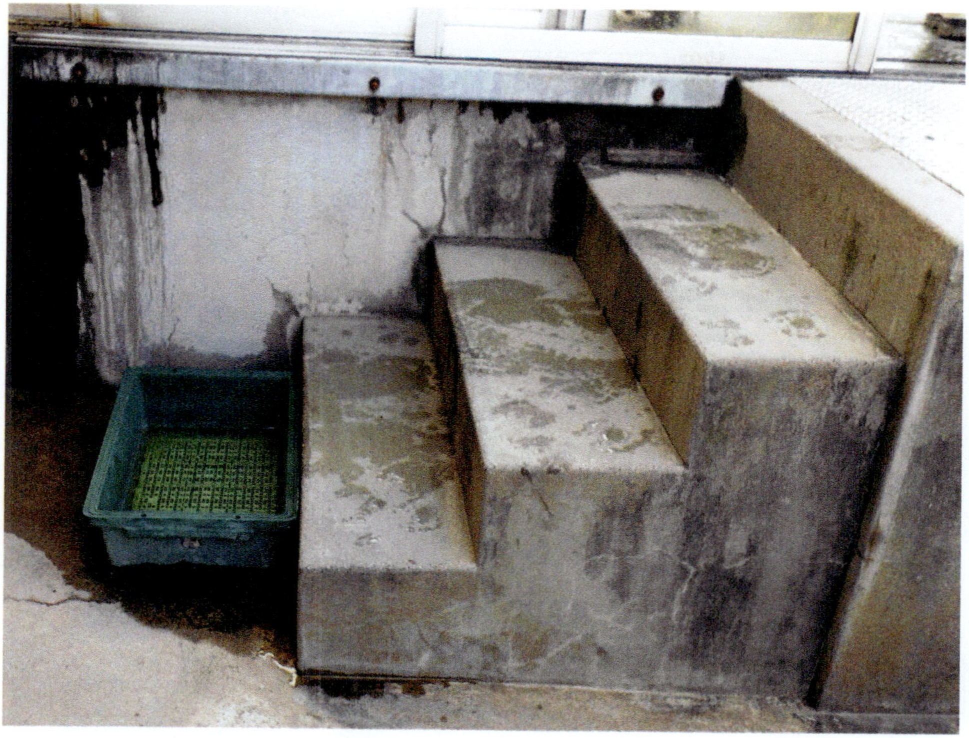

Fig. 26.2. Footbath at a Japanese Koi Farm. (Photograph by N. Saint-Erne.)

adequate disinfection. A sign stating "Footwear must be Immersed in Footbath on Exit/Entry from Quarantine Area" should be appropriately displayed. Only the provided isolation boots and shoe covers should be used to cross through this foot bath (Rashid *et al.*, 2016). Buckets of disinfectant with scrub brushes should be provided at the exit. Upon leaving the quarantine facility, all dedicated footwear should be scrubbed to remove organic debris prior to entering the foot baths (Steneroden, 2012).

10. Lockers and hangers should be provided for protective clothing. Multiple sizes and styles of protective coats or coveralls should be provided with a changing area for those when indicated. This clothing is restricted for use within the quarantine area and should be laundered separately from other laundry within the facility.

11. All holding tanks for aquatic animals should:

- be identified with permanent numbers so that individual tank records can be correlated to them;
- be fitted with lids or other approved coverings to prevent transmission of pathogens between adjacent tanks due to splash from the aeration/filter system, and to prevent the escape of aquatic animals (Fig. 26.3);
- have water intake lines equipped with automatic shut-off valves;
- be arranged in a manner that permits ready access for inspection purposes; and
- have their own set of labeled nets, buckets, and other items associated with the tank (OATA, 2023).

12. All aquatic animals within the facility should be considered to have the same quarantine status. The use of a shared water recirculation system is permissible but not advisable, as it may facilitate the spread of pathogens between tanks.

13. All entry and exit points to the quarantine facility should prominently display a permanently affixed quarantine sign (Fig. 26.4) that states "Quarantine Area–Authorized Personnel Only."

14. A suitable sink should be present for the cleaning and disinfecting of equipment. An approved disinfectant should be available at the sink. A suitable draining rack should be provided for air drying of equipment.

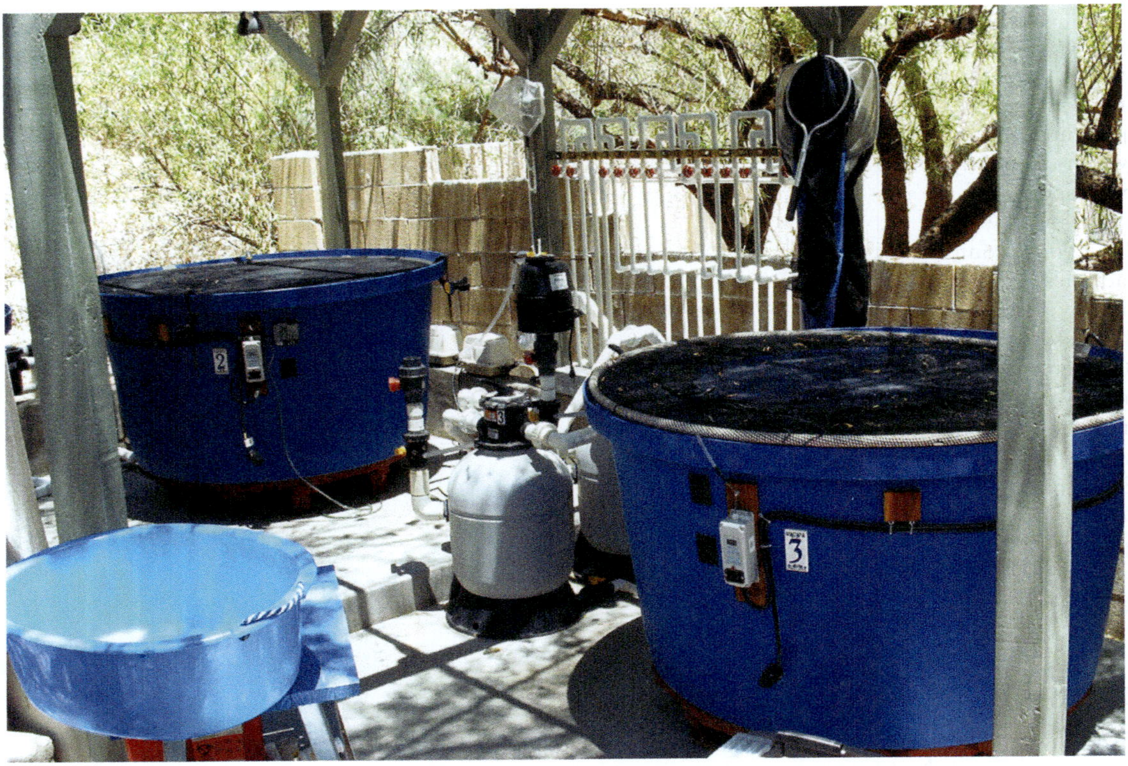

Fig. 26.3. Quarantine tanks with individual filtration, cover netting, and a shade cloth over the top is being used for quarantine of new koi fish by a home pond keeper. (Photograph by N. Saint-Erne.)

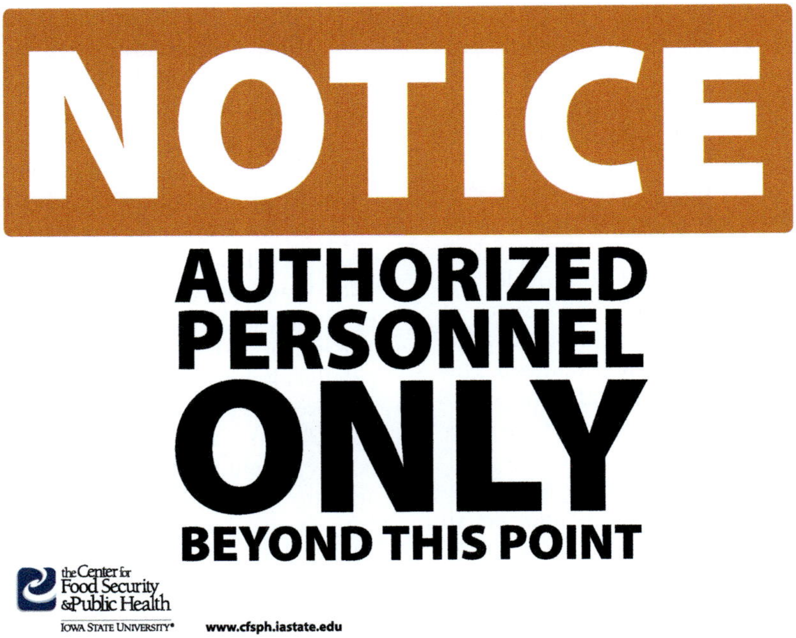
NOTICE
AUTHORIZED
PERSONNEL
ONLY
BEYOND THIS POINT
the Center for Food Security &Public Health
IOWA STATE UNIVERSITY®
www.cfsph.iastate.edu

Fig. 26.4. Quarantine Area Signage. (The Center for Food Security and Public Health.)

15. A designated refrigerator or freezer should be provided solely for the storage and preservation of dead aquatic animals. The refrigerator or freezer should be clearly identified for animal and quarantine use only, be lockable, and be located within the quarantine area. Dead animals should be disposed of in a proper manner following applicable laws.
16. Food should be stored in secure storage facilities preventing contamination or infestation by pests.
17. Before removal from the quarantine area and before any restocking, all tanks and equipment must be thoroughly cleaned and disinfected with hypochlorite solution (HClO) at 200 mg/l concentration for at least 5 min. Equipment or other material should not be removed from the quarantine area during the quarantine period.
18. All nets and other equipment should be regularly disinfected by an approved method.

26.2 Record Keeping

A logbook for quarantined animals should be created, either on paper or computerized (Fig. 26.5). A complete history of the aquatic animals being contained in the quarantine area should contain the following information:

- supplier, country of origin, and waybill
- date of arrival of stock
- total number of animals in original shipment(s) and total mortalities in each shipment upon arrival
- original number of animals stocked in each tank
- details of any clinical signs of disease and number of affected individuals, by tank
- details of any mortalities, by tank
- details of any health certificates
- details of any diagnostic tests and examinations
- details of treatments and testing occurring while in quarantine
- date(s) of release from quarantine

Freshwater Teleost Quarantine Schedule Erdman, 2020

Fish species: ____ number of individuals: ____ tank location: ____ stocking density: ____

identification: ____ source: ____ tank volume: ____ cautions: ____

Day	1	2	3	4	5	6	7	8	9	10	11	12	13	14	15	16	17	18	19	20	21	22	23	24	25	26	27	28	29	30	31	32	33	34	35	36	37	38	39	40	41	42	43	44
Date																																												
Treatments																																												
Salt water dip																																												
Praziquantel																																												
Metronidazole																																												
Fenbendazole																																												
Formalin																																												
Testing																																												
Physical exam																																												
Fecal exam																																												
skin scrape																																												
fin clipping																																												
gill biopsy																																												
General care																																												
Temperature																																												
H_2O change (%)																																												
Water testing																																												
Staff initials																																												

Notes (behavior changes, appetite changes, observations, carbon filter added/removed, testing results, etc.):

Fig. 26.5. Quarantine Log used for record keeping. (Spreadsheet created by Azureen Erdman.)

26.3 Quarantine Protocol for Aquatic Species

Access to quarantine areas should be controlled to prevent unauthorized staff and visitors from entering the biosecure area (WOAH Aquatic Animals Commission, 2024). Designate staff to handle newly arrived species. By limiting the number of people caring for quarantined species, a facility can ensure better continuity of care while allowing more accurate comparative observations throughout the quarantine period. These individuals should have limited or no access to other exhibits while working in quarantine. If limited access is not possible with smaller working teams, individuals dedicated to quarantine should support with cleaning and caring for assumed healthy exhibits before moving into quarantine. Once having entered quarantine, individuals should not enter back into general population without fully showering and changing their clothing.

Quarantine tanks should be housed in a separate room away from other animals and exhibits. To ensure proper disinfection, quarantine tanks should contain minimal gravel and hiding structures. The barer the tank, the easier it is to clean, while also allowing good visualization of changes in behavior or active lesions. However, it should be noted that many diseases become pathogenic when physiologic stress is placed on an individual and therefore efforts should be made to mitigate stressful situations while offering the ability to manage disease (Boerman *et al.*, 2006). Offering some tank "furniture" can help certain species acclimatize. Hiding areas need to be provided for welfare and security and to allow for normal behavioral activity. Hides should be smooth and not porous and must be easy to remove and scrub to disinfect between tank uses. Materials like PVC tubes make good hides that are easy to clean between uses (Fig. 26.6).

When possible, as addressed above, tanks should each have a separate life support system. If this is not possible, filtration units with both mechanical filters and UV lights could be installed between tanks to decrease pathogen load and to prevent spreading of pathogens throughout the entire facility. Tanks should be far enough apart to prevent cross-contamination by water splashing. If this is not possible, tanks should have a solid cover that

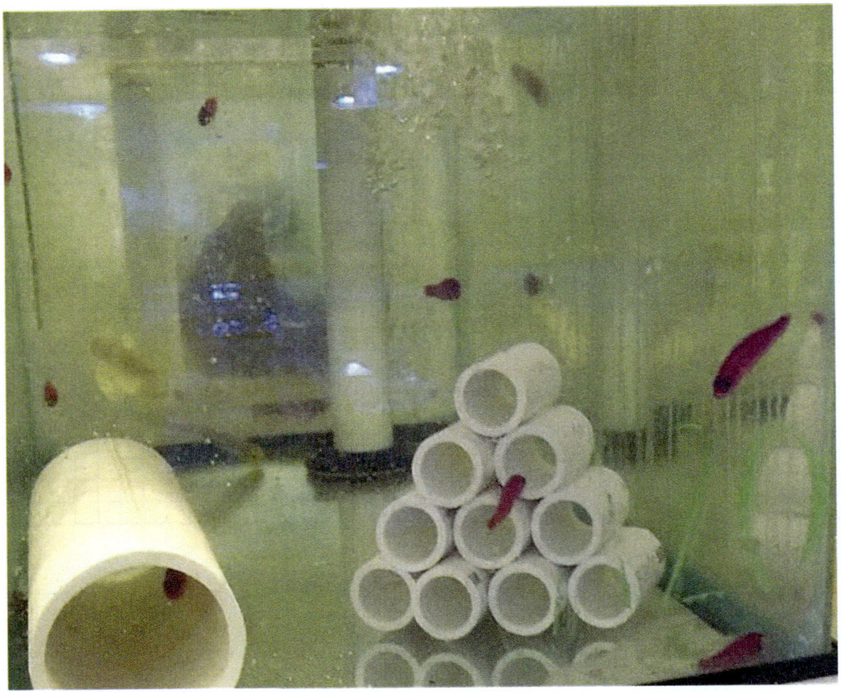

Fig. 26.6. Polyvinyl chloride (PVC) plastic tubes used for shelter in a quarantine aquarium. (Photograph by N. Saint-Erne.)

can be disinfected before removal with every handling. To reduce stress, there should be the capacity for lights to be turned off or dimmed for 12–24 h after arrival to allow the fish to rest.

The quarantine length will be dependent on the species involved, facility setup, staffing, and ability to transport a healthy animal to its future housing. Quarantine is generally 2–4 weeks in length but will be longer with sensitive species or species with active disease present upon arrival. Each tank is considered its own system and any new animals added to a tank will reset the quarantine timing and testing back to day one.

During the quarantine period, daily observations need to be made with all individuals. Notes and records should state behavior and physical changes. Appetite needs to be notated. Diagnostic and water quality testing should routinely be performed. Once the fish arrive, they should be allowed 3–4 days to acclimatize and rest prior to any further handling and stress. If there are losses within this timeframe, testing of any moribund fish can occur to facilitate treatment and minimize further losses. Water quality testing should be performed every 2–3 days for the first 2 weeks. After the initial 2 weeks, testing should occur weekly, or sooner if there is concern for the water quality. There should be a detailed log containing water temperature and water test results within the medical record.

After the initial 3 days of rest, a physical examination and diagnostic tests should be performed. Testing for large teleost and elasmobranch species should be performed on each individual. Testing for small teleost and invertebrates should be performed on a representative 5–10% subset of the population. The following testing is recommended and should be repeated at the recommended intervals listed below:

- Visual examination with behavior observation only should be performed daily
- Physical examination and diagnostic testing should occur three days after arrival with recheck physical exams as needed during the quarantine and then a final recheck exam at the end of the quarantine. Routine exam and diagnostics include:
  - Assessing body condition score (BCS) to determine if they are underweight, normal, or overweight
  - Note any wounds or lesions
  - Skin scrape biopsy—during initial physical exam and prior to transfer to display tank (Campbell, 2015)
  - Gill filament biopsy—during initial physical exam and prior to transfer to display tank (Reavill and Roberts, 2007)
  - Fin edge biopsy—during initial physical exam and prior to transfer to display tank
- Fecal examination—during initial physical exam, after treatments given for internal parasites, and prior to transfer to display tank
- Blood tests—if needed, as this is not routinely done and is very species dependent (Zang *et al.*, 2013; Campbell, 2015)
- Necropsy all mortalities—in the case of a high mortality event, a subset of individuals (10% of the deaths) can be necropsied
- Perform histopathology in cases with unknown cause of death or with large population losses (Wolf *et al.*, 2014)

26.4 Treatment Protocols for Specific Fish Groups

Treatment is based on diagnostic results and observations. When performing medicated water treatments, remember to remove the carbon from the filter system. It may be necessary to turn off UV lights and ozone during water treatment (Thomas *et al.*, 2016) to prevent breakdown of the added medications. The following is a list of aquatic species groups, and some regularly performed quarantine treatments, along with notes and recommendations on how to perform these treatments (Carpenter and Marion, 2018; Hedley, 2020). Every facility will have to manage and create a protocol suitable for its distinct setup, staffing, and incoming populations. Some facilities will prefer baths or oral dosing. Some will use dips over medicating the tank water. It is also important to use medications judiciously and with good stewardship in mind. Priority should be placed on preventing resistance and mitigating environmental contamination.

This list of recommendations contains ranges of medication doses but does not encompass all reported dose regimens for every species. Clinicians are encouraged to research and identify if there are any reported doses specific to the species entering into their care.

26.4.1 Freshwater teleosts

- Saltwater dip
  - Both dips or water treatments can be used to treat *Columnaris* bacteria and protozoan ectoparasites.
  - For a concentrated dip, create a solution of salt water with a goal of 10 to 30 g/l sodium chloride, or 1–3% sodium chloride (Roberts *et al.*, 2009). Dip the freshwater fish for 5–10 min and repeat once every 3–5 days for three dips. Remove from the water sooner if the fish becomes lethargic.
  - For a prolonged immersion add 3–6 g/l in tank water (Mashima and Lewbart, 2000).
- Fenbendazole
  - This is used to treat intestinal parasites.
  - A medicated bath can be performed at 2 mg/l tank water once every seven days for three treatments (Noga, 2011).
  - 0.2% fenbendazole can be added to the feed once daily for three days and then repeated in 14–21 days.
  - An oral dose can be given at 50 mg/kg once every 24 h for two days and then repeated in 14 days.
- Praziquantel
  - Can be used to treat cestodes, monogenean, and digenea infestations (Justine *et al.*, 2009; Francis-Floyd *et al.*, 2023).
  - For a medicated bath, aim for 5–10 mg/l for 1–5 h, repeating every 7 days as needed (Morales-Serna *et al.*, 2018).
  - For an oral treatment option, a 50 mg/kg dose can be given once by mouth.
  - As a dip, create a 100 mg/l solution of praziquantel and immerse the animal for 4 min (Noga, 2011).
- Metronidazole
  - Metronidazole is used to treat intestinal flagellates (*Spironucleus*, *Hexamita*), protozoal infections, and anaerobic bacterial infections.
  - Oral dosing is recommended at 50 mg/kg by mouth every 24 h for 3 days.
  - A medicated bath can be created but adding metronidazole at 7–15 mg/l to the tank water for 3 days.
- Formalin
  - This is used to treat ectoparasitic protozoa, metazoan, and monogenean infestations. It also has antifungal (Scholz, 1999) properties. Formalin comes as a 37% formaldehyde solution, which is very toxic in concentrated form. The following doses are based on this concentration of formaldehyde. It is important to increase aeration while treating with formalin as the oxygen levels will decrease during treatment.
  - For a concentrated dip: Mix 0.12–0.25 ml formalin per liter of water and place the animal in solution for 60 min. Repeat daily or every other day for three doses.
  - For a medicated bath: Add 0.015–0.025 ml/l to the tank water every 48 h for three treatments. There should be 50% water changes daily during this treatment.
- Use of antibiotics should be based on clinical testing and observations.

26.4.2 Saltwater teleosts

- Freshwater dip
  - This is used to treat protozoa, monogenea, and some crustacea (Mashima and Lewbart, 2000). When using a freshwater dip, set the dip up with dechlorinated water and adjust the temperature to match the marine tank water temperature. Use sodium bicarbonate to bring the pH of the freshwater to within 0.1–0.2 pH units of the marine tank water. Once ready, dip the marine fish for 5–10 min. Transfer back to salt water sooner if signs of distress occur. Repeat this dip every 3–7 days for three treatments.
- Copper sulfate (Yanong, 2010)
  - Copper sulfate baths are used to treat gill and skin protozoa, monogeneans, flavobacteria, and some molds (Calado *et al.*, 2017). One can use copper baths for eels, but they are more sensitive than other teleosts and have been reported to decrease feeding after treatment.
  - Caution: Any decrease in pH will release the bound copper from the substrate and other surfaces in the system. This risks releasing free copper into the water and raising the levels of active copper ion to potentially lethal levels. With this in mind, monitor the copper levels with water quality tests for at least 4 weeks post-copper treatment, as any of the copper bound to substrates and the filters will gradually release into the system over time.

- Remember, as discussed in the water quality section, any concentration of active copper over 0.3 mg/l will cause the bacteria within the nitrification cycle to stop functioning and there will be loss of the biofilter. If this concentration of active copper is seen, monitor the water quality parameters very closely every 2–3 days for at least 2 weeks as the biofilter re-establishes.
- To use a concentrated dip, animals can be submersed in a 100 mg/l solution for 5 min.
- To create a medicated bath, the goal is to dose at 0.15–0.2 mg/l Cu^{+2} ions, also known as active free copper. This can be maintained for 3–4 weeks. It is important to remove any activated carbon from the filter, as this will adsorb copper from the water and reduce the concentration during treatment.
  - Calculating the weight of copper to add:
    - in gallons: (volume of tank) × (0.0038) × (concentration of desired Cu in mg/l) × (3.92) = g of free Cu to add
    - in liters: (volume of tank) × (desired [copper] in mg/l) × (0.00392) = g of free Cu to add
  - Monitor pH carefully before starting treatment and then twice daily throughout the treatment period.
  - It is recommended to create a stock solution and then continue to add the stock solution to the tank as needed when the level of copper begins to fall below therapeutic levels.
    - To create a stock solution: Add 1 g of copper sulfate pentahydrate to 250 ml of distilled water. This creates a stock solution concentration of 1 mg of copper/ml. To calculate the volume of stock solution that needs to be added:
      - in liters: (# liters) × (desired concentration of copper) = mg of copper needed, which equals the ml of stock solution to add.
      - in gallons: (# gallons) × (3.78) × (desired concentration of copper) = mg of copper needed, which equals the ml of stock solution to add.
- Once the treatment period is over, cycling the tank water through an activated carbon filter will remove the copper. However, just like with the tank substrate, the carbon filter will collect bound copper molecules. It is recommended to change the filter media once testing shows the copper has been filtered out. This prevents future release of large levels of copper back into the tank.

- Fenbendazole
  - This is used to treat intestinal parasites.
  - A medicated bath can be performed at 2 mg/l tank water once every seven days for three treatments.
  - 0.2% fenbendazole can be added to the feed once daily for three days and then repeated in 14–21 days.
  - An oral dose can be given at 50 mg/kg once every 24 h for 2 days and then repeated in 14 days.
- Praziquantel
  - Can be used to treat cestodes, monogenean, and digenea infestations.
  - For a medicated bath, aim for 5–10 mg/l for 1–5 h repeating every 7 days as needed.
  - For an oral treatment option, give 50 mg/kg once by mouth.
  - As a dip, create a 100 mg/l solution of praziquantel and immerse the animal for 4 min (Noga, 2011).
- Metronidazole
  - Metronidazole is used to treat intestinal flagellates (*Spironucleus*, *Hexamita*), protozoal infestations, and anaerobic bacterial infections.
  - Oral dosing is recommended at 50 mg/kg by mouth every 24 h for 3 days.
  - A medicated bath can be created but adding 7–15 mg/l of metronidazole to the tank water for 3 days.
- Use of antibiotics should be based on clinical testing and observations.

26.4.3 Seahorses/syngnathids

Important notes: Seahorses can arrive having prolonged periods of time in transport. It is not uncommon for them to show delayed signs of stress. This can occur days after arrival, once they are already thought to be acclimatized. When performing their exams, a gill biopsy will not be able to be performed due to that brachial plate overlying the gills. In these species, perform a brachial wash by gently flushing sterile saline over the gills and collecting the fluid to observe for pathogens.

Syngnathids are copper-sensitive and should not be housed with species requiring copper treatments. Seahorses are at high risk for *Vibrio* and *Mycobacterium* infections, as well as fungal infections. Some institutions report using dip protocols with *Vibrio* bacterin vaccines for their Syngnathidae population (Koldewey and Mulligan, 2005).

- Formalin
  - For a medicated dip, create a 200 mg/l solution and place the animal in the bath for 45 min.
  - For a longer medicated bath, add formalin to the tank water to create a 15 mg/l solution every 48 h.
    - Formalin comes as a 37% formaldehyde solution, which is very toxic in concentrated form. To create the 15 mg/l solution, add 0.015 ml/l of 37% formaldehyde to the tank water every 48 h for three treatments. There should be 50% water changes on the day after treatment.
- Freshwater dip
  - Create a dechlorinated freshwater solution with matching temperature to the current animals, housing. Use sodium bicarbonate to buffer the water so that the pH of the two systems match within 0.1–0.2 pH units. Submerse the animal in the freshwater dip for 10 min.
- Praziquantel
  - Create a medicated bath for Syngnathids using 1–2 mg/l in the tank water for at least 24 h.
- Fenbendazole:
  - Feed the fish *Artemia* soaked in fenbendazole for treating intestinal parasites.
  - Add a 25 g/l fenbendazole solution to the Artemia. Allow syngnathids to feed for 1 h while the filtration system is turned off. Repeat once daily for three days and then repeat the 3-day regimen two weeks later.

26.4.4 Elasmobranchs

Important considerations must be given to sharks and rays as they are copper-sensitive species, and copper treatments should be avoided (Smith *et al.*, 2004). If copper treatment of a multi-species tank is required, it is recommended to remove sharks and rays during treatments (Cardeilhac and Whitaker, 1988). Sharks undergoing dip treatments need to be maintained in a horizontal position as being positioned vertically in the water column can cause a rupture of the hepatobiliary ligament. Also, note that sharks arriving to quarantine facilities stiff from transport are likely suffering from lactic acid buildup. These individuals can be given one Dexamethasone SP injection if in distress. If not in distress, hold off giving an immunosuppressant drug and plan to house the animal in a low noise, low lighting, and higher oxygen state for at least 24 h.

- Freshwater dip
  - This is used to treat protozoa, monogenea, and some crustacea (Mashima and Lewbart, 2000). When using a freshwater dip, bring the temperature of dechlorinated freshwater equal to the housing tank temperature. Use sodium bicarbonate to bring the pH of the freshwater to within 0.1–0.2 pH units of the marine tank. Once set up, dip the animal for 5–10 min. Transfer back to salt water sooner if signs of distress occur. Repeat this dip every 3–7 days for three treatments.
- Praziquantel
  - For a medicated dip treatment, aim for 5–10 mg/l for 1–5 h, repeating every seven days as needed (Morales-Serna *et al.*, 2018).
  - Use a medicated bath of 4–6 mg/l of praziquantel maintained for three days.
  - For an oral treatment option, 50 mg/kg up to 150 mg/kg praziquantel can be given by mouth once.
- Fenbendazole
  - Use with caution: Toxicities have been reported in some species (Myers *et al.*, 2007). Clinical signs include anemia, leukopenia, anorexia, lethargy, necrotic fins, and death (Garner, 2013). Research the specific species being treated prior to use of this drug.
  - Fenbendazole has been reportedly used in some species of sharks without any signs of toxicity at doses of 25 mg/kg every 48–72 h for 3 weeks. Because there is concern this medication can cause immunosuppression in these species, avoid using fenbendazole if there is an active infectious disease affecting the animal.
- Antibiotics should only be used if indicated with examination and diagnostics.

26.4.5 Invertebrates

Important notes: There are only a few resources regarding invertebrate quarantine protocols

(Lewbart, 2012). Some resources are from informal hobbyist and aquarist groups (Reef2reef, 2017). Invertebrates will often arrive covered in large volumes of mucus and debris. Once arriving, most authors report not using an acclimatization period and just focusing on removing these animals from their transport containers as soon as possible. It is recommended to then place them in a saltwater bath to clean them off before entering their quarantine tank. If an animal appears swollen, this can be a sign of low oxygen levels occurring during transport and the animal will need to be housed in a higher oxygen state for 48–72 h upon arrival. Ideally, invertebrates should not be treated with any chemicals or medications unless clinically indicated during their quarantine period. These animals are copper-sensitive and should not be cohoused with any species requiring copper treatments.

Studies have shown that certain invertebrates and substrates can act as fomites, introducing the trophont stage of fish parasites into a system and infecting the fish within the tank. It was shown that the sea urchin and starfish are resistant to attachment of the *Cryptocaryon* trophonts (Burgess, 1992). Further studies will need to be performed to assess different classes of aquatic invertebrates and their risk of introducing a variety of diseases. Until further research is performed, it is recommended to house invertebrates in a fish-free tank system for 80 days. *Cryptocaryon* can survive on substrates and tank surfaces for up to 72 days (Colorni and Burgess, 1997). By housing the invertebrates in a fish-free environment for 80 days, any trophonts living on the invertebrates will complete their life cycle with no ability to reproduce and the parasite will die off (Wilson, 2016; Reef2reef, 2017).

- Saltwater dip
  - Upon arrival to the quarantine facility, animals should be placed in a saltwater dip that matches the salinity, pH, and temperature of the future quarantine tank. Allow animals to rest here for at least 15–20 min. This allows rinsing off debris and mucus that accumulated during transport and prevents introduction of this debris into the long-term quarantine tank.
- Freshwater dips
  - CAUTION: This has been reported to cause mortalities in sea stars, corals, and urchins.
  - Though reports have shown safe use on some species of corals and snails, it is highly recommended to research the species being kept prior to use and consider the risks versus benefits of placing them in a freshwater bath.
  - When using a freshwater dip, prepare dechlorinated freshwater and bring the temperature equal to the marine tank temperature. Use sodium bicarbonate to bring the pH of the freshwater to within 0.1–0.2 pH units of the marine tank. Once set up, dip the animal for 2–5 min and then transfer them back to their saltwater housing.

26.5 Conclusion

This final chapter summarizes the concepts of biosecurity, quarantine, facility management, and disease treatments for a variety of fish species commonly encountered in public aquariums, fish wholesale and retail facilities, and hobbyist fish keepers' tanks and ponds. As stated in previous chapters, proper fish husbandry and welfare depend on disease prevention and treatment, good water quality, adequate space, proper nutrition, and only housing compatible species together. Providing proper welfare to fish not only helps them thrive, rather than just survive, but makes keeping ornamental aquarium fish a more enjoyable and satisfying experience.

References

Arthur, R., Subasinghe, R. and Bondad-Reantaso, M. (2008) *Procedures for the Quarantine of Live Aquatic Animals*. FAO Fisheries Technical Papers 502.

Boerman, I., Jansen, C.H.M. and Suselbeek, L. (2006) *Quarantine Protocols for Fishes Research on the Use and Extensiveness of Quarantine Protocols among EUAC and EAZA Members*. Van Hall Larenstein Hogeschool, Wageningen, Netherlands.

Burgess, P.J. (1992) *Cryptocaryon irritans* Brown, 1951 (Ciliophora): Transmission and immune response in the Mullet *Chelon Labrosus*. Available at: http://hdl.handle.net/10026.1/2632 (accessed 24 April 2024).

Calado, R., Olivotto, I., Oliver, M.P. and Holt, J. (2017) *Marine Ornamental Species Aquaculture*. Wiley, Chichester, UK. Available at: https://www.wiley.com/en-us/Marine+Ornamental+Species+Aquaculture-p-9780470673904 (accessed 1 December 2019).

Campbell, T. (2015) Blood sample collection and preparation in fish. In: Campbell, T.W. and Grant, K. (eds) *Exotic Animal Hematology and Cytology*. Wiley, Ames, Iowa, pp.183–186.

Cardeilhac, P.T. and Whitaker, B.R. (1988) Copper treatments: uses and precautions. *Veterinary Clinics of North America: Small Animal Practice* 18(2), 435–448. doi:10.1016/s0195-5616(88)50041-4.

Carpenter, J.W. and Marion, C.J. (2018) *Exotic Animal Formulary*. 5th edn. Saunders, St. Louis, Missouri.

Colorni, A. and Burgess, P. (1997) *Cryptocaryon irritans* Brown 1951, the cause of "white spot disease" in marine fish: an update. *Aquarium Sciences and Conservation* 1, 217–238.

Francis-Floyd, R., Reed, P., Klinger, R.E. and Petty, D. (2023) *FA28/FA033: Monogenean Parasites of Fish*. Available at: https://edis.ifas.ufl.edu/publication/fa033 (accessed 1 August 2024).

Garner, M.M. (2013) A retrospective study of disease in elasmobranchs. *Veterinary Pathology* 50(3), 377–389. doi:10.1177/0300985813482147.

Hadfield, C.A. and Clayton, L.A. (2011) Fish quarantine: current practices in public zoos and aquaria. *Journal of Zoo and Wildlife Medicine* 42(4), 641–650. doi:10.1638/2011-0034.1.

Hedley, J. (2020) *BSAVA Small Animal Formulary, Part B: Exotic Pets.* British Small Animal Vet, Gloucester, UK.

Justine, J., Leblanc, P., Keller, F. and Lester, R. (2009) Turbellarian black spot disease in bluespine unicornfish *Naso unicornis* in New Caledonia, caused by the parasitic turbellarian *Piscinquilinus* sp. *Diseases of Aquatic Organisms* 85, 245–249. doi:10.3354/dao02082.

Koldewey, H. and Mulligan, M. (2005) *Syngnathid Husbandry in Public Aquariums 2005 Manual*. Zoological Society of London, Regents Park, London. Available at: https://www.theseahorsetrust.org/wp-content/uploads/2020/12/2005-Syngnathid-Husbandry-Manual.pdf (accessed 21 April 2024).

Lewbart, G. (2012) *Invertebrate Medicine*. Blackwell, Ames, Iowa.

Mashima, T.Y. and Lewbart, G.A. (2000) Pet fish formulary. *Veterinary Clinics of North America: Exotic Animal Practice* 3(1), 117–130. doi:10.1016/s1094-9194(17)30097-x.

Morales-Serna, F.N., Chapa-López, M., Martínez-Brown, J.M., Ibarra-Castro, L., Medina-Guerrero, R.M. and Fajer-Ávila, E.J. (2018) Efficacy of praziquantel and a combination anthelmintic (Adecto®) in bath treatments against *Tagia ecuadori* and *Neobenedenia melleni* (Monogenea), parasites of bullseye puffer fish. *Aquaculture* 492, 361–368. doi:10.1016/j.aquaculture.2018.04.043.

Myers, G.E., Garner, M.M., Barrie, M.T., Yach, C.E. and Pribyl, G.L. (2007) Fenbendazole toxicity in sharks. In: *Proceedings of the American Association of Zoo Veterinarians Conference*, AAZV, Knoxville, Tennessee, pp. 64–65.

Noga, E.J. (2011) *Fish Disease: Diagnosis and Treatment*. Wiley, Ames, Iowa.

OATA (2023) *Biosecurity and the Ornamental Fish Industry.* Ornamental Aquatic Trade Association, Westbury, UK. Available at: https://ornamentalfish.org/wp-content/uploads/Biosecurity-and-the-ornamental-aquatic-industry-May-2023.pdf (accessed 21 April 2024).

Rashid, T., VonVille, H.M., Hasan, I. and Garey, K.W. (2016) Shoe soles as a potential vector for pathogen transmission: a systematic review. *Journal of Applied Microbiology* 121(5), 1223–1231. doi:10.1111/jam.13250.

Reavill, D. and Roberts, H. (2007) Diagnostic cytology of fish. *Veterinary Clinics of North America: Exotic Animal Practice* 10(1), 207–234. doi:10.1016/j.cvex.2006.11.002.

Reef2reef (2017) How to quarantine coral and inverts. REEF2REEF Saltwater and Reef Aquarium Forum. Available at: https://www.reef2reef.com/ams/how-to-quarantine-coral-and-inverts.228/ (accessed 24 April 2024).

Roberts, H.E., Palmeiro, B. and Weber, E.S. (2009) Bacterial and parasitic diseases of pet fish. *Veterinary Clinics of North America: Exotic Animal Practice* 12(3), 609–638. doi:10.1016/j.cvex.2009.06.010.

Scholz, T. (1999) Parasites in cultured and feral fish. *Veterinary Parasitology* 84(3–4), 317–335. doi:10.1016/s0304-4017(99)00039-4.

Smith, M., Warmoults, D., Thoney, D. and Hueter, R. (2004) *The Elasmobranch Husbandry Manual: Captive Care of Sharks, Rays and Their Relatives*. Ohio Biological Survey, Columbus, Ohio.

Steneroden, K. (2012) Sanitation. In: Miller, L. and Zawistowski, S. (eds) *Shelter Medicine for Veterinarians and Staff*. Wiley, Ames, Iowa, pp. 37–47. doi:10.1002/9781119421511.ch4.

Thomas, A., Dawson, M.R., Ellis, H. and Stamper, M.A. (2016) Praziquantel degradation in marine aquarium water. *PeerJ* 4:e1857. doi:10.7717/peerj.1857.

Wilson, A. (2016) *Comprehensive Marine Quarantine—Transfer Method II and Hyposalinity*. Reefs. Available at: https://reefs.com/magazine/comprehensive-marine-quarantine-transfer-method-ii-and-hyposalinity/ (accessed 24 April 2024).

WOAH Aquatic Animals Commission (2024) *Aquatic Animal Health Code*. World Organisation for Animal Health. Available at: https://www.woah.org/en/what-we-do/standards/codes-and-manuals/aquatic-code-online-access/ (accessed 21 April 2024).

Wolf, J.C., Baumgartner, W.A., Blazer, V.S., Camus, A.C., Engelhardt, J.A. *et al.* (2014) Nonlesions, misdiagnoses, missed diagnoses, and other interpretive challenges in fish histopathology studies. *Toxicologic Pathology* 43(3), 297–325. doi:10.1177/0192623314540229.

Yanong, R.P. (2010) Use of copper in marine aquaculture and aquarium systems. *EDIS* 2010(2). doi:10.32473/edis-fa165-2009.

Zang, L., Shimada, Y., Nishimura, Y., Tanaka, T. and Nishimura, N. (2013) A novel, reliable method for repeated blood collection from aquarium fish. *Zebrafish* 10(3), 425–432. doi:10.1089/zeb.2012.0862.

Recommended Reading

Here are some other fish disease books written by veterinarians. Multiple dates in parentheses indicate subsequent editions.

Brown, E.E. and Gratzek, J.B. (1980) *Fish Farming Handbook*. AVI Publishing, Westport, Connecticut.

Brown, L. (1993) *Aquaculture for Veterinarians: Fish Husbandry and Medicine*. Pergamon Press, Oxford.

Butcher, R.L. (1992) *Manual of Ornamental Fish*. British Small Animal Veterinary Association, Gloucestershire, UK.

Carpenter, J.W. (1996/2001/2005/2013/2018/2023) *Exotic Animal Formulary*. Elsevier, St. Louis, Missouri.

Dulin, M.P. (1976) *Diseases of Marine Aquarium Fishes*. TFH Publications, Neptune City, New Jersey.

Dulin, M.P. (1979) *Fish Diseases*. TFH Publications, Neptune City, New Jersey.

Fowler, M. (1978/1986/1991/1999/2003/2008/2012/2015/2019/2023) *Zoo and Wild Animal Medicine*. 10 Vols. (not all include Fish Medicine). Elsevier, St. Louis, Missouri.

Gratzek, J.B. and Matthews, J.R. (1992) *Aquariology: The Science of Fish Health Management*. Tetra Press, Morris Plains, New Jersey.

Hadfield, C. A. and Clayton, L.A. (2021) *Clinical Guide to Fish Medicine*. Wiley, Hoboken, New Jersey.

Jepson, L. (2001a) *Koi Medicine*. Kingdom Books, Hants, UK.

Jepson, L. (2001b) *A Practical Guide to Keeping Healthy Fish in a Stable Environment*. Barron's Educational Services Publishing, Hauppauge, New York.

Jepson, L. (2004) *The Super Simple Guide to Common Fish Diseases*. TFH Publications, Neptune City, New Jersey.

Johnson, E.L. (1996) *Koi Health and Disease*. Reade Printers, Athens, Georgia.

Johnson, E.L. (2006) *Koi Health and Disease 2*. Lulu Publishing, Marietta, Georgia.

Johnston, D.E. (1986) *Exotic Animal Medicine in Practice*. Veterinary Learning Systems, Lawrenceville, New Jersey.

Lammens, M. (2004) *The Koi Doctor.* Drukkerij Paesen, Oudsbergen, Belgium.

Lewbart, G.A. (1998) *Self-Assessment Color Review of Ornamental Fish*. Iowa State University Press, Ames, Iowa.

Lewbart, G.A. (2017) *Ornamental Fishes and Aquatic Invertebrates*. CRC Press, Boca Raton, Florida.

Loh, R. (2012) *Fish Vetting Medicines: Formulary of Fish Treatments*. Richmond Loh Publishing, Perth, Australia.

Loh, R. and Landos, M. (2011) *Fish Vetting Essentials*. Richmond Loh Publishing, Perth, Australia.

Mitchell, M. and Tully, T. (2016) *Current Therapy in Exotic Pet Practice*. Elsevier, St. Louis, Missouri.

Noga, E.J. (1996/2010) *Fish Disease—Diagnosis and Treatment*. Mosby, St. Louis, Missouri.

Reddacliff, G.L. (1985) *Diseases of Aquarium Fishes: A Practical Guide for the Australian Veterinarian*. The University of Sydney, New South Wales, Australia.

Roberts, H. E. (2010) *Fundamentals of Ornamental Fish Health*. Wiley, Ames, Iowa.

Roberts, R.J. (1978/1989/2001/2012) *Fish Pathology*. Wiley, West Sussex, UK.

Rosenthal, K.L. (1997) *Practical Exotic Animal Medicine*. Veterinary Learning Systems, Trenton, New Jersey.

Saint-Erne, N. (1994) *Diseases of Koi*. Koi Rx, Las Vegas, Nevada.

Saint-Erne, N. (2002/2010) *Advanced Koi Care*. Erne Enterprises, Glendale, Arizona.

Saint-Erne, N. (2024) *Handbook of Ornamental Fish Health and Welfare*. CAB International, Wallingford, UK.

Smith, S.A. (2019) *Fish Diseases and Medicine*. CRC Press, Boca Raton, Florida.

Stoskopf, M.K. (1988) Tropical fish medicine. *The Veterinary Clinics of North America—Small Animal Practice*. WB Saunders, Philadelphia, Pennsylvania.

Stoskopf, M.K. (1993/2011) *Fish Medicine*. Saunders, Philadelphia, Pennsylvania.

Urdes, L., Walster, C. and Tepper, J. (2022) *Fundamentals of Aquatic Veterinary Medicine*. Wiley, Hoboken, New Jersey.

Urdes, L., Walster, C. and Tepper, J. (2023) *Pathology and Epidemiology of Aquatic Animal Diseases for Practitioners*. Wiley, Hoboken, New Jersey.

Wallach, J.D. and Boever, W.J. (1983) *Diseases of Exotic Animals*. WB Sanders, Philadelphia, Pennsylvania.

Wildgoose, W.H. (2001) *BSAVA Manual of Ornamental Fish*. British Small Animal Veterinary Association, Gloucester, UK.

Yanong, R. and Lewbart, G. (2024) *The Aquarium Fish Medicine Handbook*. CRC Press, Boca Raton, Florida.

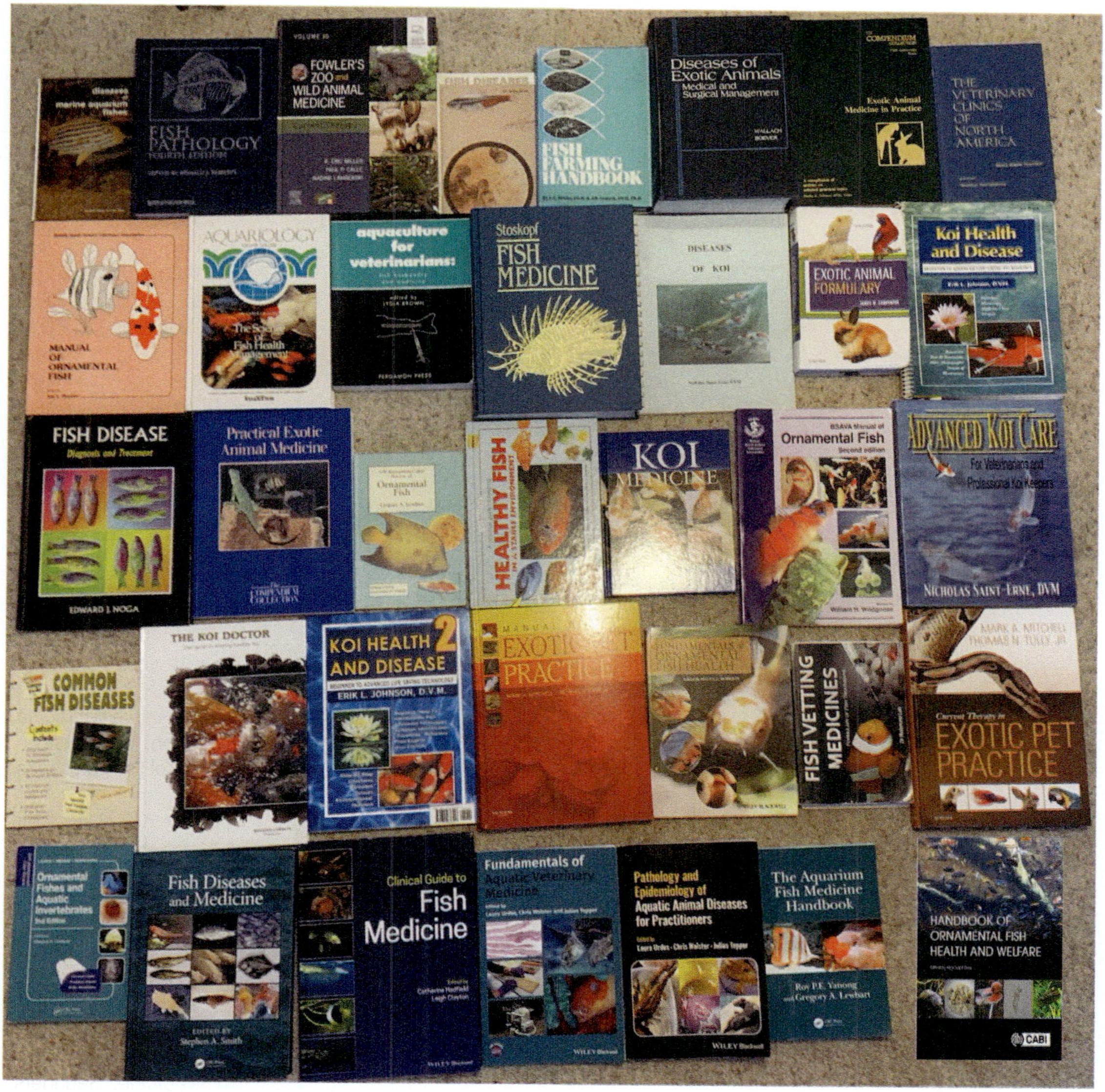

Fish health books written by veterinarians, arranged in chronological order of publication. (Photograph by N. Saint-Erne.)

Glossary

A

Abrasion—a superficial skin scrape that does not penetrate through the epithelium
Abscess —a fluid-filled cyst, usually containing pus due to infection
Acclimatization—the habituation of an organism to a different climate or environment
Acid/acidity—a solution with pH below 7 that has a buffering capacity against bases
Acidosis—a morbid condition caused by exposure to a large sudden decrease in pH, or exposure to a pH level below the tolerance range of the species
Acute—recent occurrence of clinical signs of a disease
Adenocarcinoma—a malignant neoplasm derived from glandular tissue
Adenoma—a benign tumor of glandular tissues
Adhesion—fibrous attachment of two tissues that would normally be separate, due to inflammation
Adipose—fatty tissue
Adipose fin—a soft fin composed of fatty tissue on the dorsal caudal peduncle
Adsorption—the attraction of atoms or molecules to surfaces of solids or liquids
Aerobic—requires the presence of oxygen
Alimentary canal—the entire digestive tube (mouth, esophagus, stomach, and intestines) collectively
Alkaline—describing alkali metal ions that form hydroxide ions (OH^-) when dissolved in water
Alkalinity—also referred to as carbonate hardness (KH), this is the buffering capacity of the water against acids due to dissolved bicarbonate and carbonate ions in the water
Alkalosis—a morbid condition caused by the exposure to a large sudden rise in pH, or a pH which is above the tolerance range of the species
Allostasis—the process the body uses to maintain homeostasis in response to stressors
Amino Acid—the basic unit of proteins, made of carbon, hydrogen, oxygen, and nitrogen, with a basic structure of $R\text{-}CH(NH_2)\text{-}COOH$, where R is a specific side chain for that amino acid
Ammonia (NH_3)—a pungent, colorless, alkaline gas made from nitrogen and hydrogen that is the primary end product of protein metabolism in living organisms, and is released from organic matter as it decays
Ammoniotelic—an organism that excretes nitrogenous waste mainly as ammonia
Anabolism—constructive metabolism, the building up of more complex organic molecules from simpler ones.
Anadromous—adult fish that leave the sea to spawn in freshwater
Anaerobic—occurs in the absence of oxygen
Anal—pertaining to the anus or vent
Anal fin—a fin located on the lower surface of the body of a fish caudal to the anus that stabilizes the fish while swimming
Analgesia—reducing the sense of pain without loss of consciousness
Anemia—a deficiency of hemoglobin or red blood cells
Anesthesia—loss of sensation to a specific area (local anesthesia) or complete loss of consciousness (general anesthesia) induced by an anesthetic drug that blocks the impulses along nerve pathways to the brain
Angioma—a tumor consisting of blood vessels or lymph vessels
Anorexia—lack of appetite for food
Anoxia—total lack of oxygen
Anterior—toward the front of the body or nearer to the head
Anthelmintics—drugs that are used to treat helminth parasite infestations
Antibiotic—drugs used to inhibit the growth of or kill bacteria
Antibody—a specific serum protein (immunoglobulin) that is produced by an organism's immune system in response to the presence of an antigen
Antigen—a foreign substance that evokes a specific immune response in an animal
Antimicrobial—a substance that is effective in treating microbial infections
Antiseptic—a topical chemical used to inhibit or kill microorganisms
Aquaculture—the growing of aquatic organisms for human needs, this includes fish farming

Aquarist—a person who maintains an aquarium
Aragonite—a naturally occurring porous mineral that is high in calcium carbonate and dissolves slowly in water at pH below 8.2
Ascites—The abnormal accumulation of serous fluid in the peritoneal or coelomic cavity
Aseptate—without any septum (internal walls)
Asexual reproduction—a reproductive method that does not involve the production of gametes
Asphyxia—the condition of suffocation
Ataxia—abnormal movements due to muscle incoordination
Atresia—congenital absence of a normal body opening or tubular structure
Atrophy—a decrease in the normal size of a tissue or organ
Autotrophic—organisms that synthesize nutrients from solar radiation (photosynthetic) or from inorganic substances (chemosynthetic)

B

Bacteremia—presence of bacteria in the blood
Bacteriostatic—having the ability to inhibit the growth or reproduction of bacteria
Barbels—slender, tactile, chemical-sensing organs around the mouth or snout of some fishes
Base—any ionic salt of an alkali metal that is soluble in water and forms hydroxide ions
Basic—a solution with pH above 7 that has a buffering capacity against acids
Bath—a method of administering medications by dissolving the treatment in the water that surrounds the fish
Benign—a tumor that is not cancerous (does not spread to other tissues)
Benthic—living at the bottom of a body of water
Benthos—the bottom of the sea
Bicarbonate ion (HCO_3^-)—the main buffer in water below pH 9; over pH 9 carbonate becomes predominant
BID—"*bis in die*," twice in a day
Bilateral—occurring on both sides
Binary fission—asexual reproduction by an organism that results in two progenies
Biofilter—filtration that uses nitrifying bacteria to detoxify nitrogenous wastes in aquarium water
Bioload—the living organisms present in an aquarium
Biopsy—taking a small sample of a tissue for diagnostic analysis
Biosecurity—a strategic and integrated approach to analyzing and managing relevant risks to human, animal (including aquatic), and plant health by preventing the introduction or transmission of pathogens (bacteria, viruses, fungi, and parasites) within an environment
Brackish—natural water that is less saline than seawater; occurs where a river runs into the sea
Branchial—pertaining to the gills
Buccal cavity—the mouth cavity ahead of the gills, the space behind the gills is the opercular cavity.
Buffer—a substance capable of neutralizing both acids and bases added to a solution, maintaining the original pH of the solution
Buffering capacity—the ability of a solution to neutralize acids and minimize changes in pH
BW (body weight)—the measured weight of an organism

C

Calcinosis—an abnormal condition of deposition of calcium salts in nodular foci within tissues
Calcium (Ca^{2+})—one of the major cations (positively charged ions) in water and a principal component of hardness
Calcium carbonate ($CaCO_3$)—the main mineral contributing to water hardness and alkalinity; the major component of limestone, seashells, and bones
Cancer—an uncontrolled growth of tissue cells and the ability of these cells to migrate from the original site and spread to distant sites in the body
Capillary—the smallest blood vessels, just big enough for passage of red blood cells
Carbohydrates—organic compounds that contain only carbon, hydrogen, and oxygen, that include sugars, starches, cellulose, and gums, and are produced by photosynthetic plants and consumed as an energy source by animals
Carbon dioxide (CO_2)—a product of carbon oxidation in aerobic metabolism and combustion; and is soluble in water to form carbonic acid and bicarbonate ion
Carcinoma—a malignant tumor derived from epithelial cells
Carnivore—an animal that primarily or exclusively feeds on other animals
Carrier—an organism harboring a pathogen that is not showing signs of disease
Cartilage—firm, elastic skeletal tissue in which chondrocyte cells are embedded in a matrix of collagen fibers

Catabolism—destructive metabolism, the breakdown of organic molecules into simpler forms
Catadromous—an adult fish that leaves freshwater and migrates to the sea to spawn
Cataract—a clouding of the normally clear lens of the eye
Caudal—pertaining to the tail, or a direction toward the tail
Caudal fin—the tail fin at the rear end of a fish
Caudal peduncle—the narrow part of the fish's body cranial to the caudal fin
CBC—complete blood count, an analysis of the cells in the blood
Chondroma—tumor of the cartilage cells
Chromatophores—dermal cells that contain pigments, imparting a hue to the skin
Chronic—persistent state of a disease for a long time
Cilia (singular cilium)—a short, hair-like locomotory organelle
Clean—removal of organic and nonorganic materials from a surface
Clinical sign—observable evidence of a disease
Coelom—the epithelium-lined space between the internal body wall and the digestive tract
Commensals—organisms that live together without harm and to the benefit of one another
Communicable—capable of being transmitted from one organism to another (contagious)
Congestion—abnormal accumulation of blood within an organ or peripheral blood vessel
Contusion—a bruise, the rupture of skin capillaries without breaking the epidermis
Cranial—pertaining to the head, or a direction toward the head
Crepuscular—organisms which are active in the twilight hours (dawn and dusk)
Cutaneous—pertaining to the skin
Cuticle (or Glycocalyx)—the mucus or slime (mucopolysaccharides and glycoproteins) that is secreted by epithelial cells and goblet cells in the epidermis covering the fish's skin and scales
Cyanophore—a chromatophore containing blue pigments
Cyst—a non-motile, resistant stage of an organism that is covered by a protective capsule

D

Debride—to clean a wound of all foreign material and injured or infected tissue
Definitive host—the host that harbors the sexually reproducing adult stage of a parasite
Deformity—distortion or malformation of any part of the body
Demersal—living and feeding on or near the bottom of seas or lakes (the demersal zone)
Demersal spawners—fish that mate and lay eggs on a fixed surface at the bottom of their habitat
Denitrification—the process where a nitrogen-based compound is broken down into its basic elements
Dermatitis—inflammation of the skin
Detritivore—an organism that feeds on decaying plant or animal protoplasm
Detritus—decomposing organic material in an ecosystem
Diagnosis—the determination of the cause of a disease
Diarrhea—the profuse discharge of fluid feces
Digestion—the process of breaking down food in the alimentary canal to aid assimilation
Dip—the treatment of a fish where it is dipped into a medicated solution for a short time
Direct Veterinary Supervision—written or oral guidance and oversight to a facility or persons provided by a veterinarian who is physically present on the premises
Disease—any deviation from the normal structure or function of any part of the body
Disinfect—the use of chemical to destroy microorganisms on a surface
Distal—away from the center; or away from the body when referring to an extremity or limb
Diurnal—animals that are active during the daytime
Dorsal—relating to the back or to the upper surface of an animal
Dorsal fin—single fin or a series of multiple fins on the back of a fish
Dropsy—swelling of the coelom of a fish due to fluid accumulation (ascites); the swelling may cause the scales to protrude from the body (lepidorthosis, or pinecone disease)
Dysfunction—abnormal or imperfect functioning of an organ

E

Ecchymosis—a small hemorrhagic spot on the skin or mucous membrane, larger than petechia

Ectoparasite—a parasite that lives on the outside or surface of its host
Ectothermic—an animal that has a body temperature of the surrounding environment
Edema—swelling of tissues caused by fluid accumulation
Emaciation—deficiency of muscles and fat caused by malnutrition
Embolism—an arterial blockage caused by a blood clot, air bubble, fat, or other materials
Endemic—something that is common in a specific geographic area
Endocrine—glands that release their secretions into the blood or lymph system
Endogenous—produced within the organism
Endoparasite—a parasite that lives within its host's body
Enophthalmia—eyes that are abnormally sunken into their sockets
Enteral—giving a medication by mouth so it enters the intestines
Enteric—affecting the intestines
Enteritis—inflammation of the intestines
Environment—all the external conditions, circumstances, and influences surrounding and affecting the development of an organism
Epidemic—a sudden increase in the number of cases of a disease in a particular geographic area
Epidermis—the outer layer of the skin
Epithelium—the surface layer of cells covering cutaneous, mucous, and serous surfaces
Erosion—the superficial destruction of a tissue surface by inflammation or trauma
Erythema—abnormal reddening of the skin due to blood vessel congestion
Erythrocyte—a red blood cell
Erythrophore—a chromatophore that contains large amounts of red/orange carotenoids
Estuary—an area where fresh water flows into the ocean and is subject to tidal variations
Etiology—the specific cause of a disease
Euryhaline—a wide tolerance for environmental salinity; the ability to move from fresh water to salt water and back again
Euthanasia—ending the life of an animal in a way that minimizes or eliminates pain and distress
Eutrophic—an aquatic habitat with abundant organic matter
Excretion—the process of eliminating waste products from metabolism
Exocrine—a glandular secretion that is released through a duct
Exophthalmia—the swelling or protrusion of one or both eyes, commonly called pop-eye
Exotic—originating on a foreign continent other than the continent where it is currently found
Exudate—fluid entering a tissue due to inflammation

F

Fecundity—capability of producing offspring; highly fecund fish produce many offspring
Fibroma—a benign tumor composed of fibrous tissue
Fibrosarcoma—a malignant tumor composed mainly of fibrous connective tissue
Filament—a paired series of filaments branch off each gill arch, each filament has two rows of lamellae through which chemical exchange occurs across the blood/water interface
Filter feeders—feeding on suspended particles from the water by passing the water over modified gill rakers to strain out food particles
Final host—the definitive host that harbors the sexually reproducing adult stage of a parasite
Fins—flattened limb or tissue surfaces used by fish for stability and to produce lift, thrust, or steerage in water
Fishes—the plural of "fish" when referring to more than one species of fish
Flagella (singular flagellum)—whip-like extensions of cells that facilitate movement
Flashing—a quick motion of a fish to rub its side against an object, such as gravel or an aquarium ornament, where the lighter underbelly color is visibly flashed to the observer
Fomite—a physical object that may be contaminated with infectious agents and serve in their transmission
Fry—free-swimming, juvenile life stage of fishes that have become reliant on external sources for nutrition

G

Gametes—the mature haploid sex cells: ova or sperm
Gametogenesis—gamete (sperm in males, eggs in females) formation within the gonads
Gastritis—inflammation of the stomach
Gender—having either a male or female reproductive system
Genotype—the inheritable genetic code of an organism

Gill arches—the branchial arches are a series of bony structures on each side of the pharynx, within the gill covers (opercula) of fish, that support the gill filaments
Gill cover—also known as the opercula (singular, operculum), a hard bony plate covering and protecting the gills in most fishes, comprising four fused bones, on each side of the fish's head
Gill rakers—filamentous cartilaginous or bony extensions of the gill arches, generally used for trapping food particles or holding food in the mouth before it is swallowed
Gills—the respiratory organs of fish, consisting of thin lamellae in rows on either side of paired filaments that are arranged in rows on gill arches in the back of the oral cavity (pharynx)
Gland—an organ or tissue that produces and secrets fluids that serve a specific function
Glycocalyx—the glycoprotein and polysaccharide covering on some cell types
Gonads—the testes in males and ovaries in females
Gram (g)—the weight of one cubic centimeter (1 cm^3 = 1 ml) of water at 4°C, the temperature of maximum density of water
Granulocytes—leucocytes that contain granular cytoplasmic material
Granuloma—a non-neoplastic tumor due to chronic inflammation and proliferation of macrophages
Guanine—a pigment that imparts the reflective, silvery color to the skin of the fish

H

Hardness—also referred to as General Hardness (GH), this is a measure of all bivalent mineral cations (mainly Ca^{2+}, Mg^{2+}, but also Fe^{2+}, Cu^{2+}, Zn^{2+}) in the water
Hazard—anything that has the potential to cause injury, illness, or death
Hematocrit—also called packed cell volume (PCV), it is the proportion of blood volume that is occupied by red blood cells, expressed as a percentage
Hematopoiesis—the formation of blood cells
Hemoglobin—the oxygen-carrying pigment found in red blood cells
Hemorrhage—the abnormal loss of blood from a blood vessel
Hepatic—pertaining to the liver
Herbivore—an organism that feeds mostly on plants
Hermaphrodite—an organism possessing the sexual organs of both genders
Heterotrophs—organisms that obtain energy from preformed organic compounds
Histology—the microscopic study of cellular and sub-cellular tissue
Homeostasis—the maintenance of relatively stable conditions inside an organism despite a changing environment
Hormone—a chemical secreted by a ductless gland into the bloodstream or lymphatic system that controls physiological processes in the body
Host—a plant or animal that harbors or nourishes another organism
Humane—showing compassion or benevolence
Hyperemia—excess blood in an organ or tissue
Hyperplasia—an abnormal increase in the number of cells of an organ or tissue
Hyphae—thread-like filaments that are the vegetative stage of a fungus
Hypertrophy—an abnormal enlargement of the individual cells of an organ or tissue
Hypodermis—the layer of tissue immediately under the skin (subcutaneous)
Hyporexia—a reduction in appetite
Hypoxia—a deficiency of oxygen below physiologically required levels

I

Idiopathic—a disease of unknown causation
Immunity—resistance to an infectious agent or toxin
Indirect Veterinary Supervision—written or oral guidance and oversight to a facility or persons provided by a veterinarian not physically present on the premises
Infection—invasion and multiplication of pathogenic microorganisms in body tissues
Infectious—a disease capable of being transmitted from one organism to another
Inferior—relating to the downward orientation of the mouth, common in bottom-feeding fish
Infestation—invasion of the body tissues by parasites (protozoa, helminths, arthropods)
Inflammation—a response to tissue injury to effect removal of the cause of the injury
Intermediate host—a necessary host that harbors a larval stage of a parasite
Intracardiac (IC)—an injection given into the heart
Intracoelomic (ICoe)—an injection given into the visceral body cavity (coelom)

Intramuscular (IM)—an injection given into the muscle tissue
Intraperitoneal (IP)—an injection given into the peritoneal cavity, which in fish is actually the coelomic cavity
Intravenous (IV)—an injection given into a vein
Invasive species—a species introduced beyond its native range that can establish self-sustaining populations that potentially threaten native species in the ecosystem
Invertebrate—an animal without a backbone (spine)
Ionized—a molecule that has had an electron removed or added so that it has a positive or negative charge
Iridophores (guanophores)—chromatophores that reflect light using plates of guanine crystals

K

Keratitis—inflammation of the cornea of the eye
Kilogram (kg)—the weight equal to 1000 g; equivalent to 2.2 pounds
Kype—the hooked lower jaw of salmonids that develops prior to spawning

L

Laceration—a wound made by tearing a tissue
Larva—the early stage of an animal that is unlike the adult stage and must metamorphose to adult characteristics
Lateral—relating to the side
Lateral line—pressure-sensing organs along the flanks of most fish species, helping them detect movement, vibrations, and pressure waves in the surrounding water
Lepidorthosis—abnormal condition of scales extended from the body
Lesion—any visible abnormal change in a body tissue or organ
Lethargic—deficient in alertness or activity
Leucocyte—any of the white blood cells
Leucophore—a white hued chromatophore
Lipid—fats or oils
Lipoma—a benign fatty tumor
Littoral—the shallow area of water around the shoreline
Lordosis—an abnormal inward or downward (dorso-ventral) curve of the spine
Lymphoma—a tumor of the lymph system

M

Macronucleus—the larger of the two types of nuclei found in ciliated protozoa
Macrophage—a phagocytic cell belonging to the reticuloendothelial system
Malignant—a tumor that contains cancerous cells that spread to other tissues
Maxillary—relating to the upper jaw
Melanin—a tyrosine-derived pigment responsible for the black hue in fish tissues
Melanophore—a chromatophore containing black or brown melanin granules
Metastatic—the spread of cancer cells from the initial site to another part of the body
Metazoan—animals having the body cells differentiated into tissues and organs
Methemoglobin—Hemoglobin with the iron in the ferric state so that it is unable to bind oxygen
Microbe—a living organism that is too small to see without magnification, especially bacteria, fungi, or viruses
Micronucleus—the smaller of the two types of nuclei found in ciliated protozoa
Milligram—mg (1/1000 of a gram)
Milt—a white seminal fluid that contains the spermatozoa of male fish (semen)
Monoecious—having both male and female reproductive structures in the same individual
Morbidity—suffering from a disease
Moribund—dying from a disease
Mortality—having died from a disease
Motile—an organism capable of locomotion
Mucosa—epithelia covering of internal cavities
Mucous—(adjective) describing something that contains or produces mucus
Mucus—(noun) a slippery aqueous secretion produced by glands in mucous membranes
Mycosis—a disease caused by an infectious fungus
Myomere—one segment of the lateral muscle mass
Myopathy—a wasting condition of muscle tissues

N

Nares—the openings of the nasal cavity
Necropsy—the examination of a dead body to ascertain the cause of death
Necrosis—damage and death of cells or tissues within a living body

Neoplasm—abnormal growth of new tissue
Neotenic—an organism that never develops into the adult stage of the life cycle, but is capable of reproduction in its larval form
Neural—relating to the nervous system
Neutral—a solution of pH 7 that has an equal number of hydroxide ions (OH^-) and hydrogen ions (H^+)
Nitrification—the oxidation of ammonia to nitrite and then nitrate, mediated by bacteria
Nociceptors—neurons that originate in the spinal cord and end as thin fibers in the skin that reflexively respond to painful stimuli
Nocturnal—animals that are active at night
Non-infectious—a disease not capable of being transmitted from one organism to another
Non-motile—not capable of moving on its own
Nuptial (spawning) tubercles—a male secondary sex characteristic of some fish (e.g., carp and minnows) where keratin protrusions on the skull, operculum or pectoral fin spines develop during spawning time
Nutrition—the processes where an organism takes in and utilizes food

O

Olfactory—relating to the sense of smell
Oligotrophic—a nutrient-poor body of water
Omnivore—an animal that can eat and survive on both plant and animal matter
Oogenesis—the development of the ovum (egg) in the female's ovary
Operculum—plural opercula; the bony plate covering the gills of fishes
Opportunistic—a pathogen that only affects a weakened host
Oral—pertaining to the mouth, or administration by mouth
Osmoregulation—the maintenance of the osmotic pressure of a body fluid by controlling the amount of water and salts in the body
Osmosis—the passive movement of water through a semipermeable membrane from a side of lower concentration of dissolved solids to the side of higher concentration until the two sides are equally dilute
Osseous—bony tissue
Ossification—formation of bone
Osteosarcoma—malignant tumor of bony tissues
Otoliths—calcified structures within the inner ear
Ovary—part of the female reproductive system and the site for oogenesis
Oviparous—reproduction by egg laying
Ovipositor—a tube extending from the vent in some female fish species that is used to deposit eggs
Ovoviviparous—the egg is retained in the mother's body until hatching, but the female does not supply any nutrients to the embryo, only oxygen. The embryo develops on the energy in the egg yolk and is released from the female after hatching from the egg
Ovum—plural ova; the egg produced by the female, prior to fertilization
Oxidation—the chemical process where oxygen is added to an element or compound

P

Parasite—an organism that lives upon or within another living organism (the host) at whose expense it obtains some advantage
Paratenic host—an intermediate host in a parasite's life cycle in which the parasite lives without undergoing further development, and is not a necessary host in the parasite's life cycle
Parenteral—administration of a medication by a route other than oral
Parts per billion (PPB)—1 microgram per liter (1 µg/l)
Parts per million (PPM)—1 milligram per liter (1 mg/l)
Parts per thousand (PPT)—1 gram per liter (1 g/l)
Pathogen—any disease-producing microorganism (viruses, bacteria, fungi)
Pectoral fins—paired fins located on each side of the body behind or below the gill covers, used for steering and lift when the fish is swimming
Pelagic—living in the middle or surface levels of a body of water, away from the shore
Pelagic spawners—fish that mate while swimming and release eggs that float away
Pelagic zone—the open, free waters away from the shore or bottom of a body of water
Pelvic fins—also known as ventral fins, paired fins located ventrally behind the pectoral fins but before the anus
Per os (PO)—by mouth, referring to medications given orally
Percent (%)—parts per hundred
Personal Protective Equipment (PPE)—equipment worn to minimize exposure to hazards that cause serious injuries or illnesses
Perturbation—an upset in the natural balance of an ecosystem

Pet—an animal kept for pleasure or companionship, rather than for utilitarian purposes
Petechiae—very small spots of hemorrhage in tissues
pH—the letters pH (with lowercase "p" and uppercase "H") are initials for *potentii Hydrogenii*, or the "power of Hydrogen." The pH is a measure of the hydrogen ion concentration in the solution using a logarithmic equation: $pH = -\log_{10} [H^+]$, giving a value that can range from 1.0 to 14.0, with 7.0 being neutral, and below 7.0 is acidic, and above 7.0 is basic
Pharyngeal teeth—teeth found in the throat of fishes that lack teeth in the jaws
Pharynx—the part of the throat behind the mouth and before the esophagus
Phenotype—the physical characteristics of an organism
Photoperiod—the duration of daily light exposure to an organism
Photosynthesis—the process by which green plants and some other organisms use sunlight to synthesize carbohydrates from carbon dioxide and water
Physoclistous—a swim bladder lacking a connection to the pharynx
Physostomous—having a pneumatic duct between the swim bladder and the pharynx
Phytoplankton—the autotrophic (self-feeding), photosynthetic plants and algae of the plankton community
Piping—fish at the surface of the water attempting to breathe the air
Piscivore—a fish or other animal that lives by eating fish
Planktivore—an animal that eats plankton suspended in the water
Plankton—small organisms that float or are suspended in the water column, carried along by tides and currents
Platelet—thrombocyte; a blood cell associated with clotting
Poikilothermic—vertebrates whose body temperature fluctuates with the ambient temperature
Posterior—further back in position; or nearer the rear or hind end of the body
PPB—parts per billion, or 1 microgram per liter (µg/l)
PPM—parts per million, or 1 milligram per liter (mg/l)
PPT—parts per thousand, or 1 gram per liter (g/l), or 1 milliliter per liter (ml/l)
Predator—an organism that lives by eating other organisms
Prey—an organism that is captured and consumed by a predator
Primary Host (Definitive host)—an organism in which the parasite reaches the adult stage and reproduces sexually
Prolapse—abnormal protrusion of an organ or tissue
Protozoa—a single-celled, eukaryotic microorganism
Proximal—nearer to the center
Pyriform (also Piriform)—pear-shaped

Q

QID—"*quater in die*," four times a day
Quarantine—from the Latin word "*quarant*" meaning forty, the period of days that one was originally isolated to prevent the spread of bubonic plague; this is the isolation of new or sick fish in a separate quarantine tank until such a time as they are free from contagious diseases

R

Rays—soft, branching, cartilaginous structures supporting the fins
Relapse—return of disease after a patient had previously recovered
Renal—pertaining to the kidneys
Resistance—the natural or acquired ability of an organism to overcome processes of a disease
Respiration—oxygen uptake for use in cellular activities
Roe—the eggs (ova) in the abdominal cavity of a female fish

S

Saline—a solution of sodium chloride (salt) at the physiological concentration of an organism
Salinity—the measurement of salt in a solution
Sanitize—a combination of cleaning followed by disinfection
Scales—hardened bony plates on the surface of a fish
School—fish that are swimming together in a loosely formed group
Scoliosis—abnormal curvature of the spine in a lateral deviation from normal

Secretion—the process of discharging a substance from a cell or gland
Sedation—reducing agitation and pain by depressing consciousness with sedative drugs
Selective breeding—a breeding program where the breeder chooses which animal to breed based on some predetermined criteria
Septicemia—the presence of bacteria living and reproducing in the bloodstream
Serum—the fluid portion of the blood after the cells have clotted and are removed
Sexual reproduction—mating and reproduction that involves the production of gametes
Shimmying—a disease sign where fish stay in one place and wiggle or shake
Shoal—fish swimming together in a distinctly structured formation with fish swimming equal distances apart and responding as a group
SID—"*semel in die*," once a day
Sign—a visible manifestation of a disease
Slough—separation of necrotic (dead) tissue from a wound or inflamed site
Sodium Bicarbonate—baking soda, used to buffer the pH of the water
Sodium Carbonate—soda ash, used to buffer the pH of the water, especially in marine aquariums
Specific gravity (SG)—the ratio of the density of a substance compared to the density of pure water (SG = 1.000); often used as a measurement for salinity, seawater at 3.5% salinity has an SG of 1.025
Spines—bony projections stiffening the anterior portion of the fins in some fish species
Standard Length (SL)—the measurement of a fish from its snout to the base of the caudal fin where it is attached to the caudal peduncle
Sterilize—the destruction of all microorganisms and their spores on an object
Stress—the sum of all biological phenomena elicited in an organism by adverse external influences
Subcutaneous—located under the skin
Submucosa—the tissue lying beneath the mucous membrane
Superior—relating to an upward orientation of the mouth, common in fish that are surface feeders
Swim bladder—also called the gas bladder
Symbiosis—the relationship between two species of organisms living intimately together so that each obtains some benefit from the other organism
Systemic—involving the whole body

T

Tail fin—the caudal fin
Telangiectasis—dilatation of the capillaries in the gill lamellae with pooling (microthrombi) of the red blood cells
Terminal—a location related to the end of something; also refers to a disease that leads gradually to death and cannot be cured
Testes (singular testis, or testicle)—the male reproductive organ for gametogenesis
TID—"*ter in die*," three times a day
Topical—the application of a treatment directly onto the lesion
Torpid/torpor—a slow or inactive state
Total Length (TL)—the measured length of a fish from the tip of its snout to the end margin of the tail fin held in a natural position
Toxin—a chemical that causes disease or death when introduced into the body tissues of an organism
Tranquilization—to make calm or relieve anxiety by the administration of a drug (tranquilizer) that depresses physiological or psychological activity
Tubercle—a small nodule or raised area on a surface
Tumor—an abnormal swelling of tissues that may be benign (does not spread), malignant (spreads aggressively to surrounding tissues) or metastatic (spreads via blood or lymph to other organs of the body)

U

Ulcer—a deep break in skin or mucous membranes with loss of surface tissue, disintegration, and necrosis of epithelial tissue
Unilateral—having an effect on only one side
Ureotelic—excreting nitrogenous waste as urea
Urolithiasis—the formation of mineral calculi in the urinary tract

V

Vaccine—a substance that stimulates antibody production to provide immunity against a disease
Vector—a temporary host that is responsible for transmitting a parasite between primary hosts
Ventral—on or toward the lower part of the body
Ventral fins—also known as pelvic fins, paired fins located ventrally behind the pectoral fins but before the anus
Vertebrate—an animal with a backbone

Veterinarian—an individual holding a professional degree in veterinary medicine and a license as required to practice medicine on animals
Virulence—the disease-producing power of a microorganism
Virus—a submicroscopic infectious agent that replicates only inside the cells of a host organism
Viscera—the internal organs
Vitellogenesis—egg yolk formation
Viviparous—live-bearing, where the female supplies nutrients to the developing embryos
Vomer plate—a bony plate on the roof of the mouth of some fish species, formed through the fusion of dental plates belonging to the bucco-pharyngeal denticulate bones
Vomerine teeth—small patches of teeth found on the front part of the roof of the mouth in some fish species

W

Welfare—promoting all aspects of an animal's physical and mental well-being
White Blood Cells (WBC)—nucleated leukocytes that can be granulated (neutrophils, heterophils, eosinophils, basophils) or agranular (lymphocytes, monocytes, and thrombocytes)

X

Xanthoma—a cutaneous deposition of yellowish cholesterol-rich material that can appear anywhere in the body and are manifestations of lipidosis in which lipids accumulate in large foam cells within the skin
Xanthophore—a chromatophore containing yellow pteridine pigments

Z

Zoonosis—any animal disease that can be transmitted to humans
Zooplankton—small animals suspended in the water column
Zygote—the fertilized ovum that divides into an entire organism

Index

Page numbers in **bold** refer to figures and tables. The index does not include terms listed separately in the Glossary.

P

T

Printed and bound by CPI Group (UK) Ltd, Croydon, CR0 4YY

13/09/2026

14961109-0008